PERU
History of Coca
"THE DIVINE PLANT"
OF THE INCAS

AMS PRESS
NEW YORK

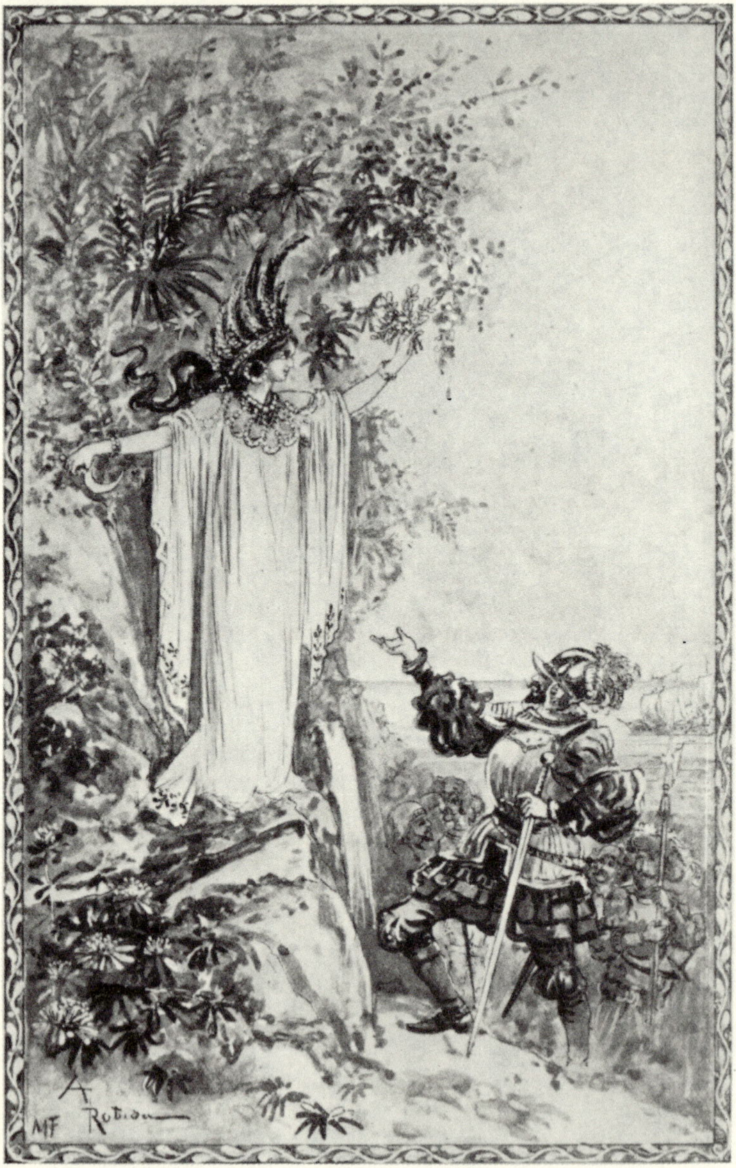

Mamma Coca Presenting the "Divine Plant" to the Old World.
[*From an Aquarelle by Robida.*]

PERU

HISTORY OF COCA

"THE DIVINE PLANT" OF THE INCAS

WITH AN INTRODUCTORY ACCOUNT OF THE INCAS, AND OF THE ANDEAN INDIANS OF TO-DAY

BY

W. GOLDEN MORTIMER, M. D.

FELLOW OF THE NEW YORK ACADEMY OF MEDICINE; MEMBER OF THE MEDICAL SOCIETY OF THE COUNTY OF NEW YORK; MEMBER OF THE NEW YORK ACADEMY OF SCIENCES; MEMBER OF THE AMERICAN MUSEUM OF NATURAL HISTORY; FORMERLY ASSISTANT SURGEON TO THE NEW YORK THROAT AND NOSE HOSPITAL, ETC.

WITH ONE HUNDRED AND SEVENTY-EIGHT ILLUSTRATIONS

NEW YORK

J. H. VAIL & COMPANY

1901

Library of Congress Cataloging in Publication Data

Mortimer, William Golden.
Peru: history of coca, "the divine plant" of the Incas.

Reprint of the ed. published by J. H. Vail, New York.

Bibliography: p.
Includes index:

1. Coca. 2. Incas. 3. Peru—Description and travel.
I. Title. II. Title: History of coca.
RS165.C5M8 1978 394.1 74-15120
ISBN 0-404-11980-8

First AMS edition published in 1978.

Reprinted from the edition of 1901, New York. Trim size has been slightly altered in this edition. Original trim size: 15.5 × 23.2 cm. Text area of the original has been maintained.

MANUFACTURED
IN THE UNITED STATES OF AMERICA

TO

Angelo Mariani

PARIS FRANCE

A RECOGNIZED EXPONENT OF
THE "DIVINE PLANT"

AND THE

FIRST TO RENDER COCA AVAILABLE TO
THE WORLD

PREFACE

This work, although of a scientific nature, has not been written exclusively for scientists, for the theme is of so universal a scope as to be worthy the attention of all who are concerned in lessening the trials of humanity, or who wish to shape the necessities of life through a more useful and consequently a more happy being.

Presuming that such a subject suitably presented will awaken popular regard in a matter of common interest, I have endeavored to surround a myriad of authentic facts with sufficient associate detail that is entertaining, and to present the data without the dryness usually attributed to scientific utterance, in a manner, as I trust, that shall maintain the attention of the general reader.

Centuries before the introduction of cocaine to anæsthetic uses, the world had been amazed by accounts of the energy creating properties ascribed to a plant intimately associated with the rites and customs of the ancient Peruvians, and first made known through the chroniclers of Spanish conquest in America. The history of this plant, known as Coca, is the history of the Incan race and is entwined throughout the associations of the vast socialistic Empire of those early people of Peru. The story of that remarkable people has been adequately told through the voluminous writings of a host of historians, and more connectedly related for English readers in the admirable works of Helps and of Prescott. But the true story of Coca, which the Incas regarded—because of its property of imparting endurance—as the "divine plant," has hitherto never been fully set forth. Indeed, the "authoritative" literature of Coca—such as contained in text books—is so filled with inaccuracies and contradictory statements that the opinion of a reader seeking information from such a source, must fluctuate between the account he might last have read and some former utterance which was diametrically opposite in conclusion. As a result of this want of knowledge, much that has been supposed must be forgotten, before the mind can be receptive for the truths of Coca which are built upon facts.

This uncertainty of detail has been the outgrowth of an inability on the part of certain experimenters, to obtain from the Coca used by them, similar effects to those that had been described by South American writers. In some instances, this was owing to the speedy deterioration of the leaves and their consequent inert condition when experimented with, but it is probable that many of these negative results were more especially due to a want of understanding of the true nature of the plant. Thus, from an expectancy of some marvelous instantaneous effect, when no phenomenal influence was immediately apparent the leaves were condemned and their properties declared to be legendary. The facts all indicate that, the action of Coca is so unique and subtle that it cannot be judged by comparison with any other natural product similarly employed. This truth is embodied by Dr. Searle in the following statement:—"It is not a little remarkable that while no other known substance can rival Coca in its sustaining power, no other has so little apparent effect. To one pursuing the even tenor of his usual routine, the chewing of Coca gives no especial sensation. In fact the only result seems to be a negative one, viz.: an absence of the customary desire for food and sleep. It is only when some unusual demand is made upon mind or body that its influence is felt. And to this fact is to be attributed much of the incredulity of those who have carelessly experimented with it and who, expecting some internal commotion or sensation, are disappointed."* Just why this is so cannot be briefly told. It is for this reason that the associations, the necessities, the uses and the characteristics of the plant are here so fully discussed.

That Coca has not only not been well known, but barely known indirectly among a majority of those who presumably should know it—physicians who should use it, and teachers

* Searle, p. 123, 1881.

who should instruct as to its properties—is emphasized by the result of an inquiry instituted for the purpose of compiling a collective investigation. Upward of ten thousand letters were sent to a representative class of practitioners and teachers, and a majority of those from whom replies were received wrote in a frank way, that they knew absolutely nothing about Coca. Others had not employed it because they believed it to be inert through a confusion of its name with cocoa, or from confounding it with other products. A few, more liberal, expressed a belief that a substance with such traditional qualities as those surrounding the "divine plant," was probably possessed with properties which when better understood, might be made a valuable boon to humanity.

The present work has been constructed in view of these contradictions and uncertainties, and undertakes to trace the associations and uses of Coca, from the earliest accounts which are to be found. The story which necessarily commences with the dynasty of the Incas, embodies sufficient of the doings and the trials of that mighty Empire and its overthrow by the Spanish, as is essential to show the intimate connection between those people and the history of Coca. This has been epitomized from sources of authority and tells of the industries, science, arts, poetry, dramas, laws, social system and religious rites of the Incas as gleaned from tradition and witnessed in their relics, through all of which is interwoven the uses and applications of Coca. The history of that people is sufficiently full of life and color to absorb profound admiration. To this is added the accounts of contemporary travellers and scientists who have further detailed the continued dependence of the Andeans upon this Incan plant, and who tell of their own personal uses of Coca to support them under similar trials to those which the Incas experienced, and to which the present Peruvian Indians are still subjected. To a better understanding of the necessities for such support, the physical aspect of the Andes, together with a description of the life and customs of the modern Andeans is given, and advances our story to the Peru of today, a marvelous country of untold wealth and unearned possibilities. The characteristics and botanical peculiarities of Coca, and the economic uses of plants of the family to which it belongs are described, and an effort is made to harmonize the early uses of the substance—which are now shown to have been of necessity and not of luxury—with its present employment, through facts of modern physiology. The possible causes which may provoke the energy yielding properties of plants are considered, and are compared with analogous processes in the human body. The chemical problems involved in the study of the products of the Coca leaf and an account of the isolation of its various alkaloids is concisely told, and the possible advantage of Coca to the benefit of nerve, to muscle and to better blood are discussed from the results of careful investigation by a long list of experimenters. The utility of Coca to provoke endurance, its influence in voice production and its adaptability as an adjunct to a popular dietary is suggested.

No effort has been made to make this work in any sense a book of Coca therapy, but a study of the early necessities and the hypothesis here advanced as to the rationale of its empirical uses will doubtless be ample to impress the true status of Coca, and will suggest its application in the affairs of modern life for conditions similar to those which originally demanded it. This is rendered still more practical by a collective investigation on the physiological action and therapeutic uses of Coca among several hundred physicians, which is tabulated in detail.

In the liberal presentation of any complex problem, it is difficult to review all sides of the question without a large accumulation of data. This subject therefore has necessitated the collection of a vast amount of testimony pro and con, which as here introduced forms a compilation convenient for reference. The facts of Coca history are widely separated, through an immense range of literature not readily available to the general reader. Much difficulty has beset the gathering of even the most trivial details, but to build up a work which shall be accepted as authoritative—because embracing the truths of the matter dealt with—has required a deep research and the repeated verification of thousands of notes. What was collected one day was denied the next; for that reason I have been very precise in quoting my authorities, and the appended bibliography embraces nearly six hundred titles. No attempt has been made to include in this all papers upon Coca, but only those consulted or alluded to in the text. It will be appreciated that this work deals specifically with the parent plant and its several alkaloids and not with merely one of these. A relative prominence is given to cocaine, however, and its physiological action and therapeutic uses is discussed. Cocaine is an alkaloid of Coca that has excited a prodigious amount of writing all over the world; the list of its papers as catalogued in the library of the Surgeon-General of the United States Army, between 1885 and 1898, extends over eighteen columns of large quarto pages, printed in small type.

The result of my labor—continued through nearly four years—must now depend upon whether the subject has been treated clearly and made convincing to the reader. As to the value of Coca, there cannot be the slightest doubt. As to its utter harmlessness there can be no question. Even cocaine, against which there has been a cry of perniciousness, is an ally to the physician of inestimable worth, greatly superior—to compare it to a drug of recognized potency, not because of any allied qualities—to morphine. The evils from cocaine have arisen from its pernicious use, in unguarded doses, where used hypodermatically or locally for anæsthesia, when an excessive dose has often been administered, without estimating the amount of the alkaloid that would be absorbed, and which might result in systemic symptoms. Medicinally employed, cocaine in appropriate dosage is a stimulant that is not only harmless, but usually phenomenally beneficial when indicated.

There has been a looseness of interpretation regarding the term stimulant, which has engendered a dread unfounded in fact. There is a vague belief that any substance capable of producing stimulation, first elevates the system and then depresses it by a corresponding fall. The physiological law that stimulants excite to action, and that all functional activity is due to stimulation is forgotten or not generally appreciated. The name stimulant has commonly suggested alcoholics, while alcoholics suggest intoxication and a possible degradation. It recalls a thought of De Quincey when told that an individual was drunk with opium, that certain terms are given too great latitude—just as intoxication has been extended to all forms of nervous excitement, instead of restricted to a specific sort of excitement. As expressed by him: "Some people have maintained, in my hearing, that they have been drunk upon green tea; and a medical student in London, for whose knowledge in his profession I have reason to feel great respect, assured me, the other day, that a patient in recovering from an illness, had got drunk on beefsteak."*

It will be shown by ample testimony that Coca is not only a substance innocent as is tea or coffee—which are commonly accepted popular necessities—but that Coca is vastly superior to these substances, and more worthy of general use because of its depurative action on the blood, as well as through its property of provoking a chemico-physiological change in the tissues whereby the nerves and muscles are rendered more capable for their work. Strong as may appear this assertion, I believe that the facts here presented will amply indicate that sufficient has not been said upon the benefits to accrue from the liberal use of Coca. Indeed, our knowledge of it is yet in its infancy, and if this present writing will but excite others to continue these investigations and experiments, Coca will achieve the position it should maintain as an aid and support to humanity worthy the greatest popularity and the highest possible respect.

As a book of reference can be of little practical value when its facts may not be readily turned to, I have carefully prepared an extended index, embraced in which is a glossary of Incan or Quichua terms. There is a wide variance in the spelling of such words in the writings on Peru, in consequence of which there is an uncertainty of meaning when these con-

* Confessions.

fusional terms recur. This is due to the fact that the Quichua tongue, as spoken by the Incas, was written by the early Spanish historians phonetically, and words were consequently variously spelled. Whenever the Peruvian terms herein employed are not assured by local usage, I have taken the *Standard Dictionary of the English Language* (Funk & Wagnall's), as my authority. In that volume a greater number of words pertaining to this work are found than in any other reference book that I have consulted.

In the furtherance of this investigation I am indebted to the kindness of those medical confrères who have replied to my inquiries. These correspondents have been in sympathy with the importance of the research, and my thanks are here expressed for their cordial support. Indeed, while engaged in this work, I have been so long under obligations to so many, with some of whom a warm intimacy has developed, that though I may feel much time and persistent effort has been spent, the pursuit of this has not been unalloyed with pleasant associations, the memories of which shall long endure.

I desire to specially acknowledge an indebtedness, for courtesies and assistance, to the following gentlemen: To Mr. Wilberforce Eames, Librarian of Lennox Library, for suggestions in Historical Research; to Mr. Morris K. Jesup, President of the American Museum of Natural History, for privileges in the Museum; to Mr. Anthony Woodward, for assistance in the Library of that Institution; to Dr. Franz Boaz, for advice in Archæological Matters; to Mr. Marshall H. Saville, for access to Peruvian Relics; to Mr. Charles Balliard, Metropolitan Museum of Art, for Photographs; to Mr. Stansbury Hagar, for notes on his Research in Incan Astronomy; to Mr. Samuel Mathewson Scott, London, England, for Photographs and details of personal experiences in Peru; to Professor H. H. Rusby, for details of personal experiences in the Coca region of Bolivia; to Professor Ralph Stockman, University of Glasgow, for reprints and details of his research on the Coca Alkaloids; to Professor A. B. Lyons, for Analytic Tables and Processes of Coca Assay; to Mr. R. L. Daus, for suggestions in comparison of Incan Architecture; to

Messrs. Parke, Davis & Co., for details of Coca selection and Assay; to Messrs. Mariani & Co., for details regarding Coca, and for other kindliness; to Messrs. Boehringer & Soehne, for specimens of Cocaine; to Messrs. Merck & Co., for specimens of Coca Products; to Professor Lucien M. Underwood, Columbia University, for advice in Botanical Research; to Captain E. L. Zalinski, U. S. A. (retired), for details of personal experiences on the Andes; to Dr. Carlton C. Curtis, Lecturer on Physiological Botany, at Columbia University, for assistance in Histological Research in the Laboratories of that Institution, and for reviewing the Botanical Chapters; to M. Angelo Mariani, Paris, France, for ten Coca plants and for details of Coca cultivation in conservatory; to the Bureau of American Ethnology, Washington, D. C., for Books and Ethnological details; to Mr. J. N. Jaros, for Photographs and for many courtesies; to Mr. Herbert Tweddle, for access to an extensive and unique Peruvian Collection, for Photographs especially made for this work, for Coca Leaves, and for reviewing the portions of text relating to Peru.

Finally I wish to express my appreciation to the publishers who have carried out the mechanical construction of this book; they have been not only generous, but indulgent in completing the work in accordance with my wishes.

New York, April, 1901.

TABLE OF CONTENTS

CHAPTER I.

AN INTRODUCTION TO THE HISTORY OF COCA.

CHAPTER II.

THE STORY OF THE INCANS.

CHAPTER III.

THE RITES AND ACTS OF THE INCANS.

CHAPTER IV.

THE CONQUEST OF THE INCANS.

CHAPTER V.

THE PHYSICAL ASPECT OF PERU.

CHAPTER VI.

THE HISTORY OF COCA.

CHAPTER VII.

THE PRESENT INDIANS OF PERU.

CHAPTER VIII.

THE BOTANY OF COCA.

CHAPTER IX.

IN THE COCA REGION OF PERU.

CHAPTER X.

THE PRODUCTS OF THE COCA LEAF.

CHAPTER XI.

THE PRODUCTION OF ALKALOIDS IN PLANTS.

CHAPTER XIV.

THE PHYSIOLOGICAL ACTION OF COCA.

CHAPTER XV.

ADAPTATION OF COCA TO VOICE PRODUCTION.

CHAPTER XVI.

THE DIETETIC INFLUENCE OF COCA.

APPENDIX.

A COLLECTIVE INVESTIGATION UPON THE PHYSIOLOGICAL ACTION AND THERAPEUTIC APPLICATION OF COCA.

PHYSIOLOGICAL ACTION OF COCA.

[*Collective Investigation.*]

THERAPEUTIC APPLICATION OF COCA.

[*Collective Investigation.*]

RESUME.

FOOD USES OF COCA.

PREPARATIONS OF COCA USED.

LIST OF CORRESPONDENTS

BIBLIOGRAPHY.

LIST OF ILLUSTRATIONS

Cover design by the Author.

CHAPTER I.

AN INTRODUCTION TO THE HISTORY OF COCA.

"He that has once the "Flower of the Sun,"
The perfect Ruby which we call *elixir*,
. . . . . by its virtue
Can confer honour, love, respect, long life,
Give safety, valour, yea and victory,
To whom he will. In eight and twenty days
He'll make an old man of fourscore a child."
—Ben Jonson, *The Alchemist;* ii. [1610].

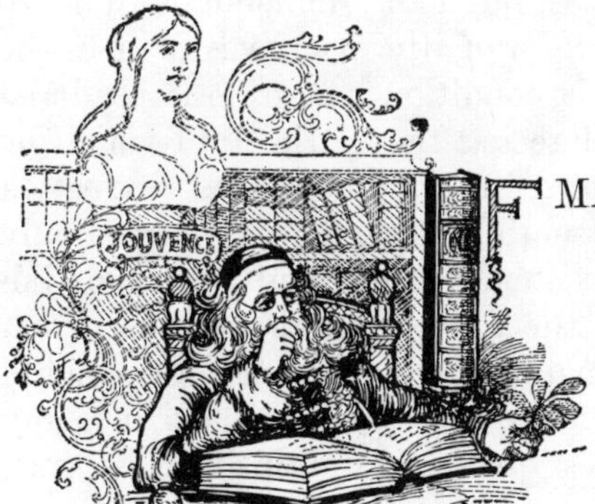

IF MAN were asked what one boon he would prefer of all Earth's bounties or Heaven's blessings, his response must be—the power of endurance. The capability to patiently and persistently do best that which the laws of life or the vagaries of association necessitates. Search for this one quality has been the impetus to inspire poet and philosopher since man's first appreciation of his mortal frailty. A something which shall check, within himself at least, the progress of time, the ravages of age, and the natural vacillation of conditions or environment. Wealth, and power, and greatness, and skill, must alike fall into insignificance without this one essential attribute to success. The artist in impressionistic work, the poet in soulful muse, the musician in celestial chords, the soldier in the mad rush of battle, the artisan in the cleverness of device, the merchant in the intricacies of commercial problems—even the most prosaic delver in life's plodding journey—each hopes to display a virility from which the slightest weakness is deprecated as humiliating. Work, indeed, is necessary to existence. It is the price—as the ancients considered—which the gods set on anything worth having. It is the power to do this work—to gain happiness for ourselves, which is the demand of modern necessity. To be enabled to keep active until the human machine may wear out as did the "wonderful one-hoss-shay," rather than rusting into a state of uselessness.

Human endurance, bounded by natural limitations, is still more closely environed by the results of a higher civilization, which presents the remarkable anomaly of two opposite conditions. While increasing, through the refinements of hygienic resources, the average term of life, it crowds man in the struggle for existence, into a condition where he is rendered less capable physically for fighting the battles into which he is thrust. So, from a natural life of pronounced perfection where his trials have been essentially muscular, he is gradually evolving into an artificial existence of eminently nervous impulse. If this be so, then the interest in any means which shall tend to establish and maintain a balance of force, should not be merely casual, but must be earnest and persistent to any who have regard for life's best qualities, and this interest must constantly increase with the requirements of time.

Even though others may point the way, everyone must fight his own battles. To each of us the world will appear as we may shape it for ourselves—a thought poetically expressed by the composer Wagner, who said: "The world exists only in our heart and conception." This shaping, if done by weakly hands or influenced by troubled brain, may not always prove symmetrical. A sensitive imagination, sharply atune, jars discordantly amidst inharmonious surroundings, which will be all the more harshly apparent if made possible through a known impotence.

There is a fund of force communicated by the Creator

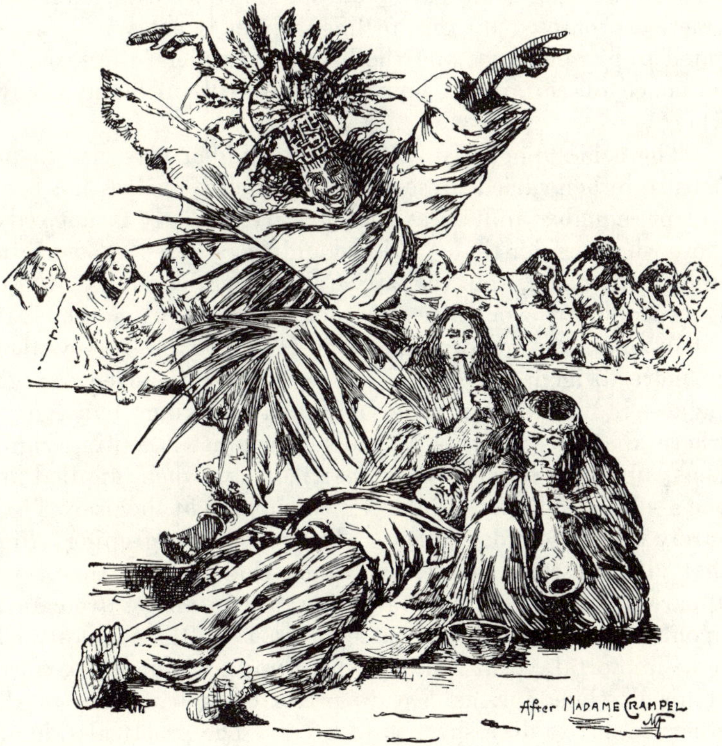

MEDICINE MAN, ARHOUAQUE INDIANS, COLOMBIA. [*Brettes*; 1898.]

to all things. It is the primal factor not only of man's existence, but of his continued being, and the activity which it generates is necessary to life, just as a cessation of energy means death. This fact has ever been so much a portion of the human mind that it requires no philosophic training to implant. It is not alone the savage who regards examples of vigor and prowess as ennobled emblems of a supreme being, while the sick or even the weak are looked upon as possessed of some evil spirit to be exorcised by priest or medicine man. This belief, whether superstitious or not, is pre-eminent and widespread. It is not only manifested by the ignorant, but often by the educated as well. The effort to ward off disease through wearing some particular substance as a talisman is a practice prompted by this feeling, which is not wholly relegated to bygone days, and the belief in amulets, rings, or the influence of certain precious stones is still prevalent everywhere.

There is supposedly some deeply hidden mystery about Nature in her varied presentations, which if it does not control presumably influences the curative art. It is not only those who consider that "yarbs should be gathered at a certain time of the moon," but the laity quite generally suppose there is a specific for every disease if not every condition, which if not immediately forthcoming upon inquiry must be revealed by more diligent search.* Nor is this belief—even though vague—indulged in merely by the unthinking, but everywhere about us there is a tendency against accepting rigid facts, and inevitable truths, particularly when applied to one's self. "All men think all men mortal but themselves" is surely a well founded adage. The result is a groping after that all necessary something, which shall supply this very apparent want, a craving for endurance in all we are called upon to bear. As Cicero has expressed it: "If not destined to be immortal, yet it is a desirable thing for a man to expire at his fit time, for, as Nature prescribes a boundary to all other things, so does she also to life." The practical side of this idea was once advanced to me by an elderly patient who said: "I don't want to controvert Nature, but I do want to be as comfortable as possible while I am here."

There has been a numerous order of philosophers not

* The Druids, who were both priests and physicians, cut the mistletoe with a golden knife only when the moon was six days old, and being afterward consecrated, it was considered an antidote to poisons and a preventive of sterility. [Pliny; *lib.* xvi, 44.]

content with simple well being, who sought for that perpetual youth—that *elixir vitæ*—which might give at least prolonged existence even if not rejuvenation. These did not commence with Faust nor end with Brown-Séquard. Happily the search for this substance—even though originating in a sanguine imagination—has often ended in findings that have been extremely important. Just as when Juan Ponce de Leon sought the *Fontaine de Jouvence* in the Island of Bimini, though he failed to locate the fountain, he did discover a land

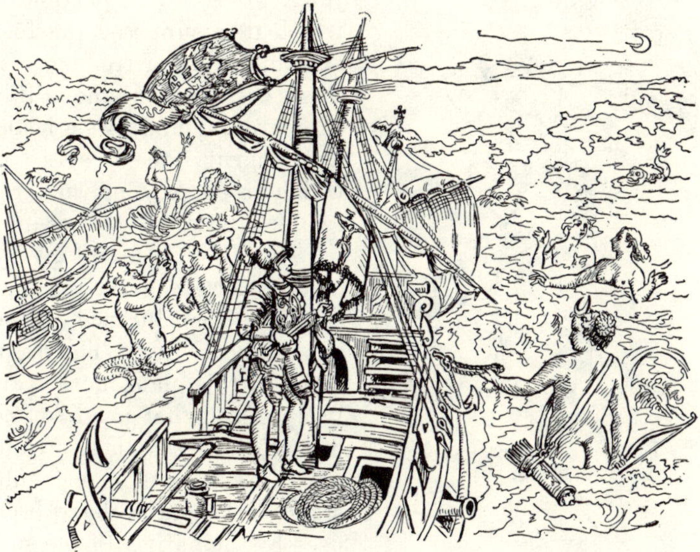

AN EARLY IDEA OF THE DISCOVERY. [*De Bry,* 1600.]

of perpetual youth, if we may so entitle the ever-blooming peninsula. Possibly it was because of some such spirit of inquiry into the vague depths of the unknown, where was presumed there might be some revelation to this knowledge of a perpetual vigor, which prompted a desire for exploration. Nature has always been ready to answer such seeking by her munificence, which, if not in the direction at first wished, has at least encouraged man to new desires.

The discovery of the Western Continent, whether due to the forethought or ignorance of Columbus, or to the hardihood of the Norsemen several centuries before his time, brought a multitude of bounties to humanity.[1] Among these none is greater than the countless plants which have been gradually unfolded to usefulness by the processes of science. Particularly is this true of the economic and medicinal plants of South America, which on the eastern declivity of the Andes and towards the valley of the Amazon, spring forth in all the luxuriance of the tropical jungle, over a vast portion of which it is supposed the foot of man has never trodden. In this locality—and among this wild profusion, grows a beautiful shrub, the leaves of which in shape somewhat resemble those of the orange tree, but in color are of a very much paler green, having that exquisite translucence of the most delicate fern. The properties of this plant more nearly approach that ideal source of endurance than is known to exist in any other one substance. Its leaves have been used by the natives of the surrounding country from the earliest recollection, as a masticatory, as a medicine, and as a force sustaining food. Its use is not confined to emergency, nor to luxury, but as an essential factor to the daily life work of these people. As a potent necessity it has been tenderly cared for and carefully cultivated through the

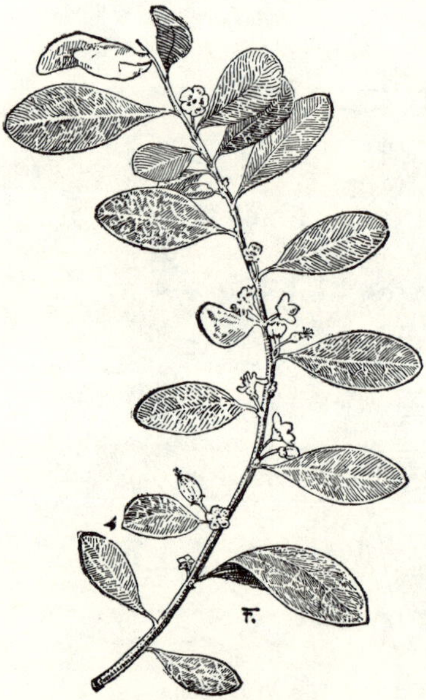

A COCA SPRAY.
[*Drawn from Nature.*]

[1] Charles Christian Rafn: *Antiquitates Americanæ*, describes the first voyages of the Scandinavians to America in the tenth and eleventh centuries. Leif, son of Eric the Red, is said to have reached the coast of *Helluland*—now New Foundland, which had been previously discovered by Bjame; he also found *Markland*—Nova Scotia, as well as the eastern coast between Cape Sable and Cape Cod.

struggles, trials and vituperation it has been the occasion of during so many hundreds of years, until to-day its cultivation forms the chief industry of a large portion of the natives and a prominent source of revenue to the governments controlling the localities where it is grown.

During the early age, when this nature's garden was unknown to the rest of the world, the Incas, who were then the dominant people of this portion of the continent, regarded this shrub as "the divine plant," so all important and complete in itself, that it was termed simply *khoka,*[2] meaning the tree, beyond which all other designation was unnecessary. This plant, which has been described under a variety of names but now known as Coca, has appealed alike to the archæologist, the botanist, the historian, and traveller as well as to the physician. Its history is united with the antiquity of centuries, while its traditions link it with a sacredness of the past, the beginning of which is lost in the remoteness of time. So intimately entwined is the story of Coca with these early associations—with religious rites, with superstitious reverence, with false assertions and modern doubts—that to unravel it is like to the disentanglement of a tropical vine in the primitive jungles of its native home.

Antedating historical record Coca was linked with the political doings of that most remarkable people of early American civilization who constituted the Incan dynasty. Since the conquest of Peru it has continued to form a necessary factor to the daily life work of the Andean Indians, the descendants of this once noble race. So important has it been held in the history of its native land that it has very fittingly been embodied in the escutcheon of Peru, along with the vicuña and the horn of plenty, thus typifying endurance with the versatile riches which this country affords.[3]

The first knowledge to the outer world concerning Coca followed Pizarro's invasion of Peru, though the actual accounts of its properties were not published until some years after the cruel murder of Atahualpa—commonly regarded as

[2] Dr. Weddell suggests Coca from the Aymara *khoka*, a tree, *i. e.*, the tree par excellence, like *yerba*—the plant of Paraguay. The Incan historian, Garcilasso, spells it *Cuca*.—Markham. [3] Marcoy; 1869.

the last Incan monarch. The effort made by the Spanish to implant their religion raised the cross and shrine wherever possible, which necessitated the founding of numerous missions, in charge of fathers of the church. These men in holy orders were often as tyrannical as those who bore arms, yet fortunately there were some in both classes less cruel, men of liberal attainments who appreciated the importance of preserving the traditions and records of this new country. To the writings of some of these more kindly disposed personages, as well as to the earnest labors of a few young nobles who were in the army of invasion, whose spirit for a conservative exploration was greater than for destructive conquest, we are indebted for the facts which form the foundation of this early history. Many of these writers had personally seen the result of the Incan civilization before its decay, and had opportunity to collect the native stories, as retold from father to son, through generation after generation, oral tradition being the early Peruvian method for continuing a knowledge of events. Unlike the Mexicans, these people had no picture writings to tell their doings in a series of hieroglyphics, nor had they a written language. But the story of this once mighty empire is told in its wonderful ruins, and through the relics of skilfully moulded pottery, and textile fabrics in exquisite designs, which all indicate a remarkable civilization. Historical facts were related by regularly appointed orators of phenomenal memory, who on all state occasions would recount the occurrences of the preceding reign, being aided in this recital by a novel fringe-like record of colored cords, known as the *quipu*. By the aid of this, as a sort of artificial memory, they told, as a monk might tell his beads. The various knots and several colors of the contrivance designating certain objects or events. In all these relations the Coca leaf was repeatedly and reverently alluded to as a most important element of their customs, as well as of their numerous feasts and religious rites.

The Spanish idea of conquest was to establish a complete mastery over the Peruvians; the Indians were to be regarded as slaves to be bought, sold, and used as such. In view of these facts it is not difficult to understand that as Coca was constantly employed among the natives, its use was early questioned and condemned as a possible luxury, for it was not considered a matter worthy of inquiry as to any real benefit in a substance employed by slaves. So superficial were the observations made by some of the early writers that the fact of this neglect is most apparent. Thus, Cieza de Leon, a voluminous writer on Incan customs, mentions as a peculiar habit of the natives: "they always carry a small leaf of some sort in the mouth." Even so experienced an observer as Humboldt, in his writings of many years later, did not recognize the true quality of Coca, but confounds the sustaining properties of the leaf as due to the alkaline ashes—the *llipta*—which is chewed with it. He refers to the use of this lime as though it belonged to the custom of the clay eaters of other regions, and suggests that any support to be derived from it must necessarily be purely imaginary.

It is not surprising that Coca chewing, if superficially viewed, should be condemned. The Spanish considered it merely an idle and offensive habit that must be prohibited, and at one time it was even seriously suggested that the plants should be uprooted and destroyed. But it was soon seen that the Indians could not work without Coca, and when forced to do so were unequal to the severe tasks imposed on them. As, however, the local tribute to the authorities demanded from all able bodied laborers a fixed amount of work, it was soon appreciated as a matter of policy that the use of Coca must at least be tolerated in order that this work should be done. Then the Church, which was from the invasion an all-powerful force in this new country, exacting and relentless in its demands, saw an imaginative evil in this promiscuous Coca chewing. If Coca sustained the Indians, it was of course a food, and its use should not be allowed before the holy eucharist. Necessity brought forth a deliverer from this formidable opponent, and it was represented that Coca was not an aliment, and so its use was reluctantly permitted.

But now came still another effort to prohibit it, from

moral motives. The Indian believed in Coca, he knew that it sustained him without other food in his arduous work, but it had been conclusively shown that it was not a food, and so could not sustain, hence his belief was false, superstitious, even a delusion of the devil to warp the poor Indian from the way he should go. Greed, however, predominated, as gold has ever been a convincing factor, and as the Indian could do most work when supplied with Coca, its use was finally allowed unrestricted, and to-day a portion of Coca is given to all Andean laborers as part of their necessary supplies.

So it will be seen that like all scientific advances which have been made, since Prometheus incurred the wrath of Jove by stealing fire from the gods to put life in mortals, until the present time, Coca has not been admitted to acceptance unassailed. That spirit of antagonism which seems rampant at the very suggestion of progress has caused its allies to rehabilitate and magnify the early errors and superstitions whenever opportunity might admit, together with those newer accessions of false premises engendered through shallowness of investigation. Every department of science has been subjected to similar instances of annoyance, though it would appear that medicine is particularly more subject to such influence. At first a partisan sentimentality, with an exaggeration which provokes condemnation and often results in oblivion, or what in calmer judgment may be a true balance of worth.

It is amusing to now look back at some attacks which were hurled against substances that all the world to-day considers as necessities. The anæsthetic use of chloroform was at first regarded as unholy because it was asserted man is born unto pain as he is unto sin, and so should bear his necessary sufferings in a holy and uncomplaining manner. Every physician frequently meets with just such original and plausible opposition to suggested remedies to-day. When in 1638 Cinchona was introduced into Europe under the name of "Jesuits' powder," it was vigorously denounced as quackery. So great was the prejudice that sprang up against it, even among those eminent physicians whom we now look back upon as the fathers of medicine, that when Chiftelius, in 1653, wrote a book against "the bark," he was complimented as though he had relieved the world of a monster or a pestilence.[4] For years it was not countenanced by "the faculty," and the various arguments then advanced concerning its supposed action form curious reading. The opposition to vaccination, in 1770, was something which excited not only the protests of physicians and learned societies, but the clergy and laity as well. The College of Physicians shook its wise head and refused to recognize Jenner's discovery. The country doctor was considered something of a bore.[5] Innumerable other instances might be cited to testify to this negative spirit prompted by any advance.

Among food products, the humble potato when introduced into Scotland, in 1728, was violently denounced as unholy because "not mentioned in the Bible."[6] It was asserted that it was forbidden fruit, and as that was the cause of man's first fall, to countenance its use would be irreligious. In France, so strong was the feeling against the introduction of potatoes that Louis XVI and his Court wore the flower of the plant as a *boutonnière* to give the much opposed—but desirable—potato at least the prestige of fashion. Tea, coffee and chocolate have each been denounced, and from very high sources too. "A lover of his country," as he designated himself, in 1673, proposed to Parliament "the prohibition of brandy, rum, coffee, chocolate and tea, and the suppressing of coffee houses. These hinder greatly the consumption of barley, malt and wheat, the product of our land." Here would seem to be an ulterior motive that is almost suggestive of the commercial spirit often now displayed, which would suppress one product that another may be permitted to flourish regardless of merit.

As an argument against the pernicious and growing tendency to use tea and coffee, after they had been rendered palatable through knowing how to use them, a Dr. Duncan, of the Faculty of Montpelier, in 1706, wrote: "Coffee and tea were at the first used only as medicine while they continued unpleasant, but since they were made delicious with

[4] Baker; 1818. [5] Russell; 1861. [6] Bell; 1842.

sugar, they are become poison."[7] The *Spectator* of April 29th, 1712, urges against the dangers of chocolate as follows: "I shall also advise my fair readers to be in a particular manner careful how they meddle with romances, chocolates, novels, and the like inflamers which I look upon as very dangerous to be made use of during this great carnival." Opinion on these beverages is not unanimous to-day even, as harmless as they are commonly considered. Alcohol and tobacco of course have come in for an unusual share of denunciation, and the argument is not yet ended. From these through the entire range of stimulant-narcotics, each has excited such vigorous protests that the very term stimulant is considered by some as opprobrious. How real must be the merit that can withstand such storms of abuse, and spring up, perennially blooming, through such opposition!

Coca is unparalleled in the history of plants, and although it has been compared to about every plant that has any stimulating quality, it is wholly unlike any other. In this comparison tobacco, kola, tea, maté, guarana, coffee, cacao, hashish, opium, and even alcohol, has been referred to. It has been made to bear the burden of whatever evils lurk in any or all of these, and has unjustly been falsely condemned through such association. That Coca is chewed by the South American Indians and tobacco is smoked by the North American Indians, that Coca is used in Peru and opium or betel is used in the East—is a fair example of this comparison. It no more nearly resembles kola—with which it is often carelessly confounded, the properties of which are chiefly due to caffeine—than through the allied harmony of its first syllable. While a similarity to various substances taken as beverages is possibly suggested through the

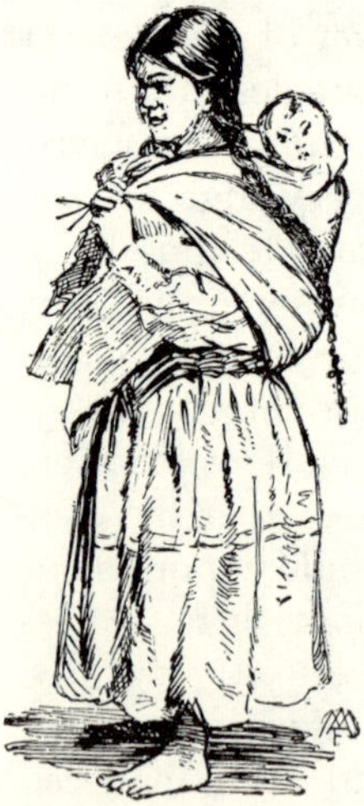

AN ANDEAN NURSE.
[*From a Photograph.*]

[7] *All About Cocoa;* 1896.

fact that Coca is sometimes drunk in decoction by the Peruvians.

The cerebral effects of Coca are entirely different from hashish or opium, and its stimulant action in no way comparable to alcohol. I do not mention these substances to decry them, but merely to illustrate the careless comparisons which have been advanced, through which imperfect conclusions must necessarily be drawn. Then again there is an unfortunate similarity between the pronunciation of the names Coca, and cocoa or cacao—the chocolate nut, and coco*—the coconut, which has occasioned a confusion of thought not wholly limited to some of the laity.

The fact remains that though Coca is used by millions of people,[8] it is not generally known away from its native country. Even many physicians constantly confound it with allied plants of dissimilar properties or with substances of like sounding name. That this is not simply a broad and hasty statement may be illustrated by the following fact. The writing of this work was prompted by the immense divergence of published accounts regarding the efficacy of Coca, in view of which an effort was made to learn the result of its use among a representative class of practitioners, each of whom it was presumed would be well qualified to express an opinion worthy of consideration. An autograph letter, together with an appropriate blank for reply, fully explaining the desirability for this data, was prepared, of which ten thousand were sent out. These were addressed to professors in the several medical colleges, and to those prominent in local medical societies—all eminent in practice. Many did not reply, while of the answers received, fully one half had—"never used Coca in any form." Of the balance, many are—"prejudiced against its use," through some preconceived notion as to its inertness, or through some vague fear of insidious danger which they were not prepared to explain, and even preferred not to inquire into, being—"satisfied it is a dangerous drug."

There are others who inadvertently confound Coca with some of the confusional drugs already referred to or with

* Egyptian *Kuku*. [8] Ten millions, Anstie, p. 35, 1865, from Von Bibra.

cocoa. That this was not merely an apparent fault, through some slip of the pen in hasty writing, is shown by direct answer to the question as to the form of Coca found most serviceable, stating so and so's "breakfast *coca*" is used in place of tea or coffee. In some instances the benefits of Coca were enlarged upon with an earnestness that was inclined to inspire confidence. The physiological action was gone into minutely and its therapeutic application extolled, only to conclude with the amazing statement that the fluid extract, the wine, or "breakfast *coca*" were interchangeably used, thus displaying a confusion worse confounded which might be amusing if not so appalling.

These confusional assertions display one source of error, yet in view of the entwined facts concerning Coca through literature and science it must emphasize the unfortunate neglect of observation, and the refusal to recognize advancement manifest even in this progressive age—among some whose duties and responsibilities should have spurred to a refinement of discernment. It is suggestive of the anecdote told by Park, who when in his Eastern travels asked some Arabs what became of the sun at night, and whether it always was the same sun, or was renewed each day, was staggered with the reply—"such a question is foolish, being entirely beyond the reach of human investigation."[9]

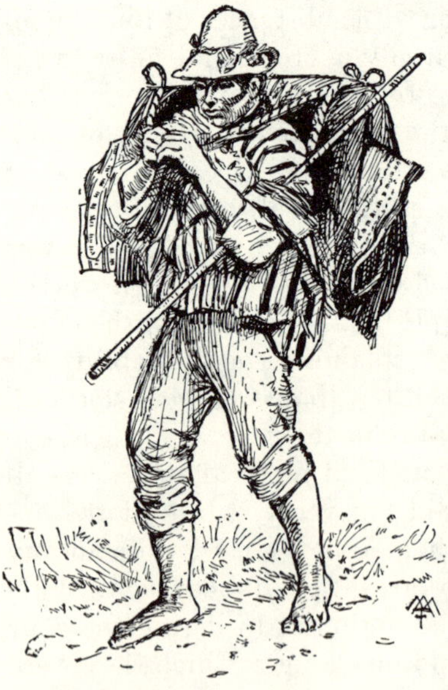

A COCA CARRIER.
[*From a Photograph.*]

Replies fully as surprising were received in this inquiry. Several have taken the "moral" side of the question quite to

[9] Sir John Lubbock.

heart, and expressed a belief that through advocating the popularizing of Coca, I was tending to contribute to the increase of a pernicious and debasing habit which was already undermining the morals of the community. Others again have tried to show me the error I had fallen into when speaking of the dietetic uses of Coca. As one gentleman emphatically expressed it: "This is some terrible mistake, you are confounding Coca with Cocoa! Cocoa is used for food, but Coca—*never*." So that even that part of my investigation pursued among modern medical men has not been as easily carried out as might at first be supposed. There has been the same or similar ignorance and error to sift apart from truth as encompassed the early historical associations of the plant.

This unfortunate confusion is probably to be accounted for because Coca was largely used empirically and without a proper appreciation of its physiological action before its properties were fully known. Writers who have described its local use among the Andean Indians have advanced statements regarding its sustaining qualities which have not been verified by some observers elsewhere located, even though these latter may have carried out a careful line of physiological experimentation. The explanation of this has only recently been determined, but is now known to be due to the extreme volatility of the associate principles of Coca.

Recent, or well cured and properly preserved Coca is wholly different from leaves which have become inert through improper treatment. Then again as our botanical knowledge of this plant has increased, it has indicated that not all leaves termed Coca are such. The family to which the classic leaves of the Incans belong has many species. Among the particular species of Coca there has only quite recently been determined several varieties. The properties of these differ materially according to the presence or absence of certain alkaloidal constituents. Some of the early experiments upon the properties of Coca were made at a time when these facts were unknown, and with this, was the added disadvantage of the impossibility of then obtaining appropriately preserved Coca in the open markets. Not only may the substance examined have been inert, but through different observers using different varieties of Coca the conclusions could not possibly agree. Unfortunately because of the apparent carefulness of research these early statements were accepted and given a wide publicity, and so from the marvelous apparent benefits of Coca among native users to the absolute inertness pronounced by some foreign observers, there has been a very wide space for the admission of much distrust. The busy physician must commonly accept the result of the provings of the experimentalist, and amidst so much doubt it may have seemed easier to set aside a possible remedy than to have personally verified the assertions. Indeed, trial has only too often depreciated hopes from a happy realization of the wonderful properties attributed to the use of native Coca on the Andes, to a realization of the uncertainty of the marketed product at command. In which connection it may not seem too astonishing to say I know of an instance where senna leaves were sold by a wholesale drug house for "fresh Coca leaves," while I doubt if any drug house would make a distinction in offering the casual purchaser any variety of Coca at hand.

It was because of "this uncertainty"—of the conflicting stories and the impossibility to unify facts—that interest in Coca, which had been stimulated in Europe by Dr. Mantegazza about 1859, soon declined until disuse almost left it in forgetfulness. About this time Niemann, then a pupil of Professor Woehler, isolated the alkaloid cocaine from the leaves, and attention was again awakened to the possible usefulness of the parent plant. It was supposed, however, that the active principle to which all the sustaining energy of Coca was due had been discovered in cocaine. Here again was a radical error, and an unfortunate one as it has since proved, to still more confound an intricate problem. This is particularly serious because it is widely accepted as truth, not only among many physicians, but also because it has been spread by this misunderstanding through the secular press, and so falsely impressed the laity. As a result, cocaine has been promiscuously used as a restorative and sustainer under the supposition that it is but Coca in a more convenient and active form. The evils which have followed this use have fallen upon Coca, which has often been erroneously condemned as the cause. It is owing to the wide spread of this belief as well as its resultant evil and because of the difficulty for the lay mind to appreciate the radical difference between Coca and cocaine—between any parent plant and but one of its alkaloids—that it must necessarily require long and persistent effort on the part of educated physicians to explain away this wrong, to reassure those who have been falsely informed as to the real merits of Coca, and so reflect credit upon themselves through the advocacy and use of a really marvelous remedy.

The truth cannot be too forcibly impressed, that cocaine is but one constituent, and no more fully represents Coca than would prussic acid—because found in a minute quantity in the seeds of the peach—represent that luscious fruit. In emphasizing this a recent investigator who passed a long period in the Coca region, studying as a scientist the peculiarities of the plant, and watching as a physician its effect upon native users of the drug, says: "With certain restrictions it may be said that the properties of cocaine, remarkable as they are, lie in an altogether different direction from those of Coca as it has been reported to us from South America."[10] So it will be seen that because of misconstruing early tales and superstitious beliefs, because inert leaves have not yielded results of the sound plant, because some different variety has not yielded the same results as the classic type, because one of its alkaloids does not represent the whole, the parent plant is condemned. Because of this ignorance of certain investigators the historical accounts of the use of Coca and its sustaining qualities among the natives, have been set down to exaggeration or absolute fabrication. As one physician replying to my inquiries would have others believe: "The Indians are great liars." Thus from ignorance, neglect or from false conception, Coca was either wholly ignored or little understood in a popular way, until in 1884 a renewed interest was awakened through the discovery of the qualities of cocaine as an anæsthetic in the surgery of the eye. Then, as though forget-

[10] Rusby; 1888.

ful of all preceding investigation or condemnation, a renewed discussion commenced regarding the asserted qualities of Coca, the failure to realize them, and the probable source of potency of the plant as represented by cocaine.

This was followed by frequently reported accounts of a new and terrible vice which was springing up everywhere—the so-called "cocaine habit." For this Coca was condemned,

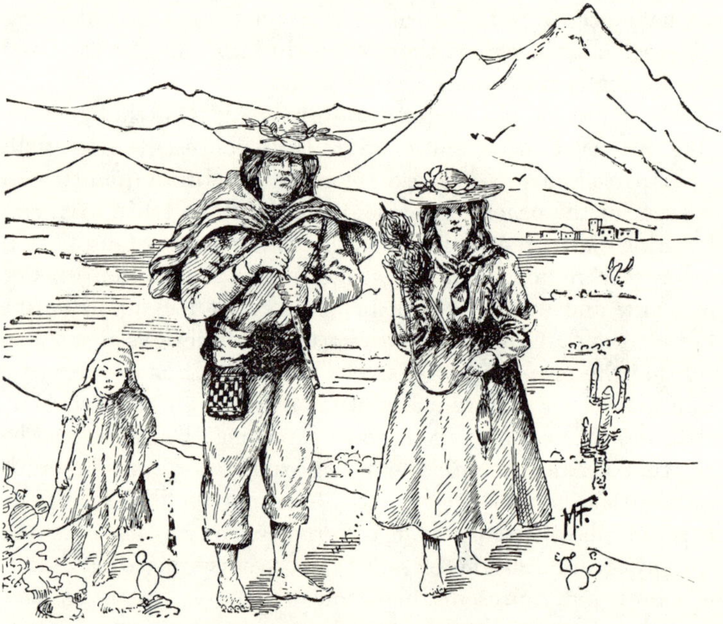

Some Descendants of the Incans.

as its enemies pretended to now see the real element of perniciousness. Yet before cocaine was ever dreamed of and during the long centuries in the history of Coca, not one case of poisoning from its use has ever been recorded. The accusation of "habit" had, however, long before been erroneously directed against the leaves. But of this, one who wrote scientifically and extensively on Peru after personal observation, sets forth his conclusions in the following positive way: "Coca is not merely innocuous, but even very conducive to health."[11] He even calculated the improbability of harm by estimating, if an Indian reached the age of one hundred and thirty years—which seems to be the only "habit" to which these people are addicted beside the "habit" for hard work—he would have consumed two thousand seven hundred pounds of leaves, an amount sufficient to have quite fully determined all pernicious possibilities. Indeed, to think of Coca as an injurious substance suggests the character in one of Madison Morton's farces who wished to "shuffle off" speedily, and determined to chew poppy heads "because poppy heads contain poppy seeds, and poppy seeds eaten constantly for several years will produce instant death."

The theory has been advanced that because cocaine is one of the chief alkaloids of Coca, it represents whatever sustaining quality the leaf can possibly have, and manufacturers base their choice of leaves upon the percentage of cocaine determined by assay. But this is not in unanimity with the selection of the native users of Coca, any more than would the quality of a choice tobacco leaf be governed by the amount of nicotine it contains. The fact is the Andean Indian selects Coca that is rich in the more volatile associate alkaloids and low in cocaine. It is what is known as the sweet in contradistinction to the bitter-leaf, which latter is made bitter by the large amount of cocaine it contains. On this very point an authority says:—"It only remains for me to point out that the relative amount of cocaine contained in native Coca leaves exerts no influence in determining the Indian's selection of his supply. As a matter of fact, the ordinary conditions to which the leaves are subject during the first two or three months after they are gathered have but little effect upon their original percentage of cocaine. The Indian, however, makes his selections from among such leaves with the greatest care, eagerly seeking the properly dried leaves from some favorite cocal, whose produce is always most readily brought out, and absolutely rejecting other leaves, notwithstanding that the percentages of cocaine may be almost identical."[12]

The absolute reliance of the Andean Indians upon Coca

[11] Von Tschudi; 1840. [12] Rusby; 1888.

not only for sustenance, but as a general panacea for all ills, has naturally led them to feel a superstitious regard for the plant. This reverence has descended to them from the Incan period, during which the shrub was looked upon as "a living manifestation of divinity, and the places of its growth a sanctuary where all mortals should bend the knee."[13] However much the Incas reverenced Coca they did not worship it; it was considered the greatest of all natural productions, and as such was offered in their sacrifices. Their ceremonial offerings were made to their conception of deity—the sun, which they held to be the giver of all earthly blessings.

The ideas of moral depravity, and the fears of debasing habit following the use of Coca, have sprung from false premises and early misconceptions as to the true nature of the plant. As a matter of fact, neither "habit," as that is understood, nor poisoning has ever been recorded against Coca among the natives where it has been continued in use for centuries. Those early writers on Andean customs who allude to Coca chewing all speak positively against any evil result following its use. One physician, after being intimately associated among the natives for nearly a year, where he had witnessed the constant use of Coca, failed to find a single case of chronic cocaism, although this one subject chiefly occupied his attention, and he searched assiduously for information. Speaking of the amount used, he says: "what it does for the Indian at fifteen it does for him at sixty, and a greatly increasing dose is not resorted to. There is no reaction, nor have I seen any of the evil effects depicted by some writers and generally recorded in books."[14]

The early objections by the Spanish against the use of Coca were rather as persecutions, intended to still further oppress this conquered race by taking from them what was looked upon as an idle and expensive luxury. But Coca-chewing could never be an expensive luxury in a country where it grows wild, and where it is given by those in charge of laborers as a regular portion of each man's daily supplies. The later cries against its perniciousness, as has been shown, were based

[13] Unanue; 1794. [14] Rusby; 1888.

wholly upon the action of cocaine following the widespread use of that alkaloid as a local anæsthetic. The reports in the medical press of injurious effects from the use of cocaine all date from the period when the entire medical world was active in the discussion of the merits of this great boon to minor surgery. It would seem that many then rushed into print without regard to method so long as something was said about the all-absorbing topic of the time, which might direct a portion of attention to themselves. A new opportunity had arisen when old tales and early prejudices might be again reiterated concerning Coca. The lay press was not slow to take up the sensational side of the subject, and the "cocaine habit" soon became a well-determined condition in theory, and a fashionable complaint. I have personally investigated a number of such reported cases and in every instance have found either that it was a condition engrafted upon some previous "habit" in a nervous subject, or else that the report was absolutely false. There is no motive—as the lawyers would say—for the offense, there is no reason for the establishment of a habit such as exists in the case of alcohol or opium. The fact is there exists a certain class of subjects who are so weak in will power, that if they should repeat any one thing for a few consecutive times they would become habituated to that practice. But such cases are the exceptions, and have no especial bearing upon Coca. In the collective investigation among several thousand physicians,* this matter was particularly impressed as an important point of inquiry and the answers sustained the facts already explained, that a Coca habit has never existed. During the early part of 1898 a case was reported very sensationally in the secular press regarding a Dr. Holmes who had died in an asylum at Ardendale, N. Y., a hopeless wreck as a result of cocaine habit. I communicated with the physician in charge of that institution and was promptly assured "Dr. Holmes did not die as a result of 'cocaine habit,' nor had he ever been addicted to it."

That Coca has survived the attacks which have been periodically hurled against it during several hundred years,

* See detailed report of physicians in Appendix.

and that its use is not only continued, but its therapeutic application constantly increasing, must suggest to the thinking mind that it is possessed of remarkable value. It has continued with the Andeans not because they have formed a "habit" for it, not because it fills their minds with that ecstatic and dreamful bliss as habit drugs would do, but because experience has taught them that they can perform their work better by its use. There is a practical utility in it which, as will be seen when detailing some of the customs of these people, is so exact that they measure their distances by the amount of Coca that they chew instead of by the rod and chain, or chronometer. Their use of this plant is continued day after day during a long lifetime, yet the amount of Coca which sustains them in young adult life is not increased in their old age. Its force product is a constant factor, just as a given amount of water under proper conditions will make a known amount of steam. The fuel taken and the work performed is always the same, other conditions being equal.

Can it be presumed for a moment that if this general and persistent use of Coca is a depraved habit, sapping the best of moral qualities, even manhood, unfitting its users to perform their duties, that these people would be capable of the immense amount of physical work which they do? It is known to be a fact by those employing large forces of workmen in the Peruvian mines, that the Indian would not and could not perform the tasks he is set to under the exposure he is subjected to without Coca. This is well shown by contrast when foreigners are compelled to work with them, and are unable to perform an equal amount of labor to theirs until they too have recourse to the use of Coca. Thus it must be seen that Coca is as worthy to-day as it was in the time of the Incas of being termed the "divine plant." It is Nature's best gift to man. It neither morally corrupts nor undermines manhood, or vitality, as is well shown in these Indians, who are long-lived and are held by those who know them best, to be conservative, respectful, virtuous, honest and trustworthy, addicted to hard work—and the use of Coca, that they may more thoroughly and successfully do that work.

That any plant or substance which has been continued in daily use by millions of people over a vast territory, for many hundreds of years, should have so long remained unrecognized by the world at large seems almost incredible. Yet the fact is undoubted, as has been shown, and Coca is even to-day unknown to a great majority of not only the masses, but of physicians. Since the date of the Conquest, the constant use of Coca leaves by the Indians has been frequently referred to by travellers, often superficially, yet commonly agreeing as to its sustaining qualities. But so wonderful have these accounts seemed that their simple relation has usually excited doubt rather than belief. They have been looked upon as "travellers' tales," relations due to an imagination, which possibly had been expanded by the conjoined influence of a rarefied atmosphere, and an exalted desire to enhance the wonders of travel. So from doubting qualities which were long looked upon as improbable or unexplainable, and from the inaccuracies recorded by those who affected scientific research on old leaves, it was but a simple step to relegate the very existence of the plant to the legendary.

It has been shown in outline how varied were the causes to account for this unbelief, and the consequent neglect which followed. Primarily to superficial observation on the part of early explorers in an unknown country, where consideration for mere existence was to the unacclimated often of the first importance. Added to this was the conservative reticence of the Indians, and their superstitious regard for this plant so intimately linked with their religious and political life. This alone was sufficient to prevent the ready acquirement by travellers of a detailed knowledge of the use of Coca, or even of native customs and the reason for them.

Here was sufficient possibility for hasty conclusions, aside from the forceful attacks of both Church and State against what they were pleased to regard as the continuance of a superstitious practice or vulgar habit, which possibly linked the desires of these people whom they hoped to Christianize, with an idolatrous past. Then, too, there existed as now, a class of zealots seeing imaginative wrong in every custom, who would have every act discontinued simply because it is done, in dread of some direful consequence which may result. In furthering each of these negative influences, theories were often advanced at variance with existent facts, and so many conflicting tales and much confusion has resulted. Absurd stories have been published, and these again, copied without apparent attempt at verification, the whole establishing a falsity from which there has grown a diversity of opinion wholly inconsistent with the exact requirements of science. Meanwhile the rapid progress of the world in exploration often engrossed attention to the exclusion of details. The demand of commercial interests, for broad facts and immediate results in the amassing of wealth, diverted attention from the tales of travellers or the disputes of scientists. But as a higher civilization demands the resources of the universe to maintain its conditions, the secret of Nature's gift to the Andean could not remain long hidden, and the means which afforded support for these simple people was recognized as of possible benefit to the rest of the plodding, toiling world. As Coca was shown to be a necessity to the Andean in his toilsome travels of exposure, its adaptability was suggested to other members of the human family elsewhere located who are comparatively as subject to privation and hardship as are these primitive people. Even in our great cities among modern resources the labor is exacting and exhaustive, and whether the work done be a strain of muscular exertion or a prolonged mental effort, the resultant wear and tear is similar, and the conditions are to be met by recourse to the most expedient means available.

Unfortunately the Spanish invasion of Peru so largely destroyed all native records that it has been difficult to readily retrace a continued history of the remarkable people of this early civilization, among whom our story of Coca must begin. But from the period of the Conquest, after it had been made known to the outer world Coca was frequently sung in poetry or recounted in the tales of travellers. It however continued, since the privilege was extended from its early users to their descendants, to almost exclusively be enjoyed by these people until less than half a century ago.

In properly determining the benefits of Coca it seems desirable to trace back its historical connections and its associations between past uses and present necessities, as well as to inquire into those surroundings which have prompted its use and called for its continuance. This must necessarily lead us through many interesting fields where the view may seem remote from our narrative, yet is essential to the full understanding of a story the first-impulse for which was generated in the horrors of the Conquest. Before entering on this more

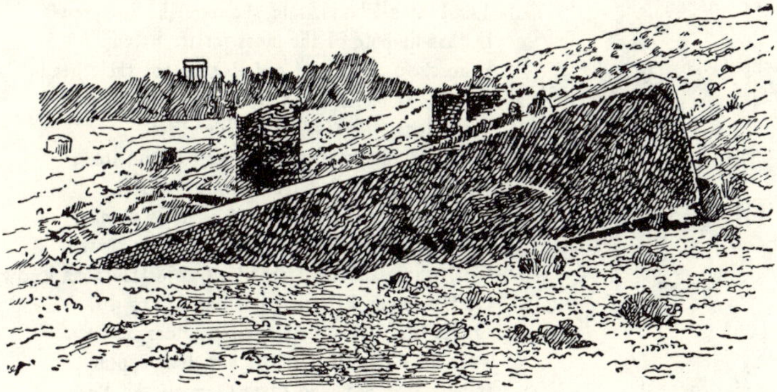

MAMMOTH STONE AT BAALBEK, SYRIA, SIMILAR TO MANY MONOLITHS IN THE LAND OF THE INCAS.

prosaic story, I wish to recall a writing of long ago that is fittingly associated with our History of Coca.

Dr. Abraham Cowley, of whom Dr. Johnson said: "In Cowley's mind botany turns into poetry"—in 1662 wove the qualities of Coca through a legendary tale so accurately and charmingly that these have scarcely been added to by the research of other scientists.

At a convention of the gods, which was presided over by Venus, to discuss various fruits, the merits of each was set forth by its god. The poem is taken up where Bacchus, in illustration of the virtues of the vine, has offered a cup of wine to a South American godling:

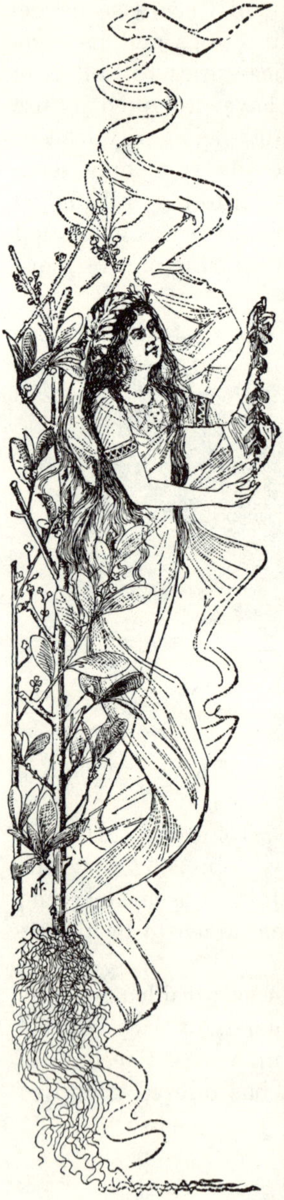

He, unaccuftomed to the acid juice,
Storm'd, and with Blows had answer'd the Abuse,
But fear'd t'engage the European Gueft,
Whofe Strength and Courage had subdu'd the Eaft;
He therefore choofes a less dangerous Fray,
And summons all his Country's Plants away;
Forthwith in decent order they appear,
And various Fruits on various Branches wear.
Like Amazons they stand in painted Arms,
Coca alone appear'd with little Charms,
Yet led the Van, our scoffing Venus Scorn'd
The shrub-like tree, and with no Fruit adorn'd,
The Indian Plants, said she, are like to speed
In this dispute of the most fertile Breed,
Who choose a Dwarf and Eunuch for their head;
Our Gods laughed out aloud at what she said.
Pachamama defends her darling Tree,
And said the wanton Goddess was too free;
You only know the fruitfulness of Luft,
And therefore here your judgment is unjuft,
Your skill in other offsprings we may truft,
With thofe Chafte tribes that no diftinction know
Of Sex, your Province nothing has to do.
Of all the Plants that any Soil does bear,
This Tree in Fruits the richeft does appear,
It bears the beft, and bears them all the Year.
Ev'n now with Fruits 'tis stor'd—why laugh you yet?
Behold how thick with Leaves it is befet;
Each Leaf is Fruit, and such fubftantial Fare,
No Fruit beside to rival it will dare.
Mov'd with his Country's coming Fate (whofe Soil
Muft for her Treafurers be expofed to spoil)
Our Varicocha firft this Coca sent,
Endow'd with leaves of wond'rous Nourishment,
Whose Juice Succ'd in, and to the Stomach tak'n
Long Hunger and long Labour can fuftain;
From which our faint and weary Bodies find
More Succor, more they cheer the drooping Mind,
Than can your Bacchus and your Ceres join'd.
Three Leaves supply for six days' march afford;
The Quitoita with this Provision stor'd
Can pass the vaft and cloudy Andes o'er,
The dreadful Andes plac'd 'twixt Winter's Store
Of Winds, Rains, Snow, and that more humble Earth,
That gives the small, but valiant, Coca birth;
This Champion that makes war-like Venus Mirth.

Nor Coca only useful art at Home,
A famous Merchandize thou art become ;
A thousand Paci and Vicugni groan
Yearly beneath thy Loads, and for thy sake alone
The spacious World's to us by Commerce Known.
Thus spake the Goddess (on her painted Skin
Were figures wrought) and next called Hovia in,
That for it's stony Fruit may be despis'd,
But for its Virtue next to Coca priz'd.
Her shade by wond'rous Influence can compoſe
And lock the Senſes in such sweet Repose
That oft the Natives of a diſtant Soil
Long journeys take of voluntary Toil,
Only to sleep beneath her branches' shade ;
Where in tranſporting Dreams entranc'd they lye
And quite forget the Spaniards' Tyranny.

—*Book of Plants.*

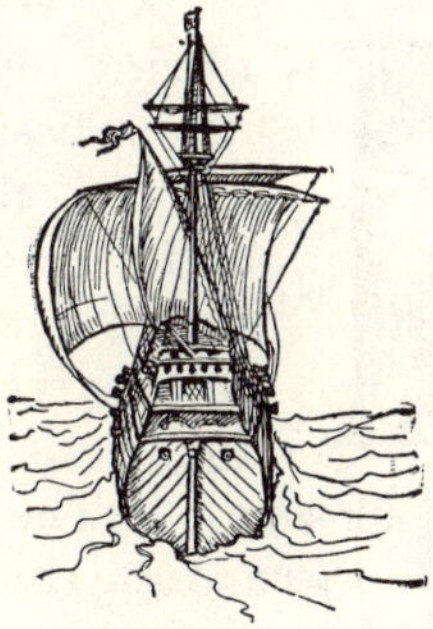

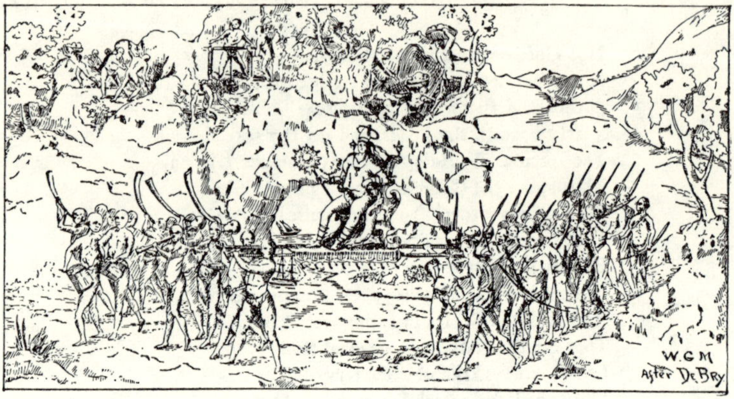

CHAPTER II.

THE STORY OF THE INCANS.

"Our *Varicocha* first this *Coca* sent,
Endow'd with Leaves of wond'rous Nourishment."
—*Cowley*.

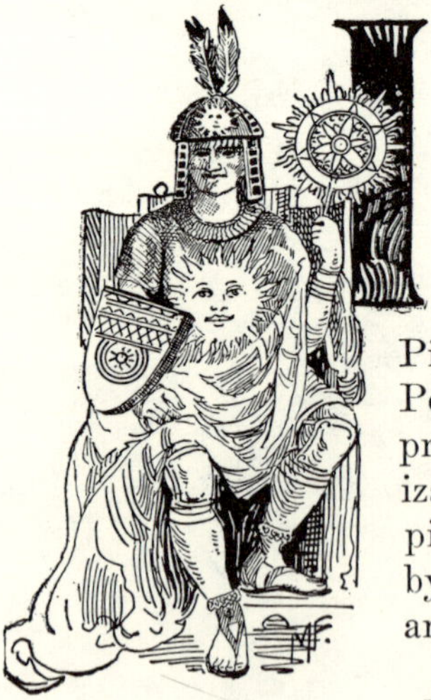

IN tracing the history of Coca from its earliest associations, we are led into that wonderland of its nativity where its discovery and even first application is lost amidst the traditions which surround the empire overthrown by Pizarro. The dominant people of Peru at the time of the Conquest comprised a race highly advanced in civilization known as Incas, a mighty empire developed from a foundation laid by the semi-legendary Manco Ccapac[1] and his sister-wife, Mama Ocllo.

We are accustomed to consider the aboriginal peoples of America as Indians, of which an accepted type is the noble red man pictured by Cooper in his classic stories of the nomadic savages

[1] The double *c* in Quichua is pronounced like *k*.

who inhabited North America; but the early Peruvians it is presumed were in no way allied to the red men of the North.[2] They were not only a race distinct in characteristics and customs, but they possessed the marked difference of a highly wrought social organization, so that we must view these early people, who are spoken of as the Incas of Peru, as a mighty monarchy quite as important—if of a less degree—as was that of the ancient Egyptians or Romans. But who these people were before they settled in Peru, where they came from and how they got there, or whether—as has been suggested—Peru was the cradle of the human race from which was peopled other continents, is an enigma, the solution of which is locked in the impenetrable mystery of the past. Antiquarians, ethnologists and archæologists have delved in vain toward unearthing this hidden past, for these people had no written language and all that has been evolved is the mute but expressive records of their works, their arts of pottery, textile fabrics, their monuments, their poetry and their traditions, through which are displayed their customs, which often speak far more concisely and forcibly than do the hieroglyphic carvings of other lands.

An attempt has been made to trace the people who established this early empire from various nations of the Old World. Montesinos,[3] an ancient Spanish chronicler, declares that they came from Armenia about five hundred years after the deluge, while other theorists connect them with the Egyptians, with the early Hebrews, and with the Chinese. It was advanced in support of this latter theory that Manco Ccapac was the son of Kublai-Khan, the first Chinese Emperor of the Yuen dynasty. Others again have supposed that the Incas may have come from what is presumed to have been an earlier civilization in Mexico and Yucatan, which with Peru had certain resemblances to the Eastern nations. Many of the Incan customs were similar to those of the Aztecs, and to the

[2] It has been asserted that the cranial and other physiological evidences indicate that the type of red man of the New World from the Arctic Circle to the Straits of Magellan is so slightly varied that all Indians may be said to constitute one race. Nadaillac: *Indigenous Races of the Earth.*

[3] A Dominican missionary who visited Peru one hundred years after the Conquest, and travelled for fifteen years through the viceroyalty. He gives a line of one hundred and one sovereigns prior to the Conquest.

Mayas, though the architecture is distinct—the first tending to temples, the latter to towered pyramids, while the arch is very rarely found among the ruins of either; yet some of the Peruvian vaulted remains indicate that the idea of the arch was known to the Incas in principle.

So stupendous is the Peruvian scenery, so wonderful the ruins that it is not surprising the founders of this mighty country should have been considered of mythical origin. Purchas, in his *Pilgrims,* relates of an early race of giants inhabiting the Peruvian coast, who were responsible for some of the megalithic remains still extant. These giants were addicted to sodomy, and as the Indians thought, were in consequence destroyed by fire from heaven. Others again would have the country originate from a lot of pigmies who were not over two cubits high, and there are not only traditions but vestiges which indicate that a race of small people really did inhabit parts of both Central America and South America. There were several traditions among the Incan people as to their origin, one of which referred to a flood and the repeopling of the world by a family of brothers who mysteriously appeared from a cave.

Gregorio Garcia, a Spanish Dominican author,

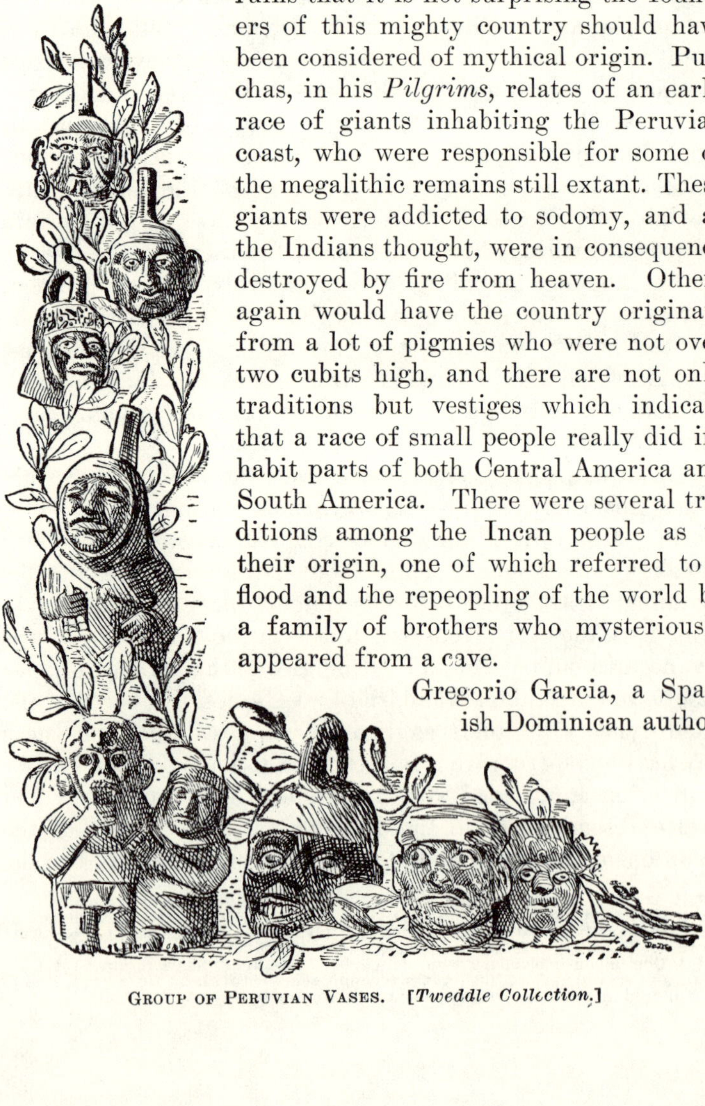

GROUP OF PERUVIAN VASES. [*Tweddle Collection.*]

alludes to a tradition,[4] according to which the Peruvians proceeded from the nine and a half tribes of Israel, whom Shalmaneser, King of Assyria, carried away captive. Humboldt has traced the origin of the Toltecs to the Huns, while Paravey, in 1844, attempted to prove that Fu-Sang, described in the Chinese annals, is the Mexican Empire which was known to the Chinese in the fifth century, and showed that at Uxmal in Yucatan, there had been found sculptured the Buddha of Java seated under the head of a Siva. Rivero considers that there is no doubt but Quetzalcoatl, Bochica, and Manco Ccapac were Buddhist priests, and that the Peruvian gods Con, Pachacamac and Uiracocha corresponded to Bramah, Vishnu and Siva. There seems certainly an intimate connection shown between the Hindu *Devadasa*—servants of the gods—and the Incan Virgins of the Sun.

In Quichua—the language of the Incas, there are many words resembling Sanscrit, as *Inti*—the sun, while *Indra* is the Hindu god of the heavens. *Raymi* was the great Incan festival in honor of the sun, and *Rama* was a child of the sun in India. *Sita* was the wife of *Rama* in Hindu mythology, and *Situ* was one of the Incan sun festivals. It would seem as though the connection is too similar to be merely accidental. There were many customs and rites followed by the Incas similar to those of the early Jews. The Incas offered their first fruits, celebrated the new moon, and divided their year into four seasons corresponding with the Jewish festivals, while their ceremonies of purification and the use of the bath and ointments, their method of fasting and manner of prayer were all somewhat suggestive[5] of the Jewish forms. Other comparisons indicate that the early Peruvians, through their architecture, resembled the Egyptians, while their pottery in shape and in design is similar to the Assyrian and to the Greek. Their features, however, and many of their customs are distinctly Mongolian. The consensus of opinion now is that these people in some prehistoric time found their way to the shores of South America from China and other

[4] Garcia; 1729.
[5] Rivero; *Memorias Antiguas Historiales del Peru. Anales o Memorias Neuvas del Peru.*

parts of Eastern Asia.[6] There are many customs among the Tibetans and throughout Chinese Tartary that closely resemble the modern customs of the Andeans.

Whatever opinions and traditions there may be on the early origin of the Peruvians, all coincide on one point, that the first appearance of the progenitors of the Incan race was in the Titicaca region,[7] and the site of their government was at the City of Cuzco.[8] The most often related legend of the Incan origin describes a pair of white people—Manco Ccapac[9] and Mama Ocllo—as mysteriously appearing on the shore of Lake Titicaca, and being possessed of a golden wand which was to act as a sort of divining rod to determine the location of the seat of the new empire wherever this rod should sink into the earth. Travelling north through the Andean garden of Eden, it was not until they reached the site of Cuzco that this golden wedge plunged into the earth and disappeared forever, and here was built the palace of the first Inca. Another legend describes a god—*Ataguju*[10]—the creator of all things, having made the first man—*Guamansuri,* who descended to the earth and there seduced the sisters of certain rayless ones or darklings—*Guachemines,* who then possessed it. For this crime he was destroyed, while the sisters gave birth to two eggs from which were hatched the twin brothers, *Apocatequil* and *Piguerao.* The former was the more powerful, and was venerated by the Indians as their maker because he released them from the soil by turning it up with a golden spade. He it was—as they supposed, who produced thunder and lightning by hurling stones with his sling, while the thunderbolts were considered to be his children. One of the principal weapons of the Incan warriors was the *huaraca* or sling, and the shaping of the hills was often considered in their traditions as due

[6] An interesting discussion and references on this point may be found in the *Narrative and Critical History of America.*

[7] *Titi*—tiger, *Caca*—rock: because of a tiger with a ruby light in its head, which legend said guarded the rock in the lake when Manco Ccapac first stepped from the sun.

[8] According to Garcilasso, in the language of the Incas, Cuzco means navel, hence the heart or centre of the Incan empire, while Montesinos considers Cuzco to be derived from the Indian word *cosca*—to level, or from the heaps of earth about that city termed *coscas.*

[9] The term "Manco" is a proper name without any significance in etymology. "Ccapac" implies rich, and the ruling Inca was known as "Sapallan," sovereign lord and king.

[10] Brinton; 1868.

to the clever hurling of monster stones by some legendary god, and so it was that *Huanacaure,* a brother of Manco Ccapac, had split the hills by some mighty throw. These stories are not wholly of Incan origin, but have rather become so through adoption in the course of centuries, for it was the habit of the

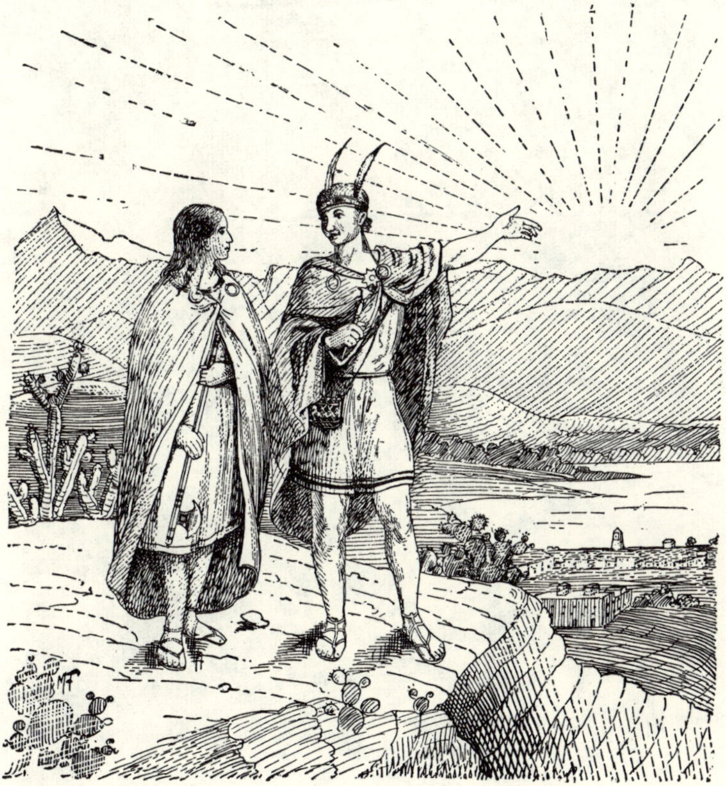

MANCO CCAPAC AND MAMA OCLLO HUACO. [*After Rivero and Tschudi.*]

Incas to blend the religion of conquered peoples with that of their own, while their traditions were continued and so ultimately looked upon as Incan.

Pachacamac, the founder of the world, was the name of an early Peruvian deity, otherwise known as *Uiracocha,* which

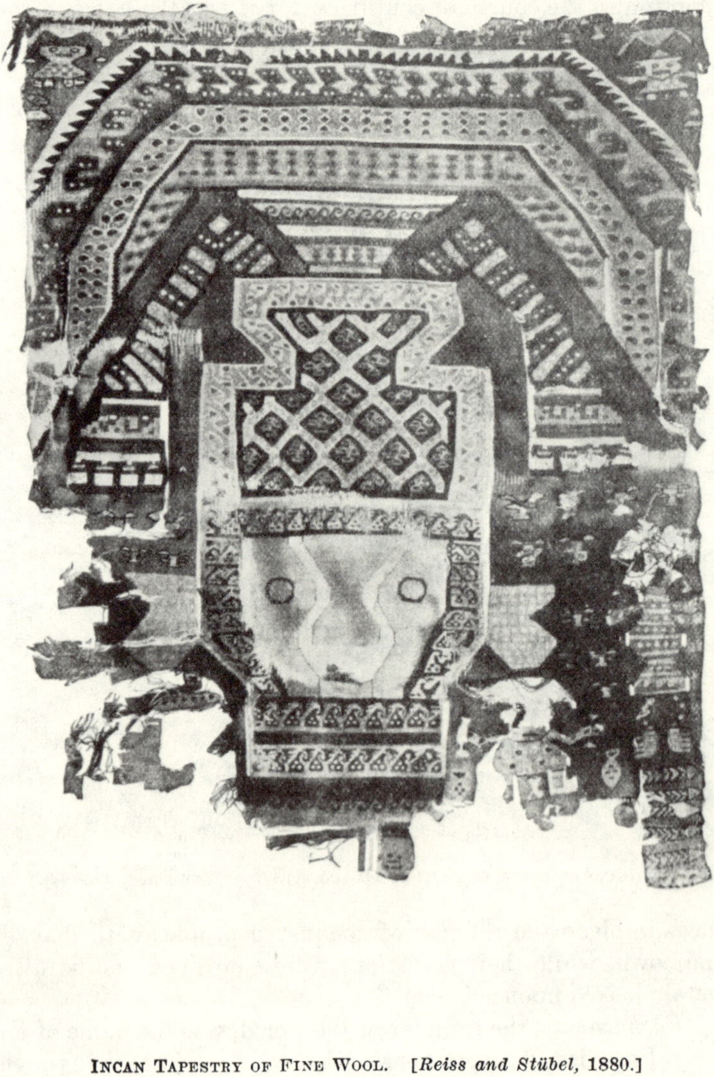

INCAN TAPESTRY OF FINE WOOL. [*Reiss and Stübel*, 1880.]

latter has been corrupted to *Viracocha*,[11] a term of varied meaning at present applied by the Indians of some provinces to all white men, while the first title it is known was adopted after the conquering of the early people about the site of the present city of Lima, where the worship of Con and Pachacama prevailed.[12] One local legend represented these two as father and son, or brothers, children of the sun. They were without flesh or blood, impalpable, invisible and remarkably swift in flight. *Uiracocha* was the culture hero of the *Aymaras* or *Collas*, who are also referred to as a portion of the *Piuras*, an early Incan tribe of the Titicaca region. In their creed he was not only the creator but possessor of all things; though offerings of lands and herds were given to other gods, none were given to him—"For," said one of the Incas: "Shall the Lord and master of the whole world need these things from us?" He it was presumably—who constructed the wondrous cities whose ruins are to be found about Titicaca. He also made the sun and moon and after placing them in the sky peopled the earth. Tradition has associated these legendary tales with real beings, of whom Manco Ccapac, the first Inca—who is supposed to have been a veritable personage—has been made the hero. However originating, it is agreed that this first sovereign founded his government, about the year 1021, at Cuzco, where, upon a hill so steep as to be practically unassailable, was established the first fortress of the Empire. But long before the time of this Incan hero this place had been the stronghold of some other race, of the origin or nature of which there is not even tradition.

In extending their dominions the Incans made no mere savage war, but their purpose was to teach the wild tribes about them, to instruct them in their religion and to elevate them to their plane. Filled with this noble purpose no depredations were permitted among the conquered and no waste of life or property was tolerated. "For," said one of the Incas, "we must spare our enemies or it will be our loss, since they and all that belongs to them must soon be ours." One of the

[11] *Viracocha* may be translated—"Foam of the sea," though Garcilasso less poetically says it is "Sea of grease."
[12] *Con*—thunder, *Ppacha*—source, *Cama*—all, the source of all things.

first things that was done after acquiring any new territory was to send a certain number of the newly conquered people into some other section of the country and these were replaced by a like number from the Incans, who were known as *mitimaes.* By this intermingling the customs of each were acquired by the other, so the transition became the easier.

In those districts east of the Andes where Coca could be cultivated, these new people were taught to raise the plant and paid their tributes in Coca to the government. Temples for worship were erected and the language of the Incas was taught, while the idols of the gods of the savages were carried to Cuzco and there set up in the Temple of the Sun. The chiefs of the conquered tribes were received in accordance with their rank and created Incan nobles, with rights little less than those of royal birth. So each new addition to the Empire was united with respect for the higher order of things because of this tribal interest in the seat of government, which was now looked upon as mutual. How far different from all this was the treatment of these noble people by those who claimed a higher civilization!

It is very probable that the Incan customs and many of their religious rites were fashioned upon the traditions of the people who preceded them as well as added to from time to time by the acquisition of newly conquered tribes. This has occasioned much historical confusion, but the fact is shown by the continuance of many Incan ceremonies which the Spanish found it impossible to wholly eradicate, and so cleverly united with their own. So that to-day, in the religious performances among the Peruvian Indians, there is frequently displayed a curious commingling of ancient ceremonies, with representations of native gods combined with the sacred images and observances of the Catholic church, which is the state religion of Peru.

As the Inca was the ruler of the four quarters of the earth, so the kingdom was divided into four parts, termed *Ttahuantin-suyu*—or the four provinces. These were *Anti-suyu*—east, *Cunti-suyu*—west, *Chincha-suyu*—north, and *Colla-suyu*—south, the people of each of these localities being distinguished by a peculiar dress, and when they were assembled in the capital city they took up their stations nearest to that part of the country to which they belonged. All the people were divided into *ayllus* or tribes, the unit of which was ten—the *Chunca,* similar to the division of government in ancient Rome. Ten families being under the command of a *Chunca camayoc.* The working members of each clan were assigned to definite occupations; the boys from sixteen to twenty were set apart for light work and were known as *Cucapallac* or Coca pickers. Above these were the *Yma-huayna* or sturdy youths, from twenty to twenty-five. Then the *Puric,* who were able-bodied men and heads of families, capable of the most trying work, finally the *Chanpi-ruccu* or elderly men, who were unfitted for labor. Ten *Chuncas* formed a *Pachaca,* ten of which were classed as a *Huaranca,* again formed into ten, making a *Hunu* of 10,000 men, each division being under an appropriate officer. The army was formed by groups of ten after a similar manner to that in which the people were divided into clans. Thus there were ten men, ten companies, and so on, extending up to a corps of five thousand, under the chief captain or *Hatun-apu,*[13] while under him was the *Hatun-apup-rantin,* and half of this number obeyed an *Apu* or captain with his *Apup-rantins* or lieutenants, while the whole army was commanded by an *Apusquipay.*

The Inca was always considered divine and as a direct descendant from the sun was regarded immeasurably beyond and superior to any others of the race. He was the source from which everything emanated, not only framing the laws, but enforcing their fulfillment. In all the ceremonies in which the sovereign participated he was surrounded with an imposing pomp, and his palaces were examples of rare magnificence. His court at all times numbered many thousand persons, including nobles of direct descent, the *curacas* or nobility of the conquered tribes, officers of the household, governors, astrologers, *amautas*—or philosophers, poets and servants.

The dress of the monarch was unique; he wore a tunic-

[13] *Hatun*—great, *apu*—captain.

like poncho, the *Ccapac-ongo*—of spotless white, bordered with precious stones. This robe was short to expose golden knee coverings. The *suntur-paucar* was a headdress of gold ornamented on each side with spurs and surmounted by two white feathers of the royal bird—*coraquenque*,[14] on its front was the figure of *Inti-churi*—the sun god. About the head was a soft turban termed *llauta*—of red, from which was suspended a scarlet fringe of wool—the *borla*—the especial badge of sovereignty, while two bandelettes dropping to the shoulders formed a frame around the face somewhat suggestive of an Egyptian headdress. On state occasions a collar of emeralds was worn, and the hair was decorated with golden ornaments. On the monarch's feet were golden *usutas*—or sandals, and a fringe of red feathers was about the ankles. From the left

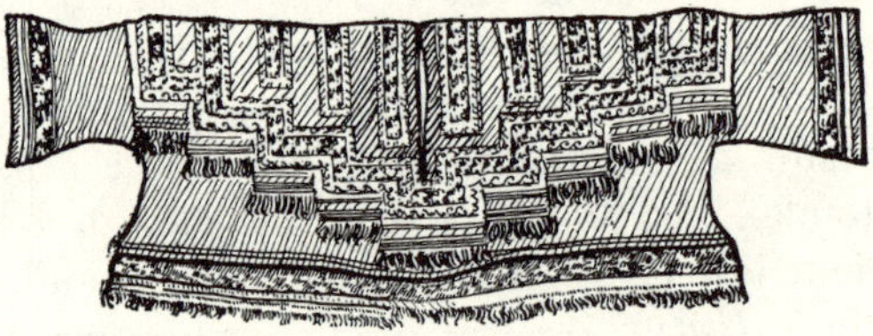

An Incan Poncho, or Shirt. [*After Wiener.*]

shoulder hung a striped mantle, while a band worn saltierwise suspended a little bag known as *chuspa*—woven in delicate patterns from the finest wool of the *vicuña*—in which the Coca leaves were carried. This bag was as important a portion of the vestments of the sovereign as was the royal headdress, or the *camppi*—sceptre, held in his right hand. The people of the Inca were distinguished by the varying colors of their headdress—that of the immediate family was yellow, while for the royal descendants it was black, and even the attendants wore some distinctive dress, the court livery being blue, while that for the guards, the army and for the nobles was all different and at once showed not only the rank, but lineage.

[14] The "Coraquenque" or "Alcamari" is a vulture-like bird of the higher Andes. It has a scarlet head, black body with long white wing feathers. The Incas believed there was but a single pair of these birds, created to supply the two white feathers in the crown of each monarch.

Usage allowed this mighty king one wife, termed *coya*, though he was privileged to maintain a royal harem formed of as many concubines as might be thought fitting to his pleasure. Usually these were maidens chosen from the Virgins of the Sun. Once they had basked in the royal sunshine, an element of grandeur clung to them ever after, even though they might be cast aside. During the most brilliant epoch of the monarchy these concubines are said to have numbered

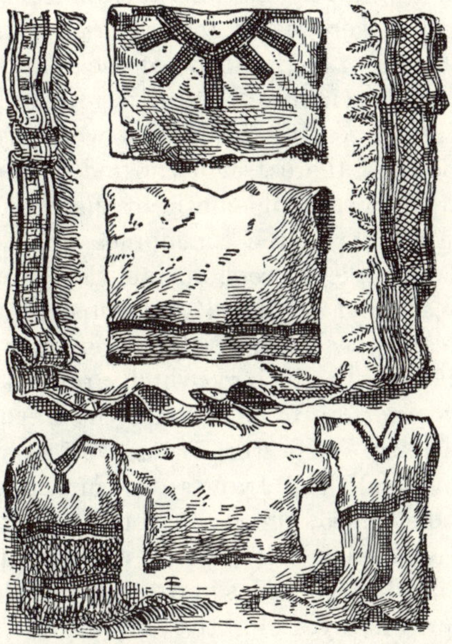

EXAMPLES OF INCAN PONCHOS. [*After Wiener.*]

fully seven hundred, each one having many servants. As may be inferred, the progeny of the sovereign was numerous, some of the Incas having left more than three hundred descendants.[15]

The daughters of the sovereign were termed *ñustas* when maidens, and *pallas* when married. While some few may have been privileged to grace the royal court, the majority were sent in childhood as Virgins to be educated in the

[15] Garcilasso; 1609.

Temple of the Sun under the supervision of a *mamacona* or mother superior. Here, tenderly guarded in chaste seclusion, they were taught to tend the sacred fires until chosen to become concubines—*huayru-aclla* for the sovereign. Thus the royal blood was continued through an exclusive descent by these incestuous unions similar to those practiced in the East.

The male children of the wife were the royal successors and formed the heads of tribes or *ayllus*. They were carefully educated in their youth by the *amautas* or learned men until such time as they were fitted for the *huaracu,* a ceremony similar to the Order of Knighthood of the Middle Ages—possibly more nearly resembling the initiation into the Ancient Mysteries. The successful candidates were accorded privileges of manhood and thereafter permitted to wear the *chuspa* and use the royal Coca, emblematic of vigor and endurance. The male descendants of the concubines, while regarded as princes, could not take succession, but they were considered as of noble lineage and entrusted with important offices.

The physical appearance of the Incan race may be surmised from the early paintings which are still preserved at Lima, and a comparison of these with the Peruvian Indians of to-day. In stature they were from five feet six to five feet ten inches, with well knit frames, the muscular system not pronouncedly developed, the limbs rounded with underlying fatty tissue, of slender form, yet capable of prolonged endurance; the head large and square, the complexion a fresh olive, nose aquiline, eyes slightly oblique, the hair straight and black. Their features were almost of a feminine cast and strongly suggestive of the Mongolian type.

The government of the Incan Empire was so cleverly planned that the sovereign had at all times the closest supervision over the minutest detail concerning his subjects. This was maintained by a sub-division of officials, who made monthly reports to their chief. Inspections were frequent and punishment, from which there was no appeal for any offense, was almost immediate and in any case within five days, while the officer who failed to enforce the appropriate punishment was himself liable to the same penalty as the guilty. The form of punishment was usually death, though not inflicted in a way of torture. The code of civil laws was very concise, embracing the following commandments:

> *Ama quellanquichu*—Avoid idleness.
> *Ama llullanquichu*—Avoid lying.
> *Ama suacunquichu*—Avoid stealing.
> *Ama huachocchucanqui*—Avoid adultery.
> *Ama pictapas huanuchinquichu*—Avoid murder.

The breaking of any law was considered not only as an offense against the community, but a sacrilege against the divinity of the sovereign.

There were special officers to oversee every industry as well as to govern every means for the public good. The various departments of agriculture—especially the cultivation of the Coca crops, were carefully supervised, while the roads, the bridges and the waterways each received direct attention. Even hospitality was governed, while rules were laid down to promote social intercourse, to insure fulfillment of which the doors of the houses could not be secured, so that everything might be free to inspection by the *Llactacamayoc*—or superintendent of towns, at any time. These several offices were usually filled by descendants of the nobility—the *aqui* or sons of royal princes, who were not only appointed governors of provinces, but led the *mitimaes* or colonists.

Agriculture was carried to a high state of perfection and the Inca as a Patron of husbandry set a worthy example at the beginning of each season by breaking the ground with a golden plough on the terraces back of Cuzco. Every available piece of earth was cultivated. Upon the barren mountains, where there was not sufficient soil, terraces—or *andenerias*, as they were termed, were built. These, of varying height and breadth according to the inclination of the mountain, were walled with rock and filled with suitable earth. In such places the early method of Coca cultivation was largely followed, some of these steps being only wide enough to maintain a single row of plants. Another method of gaining an area of suitable ground was by digging huge pits, known as *hoyas,* fifteen or twenty feet deep and often covering in area an acre of ground. These were filled with appropriate manure and soil for the local cultivation of just such form of vegetation as was desired. Some of these pits were so substantially built as to remain as examples of surprise to the modern traveller.[16]

The Incas carried their system of irrigation to the greatest perfection through a series of canals known as *acequias.* These were constructed on so substantial an order that many of them are still in existence—some in a state of decay, while others are now in use. They were built of slabs of sandstone cleverly laid together, as were all the Incan buildings, without the use of cement. They were capable of carrying a large volume of water, which was usually brought from one of the elevated lakes on the mountains, with such additions as might be made to it from smaller streams in its course. These canals were carried through all obstacles—through rocks, around mountains, across rivers and marshes—and were of very great length. One passing through the district of Condesuyu was nearly five hundred miles long.[17] *Lacarrillca*—the god of irrigation—was supposedly responsible for this great perfection of watering which the practical industry of these people carried in every direction to distribute fertility and verdure, where a higher civilization has permitted a lapse into desolate barrenness.

It was a peremptory Incan law that all must labor at something, and each subject was assigned to a certain occupation, so the various industries were followed by workers who had been trained through long experience. It is astonishing to consider how these industries were continued without what we consider appropriate appliances, for steel was unknown to the early Peruvians, and although iron was plenty about them it was not used. Their weapons and tools were made of stone or a peculiar alloy of copper—known as *champi,* made from a mixture of copper and tin, after the manner of some of the Eastern nations, the secret of which has never been learned. With this the Incans made picks, crowbars and

[16] Stevenson; 1825. [17] Prescott; 1848.

hammers, which enabled them to mine the precious ores in the mountains, and from the metals obtained they represented the various natural objects that were known to them. Gold was fashioned, molded and cut in every conceivable shape. Plates of this metal were used to line the Temple of the Sun, while statues of life size and of massive weight were neatly wrought from it. The same metal was drawn into delicate threads, which were interwoven in the royal fabrics, while small plates and variously shaped golden figures were worn upon the borders of the robes. Animals, fruits, flowers and plants were all fashioned in gold, and thin coverings of this were so cunningly put about objects as to make them appear to be of solid gold.[18] A similar merit in technical design is shown in the relics of Incan pottery, as also in the textile fabrics which these people wove from the finest wools. These each display an artistic cleverness in imitation.

The Incan architecture, while not of a very high order, had an effectual grandeur—which has been favorably compared to that of the Egyptians and early Greeks. The buildings, which were usually but one story, were commonly built of granite or porphyry, or an adobe of great hardness, the composition of which is not known. A peculiarity of the Incan buildings is the battered walls—sloping from the base upward, and straight cut doorways of a similar slant, with flat roofs or domes of thatch in some instances of great thickness. The structures often covered considerable space and were built of many courts surrounding a central opening, after a style that is pronouncedly Egyptian. The stones were laid together without cement and where timbers were used these were bound together with thongs made from the fibre of the American aloe—or maguey.

Those of the masses who were not fitted for more laborious work often became herbalists, and it is probable the Incans had an intimate knowledge of the plants about them and their application in an empirical way. The women and children were commonly employed in the Coca harvests and to this day

18 It has been suggested that gold was molded as an amalgam with mercury, which was after drawn off by heat. Yet this action of mercury is said not to have been known to the Incas.

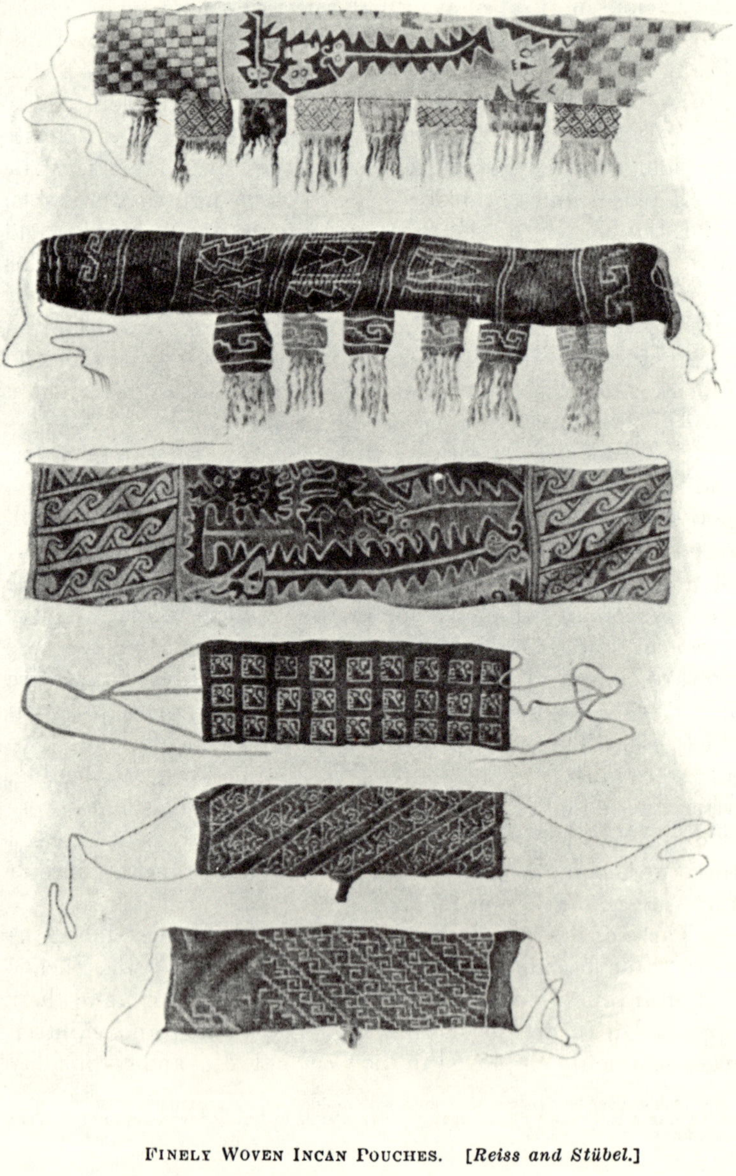

Finely Woven Incan Pouches. [*Reiss and Stübel.*]

the gathering of these leaves is best done by this class of labor. Spinning, it would seem, was hardly carried on as a separate employment, but was followed, as it is still continued by their descendants, by those nimble fingers not otherwise employed. The women were required to weave a certain amount of cloth as a portion of their contribution to the general stores of the country. All products of labor were divided between the high priest, the government, the warriors—who by their military duties were prevented from industrial pursuits—and the Inca. After these tributes had been paid, the subject was free to use his time to his individual wants. If the products of any province fell short the deficiency was supplied from some other section. Those provinces that cultivated the soil were obliged to contribute to those where only mining could be pursued, and so the earnings of the entire country were equalized by a legally arranged distribution, for money was not in use and indeed was unnecessary. So automatic had this system of equalization become at the time of the Conquest, that the Spaniards saw Incan officers noting the damages that had been done in any one province and endeavoring to make these good by assessments upon districts that had not been interfered with.

The subjects, as we have seen, were divided into small clans. It was the law that each year every male member should be allotted a certain measure of land—*fanega*—equal to an area which could be sown with one hundred pounds of maize, the cultivation of which would be sufficient not only to support him, but to provide the necessary tribute demanded by the government. No subject was permitted to leave the tribe —*ayllu*—nor the portion of land to which he was assigned. Thus there could be no roaming about in search of wealth or adventure, and no discontent, for, as has been shown, all temporal necessities, and presumably all spiritual requirements as well, were provided for by the sovereign. At a proper age —usually at twenty-four in the men and at eighteen in the women—marriage became compulsory, but a choice was permitted and the consent of the family was deemed necessary. Upon a certain day of each year the couples were joined in the public square by a representative of the Inca, and a suitable home was provided for them, an extra portion of land being at the same time allotted, while a similar grant was made at the birth of each child.

The Inca was not only the head of the temporal power, but because of his divine origin the representative of the spiritual light as well. All of the religious feasts were appointed by him, and once each year he entered the most sacred place in the Temple of the Sun stripped of his magnificence as a token of humility, to give thanks and crave for continued protection. Special sacrifices of Coca were made at these times and, in fact, it was considered essential that supplicants should only approach the altars with Coca in their mouths, and the idea was prevalent among the Peruvians that any important affair attempted without an accompanying offer of Coca could not prosper.

At stated intervals the sovereign travelled through his dominions, being carried in state over those famous roads which the Incas had constructed. The people along the way everywhere vying with each other to do homage to their sovereign, cleaned the road from every loose stick or stone and strewed flowers before the royal litter, while the places where halts were made were ever after considered as sacred. The royal *hamaca,* or sedan, was a sort of open throne emblazoned with gold and of inestimable value. It was richly decorated with plumes of tropical birds and brilliantly studded with jewels,[19] and borne on the shoulders of subjects chosen as a mark of honor, though the post was not coveted, for a fall was punished with death. Accompanying the cortege was an immense retinue of warriors and nobles.

There were two chief roadways, one built along the coast and another at an elevation on the mountains, both of which extended through the length of the domain and are estimated to have been nearly two thousand miles long. The coast road was some fifteen to twenty feet in width, carefully paved, and having a wall running at either side to prevent the accumulation of drifting sand. Wooden posts were erected to mark out

[19] Prescott; 1848.

the line of travel when crossing the desert, while in the upper road stone pillars after the manner of mile stones were set at intervals. The mountain road was the more important, and was conducted over paths often buried in snow, at other places cut through miles of solid rock, or crossing ravines and streams over frail-looking suspension bridges made of maguey fibre woven into cables. The whole construction has been pronounced worthy the most courageous engineer of modern times. Portions of these roads which still remain show a pavement of cobble stones, though some writers describe a flagging of freestone covered with an artificial cement which was harder than stone.[20] In places where the streams have washed away the substratum of earth arches of such a material are often found.[21]

Along these roadways, *Corpa-huasi,* or store houses, were erected at intervals, where Coca, quinoa, various fabrics and supplies were stored for the troops, while at shorter intervals there were post houses with relays of couriers or runners known as *chasquis,* who were at all times ready to convey messages with marvelous rapidity. These messengers, unlike some modern examples, were selected for their swiftness, and as the distance each courier ran was small, there was ample time to rest. The runners were sustained and stimulated in these efforts by the chewing of Coca leaves, each messenger being allowed a portion suited to the exertion which he might be required to perform. A despatch having been given to a *chasqui* at one end of the line, he ran to the next post house, and when within hearing commenced to shout the nature of his message, which was at once taken up by another runner, and so sent along the line. By this method it is said messages were conveyed at the rate of one hundred and fifty miles a day.[22] Montesinos relates that Huayna Ccapac ate fresh fish at Cuzco which had been caught in the sea the day before, although some three hundred miles away.

It is remarkable that we have so correct an account of the customs of the Incas when it is considered they had no written

[20] Velasco; *Historie de Quito.*

[21] Humboldt said these roads were the most useful and stupendous works ever executed by man. [22] Prescott; 1848.

language nor even a system of hieroglyphics or picture writing, as did some of the peoples contemporary with them. Their doings were handed down orally by a system of court orators known as *yaravecs,* who related at the councils before the sovereign the history of the royal race in detail. In these relations, however, it was not considered good form to speak of the achievements of the existing monarch. This ceremony was carried out on all state occasions, and intimately rehearsed not only the valorous deeds and laudatory undertakings of the preceding Incas, but also of the nobles and chiefs as well as various matters of interest to the people. In this manner all that had occurred throughout the empire was passed in review at frequent intervals, and so continued from one generation to another. They were assisted in these marvelous examples of memorizing by a knotted, fringe-like instrument, known as a *quipu.*[23] This contrivance consisted of a large cord, varying in length from two to six feet, usually woven from llama wool, from which hung cords variously knotted and of different colors. In some cases the colors were emblematic of special objects, as white—silver, yellow—gold, or green—Coca. Again they might denote abstract ideas, as white—peace, red—war, or green—the harvest, while a combination of knots usually referred to amounts. These instruments were in charge of the *quipucamayus*, or keepers of the *quipus.* By this aid they were at all times in readiness to supply the government with special information in detail.

Calculations were made from the *quipu* with the greatest rapidity, more rapidly, says Garcilasso, than could an expert mathematician cast up an account in figures. After the Conquest the Spaniards were astonished at these phenomenal exhibitions of memory, which often tended to embarrass them through the verbal exactitude in which transactions were deliberately reiterated. These orators were permitted to have recourse to Coca to strengthen, if not stimulate, their capacity for recollecting, while the *quipu* was referred to as a sort of mnemotechny, or artificial memory. This manner of recalling a thought is analogous to the *wampum* of the Indians of

[23] *Quipu*—a knot.

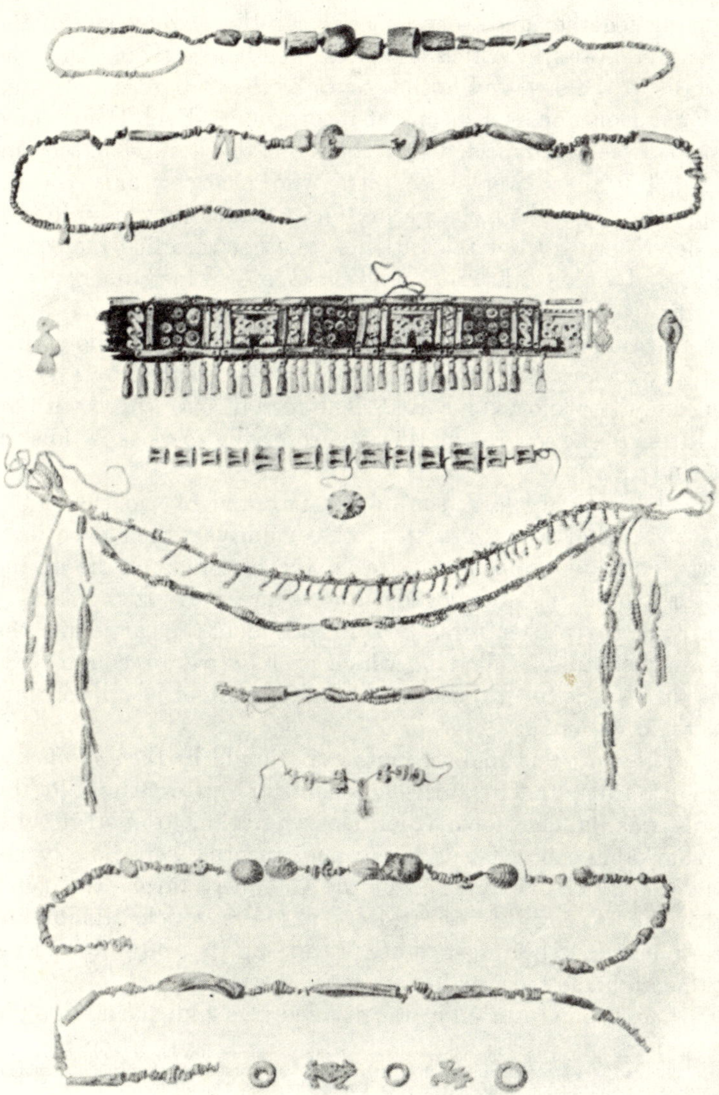

EXAMPLES OF INCAN NECKLACES. [*Reiss and Stübel.*]

the North Atlantic coast, which was composed of bits of wood strung together and worn as a belt; to the *phylacteries* of the early Hebrews, by which they preserved before their minds the words of the law, and to the *rosary* of the Catholics instituted by St. Dominic as a means of meditation. Each keeper of a *quipu* was not expected to recount all the doings of the empire, but there were specialists who recorded only certain matters. One had charge of the revenues of the state, another recorded the vital statistics, another recorded the condition and yield of the crops, and these several instruments were sent to the capital, where they constituted the national archives. When the royal orator related his account of the doings of any department of the empire, he was assisted by a reference to these knotted records. The recital commenced with an address to the sovereign; thus one referring to Coca is thus related:

"Oh, mighty lord, son of the Sun and of the Incas, thy fathers, thou who knoweth of the bounties which have been granted thy people, let me recall the blessings of the divine Coca which thy privileged subjects are permitted to enjoy through thy progenitors, the sun, the moon, the earth, and the boundless hills," following which prelude were recounted the uses and benefits of their sacred plant as might be appropriate to the occasion.

These oft-repeated accounts were taught by the *amautas* to their pupils, and by this method history in even minute details was handed down from one generation to another with remarkable exactitude. These knot records were largely destroyed by the Spanish after the Conquest through a belief that they were emblems of idolatry, so that much valuable information has been lost to us, presuming that any interpretation might now be made from such means.[24]

Cuzco, the royal city, was divided into four parts, like the

[24] It is said that before the accession of the Emperor Fo-Fli, 3,300 years B. C., the Chinese were not acquainted with writing, and used the knotted records or cords with sliding knots after the manner of the instrument known as an abacus used for teaching children numbers. These were known as *Ho-tu* and *Lo-shu*. Confucius relates that the men of antiquity used knotted cords to convey their orders, while those who succeeded them substituted signs or figures for these cords, Jaffray; *Nature*, Vol. II, p. 405; 1876. The people of Western Africa are also said to have used similar instruments. *Astley's Voyages*.

Empire, and with the same titles. The four great divisions of the country were each ruled over by a Governor, aided by his councils from the different departments. The chiefs usually resided in the capital, which was not only the royal city, but the holy city, venerated as the abode of the Incan sovereign—son of the sun, but also the lodging place for the several deities of the conquered nations. Here was the Mecca to which each subject of importance at some period of his life strove to have his duty lead him, for none could travel without the royal command.

The Incans had an especial love for music, and there were officers whose duty it was to cultivate the Muses, the subjects commonly being neglected love, or descriptive of some unfortunate event. The *haravecs* wrote the poetry, which was usually in lines of four syllables, in alternation with those of three. The poetic sentiment of this verse is shown by many examples given by Garcilasso. In one of these the moon accuses her brother, the sun, with breaking a vase and so causing a fall of snow. Here is a fragment of one of their love songs:

Caylla llapi—To the song.
Pununqui—You will sleep.
Chanpi tuta—In dead of night.
Hamusac—I will come.

There have been several cleverly written Incan plays, which are attributed to the *amautas*, who are said to have composed comedies and tragedies, in which were interwoven pastoral stories and military deeds. After the Conquest the Jesuits wrote down many of these plays, and there is some conflict of opinion as to just how much is of ancient Incan origin, and what portion later Spanish. Under the title of "Ollantay"[25] there is a very charming little drama which is supposed to date long before the Conquest. The events which are historical, are presumed to have occurred between 1340 and 1400. The following argument, which is compiled from the translations of Mr. Markham and of Mr. Squire, is an

[25] *Oll*, a corruption of the Quichua *Ull*—legend, *Antay*—of the Andes.

effort to present the imagination and poetry of these people as displayed through this little play.[26]

Ollantay, a brave general of Anti-suyu, who had carried the Incan conquests farthest east, was illegally wedded to the Princess *Cusi-Ccoyllur*—the joyful star, who was the chief beauty of the court and daughter of the Inca Pachacutec. In vain the *Villac-Umu,* or high priest, endeavored to dissuade him, and even performed a miracle by squeezing water out of a flower to divert him from his unfortunate passion, guilty alike in the eyes of religion and the law, for none but Incas could ally themselves with those of the royal blood. Pachacutec contemptuously rejected this suitor for his daughter's hand, and Ollantay fled to the mountains. Here he recounted his wrongs to his warriors, and being assured of their assistance, he arose in rebellion, determined to seek revenge. In his flight from the capital he poetically soliloquized:

"O Cuzco! Beautiful city!
From henceforth
I will be thy enemy! thy enemy!
I will break thy bosom without mercy;
I will tear out thy heart;
I will give thee to the condors!
That enemy! That Ynca!
Millions of thousands
Of Antis will I collect.
I will distribute arms,
I will guide them to the spot.
Thou shalt see the Sacsahuaman
As a speaking cloud.
Thou shalt sleep in blood.
Thou, O Ynca! shall be at my feet,
Then shalt thou see
If I have few Yuncas
If thy neck cannot be reached.
Wilt then not give
Thy daughter to me?
Wilt then loosen that mouth?
Art thou then so mad
That thou canst not speak,
Even when I am on my knee?
But I shall then be Ynca!
Then thou shalt know,
And this shall soon happen."

[26] Although the plot is very ancient, it has been asserted that this drama was composed by Dr. Valdez.

Ollantay occupied the great fortress of colossal ruins, which has ever since been called Ollantay-Tampu, where he maintained himself during ten years. Meanwhile Cusi-Ccoyllur gave birth to a child, who was named *Yma-Sumac*—"how beautiful"—for which transgression the princess was confined in a dungeon in the *Aclla-huasi,* or Convent of Sacred Virgins. Shortly after this Ollantay was captured by a clever stratagem of the opposing general, *Rumiñani,* whose name, "Stony Eye," suggests keen penetration and a cold, implacable character. Appearing before the rebel covered with blood, he declared he had been cruelly treated by the Inca, and desired to join the insurrection. Encouraging the insurgents to celebrate the festival in drunken orgies, he admitted his own troops and captured the whole party, including Ollantay, who was brought to Cuzco to suffer death. But meantime the relentless father—Inca Pachacutec, had died, and his son, whose younger heart could better appreciate the tender passions, was touched by the rebel warrior's romance, and not only pardoned him, but consented to the general's marriage with his sister. Another drama termed *Uscar-Pancar,* or the loves of the golden flower *Ccorittica,* contains many beautiful passages.

Although Montesinos gives a list of a hundred Incas, commencing long before the Christian era, the following is the more commonly accepted line of succession:

I—1021—Manco Ccapac.
II—1062—Sinchi Rocca.
III—1091—Lloque Yupanqui.
IV—1126—Mayta Ccapac.
V—1156—Ccapac Yupanqui.
VI—1197—Inca Rocca.
VII—1249—Yahnar-huaccac.
VIII—1289—Viracocha.
IX—1340—Pachacutec.
X—1400—Inca Yupanqui.
XI—1439—Tupac Inca Yupanqui.
XII—1475—Huayna Ccapac.
XIII—1526—Huascar.
XIV—1532—Inca Manco.
XV—1553—Sayri Tupac.
XVI—1560—Cusi Titu Yupanqui.
XVII—1562—Tupac Amaru.

It was said that at the death of Manco Ccapac he appointed that his treasures should be employed for the service of his body and for the feeding of his family, and from this precedent continued the custom that no sovereign should inherit the belongings of the previous Inca, so that each successor built a new palace and established a new court. The remains of some of these edifices are still to be seen, notably the palace of Manco Ccapac on Sacsahuaman Hill back of Cuzco, and at least six other palace ruins in the Incan capital. The rulers of the Incan race are said to have descended in an unbroken line, while in the latter years of the dynasty the wife was chosen from a sister of the Inca to keep the royal blood even more holy, for although legendary accounts describe the first Inca as appearing with his sister wife, such a custom of marriage seems only to have been instituted by a later sovereign.

The religious forms of the Incas are replete with interest, and it seems fitting that these should be considered in a separate review, which will recount some of the uses made by this race of the Coca they considered as divine in their rites and ceremonies.

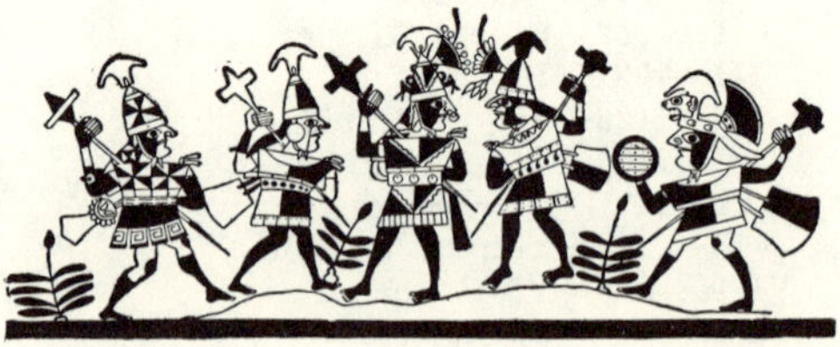

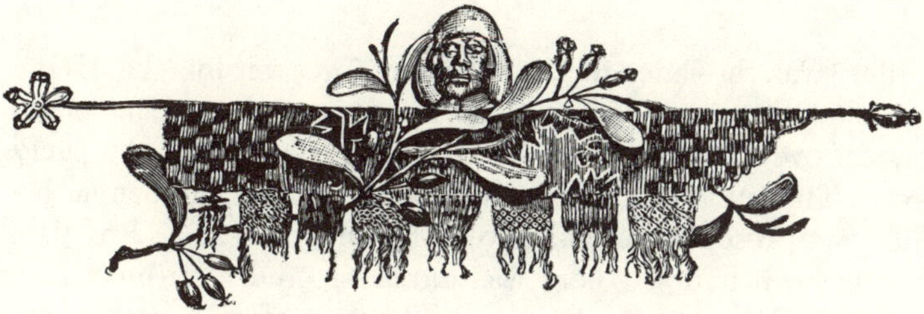

CHAPTER III.

THE RITES AND ARTS OF THE INCANS.

"The Universal Cause
Acts not by partial, but by gen'ral laws;
And makes what happiness we justly call,
Subsist not in good of one, but all."
—Pope, *Essay*, iii., i.

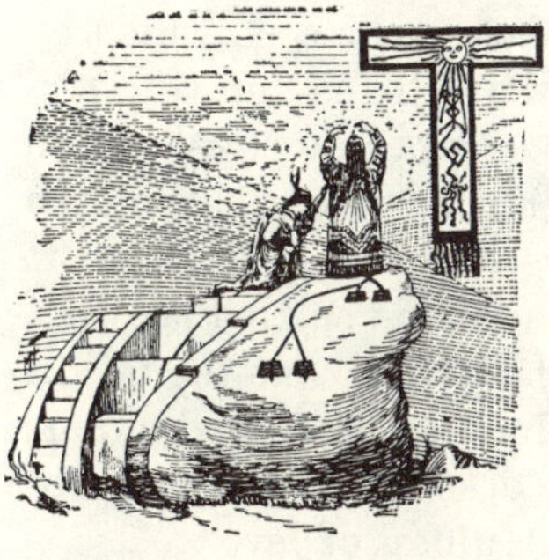

THE religion of the Incas has been commonly set down as exclusively the worship of the sun, while their traditions trace the progenitors of this race as proceeding from the sun, as children or brothers.

It is interesting in view of the supposed Eastern origin of the Incans, to compare their belief in a mythical ancestry from the sun with similar beliefs among Eastern peoples. Many of the ancient families of Hindustan claim descent from the sun, their solar dynasty numbering ninety-five successors. Every king of Egypt was styled Ze-Ra or son of the sun. The sun god of the Canaanites was Baal—lord, a title they prefixed to each deity.

Dr. Brinton, from a special study of myth-lore, suggested heliolatry was organized by the Incas for political ends, to impress upon the masses that *Inti,* the sun, their own elder brother, was the ruler of the cohorts of heaven by like divine right that they were of the four quarters of the earth.[1] Sun worship prevailed in ancient times among many of the early races. The sun was the most wonderful object the people beheld. Its presence was the giver of light, of heat and of life, while when it had set there was darkness, and a stillness suggestive of the end of all things. Thus it seems but natural that the sun should have been regarded as divine, together with those objects that were considered its representative, as the moon, the stars and fire.[2] The followers of that ancient philosopher, Zoroaster, considered fire the supreme emblem of divine intelligence. In ancient Baalbek the sun was worshiped with great ceremony. Turning toward the sun was a practice among certain Hebrews.[3] The Parsee looks toward the sun in prayer, and the custom of facing the East has been continued in the modern church. So from a regard of the sun as the creator of all things, it was but a single step to look upon the several representatives of that element as symbols of life and generation from which lesser emblems were chosen. Thus the egg as the germ of living matter, the cock which by its early morning crow seems to call forth the sun, the serpent because of casting its skin and so regaining fresh youth annually, the *phallus** and even our Easter flowers, have each been looked upon as sacred emblems suggesting creation, if not directly worshiped. It was in this same spirit that Coca was considered as the divine plant, because it was the means of force and strength as well as a stimulant to reproduction; and the Incan Venus was represented as holding a spray of Coca as typifying the power and fruitfulness of love.[4]

The Incas did not consider the sun as the Supreme Being, but only His representative. Thus at a grand religious council, held about the year 1440, to consecrate the newly built Temple of the Sun, Inca Yupanqui spoke to his subjects as follows: "Many say that the sun is the maker of all things,

[1] Brinton; 1868.

[2] The Hindus said: "God is the fire of the altar"—*Bhagavat-Gita*, p. 54. The Scriptures bear frequent reference to God appearing in a flame.—*Genesis*, iii, 24; xv, 17; *Exodus*, iii, 2; xix, 18; *Deuteronomy*, iv, 24, etc.

[3] *Ezekiel*, viii, 16.

* From *Phala*—fruit, and *Isa*—the god, hence the fructifier.

[4] Marcoy; 1869.

but he who makes should abide by what he has made. Now many things happen when the sun is absent, therefore he cannot be the universal creator; and that he is alive at all is doubtful, for his trips do not tire him. Were he a living thing he would grow weary, like ourselves; were he free he would visit other parts of the heavens. He is like a tethered beast, who makes a daily round under the eye of a master; he is like an arrow which must go whither it is sent, not whither it wishes. I tell you that he, our father and master the sun, must have a lord and master more powerful than himself, who constrains him to his daily circuit without pause or rest."[5]

Thus it will be seen that the sun, moon and lesser lights were worshiped merely as symbols, while to enforce a belief that the race descended from their sacred emblem emphasized the divine origin of the Inca, whose authority was unquestioned, for if we except the incident of Ollantay, no case of rebellion was known through the entire rule of these people up to the period when the Empire was divided between the brothers Huascar and Atahualpa, just prior to the Conquest.

The attempts to explain the various phenomena of nature and even of existence have led man to attribute to surrounding natural objects the spirit that is felt in himself with often an endeavor to typify these ideal conceptions. Darwin claimed there could be no inherent belief in God, but that it only developed after much education. There have been many races without gods, and even without words to express the idea. The Incas gave practical expression to the truth underlying the phrase: "The greatest happiness of the greatest number;" and reviewing their race in this light, we must consider they had reached a very high stage of civilization, for not only their morals but their social relations were regulated by law.

There is not only a similarity in many rites of these early Americans with the Eastern forms, but a similarity in the magnificence of the buildings dedicated to their worship. The Temples of the Sun of the Egyptian Heliopolis and the Syrian Baalbek were perhaps prototypes of the Peruvian temples.

[5] **Balboa; 1580.**

It seems fitting in the infancy of the world that ceremonies should be few and yet surrounded with a sufficient mystery as to keep the elect above the masses, a distinction which was maintained by adding new rites and ceremonies from time to time until the system of worship became more intricate. Maimonides[6] supposed the antedeluvians became sun worshipers from a belief that the heavenly bodies were placed by God, and used by Him as His ministers. It was evidently His will that they should receive from man the same veneration as the servants of a great prince justly claim from the subject multitude. This is suggestive of why throughout the world similar deities are worshiped, though under a variety of names. The sun and Noah were worshiped in conjunction with the moon and the ark, the latter pair representing the female principle, and acknowledged in different localities under the various names of Isis, Venus, Astarte, Ceres, Proserpine, Rhea, Sita, Ceridwen, Frea, etc., while the former, or male element, assumed the titles of Osiris, Saturn, Jupiter, Neptune, Bacchus, Adonis, Brahma or Odin. Thus was a gradual transition made from the helioarkite superstition to the phallic worship, while from the fact that each of these lesser deities was represented by some natural object as a symbol, these latter were often looked upon as the real objects of worship. In Egypt there was a system of taxation to defray the expense of keeping the sacred animals, just as among the Incas tribute of Coca was exacted to support the temples.

There has been frequent comparison by many writers between the Incas and the Hindus because of many similar ceremonies, many of their customs being identical. Like the Hindus, the Incas had the custom of deifying attributes instead of, like the Greeks, making gods of men. Thus the Incan sovereign was the ruler of the four quarters of the globe, while Brahma had four heads, which represent the four quarters of the earth. The origin of these four heads is explained in legend: "When Brahma assumed a mortal shape he was pleased to manifest himself in Cashmir. Here one-half of his

[6] *De Idolatria.*

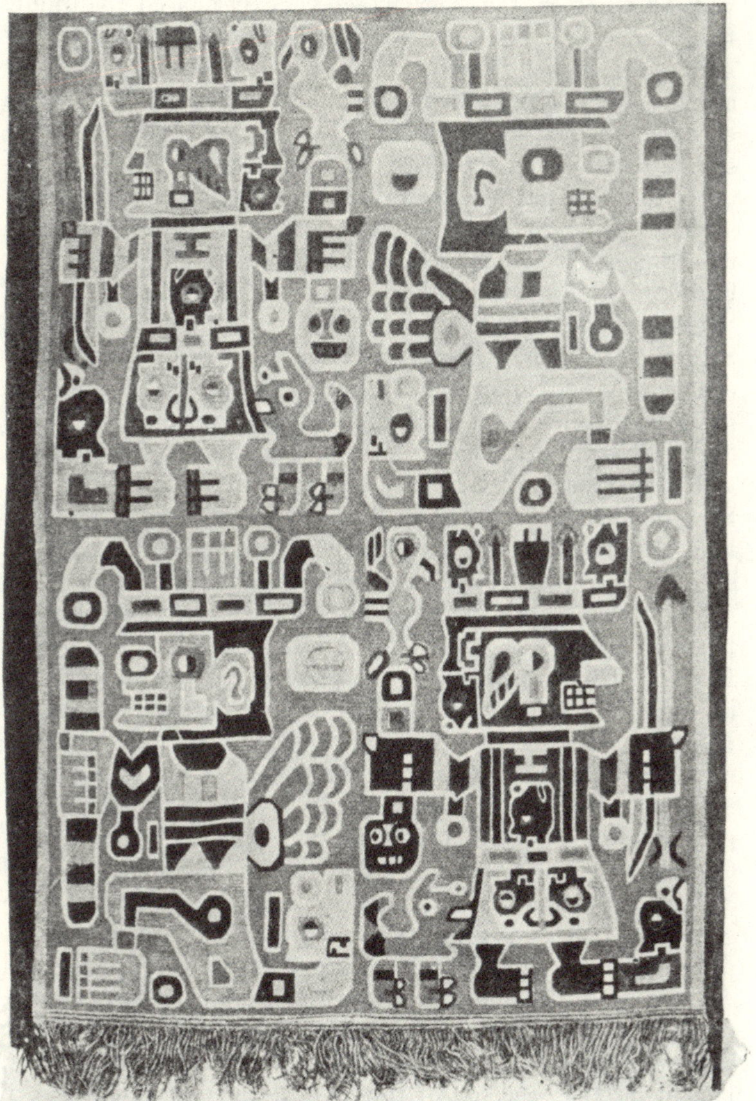

INCAN TAPESTRY OF FINE WOOL. [*Reiss and Stübel.*]

body sprang from the other, which yet experienced no diminution, and out of the severed moiety he framed a woman, denominated Iva, or Satarupa.[7] Her beauty was such as to excite the love of the god, but deeming her his daughter, he was ashamed to own his passion. During this conflict between shame and love he remained motionless, with his eyes fixed upon her. Satarupa perceived his situation, and stepped aside to avoid his ardent looks. Brahma, being unable to move but still desirous to see her, a new face sprang out upon him towards the object of his desires.[8] Again she shifted her situation and another face emanated from the enamored god. Still she avoided his gaze, until the incarnate deity become conspicuous with four faces directed to the four quarters of the world, beheld her incessantly to whatever side she withdrew herself. At length she recovered her self-possession, when the other half of his body sprang from him and became Swayam-bhuva or Adima. Thus were produced the first man and woman, and from their embrace were born three sons, in whom the Trimurtti became incarnate."[9]

Festivals were celebrated in various parts of Greece in honor of Dionysius, in which the *phallus,* as a symbol of the fertility of nature, was borne in procession by men disguised as women. Hammond has described a custom among the Pueblo Indians of New Mexico in which one of the males is rendered sexually impotent, being termed a *mujerado.* He thereafter dresses like a woman, and is set apart for the orgies practiced by these Indians after the manner of the ancient Greeks and Egyptians. A similar custom was practiced among the Incans during Sinchi Rocca's reign, when extravagant indulgence was given to every form of licentiousness. It is reported the Inca caused constant search to be made for *chutarpu*—as the male form was called, and for *huanarpu*—the female form, and these finally became so common that they were offered as presents. But just as all extremes regulate themselves, the son of this libidinous sovereign not only

[7] The female half of Brahma's body; the type of all female creatures.

[8] The triad of gods of the Hindu mythology is Bramha, Vishnu and Siva, whose attributes are Creator, Preserver and Destroyer.

[9] *Matsya Purana,* in Faber; *Pagan Idolatry,* vol i, p. 319.

forbade this practice, but set an example of celibacy by remaining single till he was an old man.[10]

Though the early Peruvians were sensual, they appreciated and respected continence in both sexes. Their virtues were indeed so many that it would be astonishing if they possessed no faults. There are frequent examples to be seen among Peruvian pottery of objects which, though carefully designed and finished, would not bear reproduction. At times

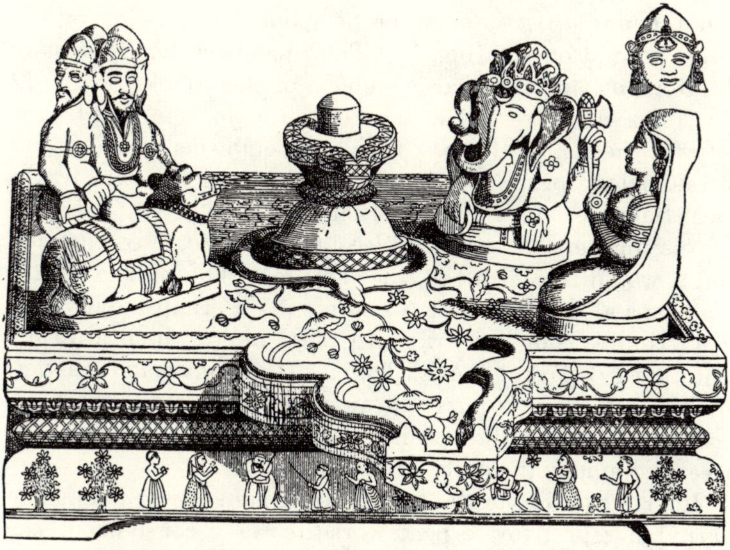

LINGAM IN INDIAN TEMPLE. [*Richard Payne Knight.*]

these assume a decided phallic form. The *huacanquis* were stone phalli, which served as love charms, for which purpose certain plants were in general use which were supposed to possess irresistible properties. Among the zodiacal constellations of the Incans two bore the name of the sexual organs. In the East the phallus was worn as an amulet against *Malocchi*—evil eye—or enchantments, as well as for its supposed aphrodisiac influence. Among the modern specimens representative of this form of worship, a clinched hand with the

[10] Santa Cruz; 1620.

point of the thumb thrust between the index and middle fingers is probably an emblem of consummation. A little shell —*concha veneris,* worn in its natural state, is evidently the emblem of the *yoni,* while another representing the half moon, usually made of some precious metal, relates to the menses. The *linga* is the symbol under which the Hindu deity, Siva, is worshiped. It is commonly represented as a conical stone rising perpendicularly from an oval-shaped rim cut on a stone platform. The *salunkha* is the top of the lingam altar, and the *pranalika* is a gutter or spout for drawing off the water poured on the lingam. The lingam is the Priapus of the Romans, and the phallic emblem of the Greeks, while the oval lines sculptured about it refer to the *yoni* or *bhaga,* symbolic of the female form. These two emblems represent the physiological form of worship which has been followed by the great Saiva sect for at least fifteen hundred years. This worship is unattended by any indecent or indelicate ceremonies, and it would be difficult to trace any resemblance between the symbols and the objects they represent. Perhaps eighty million Hindu people still worship these idols, which are common in every part of British India. It is remarkable, in view of the comparison of many Incan rites with those of the East, that numerous phallic specimens indicate that this cult was practiced among the early Peruvians.

Representations of the serpent are frequently found among Peruvian relics, for serpent worship was a conspicuous element of the Incan ritual and religion. There was an annual serpent dance in which it is asserted that the dancers held an immense golden cable, each link of which was fashioned as a serpent with its tail in its mouth, and the dancers seem to have followed a serpentine course through the streets of Cuzco. A similar dance among the Pueblo Indians has been described by the late Major Bourke, Dr. J. W. Fewkes and others. Mr. Stansbury Hagar has published an account of another serpent dance amongst the far-distant Micmacs of Nova Scotia. In Peruvian astrology the serpent rules the zodiacal sign of the Scorpion, in which position it symbolizes wisdom and, singularly enough, the diverse concepts death and immortal life;

death because of its sting, immortal life because of its annual resurrection from its discarded skin, thus displaying a wisdom in what the Peruvians considered the acme of knowledge—the evidence of life beyond the grave. As the symbol of life and the active life-giving power the serpent also attains phallic associations. Besides these relations it became from a variety of causes associated with time, the year and the zodiac.[11] The serpent appears on the ancient monuments at

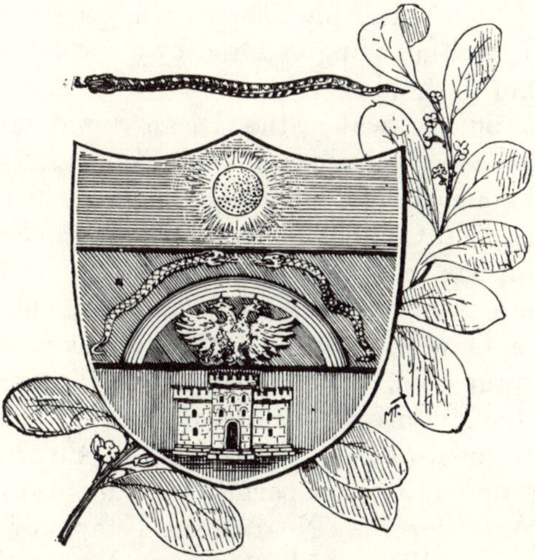

Escutcheon of the Incas.

Tiahuanaco, and in Peruvian designs wrought in gold, silver, pottery, cloth and stone and throughout many architectural ornaments. So intimately associated was the snake with the astrology and with the rites of the Incans that it was included in the escutcheon granted them in 1544 by Charles the Fifth.

Magnificent temples for the worship of the sun were erected all through the land of the Incas, the chief temple at Cuzco being on a scale of particular grandeur. It was situated in the lower part of the royal city, on the high bank of the Huatenay, probably eighty feet above the bed of that

[11] Hagar; *person. com.*, May, 1899.

stream. It was built in the same massive manner as were all the Incan structures and ornamented on a scale of unequaled magnificence, being lined with plates of gold, while all around the outside of the building ran a coronal of this metal about three feet in depth. At one end of the temple was an immense image in gold of the sun. Before this, in two parallel lines, were the embalmed—or preserved bodies of the Incas. These, arranged in the order of their succession, sat in their royal robes upon golden thrones raised upon pedestals of gold, the mummy[12] of Huayna Ccapac, who was regarded as the greatest of the line, being honored by a special position in the very front of the golden emblem.

The buildings which the Incans used for ceremonial rites were made as grand and imposing as a free use of the precious metals could make them. In the gardens surrounding the temple at Cuzco, where—as one of the Spanish chroniclers stated, the trees and even the insects were of precious metal—there were cleverly modeled representations of animals, flowers and examples of the Coca plant, all exquisitely shaped in pure gold. Cuzco was in fact the repository of the wealth of the Empire, being literally, as it was termed, *Coracancha,* the town of gold, for no gold or silver that was ever brought to the capital was permitted to leave it during the integrity of the Empire. Near to the Temple of the Sun were other structures dedicated to the moon, Venus, thunder, lightning and the rainbow, all of which were elaborately decorated with gold. Close to these was the convent—*acllahuasi,* of the Virgins of the Sun; that at Cuzco being an imposing structure some eight hundred feet long and two hundred and fifty feet broad.

In the Incan religion no women were assigned to the *huaca* of their supreme god, for as he created them, they all belonged to him, and this same idea was manifest in the royal selection. A lapse from virtue among these maidens was a crime so abominable that it was punished with death, the offender being burned or buried alive, as was also the penalty imposed among the Greeks. The male offender was not only put to

[12] The word mummy is derived from the Arabic *Mûmiâ*—bitumen.

death, but his entire family was destroyed as well as his property and effects, and his habitation was left a desert, that there might remain neither tract, trace nor remembrance of him. The Temple of the Virgins at Cuzco during the height of the monarchy is said to have contained about fifteen hundred maidens who had been selected for their physical charms.

The reigning Inca, as son of the sun, was at once sovereign and pontiff, exercising absolute authority over both temporal and spiritual matters, but the religious rites were performed by his representatives through a system of priesthood. The *Villac-umu,* or chief high priest, held office for life; he was appointed by the Inca, and was considered next in authority to him. His title, which implies "the head which gives counsel," explains his position. Priests of lower degree were appointed by him, and to preserve the faith these were usually chosen from among the nobles.

Each province had its *Villac*—or chief priest, while beneath these were others who offered sacrifices in the temples, speakers to the oracle, together with soothsayers and diviners of all kinds, each being designated in accordance with the duties of his office. Thus the one who offered Coca leaves in the fire and foretold events from certain curlings of its smoke or other signs at the time of its combustion was termed *vira-piricue.* The dress of the priests was white, emblematical of their purity in celibacy and fasts which they were required to practice. No ceremony was ever considered complete until the *Villac* had thrown Coca leaves to the four cardinal points, and from this association in every religious rite Coca was ultimately regarded by the masses as divine. Accompanying these ceremonies the priests offered prayers; examples of these which have been preserved to us by the early writers express much sentiment. One which referred to the first fruits was as follows:

"Oh, Creator! Lord of the ends of the earth! Oh, most merciful! Thou, who givest life to all things, and hast made men that they may live, eat and multiply, multiply, also, the fruits of the earth, *papas*[13] and other foods that thou hast

[13] *Papas*—potatoes.

made, that men may not suffer from hunger and misery. Oh, preserve the fruits of the earth from frost, and keep us in peace and safety."[14]

Instead of sacrificing human victims, as was the custom of early barbarous nations, the Incans presented before the golden luminary the first fruits which had come to life through his genial warmth. At some of the festivals animals were sacrificed, and because of the fact that these were offered in the names of those who gave them, as *puric*—adult man, and *huahua*—a child, it has been wrongly asserted that human offerings were made. Their laws strictly prohibited this, and Markham has suggested that the statement that servants were sometimes sacrificed by their masters is disproved through the fact mentioned in the writings of "the anonymous Jesuit" that in none of the burial places opened by the Spanish were any human bones found except those of the lord who had been buried there.

It might be supposed that as the Incas regarded the sun as their father they would have made an especial study of the heavens and been expert in astronomy, though they were not as advanced in this science as were the early Mexicans. They had a knowledge of certain constellations; the bright star *Spica* in *Virgo* they referred to as Mama Coca.* They divided their year into twelve lunar months, each distinguished by an appropriate name and usually designated as well by some festival. The months were divided into weeks, but the number of days in each is not now known. To harmonize the lunar with their solar year, observations were made by means of certain upright stones similar to the stone circles of the Druids and like those found in parts of Northern Europe and Asia. The shadows from these stone pillars formed a scale for measuring the exact times of the solstices. The equinoxes were determined by an erect stone in shape like a truncate cone, projecting above a table of solid rock from which the whole was cut. This was termed *intihuatana,*[15] or

[14] Molina; 1570.
* Hagar; *person. com.* May, 1899.
[15] *Inti*—sun, *huatana*—the place where or thing with which anything is tied up.—Squier; p. 524, 1877.

place where the sun is tied up. A line was drawn across the level platform from east to west, and observations were taken as to when the shadow of the pillar became continuous on this line from sunrise to sunset. When the shadow was scarcely visible under the noontide rays it was said "the god sat with all his light upon the column."

Similar methods for determining the seasons certainly date from the most ancient times and were known to the early people of the East, who were even considered as capable of juggling with the sun's rays. Thus, when the prophet Isaiah offered to show King Hezekiah a sign that the Lord would heal him, he asked whether that sign should be that the sun's shadow should go forward ten degrees or go back ten degrees, "And Hezekiah answered, It is a light thing for the shadow to go down ten degrees; nay, but let the shadow turn backward ten degrees," which miracle, it is related, the prophet showed.[16]

The period of the equinoxes was celebrated by important festivals, and similar festivals, differing in degree, formed an intimate part of the ceremonial worship of each month. The full moon was an occasion for honoring the deities of water and the patrons of agriculture, while her various phases were consecutively honored as having some bearing upon the crops. As the sun was their father, so the moon was to the Peruvians their *Mama Quilla,* the goddess of love and the patroness of marriage and childbirth.

Various authorities differ as to the arrangement of the Incan months and the periods when the several festivals were celebrated. Molina commences the year with the first day of the new moon in May, and Prescott describes the feast of *Raymi* as the summer solstice. The reference I have chosen fixes this feast as the celebration of the winter solstice. This confusion may have occurred among the early Spanish writings, because the word *Raymi,* which signifies to dance, is associated in several of the Quichua feasts. The succession of the Incan months, as determined by the researches of the first Council of Lima, was as follows:

[16] 2 *Kings;* xx, 10.

1.—*Yntip Raymi*—June 22d to July 22d. Festival of winter solstice or *Raymi*.
2.—*Chahuarquiz*—July 22d to August 22d. Season of plowing.
3.—*Yapa-quiz*—August 22d to September 22d. Season of sowing.
4.—*Ccoya Raymi*—September 22d to October 22d. Festival of the spring equinox or *Situ*.
5.—*Uma Raymi*—October 22d to November 22d. For brewing.
6.—*Ayamarca*—November 22d to December 22d. Commemoration of the dead.
7.—*Ccapac Raymi*—December 22d to January 22d. Festival of the summer solstice or *Huaraca*.
8.—*Camay*—January 22d to February 22d. Season of exercises.
9.—*Hatun-poccoy*—February 22d to March 22d. Season of ripening.
10.—*Pacha-poccoy*—March 22d to April 22d. Festival of the autumn equinox or *Mosoc Nina*.
11.—*Ayrihua*—April 22d to May 22d. Beginning of harvest.
12.—*Aymuray*—May 22d to June 22d. Harvesting month.

During the first month, *Yntip Raymi*, the festival of the winter solstice was celebrated, and especial attention was given to preparing the fields and arranging methods for their irrigation. Following this, during the month *Chahuarquiz,* the sovereign inaugurated the season of ploughing by turning up the soil on the royal terraces back of Cuzco with a golden plough, for, as has been shown, agriculture was taught as the favorite industry of this country, where many barren spots rendered fertile soil very precious. During *Yapa-quiz* maize was sown, from which time, until it had grown to a finger's height, the *tarpuntaes,* or special priests in charge of this harvest, fasted from drinking chicha and from chewing Coca leaves, while the songs of the people besought prosperity, to favor which, offerings of Coca, maize and sheep were made.

The festival of *Situ*—the spring equinox, was held in *Ccoya Raymi.* As much sickness commonly followed the rainy season, which was now about due, the prayers and ceremonies were designed to prevent such evil in the land. This festival was particularly imposing. The *huacas*—or sacred things, were brought to the temples, and the nobles and people assembled in the public squares for the celebration. At these times all deformed and diseased persons were forbidden to be present, for despite the extreme kindness of the Incas for the unfortunate, they superstitiously regarded sickness as a punishment for some fault, and they supposed that the presence of the ill at this time might prevent that good fortune which they craved. Even the dogs were driven from Cuzco, lest their howling might be offensive.

A curious ceremony was now performed by four hundred warriors, who were divided into groups representing the four provinces of the Empire and stationed East, West, North and South, facing the great square. After certain ceremonies in the Temple, the Inca, accompanied by his priests, came forth and exclaimed: "Oh, sickness, disasters, misfortunes and dangers, go forth from the land," when instantly the warriors ran with great speed toward the rivers Apurimac and Vilcamayo, shouting: "Go forth all evils!" Here they bathed, and the waters supposedly carried the evils away. At night bundles of straw were burned and thrown into the rivers, and so the evils of light and darkness were equally destroyed. These ceremonies were accompanied by fasting, except for the eating of a porridge termed *sancu*—a sort of sacred pudding, which was also smeared over their faces and upon the lintels of the doors. Finally this was washed away, emblematical of their desire to be free from personal sickness or from disease entering their houses. It was at this festival particularly that the bodies of the Incas were brought out into the square from the Temple, where they were set up and attended by their people, who offered them the best of everything in the way of food and drink. In the evening these bodies were bathed in the baths which had belonged to them, and the following morning offerings of Coca and various foods were set before them, and the day was concluded in feasting. *Uma Raymi*—the month following this festival, was the season of brewing. During this month the ceremonies of knighting the youths took place, followed with much rejoicing. The following month, *Ayamarca,* was the period when they commemorated their dead, and offerings of Coca were made to the mummies under the supposition that wherever the soul might be it would be fed and sustained through this emblem of strength.

The ceremony of knighthood was one of the most imposing

festivals during the Incan year. It was termed *Huaraca*—the sling, and was celebrated during the summer solstice upon the sacred hill Huañacauri, where a legend relates that a sun god had at one time been turned into stone. Here the ceremonies commenced by a prayer, offered for the perpetuation of manly vigor: "O Huanacauri! Our father, may the Creator, the Sun, and the thunder ever remain young, and never become old. May Thy son, the Inca, always retain his youth, and grant that he may prosper in all he undertakes. And to us, Thy sons and descendants, who now celebrate this festival, grant that we may ever be in the hands of the Creator, of the sun, of the thunder, and in Thy hands."

The young nobles were only initiated after they had arrived at a certain age and after they had passed through a preliminary rigorous ordeal. This was more suggestive perhaps of the severity of the initiation into the Ancient Mysteries than it was to the knighthood of the Middle Ages. The novitiates were put to very severe tests, which resulted literally in only the survival of the fittest. The first token given the applicants was a pair of breeches made from the fibre of the aloe. After this they were fitted for endurance by a severe flogging and were then given the staff, *yauri,* and *usuta*—or sandals. They then passed a night alone in the desert, and the following day continued the test of endurance by foot races at *Huaca Amahuarqui,* where tradition says there was a *Huaca* that ran like a lion. The competitors were stimulated by the encouragement of maidens along the course, who offered chicha and Coca and cried—"Come quickly, youths, for we are waiting." Those who survived the ordeal then met in an assault at arms, and those who were accepted to become warriors had their ears bored by the Inca with a golden stylet. The orifice was kept open with cotton until large enough to admit the large cylindrical earrings, the tubular support of which was pushed through the opening in the lobe, and this method of wearing these ornaments caused the lobe to elongate and occasioned an appearance which led the Spaniards to call the Incas *Orejones*—big ears. After bathing in the sacred fountain called *calli-puquio* the

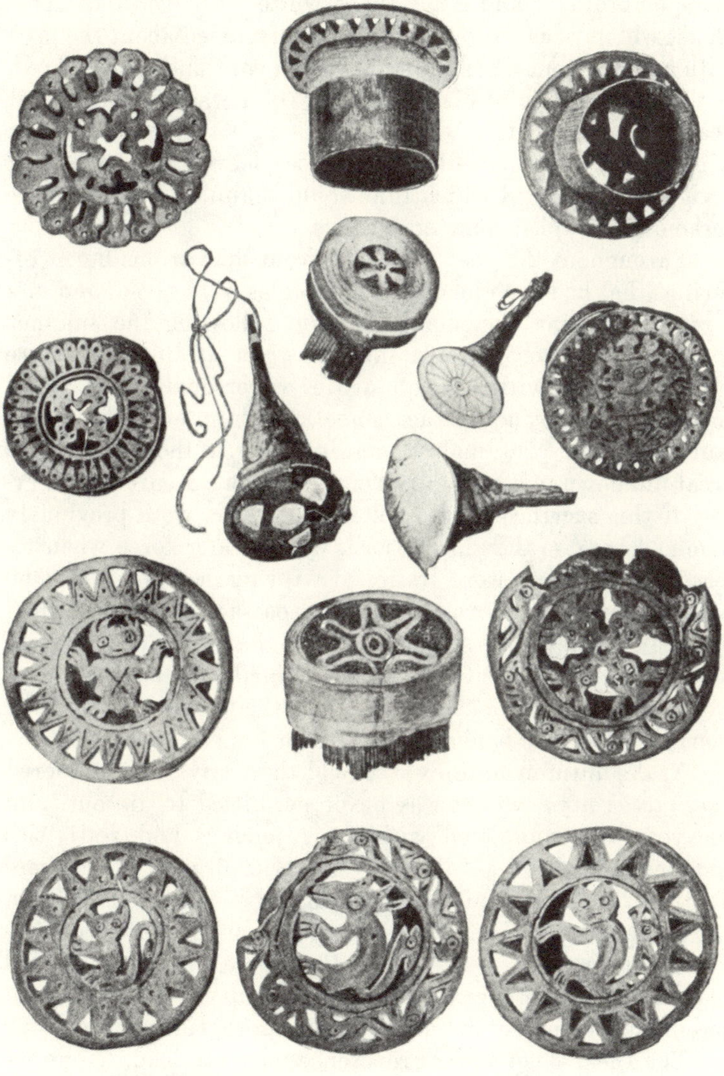

EXAMPLES OF INCAN EARRINGS. [*Reiss and Stübel.*]

Knights were given a shirt of fine yellow wool, bordered with black embroidery and a mantle of white—*supayacolla.* This cloak, which reached to the knees, was fastened about the neck with a knot, from which hung a woolen cord and tassel of red. A turban or *llauta* of distinguishing color was worn upon the head, and each Knight was now invested with the *huaraca*, or sling, and the *chuspa,* filled with Coca leaves, emblematic of a vigorous manhood which this would maintain. This entire ceremony occupied some eight days.

Throughout the year the ashes from the various burnt offerings that had been made in the temples were saved, and at a ceremony during the month *Camay,* following the summer solstice, these were thrown into the river at an hour before sunset, together with large quantities of personal effects, Coca, foods, garments, and, in fact, something from everything that had been used, presumably as an offering to the deity in the great unknown to which the river flowed. To assure the carrying of this sacrifice by the waters the rivers were previously dammed back so they might rush with greater force when released, and guards were stationed with torches to see that no part of the sacrifice was checked in passage. When all had been carried down the stream as far as the bridge of Ollantay-Tampu, two bags of Coca, termed *pilculuncu pancar uncu*, were thrown in from the bridge, and the people followed the sacrifice along the banks of the stream for two days.

At the autumn equinox was held the festival of the sacred fire, *mosoc nina,* which was never permitted to die out, and the year was completed with the rejoicings and festivities commemorative of a full harvest. Sacrifices of Coca were made in the Temple of the Sun daily, also on various hills in the valley of the Vilcamayo, the method of these offerings varying; at times the leaves were thrown to the four cardinal points, while at others they were burnt upon the altars, both ceremonies being accompanied by an appropriate prayer.

The Incans had a great reverence for their dead. Not only were the bodies of the sovereigns preserved, but it was customary for families to preserve the bodies of certain of their departed so that they might be seen. Food was set before these mummies on the occasion of all festivals, in the belief that wherever the soul might be it would return for this nourishment, while if appropriate food was withheld from the dead it would occasion disease. These bodies were termed *mallquis* or *manaos,* and were believed to extend a protection over the family, an idea not far removed from modern spiritualism.

Offerings of food to the dead was a very ancient Eastern custom; thus it is written that the Israelites in the wilderness were accused of idolatry because they ate these sacrifices.[17] The North American Indians believe in the duality of the soul, one being liberated at death, the other remaining in the body, which must be provided for.[18] The Egyptians believed the tomb of their dead was inhabited by a double—*ka,* of the deceased, and so an ante-chamber was always built where relatives might leave their offerings for this substance. In the absence of more material fare the walls of the sepulchre were profusely decorated with a semblance of good cheer.[19] In order to live in the other world, the double required a body and this was why the original body was preserved. In case the actual body was destroyed images of stone or wood were made to supply its place. Besides the double, there was the soul—*bi,* or *ba,* and the *khoo,* which was a sort of divine spark. Each of these substances had to be provided for. It may have been some similar belief which led the early Peruvians to place foods and the common objects of every-day life about the bodies of their dead, while an element of force was assured by filling the mouth of the departed with Coca leaves. Even to-day the Indians of some provinces believe that if a dying man can appreciate the taste of Coca leaves pressed to his lips his soul will enter Paradise,[20] while in the graves where mummies have been found there is always a bountiful supply of Coca in the chuspa, and many little bags of Coca leaves are distributed over the body.

At the death of an Inca, when, as it was said, he was "called home to the mansions of his father the sun," his pal-

[17] 1 *Psalms;* cvi, 28. [18] Schoolcraft; 1853.
[19] Maspero; *Historie Ancienne,* p. 55. [20] Poeppig; ii. 252, 1836.

aces were closed forever, while his estates were worked only sufficiently to support his immediate followers and servants, who continued in charge of his earthly remains, for it was supposed his soul would return to reanimate the body and all things should be left as in life ready for this reception.[21] The bowels of the dead sovereign were removed and buried, with a quantity of plate and jewels, at Tampu, five leagues from the capital, while the body was embalmed by some peculiar process which preserved it in lifelike appearance through centuries, and this, clothed in royal raiment, was set up in the Temple of the Sun at Cuzco. Posssibly it may have been a knowledge of this peculiar custom of the Incas which led Philip II. to conceive the idea of a mausoleum, in which the bodies of the Spanish sovereigns should be petrified and set up as at the Palace and Monastery of San Lorenzo del Escorial. At the festivals in the public square, when the mummies of the Incas were brought out, it was customary for their followers to invite special guests, who enjoyed the melancholy festivities with all the etiquette due the living monarch.

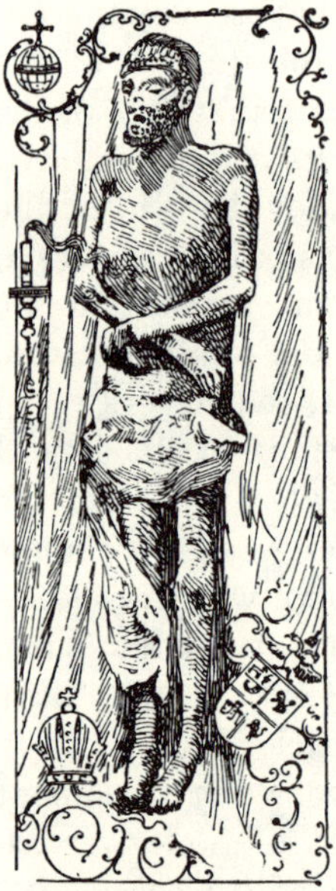

PETRIFIED BODY OF CHARLES V. OF SPAIN.

The early Peruvians had the universal myth of creation through the union of a heavenly father and an earthly mother, and though their ritual embraced many emblems, they certainly recognized a supreme being aside from this emblematic worship. Their venerated names were *Con, Illa, Ticci, Uira, Cocha*[22]—the Creator, Eternal Light, Spirit of the Abyss—together with two sacred terms which record attributes, as *Pachayachachic,* the teacher or regulator, and *Pachacamac,* the

[21] Garcilasso; 1609.

[22] *Con* is of unknown origin,. *Illa*—light, *Ticci*—foundation, *Uira*—from *Uayra*—air, *Cocha*—lake.—Markham, p. 20, 1892.

ruler of the universe, who created man and all living things. They distinguished an intelligent and immaterial soul—*runa*—from the body which the name *allpacamasca*, designated as animated earth, and throughout all their teachings the belief is manifest that he who had well employed his time would at death go to *hananpacha*—the world above—to receive its reward; or, if bad, he would descend to *ụrupacha*, the world below. Because of the reverence the Incans had for their dead they respected all burial places, displaying much anguish at the disturbance of remains, yet the only knowledge that we have of these people has come to us through the constant search that is being made in the places of their interment, for antiquities and the wealth that is supposedly buried with their bodies.

The Incan cloths, which we have had opportunity of studying from the relics found in their tombs, were woven from the coarse llama fleece, or the fine silky wool of the vicuña, the latter being reserved for the royal garments. The materials were beautifully dyed with permanent colors tastefully combined, and exquisitely woven in complicated, though tasteful, patterns, in which animals, warriors and the Coca plant were all artistically concealed in the design. The Incas excelled in their manufacture of pottery, which is little inferior to that of the Greeks. Their vases occur in every variety of form, they are commonly moulded into water bottles and represent scenes, faces, animals, vegetables; and in fact every object known to the early Peruvians was reproduced in this artistic way.

Mr. John Getz,[23] who is an expert in ceramics, spent an afternoon with me in looking over a collection of these relics, which he pronounced wonderful in design and of very great age. All such antiquities are termed by the Peruvians *huacas**—sacred. They are commonly found buried in the tombs of Incan nobles, and are much sought. The material —red, black or cream colored, is of the terra cotta order,

[23] Chief of Decoration Exhibit Departments for the Commissioner General of the United States to the Paris Exposition of 1900.

* The derivation of the term *Huaca*, Garcilasso says, is from the verb which signifies to weep.

polished and painted in design, or again rough. The examples which are known as portrait vases were doubtless excellent likenesses and would be creditable if they were done by modern artists. A keen and premeditated wit is shown in some of these designs, which is not merely the grotesque of inexperience. Many of the vases are modeled as caricatures, possibly depicting, in political satire, some local personage; others again represent various diseased conditions, as the small-pox, which has always been prevalent throughout Peru. There are others which are marked with syphilitic lesions, and some represent the swollen cheek and the agonized expression of suffering from a possibly ulcerated tooth, while others depict various ceremonies.

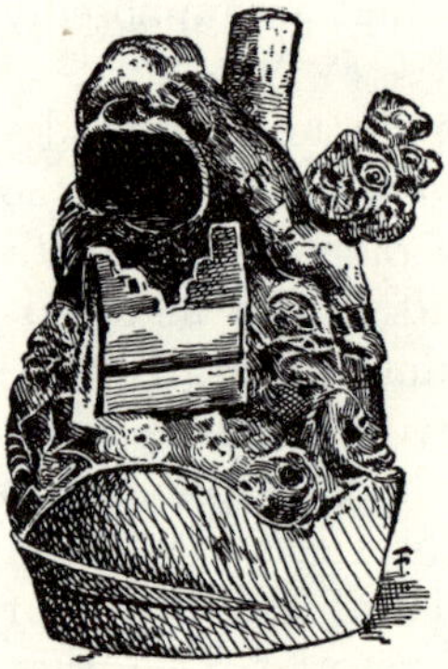

DECAPITATING ROCK VASE.
[*Tweddle Collection.*]

A curious vase in the private collection I inspected represents a rock, upon the top of which rests another rock, which seems to be capable of a lever movement, a possible instrument used in beheading victims, for a head and the headless body of a man are shown at the base, while another figure in a kneeling posture has his head bowed, as though awaiting decapitation from the fall of the small rock, which is apparently being worked by a figure standing at the side. This may illustrate some early form of capital punishment, though no mention of it is made in any of the works which I have consulted. Another form of punishment is shown by a vase representing an immense cactus of a species having digestive qualities of a phenomenal nature. Criminals placed in this gigantic plant were supposed to be literally digested and absorbed.

Some water bottles, that represent animals or birds, *silvadors*—or whistling jugs, as they are termed, were so cleverly constructed that a musical note is given in imitation of the cry as the water is poured out. A vase depicting the Coca harvest is in the form of a sitting woman with Coca branches and leaves around her. In many of the portrait vases the swollen cheek is represented as though containing the quid of Coca. Melons and gourds are common examples among these vases, as also is the llama representations of which were used as household gods, known as *conopas*.

Some of the painted vases represent scenes illustrating various rites. In the Centeno collection, at Berlin, some of the vases are over three feet in diameter. One has a painted scene, representing a battle between an Incan army using slings and savages armed with bows and arrows. Such examples suggest a knowledge of picture writing among the early Peruvians. At present there are many specimens of such pictorial work by the native artists, done on long strips of paper in flat tints, which, though crude, represent historical stories.

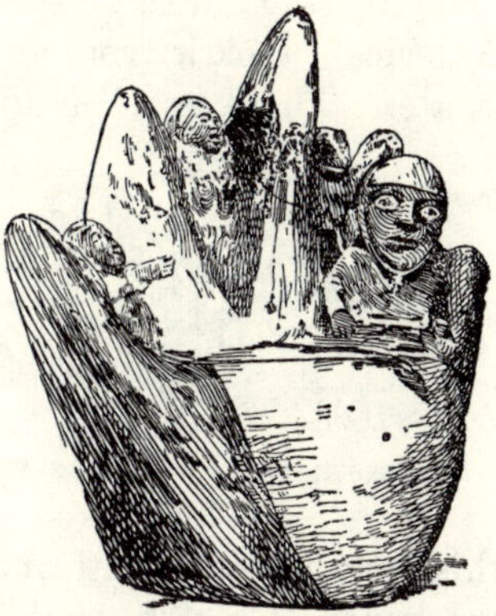

DIGESTING CACTUS VASE.
[*Tweddle Collection.*]

The Royal Ethnological Museum at Berlin possesses a rich assortment of Peruvian antiquities, and there are duplicates in the museum at Dresden, Leipzig and Karlsruhe. There is an exhibit of *huacas* in the Trocadero at Paris, and also in the British Museum, while in this country the University of Pennsylvania and the Peabody Museum in Chicago have each excellent collections. The American Museum of Natural History, of this city, has a fine assortment of water bottles, portrait vases, textile fabrics, work baskets, mummies and *chuspas* containing the leaves of Coca just as they have been taken from the tomb. The New York Metropolitan Museum of Art has also some unique specimens of household utensils made in pottery, as well as many additional examples of water bottles; for although the specimens all resemble each other, no two are exactly alike, as each was presumably modeled by hand.

There are many private collections of antiquities in Peru,

and a few in this country. It was my good fortune to have had the privilege to examine at leisure and to make copies of the very extensive collection of Mr. Herbert Tweddle, of Plainfield, N. J., which embraces many examples of relics not commonly seen. Among these is a curious tablet made of thin stone, upon which is engraved representations of the Incan warriors. It was probably worn on the royal robe. Another specimen representing a winged Puma head is almost a perfect counterpart of the early carving of the Egyptians. It is cut from a very soft stone of light amber color, and, as will be seen, greatly resembles the Assyrian lion. It was found in some diggings in the Pariñas Valley, where a Mr. Fowkes, an American, took it from an Indian grave on the La Mina Brea estate. There is no doubt of its genuineness as certified by

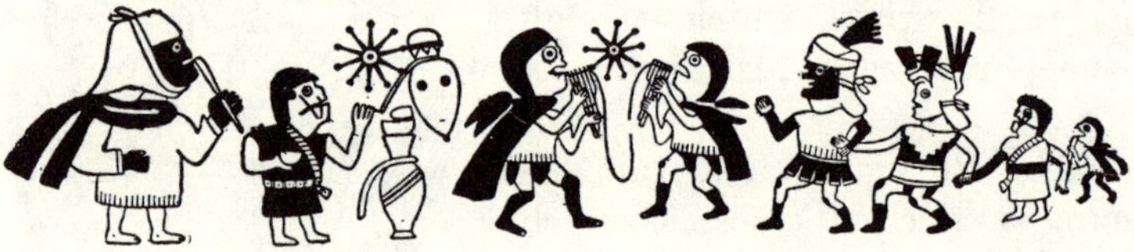

PAINTING REPRESENTING SUN WORSHIP, FROM A VASE AT CUZCO. [*Wiener.*]

this gentleman. With it were found three or four skeletons, the bones of which would indicate they were the remains of people about seven feet in height, with very large skulls. This specimen, when shown at the British Museum, was at first pronounced of Assyrian origin, but there are indications that it is distinctively Peruvian.

The puma—or *pagi* of the Peruvians is the lion of the Spanish. The Incas considered this as their most noble beast, and together with the condor, the king of vultures, they ennobled their attributes, and many families of ancient lineage still bear such titles. Thus the *Puma—cagna*—or lord of the brave lion, *Caliqui—puma*—lord of the silver lion, *Apu—cuntur*—the great condor, *Condor—canqui*—condor of excellency, or master of the order. It seems proper that these attributes should be typified in a union of both the head of the puma and the wings of the condor.

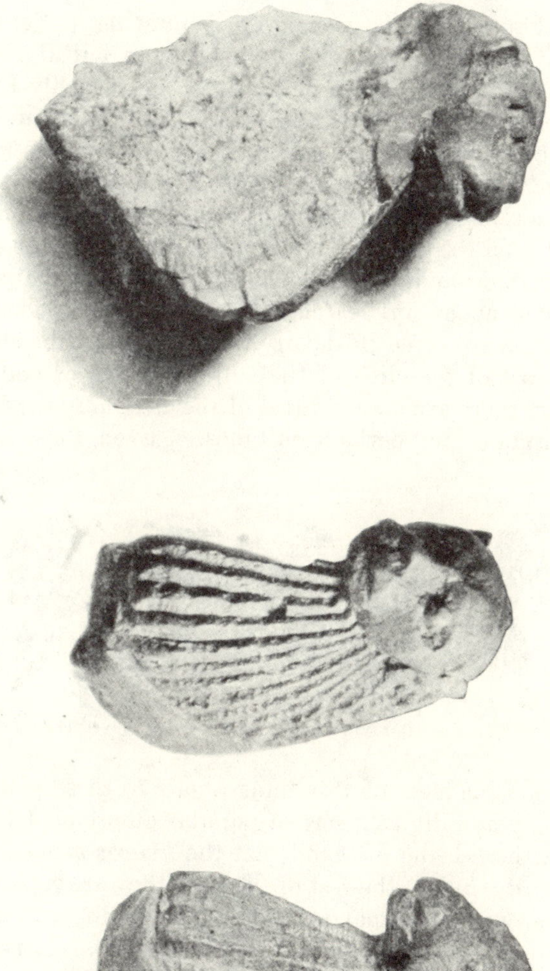

RIGHT SIDE. FRONT. LEFT SIDE.

PERUVIAN WINGED PUMA. [*Tweddle Collection.*]

Thus, it will be seen, treasure-hunting in Peru is not confined to prospecting for gold and silver, but also extends to a seeking for the riches which were presumably buried along with the bodies of the Incas; so that this much hunted race has not been permitted to rest in peace even in the grave. The *tapadas* or *huaqueros* as these relic hunters are called, constitute a class of modern adventurers. In their search for *huacas* they prod the soil with a long pole, and when a sounding indicates some underlying tomb, it is opened and the bodies are strewn about in search for antiquities. These burying grounds are often in the open desert and in the sterile soil at the foot of the cliffs of the valleys, which extend to the sea, where there are many graves of the *antiguos;* they are here by thousands and perhaps millions. Even those who do not

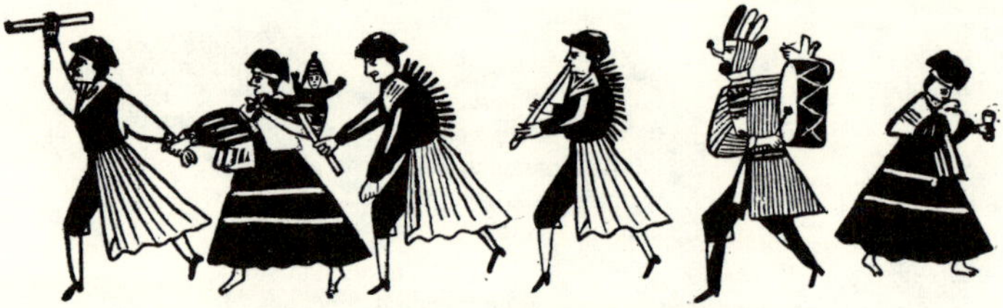

Bolivian Picture Writing. [*Wiener.*]

make a business of this hunt repair to these places on Good Friday and dig as a sort of popular amusement for that holiday, there being a legend that the *huacas* are enchanted, and while during all the rest of the year they are sunk so deeply in the ground as to make it impossible for them to be found, on Good Friday they come near the surface. It is remarkable that, though Coca is not to-day commonly used by the Indians on the coast, these graves all contain Coca among their relics. When these old graves are opened, although there is no apparent odor, those who explore them are very apt to get a very severe sore throat from inhaling the vapors or impalpable dust into which the bodies fall as they are exposed to the air. It has been long a custom to fortify against this condition by the use of Coca, thus illustrating the intuitive adaptation of a

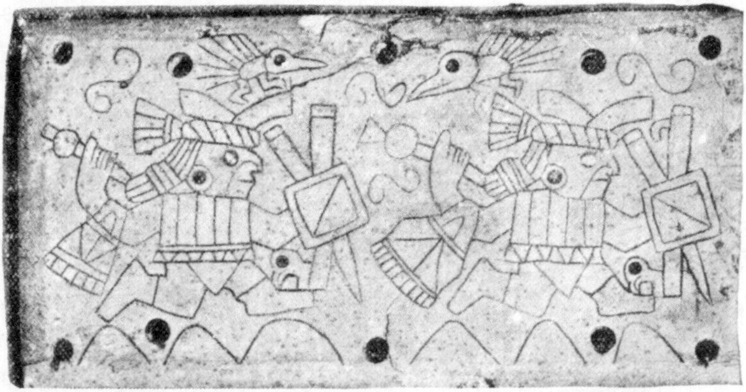

PLAQUE REPRESENTING INCAN WARRIORS. [*Tweddle Collection.*]

native remedy empirically, which it has required long years of study to since apply in a scientific way in the treatment of throat troubles.

Some of the relics that are taken out of these graves are worn as charms by the Indians. There is a supposition that many races may have been buried in these localities, as often the graves are situated directly over others of apparently different peoples. As a rule the bodies and their wrappings are well preserved, and it has been questioned whether this preservation is due to some process of embalming, or whether

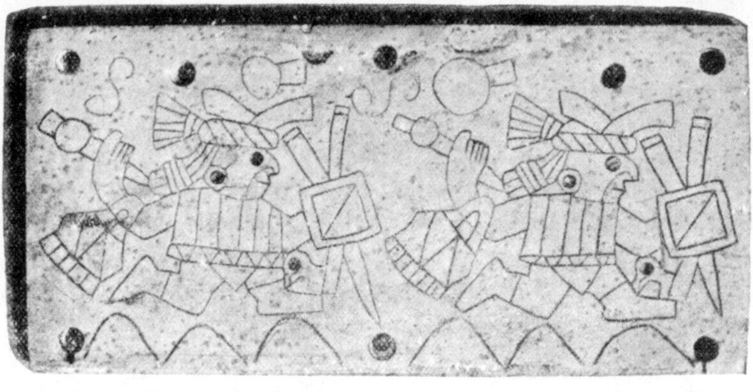

PLAQUE REPRESENTING INCAN WARRIORS. [*Tweddle Collection.*]

it is simply the result of the natron soil and extreme dryness. Various methods were followed in preparing the body for the grave. A child was usually wrapped in a coarse shroud, possibly a string of beads about the neck, with a little stick or plaything near at hand. Adults were usually buried in a squatting position, the head resting on the knees, the arms folded or supporting the head. Thus they were returned to Mother Earth in a position similar to that prior to their birth.[24] The body of the dead was covered with many wrappings—grave cloths of beautiful texture and exquisite coloring. About the mummy might be placed several pieces of pottery containing Coca or maize intended either to nourish the departed on his long journey or be ready for support on return. Near at hand were placed the implements and arms; and in the case of the women, the household utensils, spinning appliances, and the work basket filled ready for use. Commonly there were bags of netting containing a supply of wearing apparel. The fancy pieces of pottery are usually found at the head of the grave, where are also found the little woven tablets designed to keep off evil spirits.

When the wrappings of the mummy are removed, the body may not only be found well preserved, but often the flesh has a lifelike appearance. Great care seems to have been taken to wrap the bodies in the richest possible garments, so that these tombs are veritable mines of antiquities. The head of the mummy is commonly wound with a fancy turban, and the body is bound with a white tunic, elaborately embroidered with flowers and figures. The wrappings of the men are usually the richer, those of the women being more simple, but the bodies of men and women alike are found adorned with necklaces and bracelets. Although all the Indian women of to-day weave and spin, their work in no case equals that of the ancient relics found in these graves, while the antique implements are all of far superior finish to those of the present time. The *orqueta,* a crotched stick upon which is held the *copo* or ball of material for spinning, is usually to-day a natural fork cut from some tree for this purpose, but

[24] Wilson; 1876.

those which are found in the tombs are cut from solid wood beautifully carved, inlaid and polished. The modern Indian women are in the habit of plaiting thick skeins of brown cotton into braids with their hair to prevent the ends from splitting, and a similar custom is shown by these examples to have been followed by the ancients. In some of the bodies of women the lower lip has been pierced and a silver cylinder about the size of a thimble has been inserted. The crown of this is usually set with a bloodstone, surrounding which are small pieces of coral, executed with a delicacy of workmanship which would be creditable to a modern jeweler.[25]

Unlike the Egyptian mummies, those of the Peruvians do not represent the exact position of the body. They are commonly in huge square bundles, much resembling a bale of goods were it not for a headlike appearance on the top. These heads are attached to the exterior wrappings, the eyes, nose, lips and ears being fastened to the bundle in representation of a face. Often these entire bales are bound with a netting of plaited rope, two pieces of which are apparently left to lower the mummy into the grave. Some such packs have been found that are five feet high. On the shoulders, breast and back there are commonly a number of little pouches fastened together, filled with Coca leaves, while strings of such bags are often found in the tombs. Some of these mummies are found in the graves alone; in other cases there are several buried together. In some instances a large earthen vessel like a chicha jar, with the mouth broken off, is inverted over the mummy pack, evidently as a protection from the weight of earth above.

One of the largest collections of mummies was found along the coast, in the region of the Bay of Ancon, twenty-four miles to the north of Callao, where extensive excavations were made by Reiss and Stübel during 1874 and 1875. The result of this research has been exhaustively set forth in the magnificent work published by these authors in Berlin. They supposed the remains found to be of varying periods, some recent, others dating back for hundreds of years.[26] Some of the

[25] Scott; *La Goya*, also *person. com.*, 1899. [26] Reiss and Stübel; 1880.

bodies they unearthed were tattooed, a custom which was not prevalent among the Incans.

In the heights of the Western Andes there are many oven-like graves of adobe, and in the Sierra there are numerous graves found covered with huge piles of stone, some square, others oval. It is supposed that these monuments mark the resting places of important individuals or heads of families, while the graves of ordinary personages were either in rows or semi-circles, or in terraces on the mountains. Many of these stone piles are similar to the dolmans and cromlechs which may be found all over Northern Europe. They are of

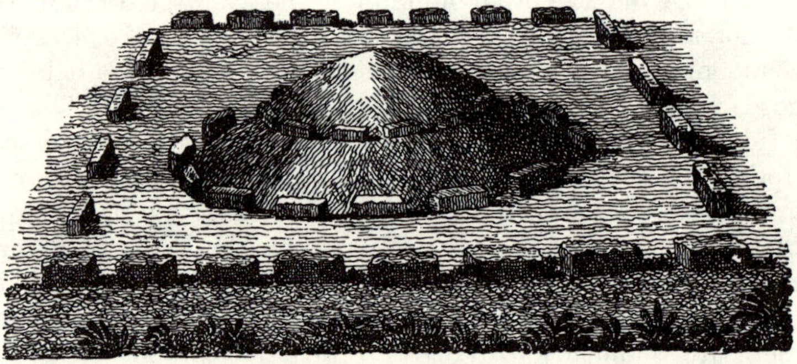

Celtic Temple, Similar to Druidical Temples and Incan Sun Circles.
[*Richard Payne Knight.*]

every variety in shape and have existed from prehistoric ages. Carnac in Brittany, Rutzlingen in Hanover, Stonehenge and Aubry in England, the stones at Orkney and at Lewis in Scotland, are but a few examples of such stone piles, which, if not belonging to one period, doubtless belonged to one form of worship. Many of these are sepulchral enclosures surrounding tumuli or uncovered cromlechs, and several mark the confines of what are termed giants' graves. These Druidical temples were similar to the Greek and Persian stone circles, in the centre of which was kindled the sacred fire. Along the Mississippi Valley, from the Great Lakes to the Gulf of Mexico, there are numerous works of stone and earth mounds, some of which cover several acres. Like the remains already cited, these are supposed to be thousands of years old. In the Titicaca region there are a great number of these stone monuments, which are known as *chulpas.* In some cases these are round, while other examples are square, in either instance looking like huge, squatty chimneys or the air shafts over an aqueduct. The tops are commonly larger than the base, extending mushroom-like beyond the sides and picturesquely overgrown with a confusion of mosses and vines. The interiors are usually of rough stone laid in clay and faced with hewn blocks of limestone, the size of the structure varying from ten to twenty feet in diameter, and from twelve to twenty-four feet high. The bodies in these tombs are usually found sewn in llama skins, upon which are pictured human features. Over this skin there are commonly wrappings, but differing from those of the mummies found along the coast.

The early Peruvians had a peculiar reverence for stones, and many of their legends refer to them. One tradition describes Viracocha as having endowed certain stones with life, from which were made the first man and woman. This is suggestive of a tale in Grecian mythology, when Deucalion and Pyrrha—the sole people left after the deluge, repeopled the earth by throwing behind their backs "the bones of their mother," which was interpreted to mean stones. So the stones thrown by the man took the shape of men, and those thrown by his wife became women.[27] The small round stones, which the Incas supposed to come from the thunderbolts, were said to have the property of producing fertility, and were regarded as love philters of remarkable efficacy. Throughout South America, between the 2° and 4° north latitude, there are thousands of rocks covered with symbolic representations, colossal figures of crocodiles, tigers and signs of the sun and moon possibly of different epochs.[28] Higgins[29] considers the examples of single unwrought stones to be emblems of generation. The Incans used to set up these single stone pyramids in their fields as protectors of their crops, and offerings were made to these as emblems—if not to propitiate a supposed

[27] Ŏvid; *Metamorphosis*, Fable x, Book i.
[28] Humboldt; *Ansichten der Natur.* [29] *Celtic Druids.*

spirit inhabiting them, as a mark of reverence or thanksgiving for guardianship. This practice is still continued, and it is in this spirit that Coca is commonly offered to such stones, because as that leaf is a prized object the Indian manifests his reverence in thus presenting something that is dear to him. Viewed in this light, such an action would seem no more idolatrous than for a Christian people to lay flowers on the tomb of their revered.

Among some specimens found among Incan relics are curious examples of trephined skulls. It is not known under what conditions this operation was performed, as similar examples have been found in various parts of the globe, and it would seem remarkable if these are merely accidental. Some of these skulls indicate that the subject had long survived the operation, while others appear to have been done after death. It has been questioned whether this operation was performed as a religious rite—a possible ordeal of initiation, or merely to make an opening to permit the imprisoned soul to escape from the dead body.[30]

At present the practice of trephining is continued among the Negritos of Papua and the natives of Australia, as well as in some of the South Sea Islands, where the operation is performed by scraping with a flint or shark's tooth, or with a piece of broken glass. Such trephining is said to have been so common with these latter people in early times that a majority of the male adults appear to have been subjected to it. An army surgeon travelling in Montenegro a few years ago said it was no rare thing to meet men who had been subjected to this operation seven, eight or even nine times.[31] Among the Kabyles, at the foot of Mt. Anrès, on the south of the Atlas, the operation is performed as a religious rite by the *thebibes*, or priests.

It is very probable that the early operations for trephining were first performed on the dead subjects with a view to obtain some mystical trophy as an amulet, which might represent some quality of the deceased. From this there was but an easy transition to the living, the operation being in the nature

[30] Broca; 1868. [31] Fletcher; 1882. Nadaillac; 1885.

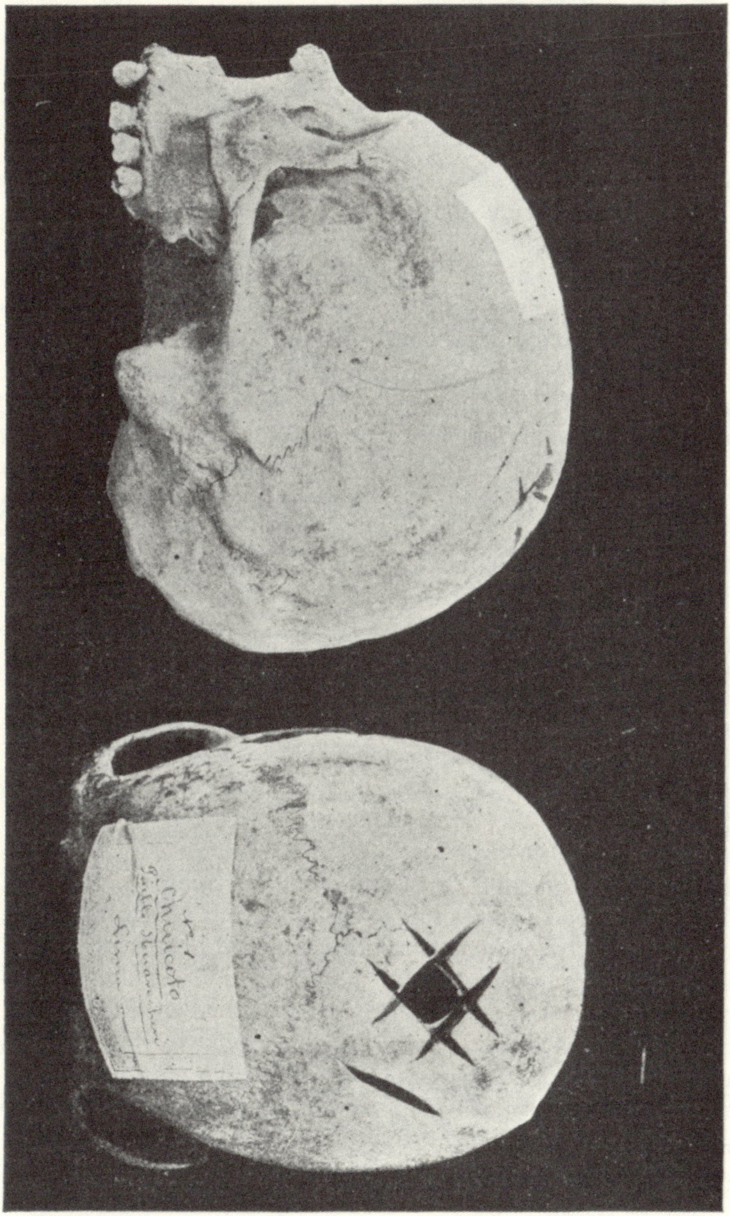

AN EXAMPLE OF PERUVIAN TREPHINING. [*Muñiz Collection.*]

of an ordeal, from which may be traced the development of the conservative methods of modern surgery.

It is supposed that the Incans had too strong a reverence for their dead to permit any mutilation for the sake of obtaining amulets. This is proven by the fact that no such fragments have been found. Dr. Muñiz,[32] formerly Surgeon-General of the Army of Peru, a few years since made an extensive collection of crania from Incan graves, mostly in the environs of Lima. Among one thousand specimens there were nineteen trephined skulls, some of which bear evidence of several distinct operations on different parts of the cranium at different periods. The percentage of trephined skulls to all crania found would indicate a ratio frequency of this operative procedure higher than that of a modern military hospital. These specimens of primitive trephining, which have been examined and discussed by many learned societies, are preserved by the Bureau of American Ethnology in the United States National Museum, at Washington, excepting one skull—showing a triple trephining, which has been placed at the United States Army Museum.

On the preceding page two views are given of a skull from a mummified body of a subject that did not survive the operation, but so perfect is the specimen—even the faintest scratches of the operation being visible—that it will serve as an indication of the method. The opening on the outer surface measures 17 by 22 mm., the dimensions being about 2½ mm. less in either dimension on the inner surface, the rectangular button having been cut by two pairs of parallel V-shaped incisions crossing at right angles. All four of the cuts penetrated both tables of the skull, while the transverse ones appear to have been deep enough to have wounded the intra-cranial tissues, probably causing death. The nature of the cuts indicate that the incision was done by a saw-like motion, accompanied with considerable pressure, the button being removed by an elevator, used lever fashion. This skull also shows wounds partly obliterated by reparative process. In some cases the rough edges of the opening have been scraped.

[32] Muñiz and McGee; 1897.

It was while the Incan Empire was at the height of its greatness that Huayna Ccapac, the twelfth Inca, after having governed for half a century, filled full of years and honors, retired to his favorite province at Quito, where he expected to spend his remaining days in peace. Realizing that the end of his career was approaching, and considering the vastness of his dominions, he determined to divide his kingdom between Huascar, his son by his lawful wife, and Atahualpa, the child of his favorite concubine. Just seven years prior to the Conquest this most mighty monarch of the line of Incas died.

The sad dissension between the two brothers, which was occasioned by this division of the Empire, and the unfortunate events which quickly follow to bring an end to this remarkable dynasty are told hereafter.

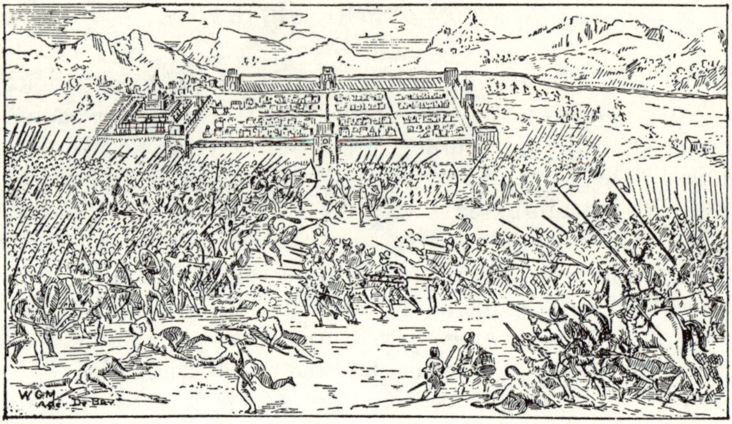

CHAPTER IV.

THE CONQUEST OF THE INCANS.

"So flits the world's uncertain span!
Nor zeal for God, nor love for man,
Gives mortal monuments a date
Beyond the power of Time and Fate."
—Scott, *Rokeby*, vi., i.

LONG before the discovery of Peru by the Spanish the Incas had so extended their empire that it reached from Chile in the south to Quito in the north. There was but one incentive to prompt this discovery, and that was gold. Indeed, gold was not only the beacon blazing from afar, but the shibboleth which led Francisco Pizarro on his voyage of conquest to the western shores of South America. Before this sordid search all else must perish; no sacrifice be too great, no device too flagrant, no torture too cruel to drag forth supposed secrets of hidden riches. The illegitimate son of a Colonel in the King's Guard, born in the town of Truxillo, in Spain,[1] and left a foundling,

[1] The date of Pizarro's birth is not positive; Prescott gives it as about 1471.

he is said to have rivaled Romulus by imbibing his early nutrition from a sow.[2] Grown to man's estate, uneducated save in the force of arms, he first appears in the history of the New World in 1509 in an expedition with Alonzo de Ojeda, who had been a companion of Columbus. Subsequently under Balboa he assisted in the establishment of the Spanish colony at Darien. Still later he was with Pedrarias, who founded Panama in 1519—and not unlike other foreign examples who readily fall into political preferment in the land of their adoption—he soon became a factor in the new city.

Rumors of fabulous wealth in some unknown country below the Isthmus had already floated toward this Spanish settlement, and proved a sufficient incentive to excite the roving nature of this adventurer into restlessness. Seeking means to further his purpose, Pizarro formed a partnership with two kindred spirits, Father Hernando de Luque, in behalf of the Licentiate Espinosa, and Diego de Almagro, the latter, like himself, an uneducated man, but a gallant soldier. Fitted out by this triumvirate, the first expedition sailed South in November, 1524, in two vessels, with a meagre crew of volunteers. One vessel was commanded by Pizarro, while the other, in charge of Almagro, was to follow with supplies. The expedition touched along the northern coast of South America, and met with an unexpected opposition from the natives, with whom the adventurers could not cope because of inadequate force. After suffering from privation, and discouraged by the dreary aspect of the country, the Spaniards wished to return to Panama; but Pizarro, made of sterner stuff, endeavored to stimulate his men by indicating the treasures that were in store for them. When their sufferings had reached almost direful straits the first part of the expedition was joined by Almagro with some sixty or seventy men. The two commanders, while appreciating the hardships before them—for Almagro had also suffered by encounter with the natives, and had lost an eye—were yet so encouraged by their discoveries that they pledged themselves to die rather than abandon their undertaking. But in view of the formidable nature of their enter-

[2] Gomara; cap. 144; 1749.

prise they thought it better to seek assistance from the government of Panama. At first the governor was not inclined to listen to what he considered the scheme of two rash adventurers, but through the plea of Father Luque, Almagro was permitted to solicit additional volunteers for the expedition. The seriousness of their prodigious undertaking was now sealed by a solemn compact made between the three—in which religion as the inspiring force, and plunder as the objective point, were commingled concerning an empire the situation and resources of which the plotters did not even know. Thus cloaked in a sincerity of religion, and with the sanction of the church, the cross was to be borne over this new land, and scathing and consuming as may have been the progress of this sign of man's salvation, it was to be enforced as the only sign by which generations yet unborn were to be rescued from perdition.[3]

It was not easy to raise a force for this second expedition, in spite of funds and the brilliant prospects of the enthusiasts; but finally two vessels set sail, each in command of one of the leaders and under pilotage of Bartholomew Ruiz, who was experienced in the southern ocean. After an uneventful voyage a landing was effected at a point somewhere on the coast of what is at present Colombia, where Pizarro and some of the men disembarked, and Almagro returned to Panama for supplies, while the other vessel under Ruiz continued south to explore the coast. This vessel soon fell in with one of the native raft-like boats, since known as *balsas,* which with a small crew displayed a rich cargo in full and tempting view upon the elevated platform raised above the deck. Here at last was a visible indication of the wealth for which the Spaniards had so long been in search. By friendly signs, and through cunningly entertaining the navigators of this novel craft, Ruiz was enabled to induce two of the people to return with him to Pizarro. His coming was none too soon, for the little band which had remained on shore was in sore distress and heartily discouraged from sickness and privation, and when Almagro arrived shortly after, the ardor of the adven-

[3] Prescott; Vol. I, p 238; 1848.

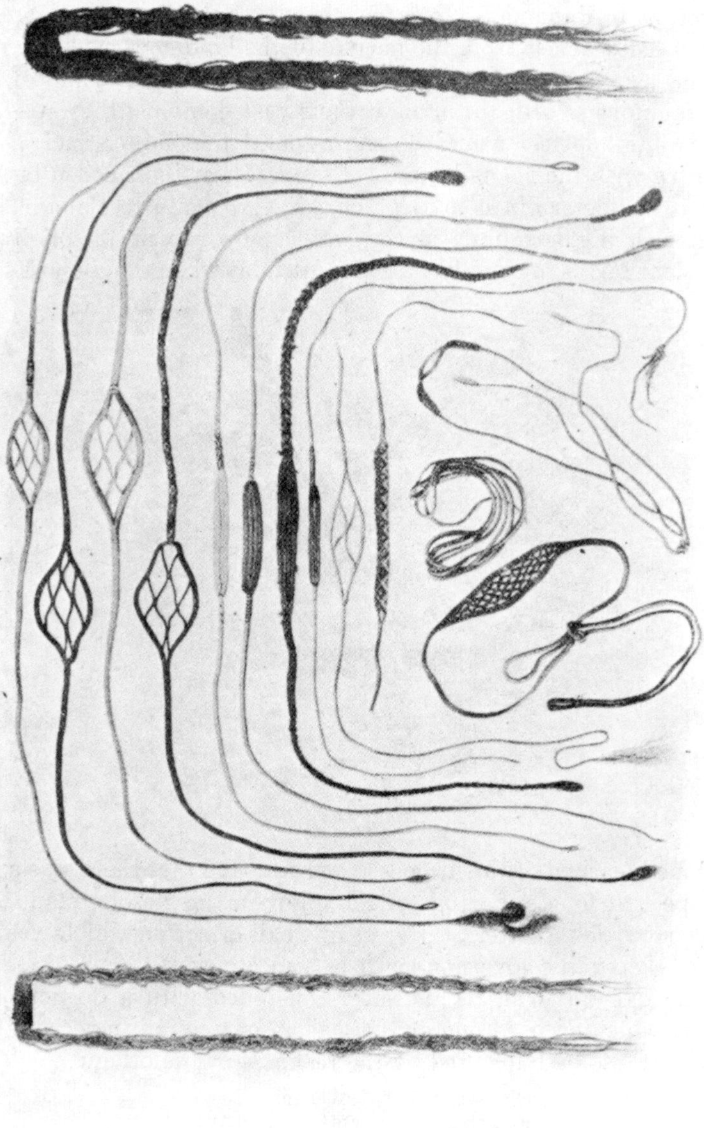

INCAN SLINGS. [*Reiss and Stübel.*]

turers had so cooled that all save the commanders were eager to return to Panama. Now, too, that the leaders of the expedition had learned from the natives of the land governed by a divine race termed Incas—descendants from the sun—and of the fabulous wealth throughout their vast domains, they realized how hopeless would be the attempt to conquer such a country with their small force. As a result of their consultation it was determined to dispatch Almagro again to Panama with such slight trophies as they might now return, to solicit sufficient forces to complete a conquest. But when the dissatis-

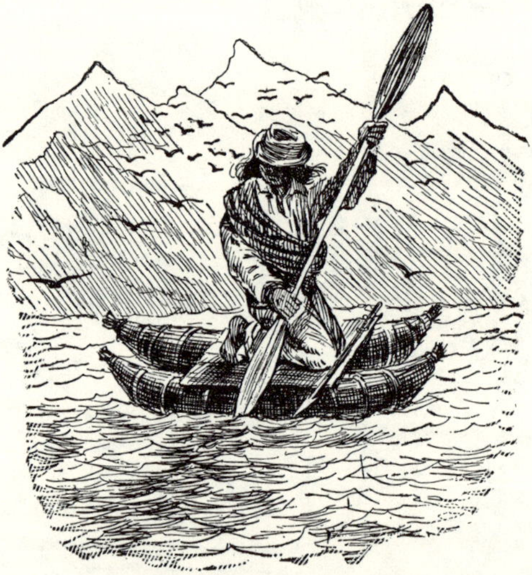

PERUVIAN BALSA. [*Marcoy.*]

fied men learned of this proposed venture, and that there was a prospect of long suffering for those left in this desolate land, they concealed a letter of protest in a ball of cotton which was to be taken to the governor's wife as a specimen of the products of this New World. This letter concluded with a doggerel verse, which accused one of the leaders of driving in recruits like cattle to be butchered by the rashness of the other:

"Look out, Señor, Governor,
For the drover while he's near;
Soon he goes to get the sheep
For the butcher who stays here."

Pizarro, in order to check all possibility of flight, soon after Almagro's sailing despatched the other vessel with some few malcontents. Those who were left experienced the extremes of suffering from privation, and when two vessels arrived from Panama with an officer of the governor to bring back the Spaniards, all were ready to desert Pizarro except some few gallant followers, who remained as the first heroes of this historic expedition. Pizarro received letters from Almagro and Father Luque beseeching him not to despair, and promising their continued aid. This faint encouragement was sufficient for so plucky an adventurer, and drawing his sword he marked a line on the sands and assured his comrades that on one side was toil, hunger, nakedness, drenching storm, desertion and death—on the other ease and pleasure. On the one side was Peru with its riches, on the other Panama and its poverty. "Choose each man what best becomes a brave Castilian. For my part, I go to the south." And he stepped across the line, being followed by "Ruiz, Cristoval de Peralta, Pedro de Candia, Domingo de Soria Luce, Nicolas de Ribera, Francisco de Cuellar, Alonso de Molina, Pedro Alcon, Garcia de Jerez, Anton de Carrion, Alonso Briceño, Martin de Paz, and Joan de la Torre."[4] But the governor's messenger refused to acknowledge such rashness, and barely consenting to leave some scanty provisions, sailed for Panama, accompanied by Ruiz, who returned in order to co-operate with Almagro and Father Luque. Their conjoined remonstrances, and protests that the expedition was for the benefit of the crown, finally induced the governor to consent that a small vessel should be fitted out for relief.

Meanwhile Pizarro was encamped with his meagre band upon the Island of Gorgona, off the northwest coast of Peru, and here they remained for seven months, and even continued their discoveries by means of a raft which they constructed, a form of navigation they were quite ready to abandon on the arrival of the new vessel. Thus favorably equipped, they at once set sail for the south, and after twenty days dropped anchor at the Island of Santa Clara, in the Bay of Tumbez.

[4] Prescott; Vol. I, p. 261; 1848.

Tumbez was then next to Quito, the most important city on the northern border of the Incan empire, and here the first exchange of visits took place between the officers of the expedition and some Incan inspectors, who ever on the alert to report to their sovereign the doings of each province, manifested a desire, through many courtesies, of learning the particulars of so mysterious a visitor to their waters. They offered fruit and game, and presented a llama, which the Spaniards termed

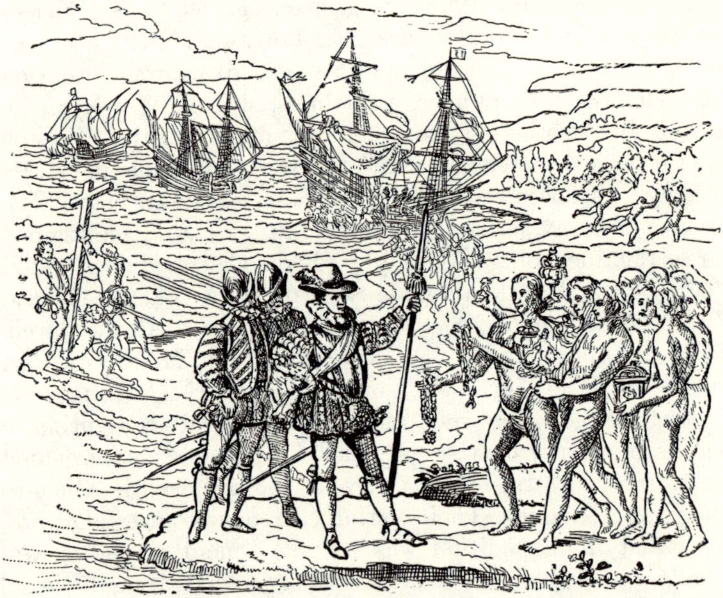

PIZARRO ON THE COAST OF PERU. [*De Bry,* 1600.]

"a little camel." Emboldened by these peaceful overtures, Pizarro continued down the coast as far as Santa, being everywhere cordially received and lavishly entertained by the natives, for hospitality was one of the first tenets of the social system of the Incas.

After an absence of eighteen months the commander was prevailed upon to return to Panama and report the result of his discoveries, which he was inclined to do in order to perfect plans which might enable him to conquer this vast territory. Two native boys were taken with him, and one of the Spaniards, at his own request, was permitted to remain at Tumbez, so that an interchange of language might add to the success of a return venture. Arrived at Panama, Pizarro excited the greatest interest as the result of his prospecting. The governor, however, refused to take the sole responsibility for so stupendous an undertaking, and it was determined that the success of the enterprise required the sanction, if not the co-operation, of the Spanish court. To assure this it was deemed advisable that Pizarro should personally explain his plan to the King, and he was despatched to the mother country to solicit the royal protection and aid.

So earnest were his representations, and so favorable were the gifts which he had taken as exhibits of the new land, that in July, 1529, permission was granted Pizarro to raise a force of not less than two hundred and fifty men with which he was to conquer this wonderful country for his king. Here the natives were to be converted and the true church established, provided a fifth of all the gold found in this new world should be sent as an allegiance to the crown for this royal privilege. To emphasize this favor Pizarro was permitted an important addition to his paternal escutcheon, was decorated with the red cross of Santiago, and appointed Governor and Captain-General over the new country in prospective. Almagro was created commander of the fortress at Tumbez, and Father Luque was made bishop of that same place, which he was never destined to see; Ruiz was given the title of Grand Pilot of the Southern Ocean, while the gallant band who had remained loyal to their leader under the privations of the expedition were made "gentlemen of coat armor."

These facts may seem a trifle dry, but as they form the framework—the anatomical basis—upon which subsequent events were shaped, perhaps their brief relation may not seem inopportune. For these invaders did not simply overthrow the existing government and permit native customs to continue under a new control, but they attempted to annihilate not only the people but their customs and traditions. That there has remained any historical data must demonstrate the firm establishment of this former empire, an endurance that is further displayed by the survival of those native products the use of which is now enjoyed throughout the world, prominent among which is Coca so intimately associated with the Incan race.

Under royal approval and with a small grant of money from the crown, Pizzaro having enlisted his four brothers, made preparations to depart from Spain. Although he had not secured a full complement of men, he hurriedly sailed from Seville, January, 1530, for Panama, where after a consultation with his associates the final preparations for his expedition were completed. Church and State went so intimately hand in hand in those days that when in the following year the temporal plans had been got in readiness, the banners were blessed, the men were consecrated to their work against the infidel, and the expedition, which now consisted of three ships, sailed with some one hundred and eighty-five men and twenty-seven horses. After thirteen days a port was made in the most northern province of Peru, where the troops were landed with orders to march south, while the vessels continued on a parallel course with them. Force of arms was now openly resorted to, the smaller coast villages being successively overcome, and the captured wealth at once despatched to Panama as the first fruits of an assured success and an indication of the fabulous treasures which might be expected to follow. It was not long before Pizarro learned of the dissension between the brothers Huascar and Atahualpa, and the weakened government occasioned by this scission. His own forces having been strengthened by an arrival of volunteers from Panama, he determined in some way to shape this opportunity to his advantage.

In November, 1532, hearing that Atahualpa, with his army, was in the neighboring mountains, Pizarro crossed the desert of Sechura, and a sort of triumphal march was continued toward the interior directly to the Inca's camp. As his troops passed on, the natives were baptized into the church, and assumed solemn vows which they could not understand, but it was sufficient that they had accepted the faith. Atahualpa learning of Pizarro's approach—presumably supposed that so small a body could only be coming upon friendly terms—so sent a messenger with greetings to inform him that the Inca would on the following day visit him in person. In the meantime the freedom of Caxamarca was extended to the invaders, and the use of the public buildings was offered for the troops.

Pizarro concealed his forces while awaiting the sovereign, who was borne in great state upon the royal litter. He was clothed in Incan splendor, a *chuspa* of Coca hung at his side, golden sandals were upon his feet, and his head bore the stately insignia of power—the *llauta* and *borla* of scarlet fringe, with the royal feathers of the sacred bird. He was accompanied by a numerous retinue of nobles of his court and thousands of followers. Friar Vicente de Valverde, the ecclesiastical head of the Spaniards, acted as spokesman, and explained through his interpreters that their little band had visited this far-off land for the sake of establishing the true religion and converting the natives. He beseeched the Inca to at once acknowledge the faith and allegiance to the king, Charles the Fifth. Authority for all this he attempted to show in a Bible which he offered to Atahualpa, but the latter, saying he recognized no other king than himself, indignantly threw the book to the ground, which the vengeful friar seemed to recognize as an affront sufficient to provoke hostilities, for he shouted, "Fall on! I absolve you," when at once the most terrible onslaught upon the unsuspecting Incas was commenced. The Spanish officers being mounted, were enabled to do some frightful work, while the troops, armed with death-dealing arquebuses, literally vomited fire upon the natives, who were massacred by thousands,[5] while not one of the invading party was injured save Pizarro, who received a slight wound from his own men while shielding the Inca, who was taken prisoner. The monarch was at first treated with courtesy, and permitted to retain his people about him. Pizarro, ever awake to some politic

[5] Ten thousand, Garcilasso said; Pizarro's secretary said two thousand.

move, hinted upon the advisability of adjusting the affairs of the brothers amicably, but the imprisoned chief, not realizing his own danger, became alarmed at such a suggestion, and secretly despatched orders to assassinate Huascar, who was then a prisoner in Atahualpa's army. Nor had his brother received very courteous treatment at the hands of the rival forces, for they put a rope around his neck and called him *Coca hachu*—Coca chewer—besides offering him many other affronts, while they gave him Chillca—*Bacchaus scandeus* leaves to eat instead of Coca. This so outraged Huascar that he raised his eyes to heaven and cried: "O Lord and Creator, how is it possible? Why hast thou sent me these burdens and troubles?"[6]

Now commenced the downfall of the Empire of the Incas. Atahualpa, chafing under restraint, suggested paying for his ransom with as much gold as the room in which he was imprisoned would hold; and as that space was seventeen feet broad by twenty-two feet long, and was to be filled to a height of nine feet, the Spaniards were only too ready to agree to his proposition. But even their most sordid expectations had not pictured the vast store of riches which, at the command of the Inca, was at once brought to them from all sections of the country. It literally poured in a golden stream of vases, vessels, utensils, ornaments, the golden Coca shrubs from the temples, immense plaques, and golden animals, and statues of life-size, and in nuggets and golden dust. All this did not seem enough to satisfy the greed of the conqueror, who determined to expedite matters by seeking the source of this golden supply for himself. Instead of freeing Atahualpa, who had shown too keen a wit to be permitted at liberty, it was decided to make away with him. He was charged with the murder of his brother, and after a hasty trial was condemned to death. In August, 1533, after receiving the last rites of the Church, he was executed in the square of Caxamarca by the *garrote,* as a distinctive torture to being burned alive in consideration for his having at the last moment submitted to baptism. The following day, amidst the most impres-

[6] Ondegardo; 1560.

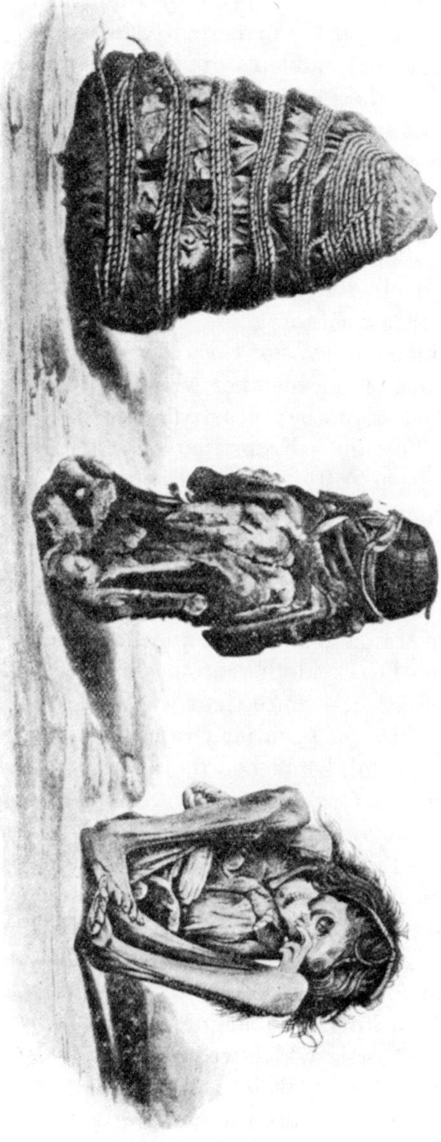

PERUVIAN MUMMIES, SHOWING POSITION OF BODY IN THE PACK.
[*Reiss and Stübel.*]

sive solemnity, the service for the dead being performed by Father Valverde, the body of the Incan sovereign was buried, Pizarro and his principal cavaliers assuming mourning as hypocritical emblems of their grief at the loss of this mighty lord. The greatest lawlessness now commenced, and booty was free among the Spaniards. Villages were destroyed, houses were ransacked, and the gorgeous temples and palaces were plundered.

Pizarro advanced rapidly to Cuzco, but little of its golden splendor was now left. The cupidity of the invaders had over-leaped itself, for as the Peruvians saw that the sole desire of the Spanish was for gold, they secreted the beautifully wrought golden emblems of Coca and other elaborate workings of the precious metal, together with the sacred vessels and the venerated bodies of the Incas which had been set up in the Temple of the Sun. From that day to this these treasures have never been fully recovered, although some years later Polo Ondegardo, while Corregidor of Cuzco, found five mummies in a tomb in the mountains, three of them men and two women. These were said to be the bodies of the Incas Viracocha, Tupac Inca Yupanqui and Huayna Ccapac, together with Mama Runtu, the queen of the first named, and Ccoya Mama Ocllo, mother of the last. Each of the bodies was well preserved, even the hair with the eyebrows and lashes remaining, while the peculiar wrappings and the sacred *llauta* about the forehead, betokened their rank. These bodies were conveyed to Lima, where they were buried with appropriate rites in the courtyard of the hospital of San Andres.

When the first vast treasure of capture was divided among the officers and followers of the conquerors, each of the invaders was allotted a fortune, and Hernando Pizarro was despatched to Spain with the royal fifth. The amount taken to the Crown proved sufficient to establish this new country in the name of the king, who magnanimously divided it into New Castile in the north, which was assigned to Pizarro, and New Toledo south of that, which was given to the control of Almagro. So gloated were the Spaniards with their newly acquired riches that the most ordinary commodities were paid for in fabulous sums, and many anecdotes are related of this prodigality of wealth. The men fell into riotous living, spent their days in lawlessness and their nights in gambling, the stakes at these bouts often being for whole fortunes. In one of these orgies the massive emblem of the Sun, taken from the Temple at Cuzco, was staked and lost at a single throw by the cavalier to whom it had fallen in the division of the spoils, from which an after allusion of arrant profligacy was referred to as: "He gambles away the sun in a night."[7]

It is recorded that when Atahualpa was imprisoned one of the priests wrote the name of God at his request upon the Inca's finger nail. This he showed to several of the guards, who, upon their pronouncing the name correctly, it excited his admiration and astonishment that characters so unintelligible to him could be read by the Spaniards. On showing the name to Pizarro—who could neither read nor write—he remained silent, and by thus displaying his ignorance provoked a contempt which his prisoner could not well conceal. It has been asserted that it was through pique at this incident that determined an approval to the Inca's death.

The Empire of the Incas being now without a chief, fell into confusion, and the governors of the several provinces each set up an independence, which Pizarro was quick to appreciate would be more difficult to overthrow than to conquer the country under one revered ruler whom he might influence through stratagem. He therefore determined to install Manco, the legitimate brother of Huascar, who had already placed himself under his protection, and he was established as the successor and sovereign Inca amidst all the ancient splendor and formality that such an occasion might demand. So much harmony had been occasioned by this shrewd course that it now seemed as though the whole country might proclaim allegiance to Pizarro's guardianship, but the avarice of the invaders had not yet been appeased by the gold they had received. Their persistent search for treasure, which did not respect even the sacred buildings and palaces, proved to the Indians the new religion was not one of peace, but rather suggested they were

[7] *Juega el Sol antes que amanezca;* Garcilasso; 1609.

to be reduced from their former freedom and happy state to become the mere slaves of a body of tyrants. A succession of internal wars now commenced, and the Incas, led by Manco, took a final stand at Cuzco, which they battled so nobly to defend that for a time it seemed the Spaniards must be routed, but the ultimate result was the complete overthrow of the Incan Empire, and Manco, chagrined and humiliated by his defeat, escaped to the mountains near Vilcabamba, where he maintained a sort of regal independence with a few loyal followers, until his death in 1544. After the overthrow of Cuzco, Pizarro, desiring a location near the coast in easier communication with Panama, established the seat of his government on

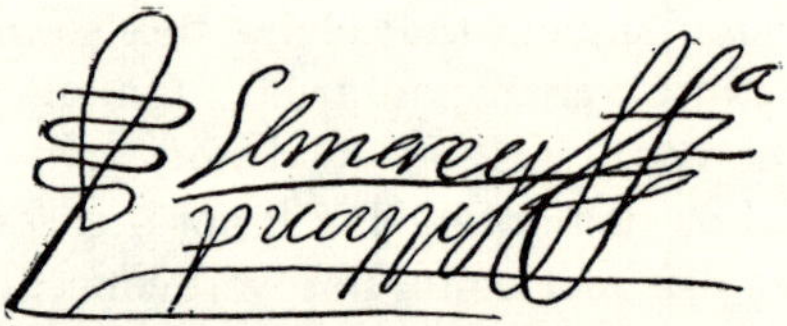

PIZZARRO'S MARK. [*El Marq Pizarro.*]
The name written by his secretary, the flourish by Pizarro.

the river Rimac, and the new capital was named *Ciudad de Los Reyes*—City of the Kings—in honor of the sovereigns of Spain, the modern name, Lima, being a corruption of Rimac.

And here the conqueror, enthroned in power, took to him Añas, the daughter of Atahualpa, by whom he had a son—Francisco, who became a schoolmate of the Incan historian, Garcilasso de la Vega, but died young in Spain. As though to unite his name more profoundly with the Incan race, Pizarro took also the sister of Huascar, who bore him two children, a son, who died young, and a daughter, Francisca, who in after years married his brother, Hernando, in Spain. As if by marriage and intermarriage the invaders might atone for the destruction of a mighty race.

But let us see how fared the partners and adventurous companions of the conqueror. Father Luque never enjoyed the fruits of the success of his partners, for he died a few months after the final expedition started from Panama; while

Juan Pizarro was killed when the Incas, under Manco, besieged Cuzco in 1536, in defense of which the several brothers were engaged. Almagro, who early fell into dissension with Francisco, was executed in Cuzco at the command of Hernando Pizarro in July, 1538; and so a bitter feud was originated between the people of Chile, who were followers of Almagro, and the people of Northern Peru, who were followers of the Pizarros—which almost rivaled the stories of the Corsican vendetta. It was not long after this that Francisco Pizarro was cruelly assassinated while dining with some friends by the cohorts of Chile, while his brother, Hernando, who had sought refuge in Spain, was imprisoned for twenty years on account of his execution of Almagro. After Francisco's death his brother, Gonzalo, placed himself at the head of a faction and assumed government, although the Crown had already sent a commissioner to take charge of Peruvian affairs. As a result of the rebellion which followed, Gonzalo was beheaded at Cuzco, in 1548, and Valverde, who had been the ritualistic light of the conquerors, was killed by the islanders of Puna.

It seems incredible how so mighty an empire could be destroyed so that the landmarks even were almost obliterated. But the solution of this is found not so much in the valor of the Spaniards as in the utter demoralization of the Peruvians through a succession of reverses. The Incans, while at first confounded by the division of their country under two heads, became almost helpless when the final loss of the leaders of both sections occurred, for they had been educated for hundreds of years to look upon their sovereign as divine and all-powerful. With the downfall of the Peruvians, Spain's interest in the new country was stimulated to excitement by the vast wealth which she had received and the still greater riches that had been reported. There, too, was the hope of finding El Dorado, that mythical city which existed somewhere in the interior of the country, where the streets were paved with gold and where the native king was every morning powdered with gold dust. This all seemed so great a treasure that the Crown determined to assume direct control by the appointment of a

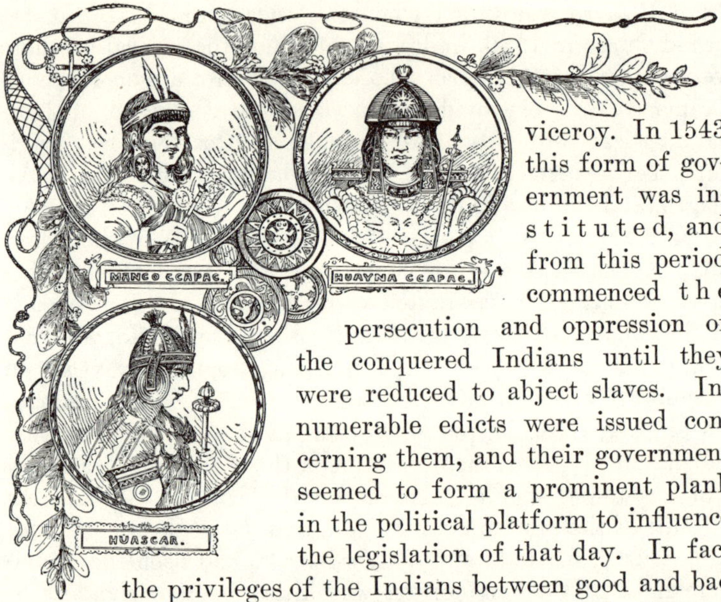

viceroy. In 1543 this form of government was instituted, and from this period commenced the persecution and oppression of the conquered Indians until they were reduced to abject slaves. Innumerable edicts were issued concerning them, and their government seemed to form a prominent plank in the political platform to influence the legislation of that day. In fact the privileges of the Indians between good and bad fluctuated in accordance with the whims or aspirations of the party in power. At one time the fact that the conquerors were deprived by edict from the personal service of the natives as slaves occasioned a rebellion, while for years the Indians were a source of perpetual warfare, of which they remained the innocent victims, their peaceable disposition not even being awakened to an uprising such as their ill treatment might have well provoked, yet kept them constantly suspicious. In the year 1560 it was supposed by the Indians that an ointment made from their bodies had been sent for from Spain to cure a certain disease for which there was no other remedy. This belief made these people very shy of the Spaniards at that time, fearing that they might be taken in and boiled down into this necessary unguent.[8] A succession of dread as a result of abuse and oppression resulted in a stolid hatred directed not only against the Spanish but toward all white persons, that is still manifest through the reticence of the Peruvian Indians of to-day.

[8] Molina; 1570.

It was during this long period of oppression that Coca was attacked because it was so esteemed by the Indians, and numerous edicts were issued by both Church and State forbidding its use and even seeking to exterminate the plant. Particularly was this so under the rule of Francisco de Toledo, the fifth viceroy, a man devoted to his sovereign, but narrow-minded and unsympathetic. During his rule there were some seventy *ordenanzes* issued concerning Coca. After his appointment in 1569 he made a tour through the country to determine the exact condition of affairs, and to study the customs of the natives. In this he was accompanied by Father Acosta, the Judge Matienzo, and Polo de Ondegardo, each of whom has left valuable works regarding the traditions and early customs of the natives upon which most of the subsequent writings have been based. Toledo seems to have determined to stamp out all Incan traditions, and to change completely the habits of the natives in conformity with his own ideas as to what Spanish subjects should be. He established the imposition known as the *mitta,*[9] a personal tax upon the Indians, which necessitated a certain number from each province to submit themselves to the control of the Governor for such work as he might assign them, at so small a pittance, $14 to $18 a year, that their labor was virtually slavery. This had grown out of the old system of common labor for the State during the Incan period. These Indians, known as *mitayos*, were assigned to service over every part of the country except the coast, where negro slaves were employed. They were compelled to work in the mines in the mountains, and in the cocals of the montaña to cultivate their precious plant for the benefit of their foreign conquerors. This enforced labor was prompted through a desire to send all possible riches home to Spain; and so brutally were the Indians driven to their tasks that in a century nine-tenths of these people had been destroyed by overwork and cruelty.[10] The owners of the *obrajes*—where the coarse cloths were woven, employed men called *guatacos* to hunt the Indians and compel them to work for a mere pittance, while the poor victims were driven into an indebtedness for necessi-

[9] *Mitta* in Quichua signifies time, or term. [10] Markham; 1892.

ties, which being advanced kept them in perpetual slavery to their masters.

In 1569 the Spanish audience at Lima, composed of bishops from all parts of South America, denounced Coca because, as they asserted, it was a pernicious leaf, the chewing of which the Indians supposed gave them strength and was hence: "*Un delusio del demonio.*"[11] The prejudice and abhorrence of the Spaniards was not only directed against Coca but against any custom of the Indians. This is shown by the following story, related by Garcilasso, the Incan historian, writing from abroad: "I remember a story which I heard in my native land of Peru of a gentleman of rank and honor named Rodrigo Pantoja, who, travelling from Cuzco to Rimac, met a poor Spaniard, for there are poor people there as well as here, who was going on foot, with a little girl aged two years on his back. The man was known to Pantoja, and they thus conversed: 'Why do you go laden thus?' said the knight. The poor man answered that he was unable to hire an Indian to carry the child and for that reason he carried it himself. While he spoke Pantoja looked in his mouth and saw that it was full of Coca, and as the Spaniards abominate all that the Indians eat and drink as though it savored of idolatry—particularly the chewing of Coca, which seems to them a low, vile habit, he said: 'It may be as you say, but why do you eat Coca like an Indian, a thing so hateful to Spaniards?' The man answered: 'In truth, my lord, I detest it as much as any one, but necessity obliges me to imitate the Indians and keep Coca in my mouth, for I would have you know that if I did not do so, I could not carry this burden, while the Coca gives me sufficient strength to endure the fatigue.' Pantoja was astonished to hear this, and told the story wherever he went; and from that time credit was given to the Indians for using Coca from necessity and not from vicious gluttony."

Salorzano,[12] a Spanish jurist, says that the *mittas* of Indians were prevented from working the cocals owing to the reported unhealthfulness of that section of the montaña by an edict of October 18, 1569. The words of the law are as fol-

[11] *Cédula* of October 18, 1569. [12] *Polit. Ind.*, lib. ii, cap. 10.

lows: "As the country where Coca is grown is humid and subject to rain, and the Indians in their work generally get wet and then fall ill from not changing their wet clothes, we command that no Indian shall commence work in that land without being provided with a change of clothes, and the master of the Coca plantation must take especial care that this be done under a penalty of paying twenty baskets of Coca for each time that he may be found to bring any Indian to this work without complying with the regulations herein set forth."[13] Finally Toledo permitted the cultivation of Coca with voluntary labor, on condition that the Indians were well paid and that care was taken of their health.

Besides the *mitayos,* some of the Indians, who were known as *yanaconas,* were bound to personal service—literally household slaves, a custom that had been continued from an

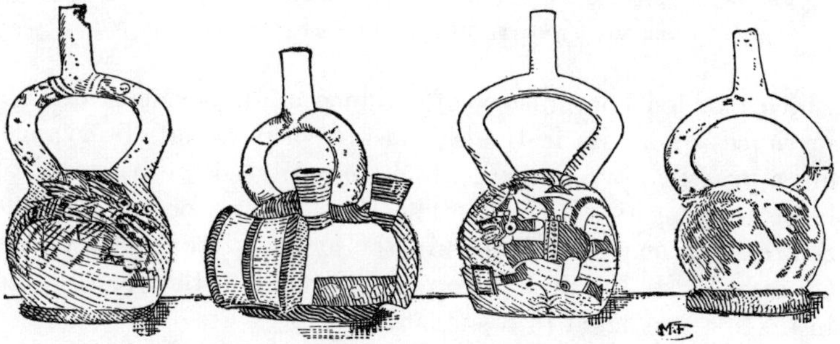

PERUVIAN VASES. [*Tweddle Collection.*]
Polished Ware with Designs in Red.

early Incan period.[14] In Toledo's time this class numbered some forty thousand who were assigned to the Spaniards as servants.

Toledo enacted some very rigorous laws affecting the In-

[13] *Porque la tierra donde la Coca se cria es húmeda y lluviosa, y los Indios de su beneficio ordinariamente se mojan, y enferman de no mudar el vestido mojado; Ordenamos que ningun Indio entre a beneficiarla, sin que lleve el vestido duplicado para remudar, y el dueño de la Coca tenga especial cuidado que esto se cumpla bajo pena de pagar veinte cestas de Coca, por cada vez que se hallare traer algun Indio contra lo susdicho, aplicados en la forma referida. Recopilación de los Indios;* tom. 2, lib. 6, tit. 14, ley 2.

[14] Inca Tupac Yupanqui granted a pardon to captive rebels at Yana-Yacu on condition that they should act as servants. These were known as *Yana-Yacu-Cuna,* which term was corrupted to *yanaconas.*

dians. Among these was one condemning any Indian who married an idolatrous woman to receive one hundred lashes, because, says the edict, "that is the punishment which they dislike most." No Indian who had been punished for such an offense, or for engaging in any infidel rites, was eligible for any public office. The poor Indians were prevented from even choosing names for their children after birds or natural objects, as had been their ancient custom. Together with this oppression from the State was the authority of the Church,

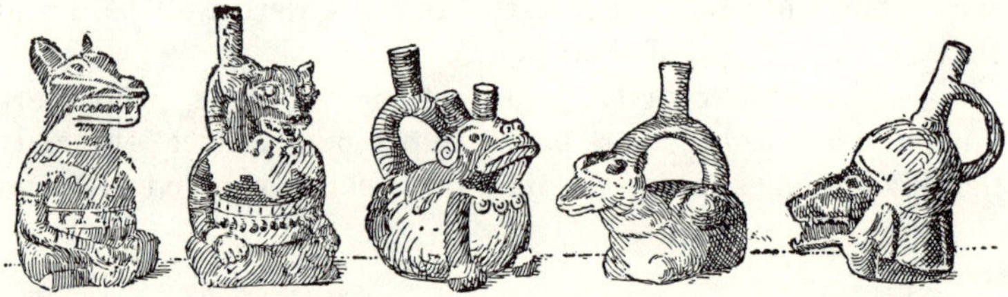

PERUVIAN ANIMAL VASES. [*Tweddle Collection.*]

which exacted compulsory attendance at its services and observances of all its festivals; not only a personal observance, but a practical one as well, which necessitated the payment of large fees for every office. The Pope had no power over the South American clergy, the king being the virtual head of the Church, while the archbishop ranked next to the viceroy and in his absence acted in his stead.

The Church, with its numerous dignitaries, had representatives in every hamlet, with absolute control over the education of the Indians. Indeed, the Spanish were not slow in educational matters, the University of San Marcos, which is the oldest in the world, being founded at Lima as early as 1551, and there were other colleges for the descendants of the conquerors, for the sons of the Incas, and for the students of the Church, with similar institutions at Cuzco, at Arequipa, at Truxillo, and Guamanga, all founded at an early date.

Among the rigorous rulings of the Church, the people were obliged to provide supplies for the several feasts in commemoration of saints, as well as offerings to the priests on Sundays, which, in lieu of money, were paid in Coca or other products of their industry. It is reported that one priest extorted in this manner two hundred sheep, six thousand fowls and fifty thousand eggs in one year. On the death of a member of a poor Indian's family, the rites of the Church were refused until a good sum had been paid for the service. In default of voluntary payment the Indian's goods were seized. The clergy lived very immoral lives; and in addition to their personal extortions from the Indians, their concubines compelled the women to work for them. There was ever a constant greed shown toward all the effects of the natives, as the following story will illustrate: An Indian stopping at a tambo, and having no money to pay for his entertainment, left as a pledge with the woman in charge a number of antique golden figures, which he promised to redeem to the extent of his indebtedness upon his return, exacting from her a promise that she would show these articles to no one. The woman subsequently being in need of money, gave the *huacas* to a priest as pledges, and when the Indian returned for them he was thrown into prison and compelled to confess that he knew of an Incan treasure, but if they dug for it, as he would indicate, the water would cover the valley where it was hidden. On search being made, it is said that a treasure of $2,500,000 was found, but the water, as he had predicted, rushed into the excavation, and the place, called Manan-Chile, is at present covered by a lake, in the centre of which is a small island.

Indians were excluded from all the higher occupations by a decree of the Count of Moncloa, who was the viceroy in 1706. No Indian, *mestizo*—half white and half Indian, negro, mulatto, or *zambo*—half Indian and half black, was permitted to have a shop for the sale of goods or even to traffic in the streets, but they were all confined absolutely to agricultural or mechanical labor. The public and military offices were all occupied by Spaniards, who maintained an insolent pride toward the creoles. The policy was to crush out all freedom of thought as well as of action in the last remnant of the Incan race. There was one redeeming feature in the Spanish cruelties, the exemption of the Indians from the jurisdiction of the Holy Inquisition, which was established in Peru in 1569 by Philip II, and which was exercised by the most terrible cruelties inflicted for often the most trivial offense.

The drain on the treasury of the home government through her countless wars necessitated a continual demand for money, and the poor *mitayos* were sent to the mines and literally worked to death in an endeavor to satisfy this constant cry for gold. The laborers were so beaten at their tasks that the punishment seemed so much a necessary part of their existence that if they did not receive it they felt that their masters no longer loved them. In the mills work was commenced before daylight, and the slaves were locked in until dark, when those who had not completed the task that had been assigned them were cruelly punished. Thus this race became gradually debased into abject slaves, and gold, which had been poetically termed by the Incas "Tears which the sun shed," might well have been corrupted into tears of darkness and toil!

At the height of its prosperity the Incan population numbered some ten million souls, but the system of serfdom so reduced its people that at the time of the census made by Archbishop Loaiza, in 1580, there were but 8,280,000, which to-day has dwindled into less than two millions. The poor Indians had a hard taskmaster under Spanish rule, and it was not until Peru was declared independent in 1821 that the system of slavery, known as the *mitta*, was forever abolished by law. There was still another abuse to which the Indians were subjected. They were compelled to buy useless things from the Spanish stores, which not only consumed any little savings they might have, but forced them into an indebtedness from which they were compelled to work in order to gain freedom. Under the pretense that they were being supplied with necessary goods at unusually advantageous prices, the most absurd things were imposed on them, such as fine silken hose for a barefooted Indian girl, silks, velvets and laces for the Indian's wife, padlocks to lock up what they never possessed, razors to shave beardless faces, and at one time a job lot of spectacles was distributed, through an edict that no Indian should appear in church unless wearing these necessary adjuncts to seeing the true light. The policy of the masters was to keep the Indians in debt to them—a custom that still continues—it being an established law that an Indian shall not leave his master so long as he shall be indebted to him; and, indeed, he could not find employment elsewhere so long as he is hampered by this incubus, so that the only way to escape from a life of continued slavery is to run away to some other part of the country, where the same system is continued and the weight of indebtedness is gradually assumed anew.

Excessive duties were also established against harvests to increase the revenue. The *alcabala* was an excise duty of two per cent. on all provisions sold in the market, which in the case

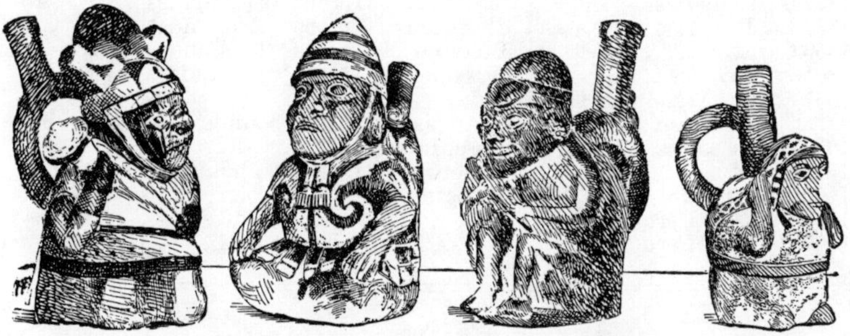

Peruvian Vases. [*Tweddle Collection.*]
Representing Incas and a Plebeian.

of Coca was extended to five per cent. Acosta wrote that in his time the Coca trade at Potosi was worth five hundred thousand dollars annually, and that in 1583 the Indians consumed one hundred thousand *cestas* of Coca, worth two and a half dollars each at Cuzco, and four dollars at Potosi. Borja y Arragon, who, by his marriage, became Prince of Esquilache, reports that in 1746 the excise of 5 per cent. imposed upon Coca yielded eight hundred dollars from Caravaya alone, while between 1785 and 1795 this Coca tariff yielded a revenue to the Peruvian vice-royalty of $2,641,487. This oppressive tax occasioned an insurrection in Quito, which was put down and the excise rigidly enforced.

The following table will give an idea of the prices which Coca leaves have brought at varying periods in different localities:[15]

Date	*Locality.*	*Authority.*	*Amount.*	*Price in Piasters.* *
1583	Cuzco..............	Acosta	Arroba (25 pounds)	2½—3
1583	Potosi................	Acosta	Arroba (25 pounds)	4½—5
1583	Potosi................	Unanue	Arroba (25 pounds)	5
1794	Vice-royalty of Buenos Ayres...............	Unanue	Arroba (25 pounds)	6
1794	Plateau of the Andes..	Unanue	Arroba (25 pounds)	3—4
1794	Mines	Unanue	Arroba (25 pounds)	7—8—9
1831	Chinchao.............	Poeppig	Arroba (25 pounds)	3½—4
1831	Huanuco..............	Poeppig	Arroba (25 pounds)	4—7
1831	Cerro de Pasco........	Poeppig	Arroba (25 pounds)	Very high
1832	La Paz...............	d'Orbigny	Arroba (25 pounds)	6
1850	Caravaya.............	Bolognesi	Arroba (25 pounds)	3½—4
1851	La Paz...............	Weddell	Cesta (24 pounds)	4½—6
1857	Salta, Argentine Confederation..........	Mantegazza	25 pounds	4½—6
1858	Santa Anna...........	Grandidier	Arroba	9
1859	La Paz...............	Scherzer	Cesta (25 pounds)	8—10
1860	Arequipa.............	Bolognesi	Arroba	4½—5
1888	Ports of Peru.........	....	Pound	16 cents
1900	Ports of Peru.........	....	Pound	24 cents

It is remarkable that during a period of several hundred years the price of Coca has remained at so uniform a rate.

During the vice-royalty of Chinchon, in 1628, the febrifuge virtue of the cinchona tree was made known through an Indian descendant of the Incas of Uritusinga, near Loxa in Quito, having given some of the fever-curing bark to a Jesuit missionary, who sent it to Dr. Diego de Torres Vasquez, by means of which he was enabled to cure the wife of the viceroy, who was ill with *tertiana*.[16] It is presumed that the Incas were long acquainted with the medicinal virtues of this bark, which, like all of their remedial measures, they kept secret.

[15] Compiled from Gosse; 1861.

* The Piaster is the Spanish silver dollar, equal to the Spanish-American golden pesos, equivalent to about 97 cents of United States money.

[16] Mr. Markham, who made a special study of the cinchona-bearing trees, has written a little work advocating the spelling of the word chinchona in conformity with its derivation.

From the speedy cure which was effected, the remedy was honored with the title "Countess' Bark," and subsequently because of being introduced into Europe in powdered form by the Jesuits of Peru it was known as "Jesuits' Powder." Linnæus gave the name of cinchona to the genus of plants which produces it, in memory of the viceroy. The bark derived from the forests near Loxa, in the ancient province of Quito, was for many years the only kind known to commerce, being exported from the port of Payta and known as Crown Bark. But various species of this precious tree are found throughout the Eastern cordillera of the Andes for a distance of two thousand miles, along the same curve where Coca is grown, though unlike Coca, it is not cultivated but is found in its native home deep in those forests and glens which are situated at an altitude of from 1,000 to 2,000 metres (3,280 to 6,560 feet). The *cascarilleros,* as the collectors are known, undergo great hardships in gathering it. They are usually half civilized Indians, and often they are cheated out of their just claims, the price of the bark being regulated by law. The forests where cinchona is gathered are extremely unhealthful; the temperature, usually about 70° F., does not vary two degrees during the day, while at night, when there are usually rains, it falls perhaps eight degrees. The cinchona tree grows slowly, it requiring a man's lifetime for it to reach perfection, while often carelessness in gathering destroys the trees, which are forever lost. The Indians who gather the bark get sick from exposure in the malarial regions into which they must penetrate, and the *cascarillero* looks to his Coca as a more ready means of sustenance and relief than is the recognized specific which he is engaged in collecting, for the Indians regard Coca as a remedy against malaria superior to quinine.[17]

After the establishment of the Bourbon kings in Spain a brisk trade, which had before then been held as a monopoly, was opened with American commerce, to which all of Europe was invited to contribute. Merchantmen were fitted out, and a flota of some fifteen vessels annually sailed from Cadiz, stopping at Vera Cruz and Havana, where the merchandise was

[17] Markham; p. 53, *et seq.;* 1880.

discharged and the vessels were loaded with the riches of the New World, which had come by way of Porto Bello from Peru. The immense wealth of the cargoes carried by the galleons below the Isthmus attracted the set of buccaneers who cruised off the Peruvian coast to prey upon this traffic, occasioning constant alarm. But as even evil may have a portion of good, so these pirates awakened considerable interest among the literary workers of that time; while remedial measures were enriched by at least one compound attributed to Clipperton's captain of marines, who is said to have first made the since famous Dover's powder. Then there was Rogers, who found Alexander Selkirk—the hero for "Robinson Crusoe," on the island of Juan Fernandez, where he had been left four years before by Stradling; and, finally, Shelboche, on whose vessel the incident of shooting a black albatross, a bird of

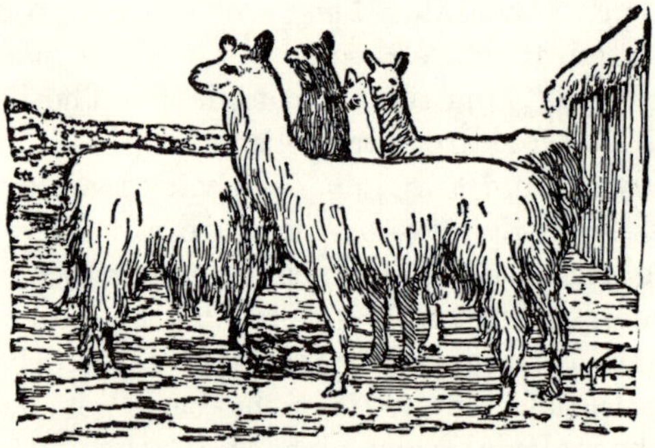

GROUP OF LLAMAS. [*From a Photograph.*]

superstitious reverence to seamen, is said to have suggested to Coleridge *"The Rime of the Ancient Mariner:"*

> "And I had done a hellish thing,
> And it would work 'em woe,
> For all averred I had killed the bird
> That made the breeze to blow."
>
> —*Coleridge;* XXIII.

The Spanish oppression in Peru, as has been seen, was

cruelly severe; the once happy and peaceful Incas were forever destroyed. The progress and advanced socialism of these early people was engulfed in an onward rush of what was supposedly a higher civilization. It is suggestive of the old fable of the boys and the frogs, for while it was a good thing for Spain, it was death to the Incans. It is even questionable whether the Spanish Conquest was advantageous to Peru,[18] though as a slight compensation in exchange for her riches—for plants and products of inestimable value, she has received from Spain the domestic animals, wheat, the vine, sugar cane, the olive, the date and many fruits. If Spain did not feel she had done an injustice, at least there were some among the conquerors who viewed matters in that light. When Marcio Sera de Lajesema, who was the last of Pizarro's original party, died he left a will which expressed this sentiment as his personal view of the Spanish invasion. This portion of the will, which was admitted to probate at Cuzco, November 15, 1589, reads: "First, before beginning my will, I declare that I have desired much to give notice to His Catholic Majesty, King Philip, our lord, seeing how good a Catholic and Christian he is, and how zealous in the service of the Lord our God, concerning that which I would relieve my mind of, by reason of having taken part in the discovery and conquest of these countries, which we took from the lords Yncas, and placed under the Royal Crown, a fact which is known to His Catholic Majesty. The said Yncas governed in such a way that in all the land neither a thief, nor vicious man, nor a bad, dishonest woman was known. The men all had honest and profitable employment. The lands and mines, and all kinds of property were so divided that each man knew what belonged to him, and there were no lawsuits. The Yncas were feared, obeyed and respected by their subjects, as a race very capable of governing, but we took away their land, and placed it under the Crown of Spain, and made them subjects. Your Majesty must understand that my reason for making this statement is to relieve my conscience, for we have destroyed this people by our bad examples. Crimes were once so little known among them that an Indian

[18] Reclus; 1886.

with a hundred thousand pieces of gold and silver in his house left it open, only placing a little stick across the door, as a sign that the master was out, and nobody went in. But when they saw that we placed locks and keys upon our doors, they understood that it was from fear of thieves; and when they saw that we had thieves amongst us, they despised us. All this I tell your Majesty to discharge my conscience of a weight, that I may no longer be a party to these things. And I pray God to pardon me, for I am the last to die of all the discoverers and conquerors, as it is notorious that there are none left but me, in this land or out of it, and therefore I now do what I can to relieve my conscience."[19]

[19] *Calancha*, lib. i, cap. 15, p. 98, quoted in Markham; *preface to Cieza*.

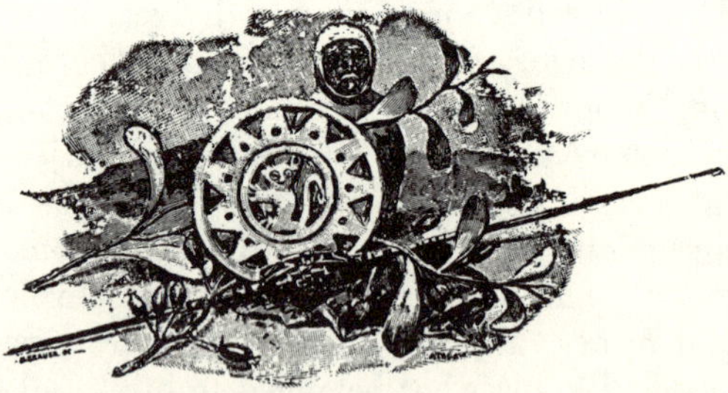

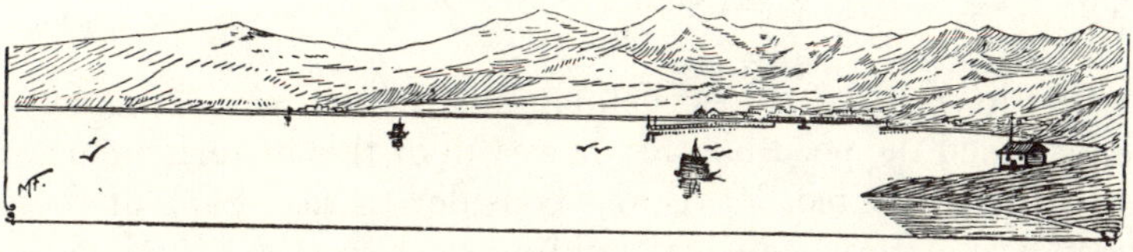

CHAPTER V.

THE PHYSICAL ASPECT OF PERU.

"The dreadful *Andes* plac'd 'twixt Winter's Store
Of Winds, Rains, Snow, and that more humble Earth,
That gives the small, but valiant, *Coca* birth."

—*Cowley.*

MANY miles and many conditions intervene between the gathering of Coca from the cocals of the montaña on the eastern slope of the Andes until its ultimate consumption by the millions of people throughout the world, who now find in it solace and power.

The physical aspect of the mighty Andes must still be much as when our first knowledge of them begun, for though time changes even these sturdy mountains their stupendousness remains, while conditions for transportation and for subsistence seem by comparison more severe. Fully as wonderful then as the associations of Coca with the arts and customs of the Incas, are the prodigious heights and sublime trials to which those who work, who gather and who transport the little leaf are subjected. Care in cultivation, the importance and perplexities of harvesting, and the problem of the final preparation for shipment, are as nothing when compared with the long, toilsome and even dangerous journey through which Coca must be conveyed to the coast.

We may perhaps better appreciate this in a review of some of the topographical difficulties which this marvelous leaf has to pass in transit; and as such landmarks and features as have determined the peculiarities or wealth of this historic home of Coca are presented, let us also consider these. Each of these factors is of importance as tending to shape the habits of the people we are studying, and may prove interesting, if not wholly essential, for a proper appreciation of the dependence placed by them on Coca as the means of surmounting every difficulty. In doing this we may best trace the path of travel from the ocean which washes the shore of this golden land, across those perilous and barren rocky steeps and lofty fertile plains, to the luxuriant fields beyond of perpetual verdure, where Coca is ever growing, ever blooming into one continuous harvest of pent-up endurance.[1]

From Panama to the equator the coast is green, but the Peruvian shores are as desolate and barren a view as ever human eyes, which have anxiously looked for land, beheld. The entire aspect of the rugged Andes, which skirt the shore of South America from the southern extremity to the Caribbean Sea, is not only absolutely uninviting, but seems to present a veritable barrier to further advance, even by land. Along a dreary stretch of reddish-yellow sand Peru has but the single harbor—of Chimbote. In places the waters are filled with angry rocks, as though so many extended roots had been thrown out from the great mountains to bind them more securely to their base, or to assert dominion even in the ocean. Here has evidently been the home of the sea fowl—pelicans and cormorants, since this New World began; they are in countless numbers everywhere, on the rocks and about the desert islands off the shore. As a result of their abiding place here through many centuries, the excrement of these birds, mixed with decomposing carcasses and eggs, has formed an accumulation to the depth, in some localities, of nearly a hundred feet, which is known as *huanu,* or guano.[2] So extensive was the accumulation of this vari-colored deposit on some of the adjacent islands that it formed lofty hills, which, being

[1] There are at least three and commonly four harvests a year, so that it is almost continuous.

[2] *Huanu* is the Quichua term, which has been converted by the Spanish into the present form. The Quichua language has no *g*, and the common terminal *u* has usually been changed to *o;* Tschudi; p. 239; 1847.

topped with a white incrustation of urates, led the Spanish invaders to name them the *Sierra Nevada,* or "Snowy Mountains."[3]

Although this source of wealth at the very portals of Peru is now greatly diminished, for a number of years it has brought an annual return to the State of nearly $15,000,000, an income sufficient to have awakened more than a neighborly interest, which finally culminated in war with Chile, well described by Mr. Clements R. Markham, a voluminous writer on Peruvian customs, to whom we are indebted for many facts.[4] An anecdote is current in Peru which emphasizes the displeasure of the Chileans at this author's account of that war, his description of which they consider rather favored the Peruvians. It is said they do not so much object to his having written they made a cruel war, in which they killed—murdered—thousands of innocent people, but to say they had stolen the Peruvians' guano, "that is too much! and makes them mad." So the name of Markham is not recalled in Chile with friendly emotions.

There has been considerable speculation as to the derivation of the name Andes. Prescott supposed the word to be a corruption of the Quichua word *Anta,* copper, while Garcilasso suggested *Anti,* from the province east of Cuzco. Others again have assumed that the title was derived from the Spanish term *anden,* the lower steps of the mountain terraces, *andenes*—or *andeneria,* where Coca is cultivated. But these are all merely fanciful suppositions, and the real derivation must be considered, as Humboldt has said: "lost in the obscurity of the past." This is a land of prodigious distances, extreme heights and gigantic proportions, so it may not seem remarkable to speak of the Andes as extending through Peru for a thousand miles, nor to allude to towering elevations for thousands of feet. The Andes are commonly described as in two ranges, but this arrangement depends wholly upon the locality. In northern Peru above the latitude of Lima there

[3] Prescott; Vol. I; p. 138; 1848.

[4] War was declared by Chile April 5, 1879, a declaration which this author said was caused "because the Peruvian ships stood no chance with the new ironclads of Chile"; Markham; p. 386; 1892.

are V-shaped projections from the cordillera which form shorter ranges, while in southern Peru a bird's-eye view of the country appears like a succession of petrified whirlpools. Spurs and knots abound in every direction, so that the whole lower country is a succession of mountains and basins and valleys. The western cordillera, sometimes termed the "maritime" or the *cordillera de la costa*—runs parallel with the coast, while separated from that by erosion is the central chain; and still further east is the *cordillera real,* which is commonly described as the Andes proper. The eastern range is broken in the north into several V-shaped formations, between which lie the forests of the northern montaña, while east of the entire range extends the low flat stretch of the Amazonian valley for thousands of miles to the Atlantic. The coast chain is a bleak, untimbered range of barren rocks, above which is a belt of some hundred miles broad, cold and desolate, known as the *puna,* across which the traveller is glad to hasten. It is to this varied configuration of mountain that Peru owes its marvels of climate.

Separated from the ocean by a narrow strip of land, the bluff fronts of the Andes rise like a mighty wall, the stupendous grandeur of which can only be partially judged by a distant view from a vessel as she lies far off.[5] At places the mountains run directly down to the water, while at others the coast varies, having an average width of twenty miles; the whole a sandy desert, or, rather, a succession of deserts, with here and there a spot capable of cultivation, if the conditions were favorable. Between these desert places, often separated by many miles, there are fertile valleys which have been reclaimed by irrigation, or which are watered by some scanty mountain stream coursing through one of the *quebra-*

[5] Hall, 1825, says at 130 miles the mountains seemed quite close.

DESCRIPTION OF SCENES IN THE ANDES ON OPPOSITE PAGE.

Near the base of the mountains may be seen the narrow mule path which winds around the hills.

1. Grove of Algarroba trees. 2. Typical scene amidst the low hills near the coast; Department of Piura. 3. Devil's Bridge, on line of Oroya Railroad. 4. Quebrada of Challape, altitude 7,507 feet, Oroya Railroad. 5. A native hut in desert near the coast. 6. Quebrada of Chicla, altitude 12,220 feet, eighty miles from Lima. 7. A Quebrada of the coast; a typical irrigation stream.

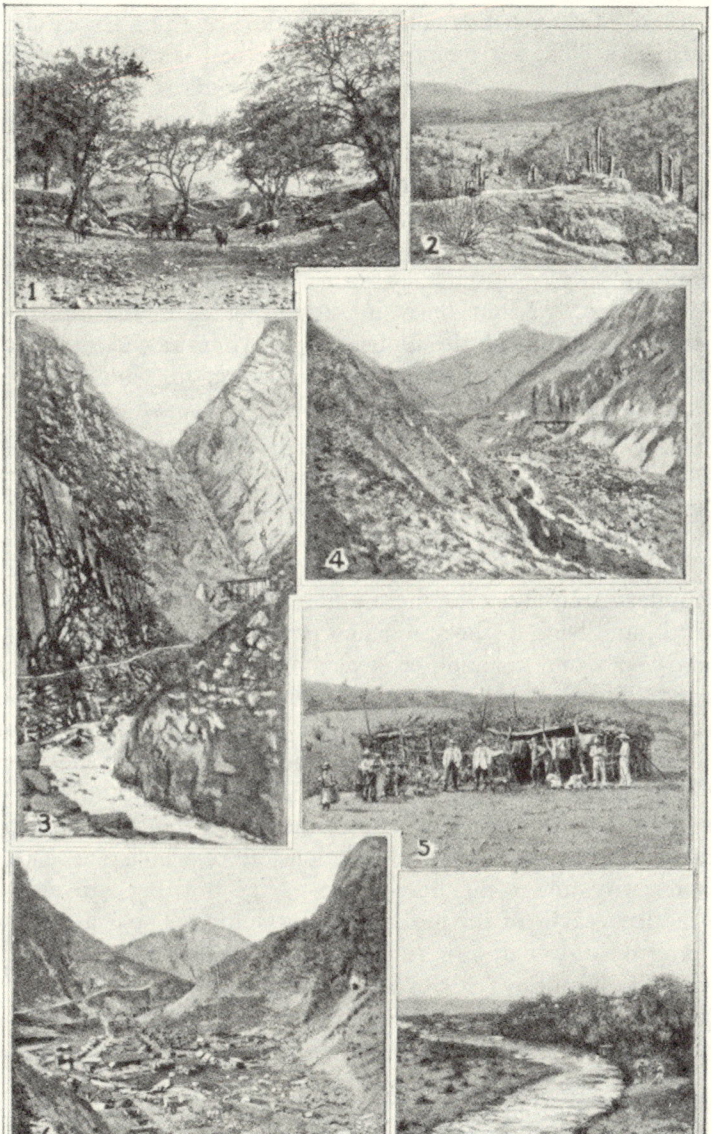

SCENES IN THE ANDES. [*From Photographs.*]
For description see opposite page.

das,[6] or gulches, which convey the waters of the western slope to the sea. The extreme fertility of the soil is shown in every favored location promptly following any effort at irrigation, when the line of demarkation—as we might say in surgery—is sharply defined against the barrenness beside it, which, from a distance, appears as though some monster green patches had been cut out by gigantic shears and set down here and there against the yellowish-red background. It never rains along this entire stretch, or so rarely that it is presumably always dry. About once in seven years, owing to some peculiar position of the globe at such times, some rain may fall. The early Peruvians used to consider this condition had originated through a quarrel between Pachacama and Con, those traditional brothers of the sun, who first possessed the coast land. Con, the thunder god, having been overpowered in the dispute, fled to the north, and in irritation at his defeat took the rain with him, leaving the arid desert behind.[7] Whether because of this quarrel or not, it never rains nor thunders from Ecuador in the north to the River Loa in the south, and back to the sun-baked outposts of the Andes, from one year's end to another, except on the phenomenal occasions alluded to, when the wild torrential rain of the tropics pours down.[8] Then, as though to be an index to the possibilities of this region, when prompted by appropriate encouragement following a septennial drought, the parched desert is transformed by Nature's magic touch into a luxuriant garden of grasses, flowers and melons, all of which as speedily melt away under the fierce rays of the broiling sun as did Aladdin's castle at the bidding of the Genie. The grasses now changed into what might be termed a natural hay, remain with the beanlike fruit of the *algarroba* trees growing in the *quebradas,* the sole pasturage for the great herds of goats, cattle and horses of the coast. But fodder is not plenty, and the best hay must be brought from Valparaiso and San Francisco, for, as a lady in emphasizing this point to me declared, "Hay is hay in Peru."

[6] These *quebradas* correspond to the deep ravines termed cañons in Colorado.
[7] Brinton; 1868. [8] At the time of this writing more than ten years had elapsed without rain on the Peruvian coast.

Nature manifests a constant activity here in all her belongings, and rumblings and quakings of the earth are of frequent occurrence, running parallel with the sea, and upon occasions too frequent a great deal of damage has been done from such disturbances. Several such attacks of unusual violence have almost destroyed the ancient capital city of Lima, once in 1586, and again in 1630, and another in 1687, but the most terrific shaking up was in October, 1746, when over five thousand people were killed, and an immense wave carried the frigate "San Fermin," which was lying off the coast, inland, and left her high and dry, as was stranded the ark of old, far above the waters. This experience was repeated more than a hundred years later, when the United States man-of-war "Waterlee" and other vessels were carried two miles inland by a tidal wave at Arica, while the city of Arequipa was destroyed by an eruption of Misti in August, 1868.

Even the winds manifest peculiarities in this land of many wonders, and persistently blow always from the south, from the sea by day and from the shore at night, carrying the light sand of the coast into great crescent-shaped shifting hillocks twenty or thirty feet high, which are known as *medanos.* This constant drifting obliterates such narrow trails as may have served for roads, and covers up everything that comes in the way. Sometimes in the stillness of the night the winds play quaint music on these sandhills, which sounds very weird, and whispers strange things to the belated traveller. In some cases whole villages have been covered over with this ever-changing sand, and so the inhabitants were literally compelled to build their homes elsewhere.

We have seen how in the time of the Incas many parts of this barren strip of coast were reclaimed by their immense system of irrigation, which carried water through canals over great distances. Some of these old aqueducts are still used to water the *haciendas,* or large plantations of the coast valleys, many of which owe their existence wholly to this possibility. Particularly is this so in the Nasca Valley, in the Province of Ica, a naturally unpropitious spot in the very heart of a desert, with forty miles of arid sand on one side and a hundred miles of barrenness upon the other, yet the stimulus of irrigation has made this a prolific centre where cotton, grapes and numerous fruits are grown in perfection. In some cases these old conduits, long since neglected, show their route by the rank vegetation which has sprung up in their course. In others, where the supply is dried up, the beds serve as roads, and often form the only available path for travel up the mountains.

Whether Con, through pique, was partly responsible or not for the total absence of rain along the coast, the physical cause from the combined action of trade winds and lofty snow-capped mountains may seem a more scientific interpretation to

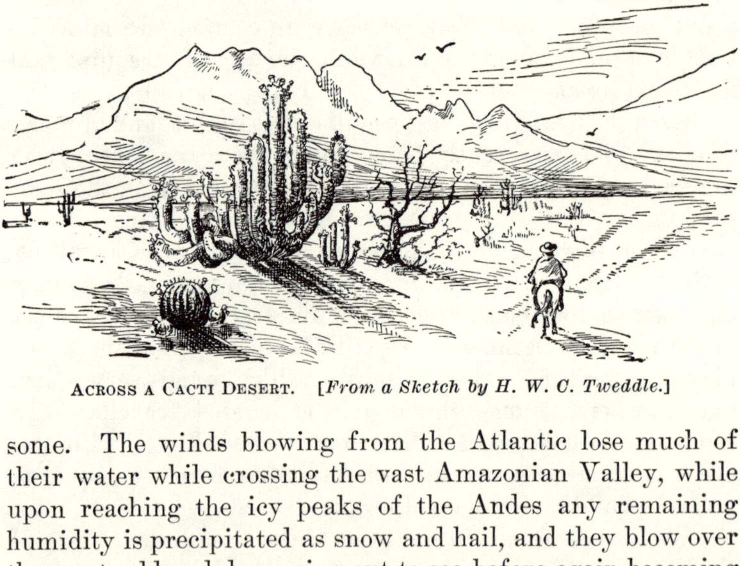

ACROSS A CACTI DESERT. [*From a Sketch by H. W. C. Tweddle.*]

some. The winds blowing from the Atlantic lose much of their water while crossing the vast Amazonian Valley, while upon reaching the icy peaks of the Andes any remaining humidity is precipitated as snow and hail, and they blow over the coast cold and dry, going out to sea before again becoming charged with moisture. To replace this absence of rain there is from June to December either a drizzle termed *garua,* or a cloudy mist known as *neblina,* as a result of which, combined with the scorching sun, malarial fever—*tertiana* as it is here termed—is very prevalent, though it is not at all known in the mountains.

Although we must consider Peru as a country of infinite

phenomena, its most remarkable feature is its climate, for it presents every variety on the globe from the Equator to the Polar regions. Here one may have a choice, from the blazing suns of the desert, through the bleak and cheerless *puna* to the delightful equable climate of the Sierra; from the heat and humidity of the tropical home of Coca to the perpetual spring of the table lands; from everlasting winter upon the mountain tops to never-ending summer in the higher valleys. These changes vary with the elevation, and are not materially affected with the seasons, but remain in each locality nearly the same throughout the year, each gradation being happily displayed by Nature in the vegetation which, through successive altitudes, represents the product of every country on the earth; so that a trip across the Andes to the cocals of the montaña does not necessitate, like some other journeys, a wait upon time, unless deterred by the swelling of mountain streams during the rains. The traveller may pass from one season to the other, through every change of heat and cold, from temperate vegetation to tropical luxuriance; from wintry storms to sunshine. Particularly in descending the Eastern slope is this transition noticeable, when one may sit down to cool off from the exertion and excessive heat of a summer's day, which a profusion of tropic flowers, gorgeously tinted butterflies and sweetly warbling birds assure as a reality, while the melting snow upon hat and shoulders drips down to recall those wintry blasts which were but shortly left above and behind.

If we commence our journeying, as did Pizarro, from the most northern end of the coast and travel south we may successively review several important industries. About sixty miles north of Payta, in the District of Piura, below the Brea or "Pitch Mountains," there is a tablazo at an elevation of some three hundred feet, which is covered with calcareous sandstone, resting on alternating strata of pudding stone and shale marl on a base of argillaceous shales. Here there bubbles up like spring water a rock oil, which, trickling over the surface, becomes filled with the sand blowing from the desert, and dries into a black tarry-like pitch. This substance is used by the people near by for making the pavement of their roads, and even the floors of the houses, just as asphaltum might be employed. In early times the Spaniards used the cleanly fired pitch as a coating for their wine jars. Some forty years ago trial borings proved that petroleum was present here in very large quantities, and Mr. H. W. C. Tweddle, who was the first refiner of this oil on a commercial basis, interested himself in this locality. It is due to the foresight of this skilled engineer and his keen appreciation of the possibilities here presented that this region has developed what has been termed the second largest field of petroleum for fuel purposes in the world.

Beyond this petroleum district, toward the south, there extends a succession of fertile valleys. Those of the Chira and Piura rivers are connected with the port of Payta by short lines of railroad. Both of these places are noted for their extensive plantations of cotton, an important product which is grown in many of the *haciendas* along the coast as far south as the Nasca Valley. There is a peculiarity about Peruvian cotton which must strike one who is only familiar with its shrub-like growth in our Southern States and who sees it here for the first time, where it grows upon trees ten to fifteen feet high, as in the East. The wool is of every variety of coloration, ranging from white to deep orange brown, and through various shades of violet. This coloring, which is presumably due to the action of some insect, affects about one plant in fifty. The Yuncas, who early inhabited the coast, considered such colored cotton sacred, and used it as a wrapping for the heads of their mummies.[9] Other important coast crops are sugar and grapes. At Pisco and Yca, in the dominion of the ancient Chimu, there are extensive vineyards, and here the native "Italia" and "Pisco" brandy is made, a rather crude distillation of grape alcohol, pure white and tasting like dilute spirits. It is put up in conical earthen jars with narrow necks, each containing about three gallons, a *pisquito,* as the jar is termed, costing about eight dollars at the vineyard. The ancient valley of Santa is rich

[9] The Egyptians also reserved their colored cotton for certain rites.

in animal and mineral productions, and with a vast buried store of treasure in pottery.

In all of the larger *haciendas,* vegetables of all kinds are raised, together with the various fruits, both indigenous as well as the adopted varieties, each of which grows best only in some certain locality. It is estimated that during the time of the Incas the population of the Chira and the Piura valleys was nearly two hundred thousand, which has diminished, as shown by a recent census to be but little over seventy-five thousand. The Incans, wherever located, were a thrifty race, expert in agriculture, and we owe to them the improvement and cultivation of many serviceable products, perhaps the two extremes of utility being shown in the domestication of the potato, which has required hundreds of years to develop from

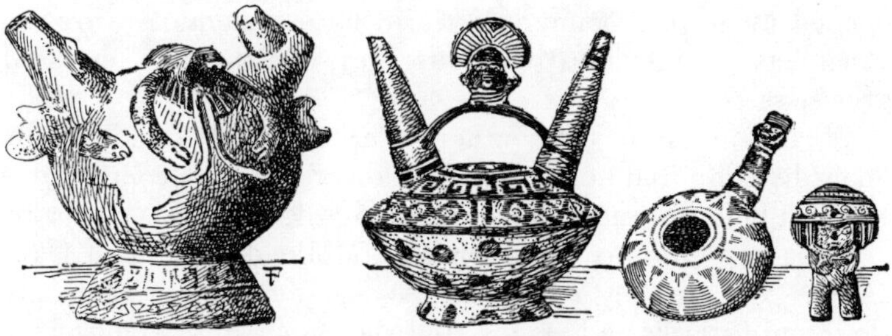

Peruvian Vases and a Doll. [*Tweddle Collection.*]
Showing Similarity in Decoration to the Grecian and Assyrian Ornamentation.

its wild state, and Coca, originally of natural selection, which has been preserved through so many centuries to its final adaptability to present usefulness.

At a short distance back from the coast are low hills known as *lomas,* which from June until December are covered with vegetation and wild flowers. Here in the early days of prosperity—"before the war," as the Peruvians are wont to say—there was a constant scene of jollity, when these places were made the camping ground of many happy families from the neighboring plantations. There are many thermal springs throughout Peru, some ferruginous, some sulphurous, which are administered as remedies in dysentery, rheumatism and cutaneous diseases. At Piura, where the air is exceedingly dry, and as a native describes it, "as hot as the infernal regions could be," the springs have considerable local repute in the treatment of syphilis. They are commonly conducted by old women, who administer mud baths and recommend a sort of sweating-out process, after the manner of the Hot Springs of Arkansas.

A very important source of Peruvian wealth has long been the immense deposits of nitrates, which some few years ago yielded an income of upwards of $17,000,000. The principal territory where this is deposited is at Tarapaca, now held by Chile, the ravines of which it is said contain a supply sufficient to last more than a thousand years. But with her newer petroleum industry, and the development of those innumerable natural resources of her land, which are only about being opened up to the commercial world by a system of railroads, Peru has an inexhaustible source of wealth and means of greatness.

From Callao to the southern Peruvian port of Mollendo, about five hundred miles, is a three days' trip in a comfortable English-built steamer. The surf along the coast is very heavy, and sea captains say the harbor of Mollendo begins at Cape Horn. On still days the water looks smooth, but there are threatening rocks and rapids, and the vessel sinks eight or ten feet between the long swells. The ships are always unloaded off shore by lighters, and when the weather is bad many days often pass before a landing can be made. Mollendo, situated on a rocky bluff, is a small coast town of bamboo and adobe huts, made somewhat modern in appearance through being the railroad terminus from the eastern montaña as well as the port of Arequipa, and principal shipping point for Coca, wool, minerals and other products of export from southern Peru. Here as we come into the volcanic region there is an immense desert covered with a dirty white dust which the natives say has been thrown out from the mighty mountain in some eruption.

From Mollendo the Southern Railroad of Peru, which is one of the marvels in engineering of the world, extends to

Juliaca, from where a branch road connects south to Puno on Lake Titicaca, and another running north is planned to be continued to Cuzco. The cars, which are English built, are divided into first and second class. Starting from Mollendo in the morning at eleven, a run is made for a hundred miles through a waterless desert, so barren not even the cactus will grow, to Arequipa,[10] at an altitude of seven thousand five hundred and fifty feet. Along this route, which ascends two hundred and twelve feet in a mile, one may look down for two thousand feet into the fertile valley of Tambo, where sugar cane is extensively grown, from which much of the Peruvian fire water is manufactured. There is a gradual rise by an intricate succession of switchbacks and curves to the tableland of La Joya, from where a fine view may be obtained of

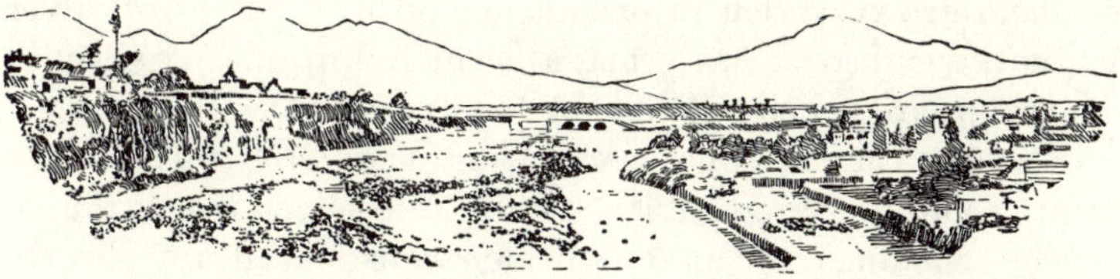

AREQUIPA FROM THE CHILE RIVER. [*From a Photograph.*]

the ancient city of Arequipa, which is reached about seven o'clock in the evening, and a stop is made to enable the traveller to secure a comfortable night's rest in a good modern hotel, which bears the conventional name of "Grand Central." The Peruvian railroads follow strictly the custom of the country, and do everything in a leisurely way, so they only travel by daylight, not necessarily because of any particular difficulty in the route, for the roads are all well equipped and have been efficiently constructed at great expense.

At Arequipa the traveller usually spends a few days to become accustomed to the change before proceeding to higher altitudes. This is the second largest city of Peru, and is the distributing centre for the whole southern country. It is

[10] Arequipa, from the Quichua *Ariquepai*, "Yes, rest here," the name given by the Incans to the station where a rest was made on the journey from Cuzco to the coast.

crowned by the lofty volcano of Misti, which, with a height of over 20,000 feet, looms up imposingly in the background, while Pichu-pichu, 17,800 feet, Charchani, 19,000 feet, and the Pan de Azúcar all seem to keep a stolid guardianship over the city. The Boyden meteorological station of Harvard is situated on the heights of Misti at 19,200 feet, where with an eight-inch Bache telescope some fine astronomical photographs have been made. From Arequipa an iron pipe line carries water to the coast, where nearly 500,000 gallons are delivered in twenty-four hours through the largest pipe aqueduct in the world. The streets of this old city are narrow, and the houses are picturesquely built of white volcanic stone, and the latticed balconies and covered façades, with everywhere the Spanish arms, serve to carry one into the quaint antiquity of long ago. The churches are numerous, and some of them are very rich in ornament and have altars of silver, while the cathedral has a magnificent pulpit of carved cedar. The shops are principally conducted by Germans, though there are many English and Americans who are interested in mining and other industries. The Chile River is a turbulent stream, spanned by an old bridge constructed by Pizarro. Along its banks are the remains of the once beautiful *alamedas*—promenades—while the former palaces which bordered it are now drinking places, where *chicha* is dispensed to a thirsty populace.

Continuing the journey east, a start is made from Arequipa in the morning, and the run to Juliaca occupies a day of hard climbing, the road circling about Misti for hours until the *Pampa de Arrieros* is reached at an elevation of twelve thousand feet, where a stop is made for breakfast. The first chain of the Andes is crossed at Alto Crucero, at an elevation of about fifteen thousand feet, and a descent is made to a great plateau, here the road winds about two small lakes—Saracocha and Cachipascana—about which are many terraces which reach to the tops of the mountains.

Juliaca—the eastern terminal of the southern road—facetiously termed the Chicago of Peru—is one hundred and eighty-nine miles from Arequipa. It is the stopping place for miners, and the junction for the road north to Sicuani, where there is a coach line to Cuzco, some two and a half or three days' journey. During early Spanish times this locality was a mining centre, and the neighboring hills are honeycombed with the ruins of abandoned mines. From Juliaca the line runs south to Puno, on Lake Titicaca, where may be found a comfortable modern iron steamboat, which affords accommodation for fifty first-class passengers. It took many years to construct this boat, which was built in Europe, and after being landed at Mollendo in pieces it was carried over the mountains on the backs of mules. Some of the pieces of machinery were lost, and it required considerable time to replace them, so that ten years was consumed before the boat was finally set up and running. But so extensive has been the traffic for this improved transportation that this steamer can earn a handsome profit while burning coal brought all the way from Australia at an ultimate cost of forty-four dollars a ton in Peruvian money. Anthracite and bituminous coal are both found in the mountains in abundance, but there is not only the difficulty of mining it, but the added problem of transportation.

Beyond Juliaca to the north the railroad is left at Pocara, which was the favorite resting place of the last Inca in his journey between the Titicaca region and Cuzco. Here mules which have been engaged in advance are in waiting with their *arrieros,* and arrangements are perfected for the long ride over the mountains to the montaña. From Pocara the first stop of the mule train is made at Azangaro. The houses here have thatched roofs, and are built of adobe. All the booths in the plaza sell alcohol and the various knick-knacks admired by the Indians. The women wherever they are met are industriously engaged in spinning, no matter what their other occupation may be, and the result of this diligence is displayed in balls of cotton which are hung in the houses. Cotton cloth is commonly used here in traffic, a yard of it being equivalent to the hire of a laborer for a day, equal to about thirty cents of Bolivian money. From Azangaro the second day's journey on mule back continues through a low valley of fair pasture land. The soil is of a red sandstone, in places very silicious, at others soft and friable, while the surrounding hills are of granite with large quartz boulders. The *hacienda* of Oggra is shortly reached, which belongs to a convent, and ignoring the good old hymn of Dr. Watts, is curiously enough noted for the raising of good fighting bulls. After a six hours' ride a stop is made at the *hacienda* Huancasayana, a ranch with some four thousand cattle and twelve thousand sheep, where *chalona,* or dried mutton, is extensively prepared. The sheep are killed, skinned and cleaned, and the carcasses split open and slashed so that the blood may drain off. About two pounds of salt is rubbed into each carcass, and these are then exposed to the frost and sun for twenty days, by which time they will have lost some two-thirds of their former weight, and are dried hard and stiff, and will keep for a long time in this rarefied atmosphere. Here at an altitude of 13,500 feet a stop may be made at the end of the day, where an adobe hut of but a single room affords gratuitous shelter to travellers.

From here an early start is made in the morning; the atmosphere is cold at this high altitude, and the ponds are covered with a thin crust of ice which the rising sun melts. Following the long narrow valley, many mountain streams are crossed, and the vegetation gradually changes from long grass to a shorter kind, while a sort of woolly lichen grows which is said to be good for cattle. A steep ascent is soon made to fifteen thousand four hundred and fifty feet, and though the air seems exhilarating, one cannot walk far without getting out of breath in consequence of the rarefied atmosphere. An occasional vicuña is to be seen here, but they are very shy, and it is difficult to shoot them. The rocks about are stratified layers of granite. Six and a half hours' ride brings the traveller to Picotani, where there is a farm of some twenty leagues in circumference, capable of supporting seventy thousand sheep. It never rains in this locality, for the air is so cold that the moisture is precipitated as snow. The rarefied air makes one feel the cold even more than the low temperature, while aside from the great loss of latent heat there is no fire to warm up by. Butter of fine quality is made in this region.

From Picotani the trail is through a rolling grass country, from where a splendid view may be had of the snow-clad tops of the Vilcañota range. Travelling parallel with these mountains and going due east, Rinconado, a small deep lake of rough water at the foot of Ananea, may be seen. At its southern end this lake is twelve hundred yards wide, narrowing at the north to four hundred yards. Here are peat bogs and a lot of ice-cold springs, while at the top of the hill is an old Spanish mountain town with a quartz mine at an altitude of over seventeen thousand feet, but too far above the line of

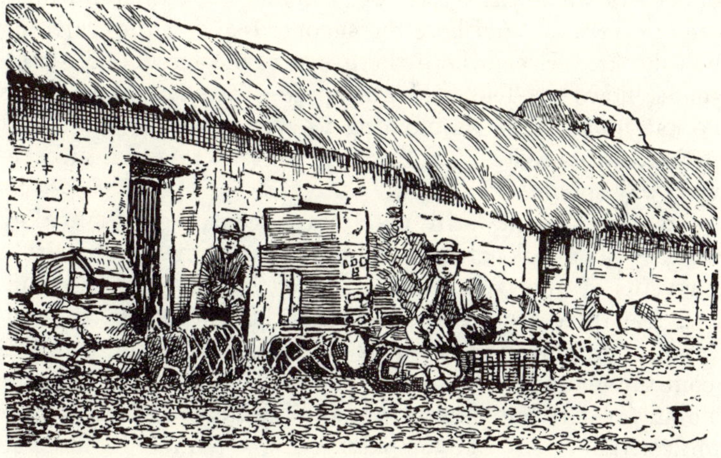

POST HOUSE AT AZANGARO. ALTITUDE 13,500 FEET. [*From a Photograph.*]

perpetual snow to prove attractive for work. A stop is made at Poto, near by, where there is a plant for gold-washing. Leaving here in the morning and riding to the northwest, the crest of the Andes, at about sixteen thousand feet, is crossed, and the abrupt descent into the montaña begins. Down between dark snow-clad hills, in beating rain to Tambillo, the descent continues through a mountain path of slate forming a sort of stairway. The scenery is now of the grandest nature. The mountains rise precipitately on either side for thousands of feet, and here and there are topped with snowy patches. A little stream which above was known as the Lata now changes its name to the River Sandia, and dashes on over a solid bed of slate, which is often stained black by organic matter. To look up against the face of the mountain it appears like a dead wall, and yet this precipitous place has been gradually circled in the descent, and far back the baggage mules may be seen slowly crawling along and appearing like so many diminutive insects as they wind around the narrow path. As the region of vegetation is reached the hillsides are terraced for grazing wherever available on account of the stony nature of the soil. Some of these terraces are only two or three feet wide. In some cases where there have been immense earth slides these also are terraced, and here the shepherds live while watching their flocks. Everywhere there are vari-colored and sweet-scented flowers. The wild pineapple—*wheenay-wheenay,* as the natives term it—is clinging to every rock, even without earth about its roots. The Indians hang up this plant to conjure away spirits.

As the descent, still precipitate, continues, the valley widens. The rocks are now crystalline and mica slate, with a few veins of quartz in places. At eleven thousand six hundred feet there are a few song birds, but no insects. Cuyu-Cuyu, at an elevation of about seven thousand feet, contains about three hundred houses of adobe and thatch, and here the Indian farmers raise vegetables, and huge cabbages are grown into veritable trees, like the palm, eight or ten feet high. The mountains about this little town are so high that the sun only reaches Cuyu-Cuyu after eight o'clock in the morning, and some parts of the valley are in shadow at a quarter past two in the afternoon. Leaving here the trail descends through a valley surrounded by high hills. At seven thousand feet the first cultivated orange trees are found, though there is not enough soil here for timber. Five leagues further on, the town of Sandia is reached, close to the heart of the Coca region. The Indians met with indicate this, as their hats are bound with sprays of Coca. The scenery here is picturesquely varied; from the surrounding heights there are magnificent cataracts, and for a thousand feet up the mountains there is a multiplicity of trees bearing peaches and other fruits, while myriads of flowering plants fill the air with sweet perfume and form a marked and delightful contrast to the previous bleakness.

Another approach to the montaña is through northern Peru. Starting at Callao, one hundred and thirty-six miles of the journey may be made over the Oroya railroad, which is a succession of switchbacks and tunnels. Beyond the fertile delta of Lima there are vast fields of sugar cane until Chosica is reached, thirty-three and a half miles from Callao, at an altitude of two thousand eight hundred and thirty-two feet. This region is above the fogs of the coast, and is so full of perpetual sunshine as to be regarded as a health resort. In all available places irrigation is carried on, and alfalfa, corn, sugar cane and large quantities of fruit are grown. From here donkeys and llamas compete with the railroad in carrying eggs, provisions, fowls, coffee and Coca to Lima. Further east beyond San Bartolomé the steepest grade of the road begins, rising four feet in a hundred and winding in horse-shoe curves about the barren rocks. At Veruggas, spanning the Rimac, a bridge is crossed which is three hundred feet high. The name is derived from a peculiar disorder occurring in this locality, caused, as the Indians believe, from drinking the *agua de Verugga* from certain springs. The symptoms are first manifest by a sore throat and general aching, accompanied by an elevation of temperature. Within a few days an eruption of pimples appears, soon becoming bloody warts, which exhausts the strength of the patient. The workmen who built this bridge died by thousands from this disease.

The Oroya railroad is unique in its consumption of petroleum as fuel, which was made practical in 1890 through the ingenuity of Mr. Herbert Tweedle, and has resulted in a saving of seventy-five per cent. Along this line in every available place are the remains of Incan terraces built upon the barren rocks, for it is all rock here, and even the road bed is of this same substantial nature. Far down in the valley may be seen a muddy little stream which is the Rimac, while here and there are small patches of pasture, with a few Indian huts. For many years the mining town of Chicla was the terminus of this road. Here are large smelting works, and silver is sent in bars to Lima, where it is minted or shipped abroad. Above 14,000 feet the crest of the cordillera is tunneled at Mount Meiggs—named after the American contractor who built the Peruvian railroads—and the descent is made to the terminus at Oroya. From here there are two highways, one a good road for hauling minerals extends to the famous mining town of Cerro de Pasco, where there are hundreds of mines still worked, and on to the Coca region of the northern montaña. The other road extends south through the valley formed by the western cordillera and the Andes proper to Jauja and Cuzco.

In the northern part of Peru, between the cordilleras the tributaries of the Amazon form broad valleys having a tropical luxuriance, which is subdued by the modulation of the great altitude into a temperature of everlasting summer. The Marañon rises in a split of the first chain of the western cordilleras, flowing north and thence through a cleft at Pongo de Manseriche, in which valley commences the northern montaña. From Oroya going east and crossing the Andes proper at about ten thousand to eleven thousand feet, the head waters of the Perené, a branch of the Ucayali, is reached, which in its upper waters is called Chanchamayo.[11] There is an English colony here, where coffee is extensively grown. At Bellavista, at an elevation of one thousand five hundred feet, the Marañon leaves the Andes. From here the river flows on through the great Amazonian plain three thousand miles to the sea, having a fall of about six inches to the mile. The valley of the Marañon is two miles wide, the river varying from a volume of a hundred yards across to a network of channels half a mile in extent. In the rainy season the river rises five or six feet and floods the lowlands. Bellavista consists of a few shabby houses of adobe surrounding the public square, in which is the cathedral and principal shops. The lands here all belong to the municipality, and are worked in community on the old Incan order, being allotted to the people rent free, who in exchange are obliged to give their services to the public good

[11] *Mayo* is Quichua for water.

in repairing roads or buildings, and acting as messengers. Some of the finest chocolate in the world comes from this region, and Coca of fine quality is grown. Wheat bread is too great a luxury for ordinary consumption here, and even the well-to-do use bananas as a substitute; indeed chocolate, bananas and Coca constitute about the only available food. Such fertile places afford an agreeable relief from the barren bleakness of the mountains, in fact to the Andean traveller there is always encouragement to struggle on to the realization of more delightful scenes beyond. In this respect the journey across the Andes, though severe and trying, so far excels the ascent of Ætna, Vesuvius, or the Matterhorn, made merely for the gratification of an idle curiosity, or simply to test the powers of endurance. In one case there is constant ascent into bleak and dreary regions, where one is obliged to sleep with the prospect of being frozen to death or precipitated into some icy crevasse for the mere hope of being enabled to see the early rising sun or to gaze into the depths of some sulphurous crater, while in the other there is the consciousness of bright and ever-blooming fields beyond, of verdant plains and fertile valleys, with a luxuriance of vegetation, which combine to amply repay for the arduous journey.

The grandeur of some of the Andean plains is unequaled elsewhere on the globe. Separating profound ravines filled with a wealth of verdure are lofty ridges, while beyond are long valleys, and surrounding all are snowy peaks backed by a sky of intense blue. In such a plateau and amidst such surroundings and advantages, at an altitude of 12,000 feet, is the beautiful valley of Vilcamayu, running northwest and southeast. Here was the site of foundation of the Incan empire—here is the city of Cuzco—and here were built the palaces of the Incas, and their terraced gardens and impregnable fortresses. In the neighboring hills may be seen vast flocks of sheep and alpacas, cropping the coarse *ychu* grass, while across the stillness comes a faint piping, which directs attention to a long train of llamas, slowly winding over the mountain bearing a cargo of Coca to the city of Cuzco. The air here, though thin, is so pure, soft and exhilarating as to at once suggest that Nature has founded an ideal sanitarium for all the world. This fertile valley extends to the Vilcañota range, a chain connecting the eastern and central cordillera, which abruptly cuts off all verdure, for south to beyond Titicaca is the bleak region known as the *Collao,* where all is

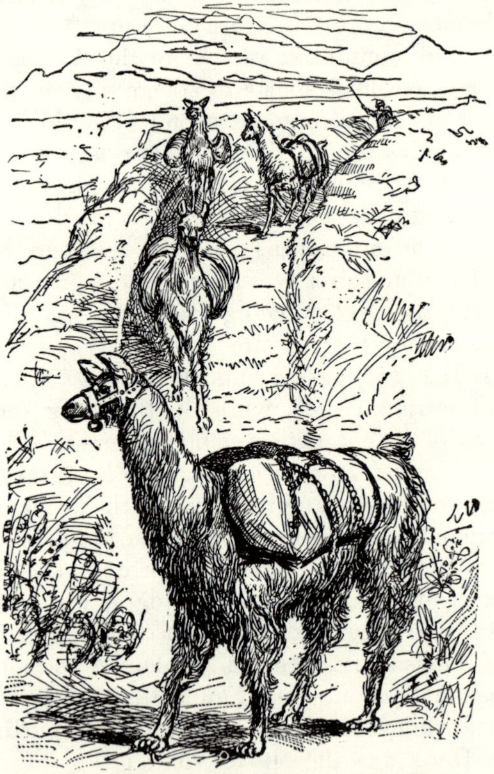

Llamas Carrying Coca. [*From a Photograph.*]
[See page 219.]

barren and desolate, through a section three hundred miles long by one hundred wide, where vegetation is about impossible and only occasional potato crops and scrawly quinoa and molle trees grow. It is always winter here, and the cattle find their scanty sustenance by feeding on the rushes of the lake, which serve many uses, from making ropes, sails and even balsas to supplying fodder. Looking east may be seen the lofty peaks of Illimani and Illampu, among the highest in South America, while amidst these barren surroundings is the historic Lake Titicaca, in the southern limit of the Peruvian Andes.

Lake Titicaca, which is situated in a basin 12,545 feet above the sea, between Peru and Bolivia, is irregular in form and almost cut in two by the Peninsula of Copacabana. It has never been accurately measured, but it is estimated to be upward of a hundred miles in length and about fifty miles broad at its widest part. Near the eastern side its water has a depth of over seven hundred feet, but the western shore slopes more shallow, affording growth for rushes, which make a home for numerous water fowl. Many rivers go to form this body of water, the largest being Ramiz, formed by the Pucara and Azangaro, entering the lake at its northwest border, while the Suchiz, formed by the Cavanilla and Lampa, flow in on the north side, together with the Yllpa and Ylave. On the east are the Huarina, Escoma and Achacache, from a low chain parallel with the Eastern Andes, while the only outlet for this great volume of water is the Desaguadero, a river one hundred and seventy miles long, flowing with great rapidity from the southern end of the lake and emptying into Lake Aullagas or Poopó, beyond which the water is lost in a marshy swamp through which it possibly percolates to some cavernous depths below, and so on out to the Pacific. Lake Titicaca is often described as the most elevated body of water in the New World, but Lake Aricoma, the bed of which is said to be full of gold, and Lake Rinconado, both of which are fed

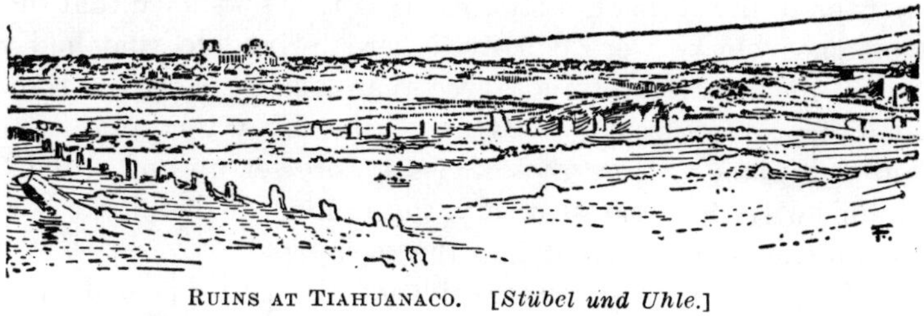

RUINS AT TIAHUANACO. [*Stübel und Uhle.*]

from the glaciers of the neighboring mountains, have their outlets here and are at greater altitudes, only exceeded in height by those lofty lakes of Tibet, situated almost diametrically opposite on the globe.

Some forty miles from the southern end of the lake is a vast field of cyclopean ruins which are only to be reached by mule back over an ancient highway. There is no tradition to link these archæological relics with the present people, or even with the Incas. Here are strewn the remains of two large quadro-lateral buildings, monolithic towers and broken

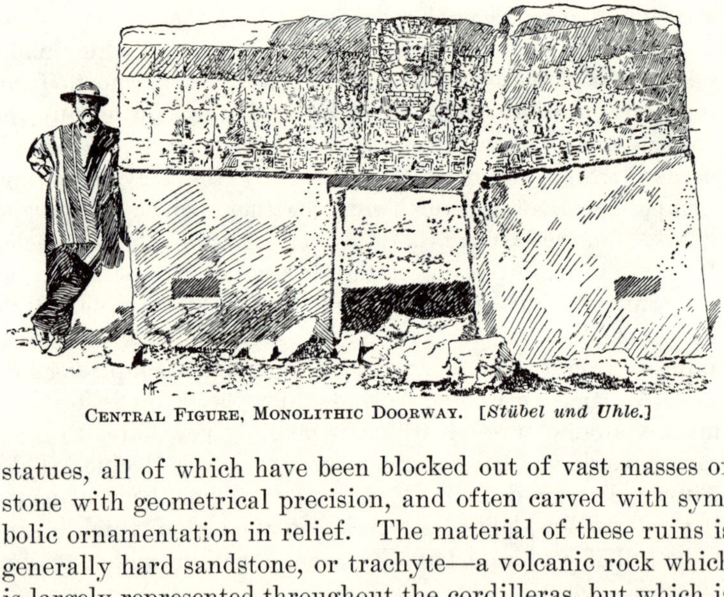

CENTRAL FIGURE, MONOLITHIC DOORWAY. [*Stübel und Uhle.*]

statues, all of which have been blocked out of vast masses of stone with geometrical precision, and often carved with symbolic ornamentation in relief. The material of these ruins is generally hard sandstone, or trachyte—a volcanic rock which is largely represented throughout the cordilleras, but which is not found in this particular locality. It is presumed that these immense blocks were conveyed here by people who had no other means of applying force than main strength, from a distance of at least twenty-five miles by water and fifteen miles by land. Here these masses were set up and fitted together with the greatest nicety, the joining of the blocks being by mortices accurately cut in the rocks.

One of the most remarkable of the ruins is a doorway

carved from a single block seven feet high, thirteen and a half feet long, and about two feet thick. There is a fracture across the lintel, but the fragment, which has settled a little, has not fallen. Above the arch is a frieze sculptured in low relief. In the centre is a figure, the head surrounded by rays representing serpents, while on either side of this there are four rows of figures, very much resembling the jacks on playing cards. A similar design occurs so often among the ancient Peruvian relics found upon the coast as to suggest a common origin. There are forty-eight of these figures, each in a kneeling posture, facing toward the central figure. All are winged and hold sceptres terminating with condors' heads, while the figures of each alternate row have either crowned human heads or condors' heads. It is supposed this relic commemorates some homage to a deity or mighty sovereign, but of what people or in what epoch is not even conjectured.

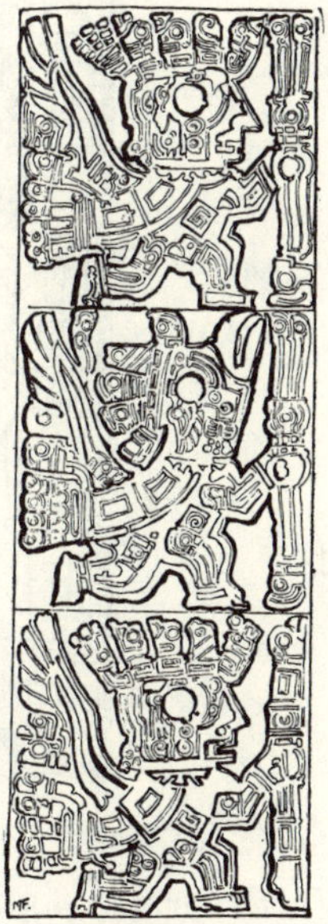

DETAIL OF FIGURES ON FRIEZE. MONOLITHIC DOORWAY. [*Stübel und Uhle.*]

These ruins are collectively spoken of as *Tiahuanaco*—a Quichua term, which tradition says originated through one of the Incan sovereigns having addressed a *chasqui*—or rapid messenger who had come to him here, *tia-huanaco*—"Be seated, O Huanaco!"—referring to the rapidity of his journey by comparing it with the swiftness of the *guanaco,* of the llama tribe. The style of the architecture and sculpture of the Tiahuanaco ruins is decidedly unique, and the exactness of squaring and joining the blocks is pronounced to be unsurpassed, even by the famous ancient works of the Old World. Many of the walls have been destroyed by treasure hunters, or to obtain material for building in the vicinity; but the early writers all agree in their description of the massiveness when intact. Among other ruins are immense hewn stones, thirty-six and twenty-six feet long, suggesting the mammoth stones of Baalbek in Syria. Here are Cyclopean walls, huge monoliths on end, and the remains of many statues, while bits of pottery indicate that the whole plain was once a burial ground. Archæologists suppose that these ruins point to the existence of a civilized race in very remote times, long antedating the Incas. Other works of a gigantic character but of

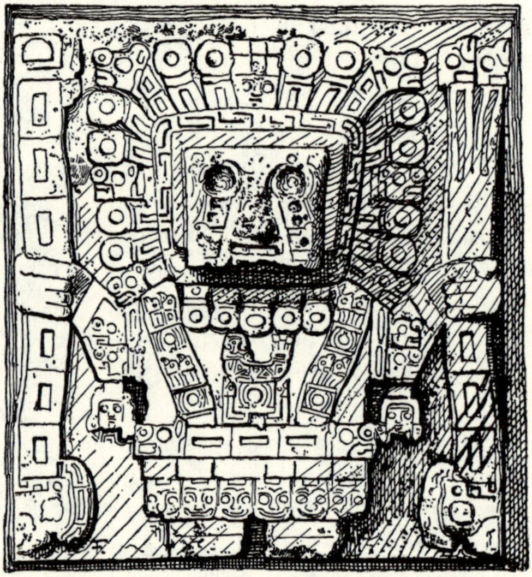

CENTRAL FIGURE, MONOLITHIC DOORWAY. [*Stübel and Uhle.*]

a different quality of architecture are to be found in many parts of Peru. Such as the ruins about Cuzco, and the megalithic remains of Ollantay-Tambo, in the Valley of Yuca, which have been told of in the drama of Ollantay, and minutely described by Cieza de Leon. Other ruins are to be found at Concacha, near the Apurimac; Huiñaque, at Chavin, and at Huaraz. At Quecap, in Chachapoyas, there is a mammoth structure which is said to belong to an early period.[12]

A trip to Cuzco may be made from Sicuani, the terminus of the southern railway, one hundred and ninety-seven miles north of Juliaca. The route is along the picturesque valley of

[12] Markham; 1892.

the Vilcamayu for about one hundred and twenty-five miles by stage. The valley is well populated by a people who represent the remains of the Incan race, and everywhere about may be seen the relics and ruins of the former empire. The Indians are industrious and delight in husbandry. They use a curious form of plough, sometimes made from the fork of a tree, or again consisting of a spear-pointed implement which they term *rejka.** This is thrust into the ground by hand while women follow and break the clods with a club. Here are still met the couriers who carry the government despatches, just as was done in early Incan times. Supported solely by Coca, they are considered capable of running a hundred miles, a feat often repeated. They are a sturdy-looking lot of fellows, who appear to be a race by themselves.

About twenty-five miles from Cuzco the road leaves the river and climbs a steep hill, from which a level valley extends to the ancient capital, which is entered through the ruins of a gateway of an old Incan wall. Whatever Cuzco may have been during the time of the Incas, it is now a wretchedly filthy city. The churches, which are numerous, are built on the foundations of the old palaces, and everywhere the relics of Incan greatness have been employed to modern advantage. The once Temple of the Sun is now the Church of the Dominican Friars; the Temple of the Virgins is a convent, while many private dwellings are constructed of stone from the various ruins. In one of the richest chapels of Cuzco is a relic which was sent by Charles V.—the crucifix of *Nuestro Señor de los Temblores*—"Our Lord of the Earthquakes," which the Indians regard with great veneration. To the north is the famous hill of Sacsahuaman,[13] the fortress of which dominated Cuzco and was pronounced by the conquerors, "The ninth wonder of the world." Whether this was of Incan structure archæologists are not agreed. The works were defended by a line of walls eighteen hundred feet long, formed in three terraces, each supporting a parapet. The Spaniards reduced these walls, but their line may still be studied. Some of the

* Illustrated on page 196.

[13] *Sacsahuaman*, fill thee, falcon! implying the vultures would feast on those who attempted its assault.

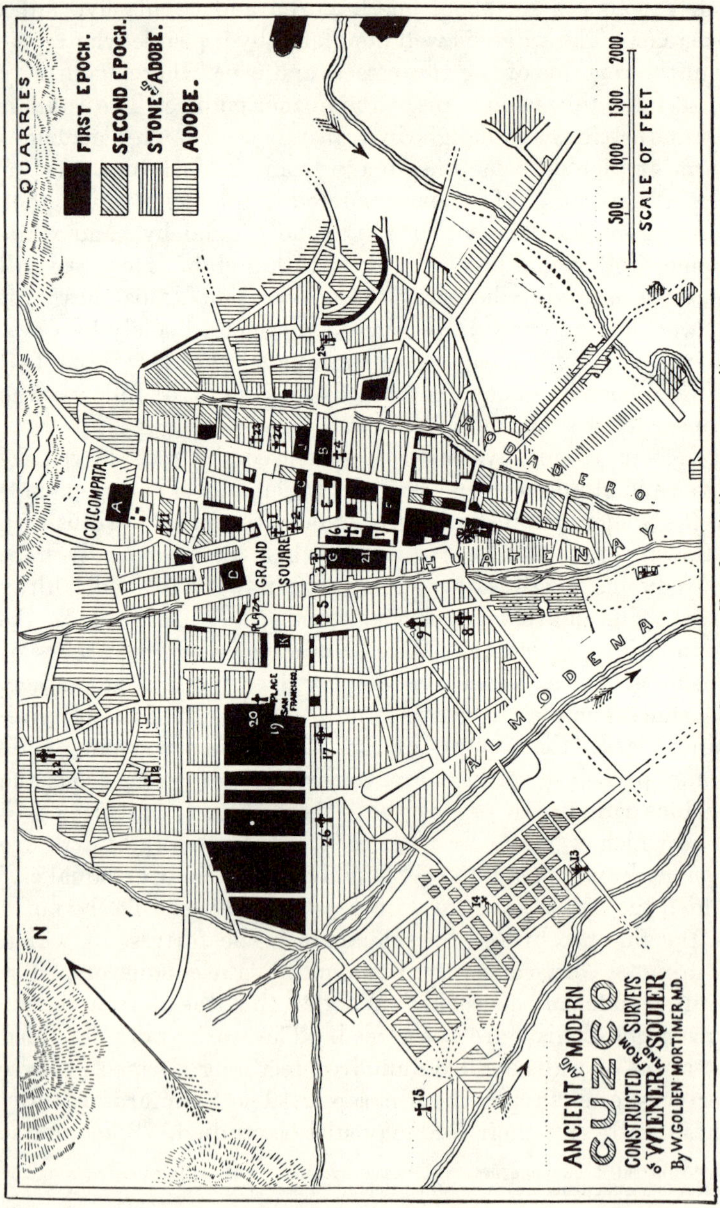

Plan of the Incan Capital. For description see opposite page.

stones forming the wall at its northeast angle were of Cyclopean size, weighing hundreds of tons. The stones were of every conceivable shape, but were cut and dressed with the greatest precision, laid without mortar, and fitted together with such exactness that a knife blade could not be thrust between them. The ruins of Ollantay at Urabamba, about a day's journey from Cuzco, are fully as wonderful as those of Sacsahuaman. The chief commerce of Cuzco, which is controlled by Germans, is in Coca leaves and other tropical produce of the valleys, and in the wools of the mountains.

DESCRIPTION OF PLAN OF ANCIENT AND MODERN CUZCO.
on opposite page.

1. Cathedral.
2. Triumphe.
3. Companía.
4. San Agustin.
5. Merced.
6. Convent Santa Catalina.
7. Santo Domingo.
8. Santa Rosa.
9. San Andres.
11. San Cristobal.
12. Arcopata.
13. Belen.
14. Santiago.
15. Panteon.
16. Convent Recoleta.
17. Hospital Santa Clara.
18. Hospital San Pedro.
19. University.
20. San Francisco.
21. Jail.
22. Santa Ana.
23. Los Nazarenos.
24. San Antonio.
25. San Blas.
26. Hospital for Men.

A. Palace of Manco Ccapac.
B. Palace of Sincha Rocca.
C. Palace of Viracocha.
D. Palace of Pachacutec.
E. Palace of Inca Yupanqui.
F. Palace of Tupac Inca Yupanqui.
G. Palace of Huayna Ccapac.
H. Temple of the Sun.
I. Palace of Virgins.
J. Palace of Yachahuasi or The Schools.
K. House of the historian, Garcilasso.

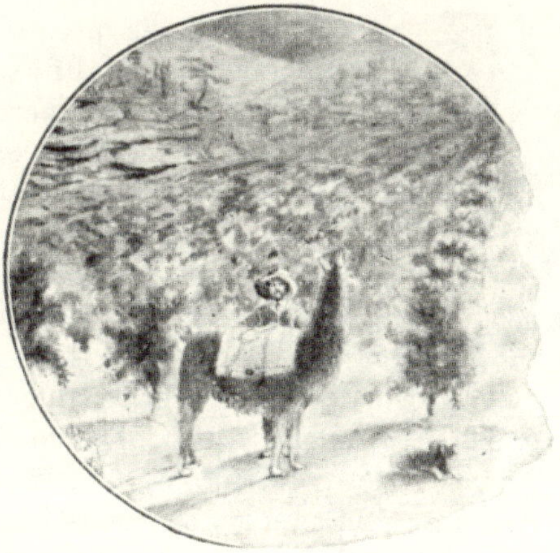

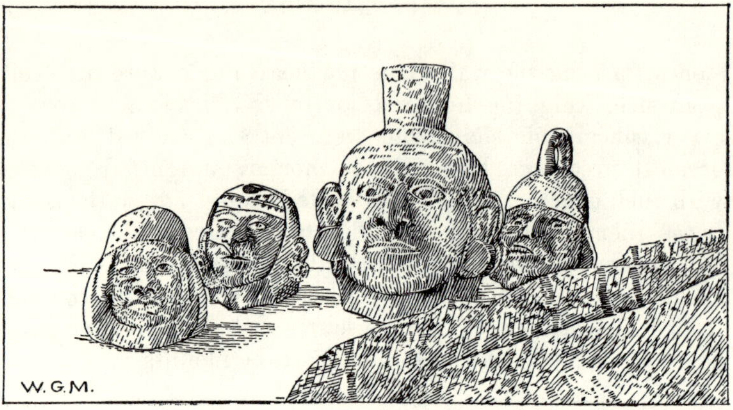

CHAPTER VI.

THE HISTORY OF COCA.

"Like *Amazons* they stand in painted Arms,
Coca alone appear'd with little Charms,
Yet led the Van, our scoffing *Venus* scorn'd
The shrub-like tree, and with no Fruit adorn'd."

—*Cowley.*

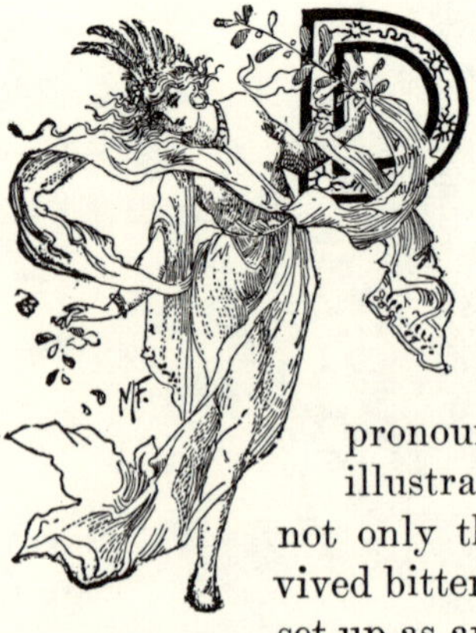

DARWIN gave prominence to the doctrine of Malthus that organic life tends to increase beyond means of subsistence, and emphasized a statement of Spencer that in the struggle for existence only the fittest survive. Among economic plants we have no more pronounced example of these laws than is illustrated in the Coca plant. It has stood not only the mere test of time, but has survived bitter persecutions wherein it was falsely set up as an emblem of superstition, in a cruel war of destruction when the people among whom it was held as sacred were exterminated as a race.

Coca has marked the downfall of one of the most profound examples of socialism ever recorded in history, and has outlived the forceful attacks of Church and State which were maliciously hurled against it as an example of idolatry and perniciousness. These attacks were the outgrowth of a shallowness of thought, intermingled with the prevalent prejudices of the several important epochs of its history. In the earliest literature concerning Peru we trace the beginning of this element of superstition toward Coca, for it was presumed there could be no good custom followed by the Indians. The entire aboriginal American race was regarded by the invaders as little more than savage devils worthy only of extermination. Thus Pedro Cieza de Leon, who wrote at the time of the Conquest, garnished his tales with pictures and stories of the Prince of Evil, with whom the Indian was inferred to be in close compact.

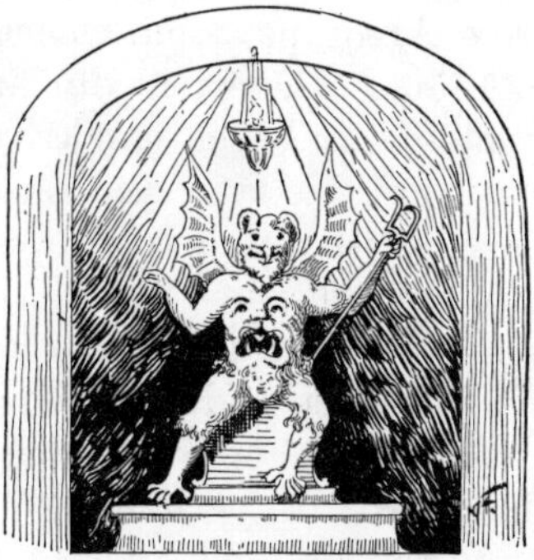

EARLY SPANISH DEVIL.
[*After De Bry*, 1600.]

Cieza was a mere boy of fourteen when he embarked with Don Pedro de Heredia, in 1532, to seek fortune in the New World. When we consider that the conceptions of this writer were only such as might be inspired by the rough and rugged opportunities which camp life offered, it certainly seems remarkable that he had the foresight to compile so acceptable a journal of the early Peruvians. The seriousness with which he undertook this task, and his exactitude in recording current events, may be appreciated from his statement: "I noted with much care and diligence, in order that I might be able to write with that truth which is due from me and without any mixture of inaccuracies."[1]

Heredia founded the city of Cartagena, in the province of Tierra Firma, as Panama was originally termed, and after

[1] Cieza; p. 15; 1550.

Cieza had spent five years of life there, he enlisted under Pedro Vadillo in a desperate exploit across the mountains of Abibe and through the valley of Cauca and Popayan. Subsequently we find this boy historian marching with Robbdo and then serving under Belalcazar, until, as the chronicler states, "he, too, became entombed in the bellies of the Indians"—for they were marching through a country of savages who were cannibals.

Cieza was first intimately associated with Peruvian affairs in the campaign with Gasca, at the final rout of Gonzalo, and he afterward travelled under this first President of the Royal Audience through the interior of Peru. Having compiled an extensive notebook of the country and the doings of the times, which was to form a connecting link between the Incas and the Spanish invaders, he returned to Lima by way of the coast from Arequipa, from whence he sailed for Spain September 8, 1550. The events during seventeen years of travel he has recounted in his chronicles with remarkable minuteness.[2]

There was a prejudice and superstitious credulity among the Spanish conquerors for all the customs of the Incas. The bigotry of the time is well illustrated in a story told of Columbus. On the return from his first voyage he took with him to Spain several Indians, who were baptized at Barcelona, where one of them shortly afterward died, and Herrera, referring to this nearly three hundred years after, tells us this Indian "was the first native of the New World who ever went to Heaven,"[3] though no intimation is made as to the probable destination of the millions of Americans who had preceded him. Amidst such prejudices, it is not surprising that the Coca plant so prized by the Indians was deemed by the Spanish unworthy of serious consideration, and that it was looked upon by them merely as a savage means of intoxication, or at best a mere source of idle indulgence among a race they so much despised.

Throughout his writings Cieza refers frequently to Coca, though he has not given any very concise botanical descrip-

[2] Part First, published in 1550; Part Second, the *Relacion* of "Juan de Sarmiento;" Parts Four and Five are supposed to still be in manuscript at Madrid.
[3] Markham; Cieza, *Introduction;* p. LVII; 1883.

tion of the plant, referring more particularly to its common use. In the first part of his chronicles of Peru, he says: "In all parts of the Indies through which I travelled I noticed the Indians delighted to carry herbs or roots in their mouths; in one province of one kind, in another another sort, etc. In the Districts of Quimbaya and Anzerma they cut small twigs from a young green tree, which they rub against their teeth without cessation. In most of the villages subject to the cities of Cali and Popayan they go about with small Coca leaves in their mouth, to which they apply a mixture which they carry in a calabash, made from a certain earth-like lime. Throughout Peru the Indians carry this Coca in their mouths; from morning until they lie down to sleep they never take it out. When I asked some of these Indians why they carried these leaves in their mouths, which they do not eat, but merely hold between their teeth, they replied that it prevents them from feeling hungry, and gives them great vigor and strength. I believe that it has some such effect, although perhaps it is a custom only suitable for people like these Indians. They so use Coca in the forests of the Andes, from Guamanga to the town of La Plata. The trees are small, and they cultivate them with great care, that they may yield the leaf called Coca. They put the leaves in the sun, and afterwards pack them in little narrow bags containing a little more than an arroba each. This Coca was so highly valued in the years 1548, '49, '50 and '51 that there was not a root nor anything gathered from a tree, except spice, which was in such estimation. In those years they valued the repartimientos of Cuzco, La Paz and Plata at eighty thousand dollars, more or less, all arising from this Coca. Coca was taken to the mines of Potosi for sale, and the planting of the trees and picking of the leaves was carried on to such an extent that Coca is not now worth so much, but it will never cease to be valuable. There are some persons in Spain who are rich from the produce of this Coca, having traded with it, sold and resold it in the Indian markets."[4]

The Incas regarded Coca as a symbol of divinity, and originally its use was confined exclusively to the royal family.

[4] Cieza; p. 352; 1550.

The sovereign could show no higher mark of esteem than to bestow a gift of this precious leaf upon those whom he wished to endow with an especial mark of his imperial favor. So when neighboring tribes who had been conquered by the Incas, acknowledged their subjection and allegiance, their chiefs were welcomed with the rank of nobles to this new alliance and accorded such honors and hospitalities as gifts of rich stuffs, women and bales of Coca might impress.

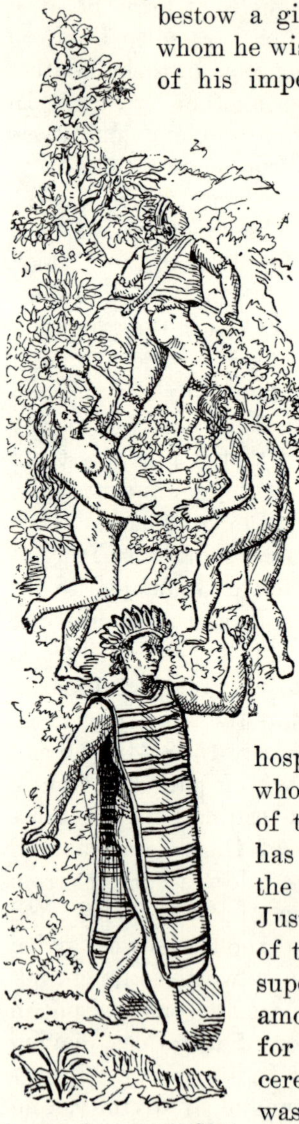

INCANS GATHERING COCA.
[*After De Bry*, 1600.]

At the time of Mayta Ccapac—the fourth Inca, his queen was designated Mama Coca — "the mother of Coca," as the most sacred title which could be bestowed upon her. From so exalted a consideration of the plant by royal favor, it was but a natural sequence that the mass of the people should regard Coca as an object for adoration worthy to be deemed "divine."

Cristoval Molina, a priest at the hospital for the natives at Cuzco, from whose work[5] we have drawn our account of the rites and festivals of the Incas, has related the method of using Coca by the high priests in conducting sacrifices. Just as Cieza, with the material instinct of the soldier, saw only the physical or superstitious element in the use of Coca among the Indians, so this priest traced for us its spiritual association with the ceremonies of the people. Thus there was early interwoven the factors of a prejudice of superstition, a popular

[5] Molina; 1570.

adoration of the masses, and a blending of these with a religious regard for Coca, for the teachings of the Church were engrafted upon existing customs in order to hold the people.

The first scientific knowledge of Coca published in Europe was embodied in the writings of Nicolas Monardes,[6] a physician of Seville, in 1565, from material possibly gained from Cieza, though it would seem that he had intimately examined the Coca shrub. A translation of this work was made a few years later by Charles l'Ecluse[7]—a botanist and director of the Emperor's Garden at Vienna—which was published in Latin at Antwerp, and this is often quoted as the earliest botanical reference to Coca. The Kew Library possesses a translation of this book, "made into English" by John Frampton and printed in black letter with the curious title: *"Joyful News out of the Newe Founde Worlde, wherein is declared the Virtues of Hearbes, Treez, Oyales, Plantes and Stones."*

As showing the discernment in this botanical description of Coca made so many years ago, it may not be uninteresting to read a paragraph translated from the very language of Monardes:

"This plant Coca has been celebrated for many years among the Indians, and they sow and cultivate it with much care and industry, because they all apply it daily to their use and pleasure. * * * It is indeed of the height of two outstretched arms, its leaves somewhat like myrtle, but larger and more succulent and green (and they have, as it were, drawn in the middle of them another leaf of similar shape); its fruit collected together in a cluster, which, like myrtle fruit, becomes red when ripening and of the same size, and when quite ripe it is black in color. When the time of the harvest of the leaves arrives, they are collected in baskets with other things to make them dry, that they may be better preserved, and may be carried to other places."

This description will hold equally good to-day. The peculiar leaf within a leaf arrangement formed by the curved lines

[6] Monardes; 1580. [7] Lat. Carolus Clusius; 1582.

running on either side of the midrib, being a marked characteristic of Coca.

When Hernando Pizarro returned to the court of his king, with the first fruits of the golden harvest from the New World, he probably took with him specimens of Coca. This plant could not have failed to have awakened at least the curiosity of the invaders, because of the numerous golden duplications of the Coca shrub and of its leaf that had been found in the gardens of the Temples of the Sun, at Cuzco and elsewhere among the royal domains of the Incas. So that whatever the prejudices may have been regarding the use to which Coca was put by the Indians, these golden images at least would prove sufficient to excite admiration and comment.

Another voluminous writer upon the early Peruvians is Joseph de Acosta, a Jesuit missionary who made a passage across the Atlantic in 1570, which he assures us:—"would have been more rapid if the mariners had made more sail." After his arrival at Lima he crossed the Andes by the lofty pass of Pariacaca to join the Viceroy Toledo, with whom he visited every province. In the higher altitudes of the mountains the party suffered severely from the effects of the rarefied atmosphere, with which he was afterwards prostrated upon three successive occasions, while he also was severely annoyed from snow blindness, for which he relates a homely remedy offered him by an Indian woman, who gave him a piece of the flesh of the vicuña, saying, "Father, lay this to thine eyes, and thou shalt be cured." He says: "It was newly killed and bloody, yet I used the medicine, and presently the pain ceased, and soon after went quite away."

Father Acosta was a man of great learning, an intelligent observer, and had exceptional opportunities for collecting his information. His work on the Natural History of the Indies ranks among the higher authorities. He has given a very extensive description of Coca, and, referring to its employment, says: "They bring it commonly from the valleys of the Andes, where there is an extreme heat and where it rains continually the most part of the year, wherein the Indians endure much labor and pain to entertain it, and often many die. For that they go from the Sierra and colde places to till and gather them in the valleys; and therefore there has been great question and diversity of opinion among learned men whether it were more expedient to pull up these trees or let them grow, but in the end they remained. The Indians esteemed it much, and in the time of the Incas it was not lawful for any of the common people to use this Coca without license from the Governor. * * * They say it gives them great courage, and is very pleasing unto them. Many grave men hold this as a superstition and a mere imagination. For my part, and to speak the truth, I persuade not myself that it is an imagination, but contrawise I think it works and gives force and courage to the Indians, for we see the effects which cannot be attributed to imagination, so as to go some days without meat, but only a handful of Coca, and other like effects. The sauce wherewith they do eat this Coca is proper enough, whereof I have tasted, and it is like the taste of leather. The Indians mingle it with the ashes of bones, burnt and beat into powder, or with lime, as others affirme, which seemeth to them pleasing and of good taste, and they say it doeth them much good. They willingly imploy their money therein and use it as money; yet all these things were not inconvenient, were not the hazard of the trafficke thereof, wherein so many men are occupied. The Lords Yncas used Coca as a delicate and royall thing, which they offered most in their sacrifice, burning it in honor of their idols." Again, when speaking of the importance of the trade in Coca, he says: "It seems almost fabulous, but in truth the trafficke of Coca in Potosi doth yearly amount to above half a million of dollars; for that they use four score and ten or four score and fifteen thousand baskets every year."[8]

This extensive mining centre in the southern part of Bolivia is some three hundred miles south of Sandia, which is today the very heart of the Coca region of Caravaya. These mines were at an altitude of seventeen thousand feet, and Garcilasso says the Indians applied the term Potosi, literally a hill, to all hills. In the Aymara tongue Potosi means, "he

[8] Acosta; Book I, p. 245; 1590.

who makes a noise," and the Indians have a legend which suggests the derivation of the name from such a source. When Huayna Ccapac caused his people to search this mountain for silver, a great noise came from the hills warning the Indians away, as the protecting genius destined these riches for other masters. Within a short time after the Incas had discovered silver here over seven thousand Indians were at work mining the precious ore.

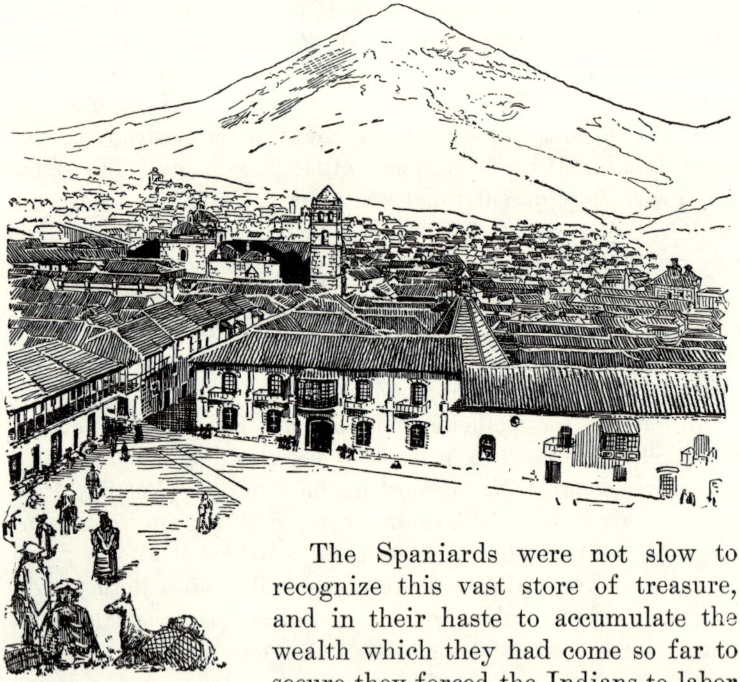

MODERN POTOSI.
[*From a Photograph.*]

The Spaniards were not slow to recognize this vast store of treasure, and in their haste to accumulate the wealth which they had come so far to secure they forced the Indians to labor in veritable slavery through an enactment which drafted a certain number from each of the adjoining provinces. This law, known as the *mitta,* instituted under Toledo, required all Indians between the ages of eighteen and fifty to contribute a certain labor, which amounted to eighteen months during the thirty-two years in which they were liable. For this they were paid twenty reals a week, and a half real additional for every league distant from the village of Potosi. During the year 1573 the draft of Indians for this labor amounted to 11,199, while a hundred years later—in 1673—it drew only 1,674, showing that cruelty and hardship had depopulated the province nearly ninety per cent.

So extensive were the mining operations at Potosi that the place had the appearance of a great city. Every Saturday the silver was melted down and the royal fifth was set aside for the Spanish crown, and although this amounted during the years 1548 to 1551 to three million ducats, it was considered the mines were not well worked. In those times the markets or fairs were important functions, and that of Potosi was looked upon as the greatest in the world. It was held in the plains near the town, and there the transactions in one day were said to amount to from twenty-five to thirty thousand golden pesos, Coca being a prominent commodity in the reckoning, owing to its absolute necessity in the arduous work exacted from the Indians.

Because of this need the highest price was obtained for Coca in this region, where every indication was presented for its use—the extreme altitude of the mines, the mental dejection of slavery, and the enforced muscular task of the Indian with insufficient food. This labor was found to be utterly impossible without the use of Coca, so that the Indians were supplied with the leaves by their masters, just as so much fuel might be fed to an engine in order to produce a given amount of work. Garcilasso tells us that in 1548 the workers in these mines consumed 100,000 *cestas* of Coca, which were valued at 500,000 piasters.

This absolute necessity was the sole reason for the Spanish tolerance to the continuance of Coca; they saw that it was indirectly to them a source of wealth, through enabling the Indians to do more work in the mines. As the demands of labor increased the call for Coca, situations for new cocals, where a supply of the plant could be raised to meet this want, were pushed further to the east of the Andes, in the region of the montaña. To make favorable clearings numerous tribes of savage Indians, who had not been previously subdued by the Incas, were driven from the Peruvian tributaries of the Amazon further into the forests.

Agustin de Zarate, who was *contador real*, or royal comptroller, under the first Viceroy, Blasco Nuñez Vela, in his history of the discoveries of Peru, in writing of Coca, says: "In certain valleys, among the mountains, the heat is marvellous, and there groweth a certain herb called Coca, which the Indians do esteem more than gold or silver; the leaves thereof are like unto Zamake (sumach); the virtue of this herb, found by experience, is that any man having these leaves in his mouth hath never hunger nor thirst."[9]

Garcilasso Inca de la Vega—as he delighted in terming himself—has very rightly been classed as an eminent authority on Incan subjects. His father, who was of proud Spanish ancestry, illustrious both in arms and literature, came to Peru shortly after the Conquest, served under Pizarro, and after the overthrow of the empire, when the Incan maidens were assigned to various Spanish officers, his choice fell upon the niece of Inca Huayna Ccapac, who in some manner had been preserved from the massacre which had followed upon the death of her cousin, Atahualpa. It seems fitting that a son of such parentage should embody in his writings facts which he had obtained from both branches of the family tree, and because of this his work is accepted as a reliable presentation.

That this Incan author was well qualified to speak upon Coca there can be no doubt, for he owned an extensive cocal on the River Tunu, one of the tributaries of the Beni—which drains the montaña for Paucartambo—where there are still numerous cocals. This plantation was started in the twelfth century during the reign of Inca Rocca, when that king sent his son with fifteen thousand warriors to conquer the savage tribes of Anti-suyu.

Lloque Yupanqui advanced to the River Paucartambo and thence to Pillcu-pata, where four villages were founded, and from Pillcu-pata he marched to Havisca, and here in the year 1197 was located the first Coca plantation of the montaña on

[9] Zarate; 1555.

the eastern base of the Andes.[10] This Incan plantation became an inheritance of Garcilasso from his father, but was forfeited by the historian because of his parent's early defection to the cause of Gonzalo.

The work of Garcilasso is interesting as embracing with the relation of others that of Father Blas Valera, whose manuscripts have since been lost, and in this embodied record we have the only available account of one who was a close observer of Incan customs during a residence of many years in Peru. To the peculiar wording of the work of this author we may trace an oft-repeated error regarding the Coca shrub, which he describes as "a bush of the height and thickness of the vine."[11] Whether this designation of vine refers to the grape, which in some vineyards is grown as a low clump resembling a bush, or whether the term vine simply alludes to the delicate nature of the Coca shrub, can only be inferred. It has introduced a source of inaccuracy among some who have since drawn their description of the plant from this record. One author has even amplified this early comparison by saying that the Coca bush twines about other plants for support.[12]

Valera, in describing the leaves of Coca, says: "They are known by Indians and Spaniards alike as *Cuca*, delicate, though not soft, of the width of the thumb and as long as half a thumb's length, and of a pleasant smell." In his day the Indians were so fond of Coca that they preferred it to gold, silver and precious stones. He has given us a careful account of the diligence which is necessary in the several stages of its cultivation and the importance of the final gathering of the leaves, which he says, "they pick one by one by hand and dry them in the sun." He, however, wrongly viewed the method of use, and supposed that the leaves were merely chewed for their flavor and that the juice was not swallowed.

Referring to the general employment of Coca for a variety of purposes, he says: "*Cuca* preserves the body from many infirmities, and our doctors use it pounded for applications to sores and broken bones, to remove cold from the body or to

[10] Garcilasso; Vol. I, p. 330; 1872. [11] Valera; in Garcilasso; 1609.
[12] Ulloa; p. 488; 1772.

prevent it from entering, as well as to cure sores that are full of maggots. It is so beneficial and has such singular virtue in the cure of outward sores, it will surely have even more virtue and efficacy in the entrails of those who eat it!" Nor did this observant author fail to recognize another important use in which this famous plant was practically serviceable. A tax of one-tenth of the Coca crop was set apart for the clergy, of which he says: "The greater part of the revenue of the bishops and canons of the cathedrals of Cuzco is derived from the tithes of the *Coca* leaves."

There is a marked contrast between the open, conscientious manner of Valera's writings with that of other Spanish authors, who displayed an abhorrence for all the customs of the Indians. Thus Cieza, reflecting this superstitious prejudice, tells us that the old men of every tribe actually conversed with the arch-enemy of mankind. Referring to the Incan rite of burying bags of Coca with their dead, as a symbol of support for the departed in a journey to the eternal home, he mockingly says, "as if hell was so very far off." The good *padre,* in his appeal for the continuance of Coca, has shown a liberality for such a period of bigotry which might be well for the consideration of others in even this more enlightened age. Thus he writes:

"They have said and written many things against the little plant, with no other reason than that the Gentiles in ancient times, and now some wizards and diviners, offer *Cuca* to the idols, on which ground these people say that its use ought to be entirely prohibited. Certainly this would be good counsel if the Indians offered up this and nothing else to the devil, but seeing that the ancient idolaters and modern wizards also sacrifice maize, vegetables and fruits, whether growing above or under ground, as well as their beverage, cold water, wool, clothes, sheep and many other things, and as they cannot all be prohibited, neither should the *Cuca.* They ought to be taught to abhor superstitions and to serve truly one God, using all these things after a Christian fashion." Surely, an impartial judgment, which is worthy of present acceptation.[13]

[13] Valera; in Garcilasso; Vol. II. pp 371-375; 1871.

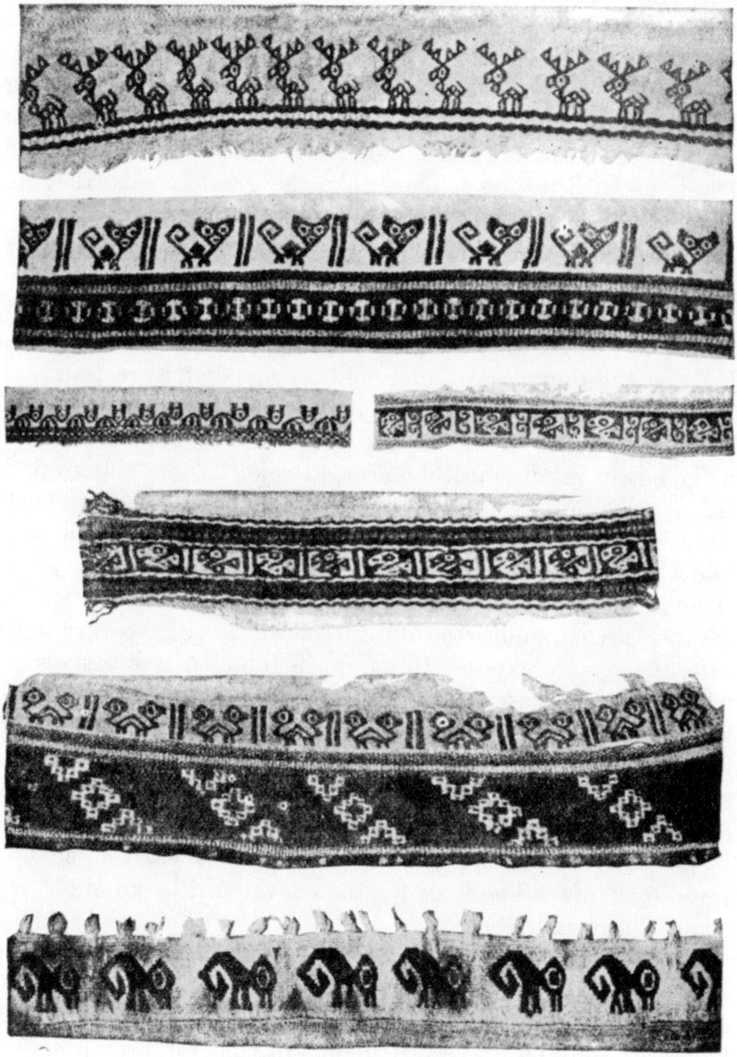

BORDERS OF INCAN TAPESTRY. [*Reiss and Stübel.*]

Garcilasso has added to this account some further particulars made familiar to him through his intimate acquaintance with the cultivation and care of Coca. In his quaint verbiage, which has possibly suffered through translation, he says of the shrubs: "They are about the height of a man, and in planting them they put the seeds into nurseries, in the same way as in garden stuffs, but drilling a hole as for vines. They layer the plants as with a vine. They take the greatest care that no roots, not even the smallest, be doubled, for this is sufficient to make the plant dry up. When they gather the leaves they take each branch within the fingers of the hand, and pick the leaves until they come to the final sprout, which they do not touch, lest it should cause the branch to wither. The leaf, both on the upper and under side, in shape and greenness, is neither more nor less than that of the arbutus, except that three or four leaves of the *Cuca*, being very delicate, would make one of arbutus in thickness. I rejoice to be able to find things in Spain which are appropriate for comparison with those of that country—that both here and there people may know one by another. After the leaves are gathered they put them in the sun to dry. For they lose their green color, which is much prized, and break up into powder, being so very delicate, if they are exposed to damp, in the *cestas* or baskets in which they are carried from one place to another. The baskets are made of split canes, of which there are many of all sizes in these provinces of the *Antis*. They cover the outside of the baskets with the leaves of the large cane, which are more than a *tercia* wide and about half a *vara* long,[14] in order to preserve the *Cuca* from wet, for the leaves are much injured by damp. The basket is then enveloped by an outer net made of a certain fibre."

Referring to the extreme care essential for its preservation, this Incan author concludes: "In considering the number of things that are required for the production of *Cuca*, it would be more profitable to return thanks to God for providing all things in the places where they are necessary than to write concerning them, for the account must seem incredible."

[14] A *vara* is thirty-three English inches.

Father Thomas Ortiz, who accompanied Alonzo Niño and Luis Guerra in their expedition in 1499, described the use of Coca by the natives along the coast of Venezuela under the term *hayo.*[15]

Antonio de Herrera, who was royal historian under Philip II, drew his facts from correspondence with the *conquistados,* and his history, which is divided into eight decades, covers the period of the Spanish discoveries. In speaking of the customs of the northern provinces, he refers to "the herb which on the coast of the sea is called *hayo.*"[16] The word *hayo* has been shown to belong to the vocabulary of the Chibchas[17] and is generally applied to Coca by several tribes bordering upon the northern coast of South America.

Among some of the earlier Spanish writings of this section Coca is alluded to as "hay," and doubt has been expressed as to whether this is identical with *hayo,*[18] presumably derived from *agu,* to chew; but the absence of the final vowel, according to a writer who is familiar with this region, does not signify, while it is absolutely certain that all the species of *Erythroxylon* which are to-day used in Venezuela and along the Caribbean Sea are termed *hayo.* Even the *Erythroxylon cumanense,* HBK, is called by this name and not that of *ceveso,* as mentioned in the description published by Kunth.[19]

The account which Ortiz gives of the plant used by the Indians of Chiribiche does not exactly correspond with the Coca shrub, though what he says of the leaves and their use among the Indians is correct. Gomara, in speaking of the customs of the *Cumana,* confirms the account given by Ortiz.[20] At present Coca is not very extensively grown through Venezuela. The ancient cocals on the peninsula of Guajira are becoming extinct on account of excessive drought, while the cultivation of tobacco has proved a more profitable industry and is better adapted to the climate.

We know that prior to the Conquest the province of the Incas extended north to Quito, having been conquered by

[15] Pierre Martyr; Chap. 6, decade 8; 1530; Ernst; 1890.
[16] *Yerva que en la costa de la mar llamen hayo;* Herrera; decade VI., Chap. 6; 1730. [17] Uricoechea; 1871. [18] Waitz; *Anthropologie,* III, 366.
[19] *Nova Gen. et Spec. Plant;* V, 177; Synopsis III, 191; quoted by Ernst; 1890.
[20] Gomara: p. 72. Chap. LXXIX; 1749.

Huayna Ccapac some years before for his father, Tupac Inca Yupanqui, by which conquest the powerful State of Quito, which rivaled Peru in wealth and civilization, was united to the Incan Empire. When Huayna Ccapac succeeded his father, this newly acquired kingdom became his seat of government, and here with his favorite concubine, the mother of Atahualpa, he spent the last days of his life.

Because of this removal of imperial influence far from the original home of the empire at Cuzco may be attributed one source of the final weakness of the Incas, for it may be recalled that at the time of Huayna Ccapac's death the kingdom, which now extended over such immense territory, was for the first time divided under two rulers, one-half being given to his son, Huasca, and the other half to his son Atahualpa. It therefore seems quite probable that as the interests of the government extended northward the customs of the people of the lower Andes should follow, and be propagated among a people where similar conditions called for whatever beneficial influence might be derived from the use of Coca. From Quito travel northward, aided by the canoe navigation of the Cauca and Magdalena rivers, would rapidly carry the customs of the people of the south to the northern coast, where, as shown by early historical facts, commerce was so extensive as to favor the adoption of the habits of the interior.

There are still many tribes along the Sierra Nevada of Santa Marta who have preserved their ancient customs and habits from prehistoric times, for it is known that the Spanish were never able to completely attain possession of this region. It has been suggested that these Indians had never been subject to a king as were the Incas, while their country was so extremely fertile that when pursued by the Spanish they merely destroyed their homes and took up habitations elsewhere, depending upon a bountiful tropical vegetation for their support. In marked contrast to the Indians of New Grenada, the Peruvians were accustomed to subjection under their Lord Inca, and at the time of the Conquest they were obliged to submit themselves to their new masters, for if they abandoned their homes and the lands which they had cultivated to flee to the barren mountains or snowy plains they must also give up their means for subsistence. Piedrahita speaks of the use of Coca along the northern coast, and says that the leaves were chewed by the Indians without lime, an addition which he suggests was carried from the Incan domains to the northern Indians by the Spaniards after the Conquest.[21]

The expedition of the French mathematician, La Condamine, which went to Quito in 1735 to measure an arc of the meridian in the neighborhood of the equator, and thus verify the shape of the earth, was made memorable through a host of important scientific discoveries, primary among which was the introduction of many new plants into Europe; among these was caoutchouc or india rubber. Accompanying this expedition was Antonio d'Ulloa, a Spanish naval officer; Godin, Bouguer and the botanist, Joseph de Jussieu, whose name is associated with the classification of Coca. Condamine was the first man of science who examined and described the *quinquina* tree of Loxa, of which Linnæus in 1742 established the genus *Cinchona*.

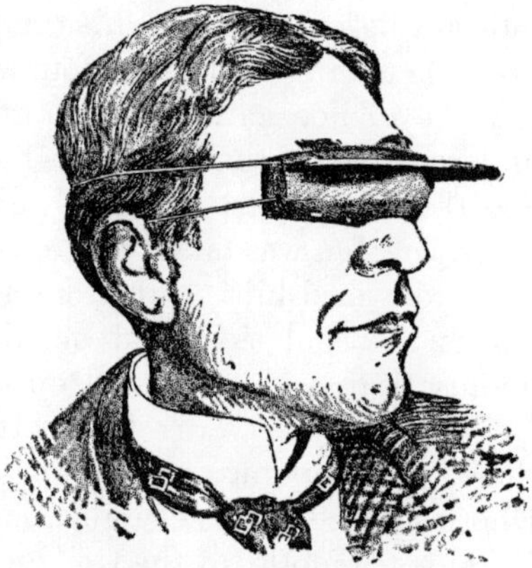

ESQUIMO SUN SHIELD.
[*A. J. Stone.*] [*From a Photograph.*]

Jussieu travelled on foot as far as the forests of Santa Cruz de la Sierra, collecting botanical specimens from the richness of the Peruvian flora. Many of his exploratory trips were hazardous in the extreme, and in 1749, while crossing the Andes to reach the Coca region of the Yungas of Coroico, he nearly lost his life. Added to the dangers of the route the glistening brilliancy of the sun reflected from the snow seemed to threaten him with blindness. In the Arctic region travel-

[21] Piedrahita; 1688.

lers are subject to a similar discomfort, and commonly wear a visor-like protector to shield their eyes. The sun shade illustrated is carved from wood with slots cut beneath the peak to permit of vision.

Jussieu sent specimens of the Coca shrub to Paris, and these, examined and described by the explorer's brother Antoine, were afterward preserved in the herbarium of the Museum of Natural History there, and have served as classic examples of many subsequent studies of the plant. But the glory of meritorious labor pursued through great trial and privation was not to be enjoyed by this explorer. Just as many another collector before and since his time has suffered the loss of treasures when work was about completed, so this intrepid botanist lost the choice gatherings of fifteen years through robbery, under the belief that his boxes contained a more merchantable wealth than plants. In 1771, after an absence of thirty-four years, Jussieu was taken home, bereft of reason, as a result not alone of hardships, but from that unfulfilled desire which makes the soul sick, and he died in France, leaving many manuscripts, which are still unpublished.

The Jussieus were a family of botanists for several generations; contemporary with them were several noted naturalists who followed their classification. Among these, Augustin Pyrame Candolle, of the College of France, and Antonio Jose Cavanilles, a Spanish ecclesiastic, each described Coca from the examples which had been sent by Joseph.

Many interesting accounts have been written of the expedition of La Condamine,[22] and as a result of these early researches several of the powers have been prompted to send botanical expeditions to the South American forests. Among these there is given in the writings of Captain Don Antonio d'Ulloa a brief account of the country of Popayan, in the jurisdiction of Timana. While following Father Valera's description of Coca, he adds: "It grows on a weak stem, which for support twists itself around another stronger vegetable like a vine. * * * The use the Indians make of it is for chewing, mixing it with chalk or whitish earth called *mambi*.[23]

[22] Condamine; 1745. [23] Spelled *manbi* by Delano; 1817.

They put into their mouths a few Coca leaves and a suitable portion of *mambi,* and chewing these together, at first spit out the saliva which that mastication causes, but afterwards swallow it, and thus move it from one side of the mouth to the other till its substance be quite derived, then it is thrown away, but immediately replaced by fresh leaves."

He confounds Coca with betel, saying: "It is exactly the same as the betel of the East Indies. The plant, the leaf, the manner of using it, its qualities, are all the same, and the eastern nations are no less fond of this betel than the Indians of Peru and Popayan are of their Coca; but in other parts of the province of Quito, as it is not produced, so neither is it used." But he was conscious of the physiological effects of Coca from its employment, and wrote: "This herb is so nutritious and invigorating that the Indians labor whole days without anything else, and on the want of it they find a decay in their strength. They also add that it preserves the teeth sound and fortifies the stomach."[24]

The early writings upon Coca were not, however, all of foreign authorship. Peru numbered among her men of letters a noted physician and statesman who drew his facts from a keen observation of the people of whom he wrote. I refer to Dr. Don Hipolito Unanue, of Tacna, whose name is intimately linked with the political and educational history of Peru. He published the *Mercurio Peruano,* the first number of which appeared in January, 1791, a paper which gave an impetus to the writings of his countrymen, in which there are many interesting details of Peruvian customs.

From his political interests in a land where insurrection was a common occurrence, Dr. Unanue could appreciate the advantage possible from the use of Coca in the army. He tells an incident of the siege of La Paz, in 1771, when the inhabitants, after a blockade of several months, during a severe winter, ran short of provisions and were compelled to depend wholly upon Coca, of which happily there was a stock in the city. This apparently scanty sustenance was sufficient to banish hunger and to support fatigue, while enabling the soldiers

[24] Ulloa; Pinkerton; Vol. XIV, p. 448; 1813.

to bear the intense cold. During the same war a body of patriot infantry, obliged to travel one of the coldest plateaus of Bolivia, found itself deprived of provisions while advancing in forced marches to regain the division. On their arrival only those soldiers were in condition to fight who had from childhood been accustomed to always carry with them a pouch of Coca.[25]

That early prejudice is difficult to eradicate, is shown in the writings of some who, having given the facts of the use of Coca, then seem to apologetically qualify their reference to its support as a mere delusion. Thus Dr. Barham, writing of Coca in 1795, says: "This herb is famous in the history of Peru, the Indians fancying it adds much to their strength. Others affirm that they use it for charms. Fishermen also put some of this herb to their hook when they can take no fish, and they are said to have better success therefor. In short, they apply it to so many uses, most of them bad, that the Spaniards prohibit the use of it, for they believe it hath none of these effects, but attribute what is done to the compact the Indians have with the devil."[26]

But if there was prejudice on the part of the Spanish against native customs, the Indians resorted in kind with an equal antipathy against all Spanish innovations. This has been exhibited in the strong objection which the Indians have made to using cinchona bark. Humboldt, who forms the connecting link between the eighteenth and nineteenth centuries in our history of Coca, has referred to this, as have several other observers. It is quite probable, however, that this was a pretended prejudice openly expressed, while secretly the Indians acknowledged the benefits of the bark, which the story of its introduction relates as having been presented to the Countess of Chinchon by a descendant of the Incas.[27]

Humboldt traveled extensively through the province of Popayan in 1801. In describing the use of Coca among the early inhabitants he asserted that several species of *Erythroxylon* were in use, chiefly *E. Hondense*. His conception of the benefit of Coca, however, was confined to a belief that it was

[25] Unanue; 1794. [26] Barham; 1795. [27] Markham; 1874.

the lime rather than the leaf which formed the element of sustenance. Since his time so many travellers directed attention to the fact that the Indians were supported by some mysterious principle, that European investigators began to question whether this was really due to the Coca leaf or some secret admixture. The popular interest at the time was well set forth by an English writer, who appreciating the importance to be expected to a modern civilization from the introduction of the method of the Andean, said: "While not yet fully acquainted with the secret with which the Indians sustain power, it is certain they have that secret and put it in practice. They masticate Coca and undergo the greatest fatigue without any injury to health or bodily vigor. They want neither butcher nor baker, nor brewer, nor distiller, nor fuel, nor culinary utensils. Now, if Professor Davy will apply his thoughts to the subject here given for his experiments, there are thousands even in this happy land who will pour their blessings upon him if he will but discover a temporary anti-famine, or substitute for food, free from all inconvenience of weight, bulk and expense, and by which any person might be enabled, like the Peruvian Indian, to live and labor in health and spirits for a month now and then without eating. It would be the greatest achievement—whatever a London alderman might think—ever attained by human wisdom."[28]

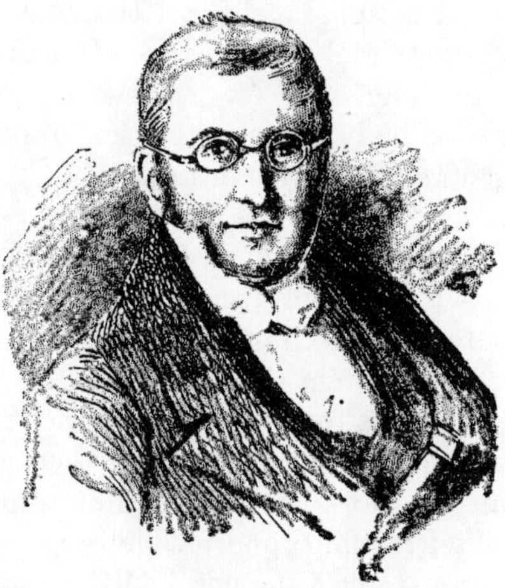

AUGUSTIN PYRAME DE CANDOLLE.

In the early days when the traveller crossed the Andes in the region of Popayan, he was carried in a chair on the back of an Indian. The roads, then dangerous at all times, be-

[28] *Gentleman's Magazine;* Vol. 84, p. 217, *et seq.;* 1814.

came practically impassable in unsettled weather; and the journey of twenty leagues from Popayan to La Plata on the Magdalena River occupied twenty to twenty-two days. The conditions were such as to call forth all reserve of endurance, and not only the Indian, but the traveller found relief and support during severe trials from the use of Coca. Bonnycastle, a captain of royal engineers, in referring to the use of Coca by the natives in these journeys, confounds it with betel, following the earlier error of Ulloa.[29]

The wonderful endurance of the guides and mail carriers travelling through passes of the Cordilleras where a mule could not go, has been a frequent topic for comment by many writers, and though so often repeated is still wonderful. Stevenson, who was for twenty years in Peru, during which period he held many political appointments under the captain-general of Quito, in describing the customs of the people, refers to the runners, or *chasquis,* carrying letters from Lima, a distance of upward of a hundred leagues, without any other provision than Coca, just as did their predecessors centuries before in the time of the Incas.[30]

The attention of the English people was particularly directed to this sustenance of the Andeans by the fact that one of their countrymen, who became a prominent participant in the Peruvian war of independence, boldly announced his belief in the support which his troops derived from the chewing of Coca. General Miller not only employed Coca in his army during the campaign of 1824, but so freely acknowledged the benefit he derived from its use that he established a warm sympathy with the natives, and it became desirable for an Englishman travelling through the interior to announce himself as a countryman of Miller, when he was sure to receive:—"the best house and the best fare that an Indian village could afford."[31]

The frequent occurrence of similar allusions in the writings of South American travellers to the sustaining influence of Coca emphasized by repetition the importance of this prop-

[29] Bonnycastle; Vol. I, p. 276, *et seq.;* 1818.
[30] Stevenson; 1825. [31] Miller; Vol. II, p. 198, *et seq.;* 1828.

erty, while happily the developments of time have removed the stigma of a fabulous or superstitious element from its use.

Among the eminent scientists who wrote of Coca during the next decade were Poeppig, Tschudi, Martius and Weddell. Eduard Poeppig was a German naturalist who travelled in Peru and Chili between the years 1827 and 1832. Poeppig was not an enthusiastic admirer of Indian customs, and endeavored to associate some pernicious after effect with the sustaining power of Coca, which he considered comparable with opium. In referring to this statement Dr. Weddell—a more careful observer, held that while possibly there had been some abuse in the intemperate use of Coca by Europeans, there was in no instance the injurious results which had been asserted. He believed, as many of the Indians had assured him, that Poeppig had been led into error through generalizing exceptional occurrences

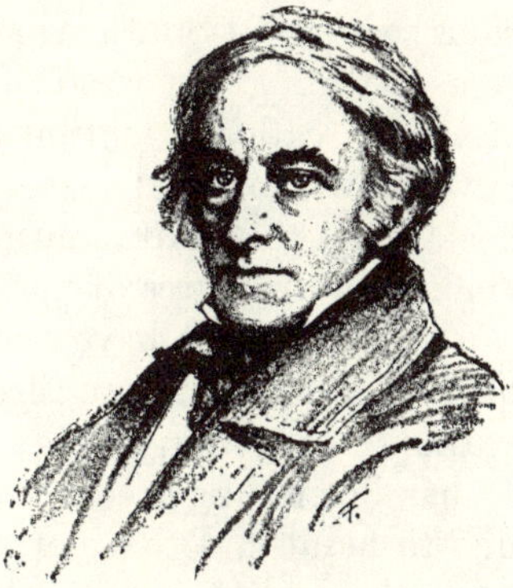

KARL VON MARTIUS.

Perhaps the Swiss naturalist, Von Tschudi, who visited South America in 1838, has been more frequently quoted in a popular way regarding Coca, than any other Peruvian traveller. Throughout his writings he testifies enthusiastically and forcibly for Coca, not only as employed among the natives, but from personal benefit in sustaining respiration when ascending to high altitudes. He tells of an Indian sixty-two years old who labored for him five days and nights without food and with but two hours' sleep each night, yet was still in condition to accompany him over a journey of twenty-three leagues, through which he jogged along afoot as rapidly as the mule carried his master, though depending wholly upon Coca for his sustenance. A similar experience has been reported by many travellers, for this custom is still practiced by the Indian guides.

Von Tschudi concluded that Coca is nutritious in the

highest degree. "Setting aside all extravagant and visionary notions on the subject, I am clearly of the opinion that moderate use of Coca is not merely innocuous, but that it may even be very conducive to health. In support of this conclusion, I may refer to numerous examples of longevity among Indians, who, almost from the age of boyhood, have been in the habit of masticating Coca three times a day, and who in the course of their lives have consumed no less than two thousand seven hundred pounds if at the age of one hundred and thirty, and they commenced masticating at ten years—one ounce a day, yet nevertheless enjoy perfect health."[32]

This testimony is repeatedly added to by observers in various sections of South America. Martius, in describing Coca as used throughout western Brazil, under the name of *ypadú,* or *ipadú,* called attention to the wonderful effect which the powder of the dried leaves has upon the nervous system, especially on the brain, and recommended the adoption of Coca among the treasures of materia medica.[33]

Many theories have been advanced, to explain the ability of the Indian to endure through long journeys and hard labor, without other support than is afforded through chewing Coca. It has been suggested that this hardihood and abstinence is due to habit and to vigorous development. But on the contrary the Indian is muscularly weak, and while training and habit may have much to do with his fortitude, he constantly requires the physical support afforded by Coca. Dr. Valdez, in writing of the use of Coca—or "*folha sagrada,*" as he terms it, has emphasized this: "The Indian is naturally very voracious, and loses his strength when abstaining from the leaves. With a handful of roasted corn and only Coca an Indian will travel a hundred miles afoot, keeping pace with a horse or mule."[34]

The researches of Dr. Weddell, a French botanist who went to South America with the scientific expedition of Count de Castelnau, sent out by Louis Philippe in 1845, not only confirmed, but harmonized the writings of those who had previously described the sustenance from this leaf.

[32] Tschudi; 1839. [33] Martius; 1840. [34] Valdez; 1844.

Though his researches were chiefly directed to the study of cinchona, his travels necessarily took him through the Coca regions. He visited the forests of Caravaya and Sandia, and the valley of Santa Ana, near Cuzco, all prolific Coca districts, where he had favorable opportunity for carefully examining the method of raising and preparing the leaf for the market. The commendations and carefully written details of this scientist gave a marked and added interest abroad to the economic use of Coca.[35]

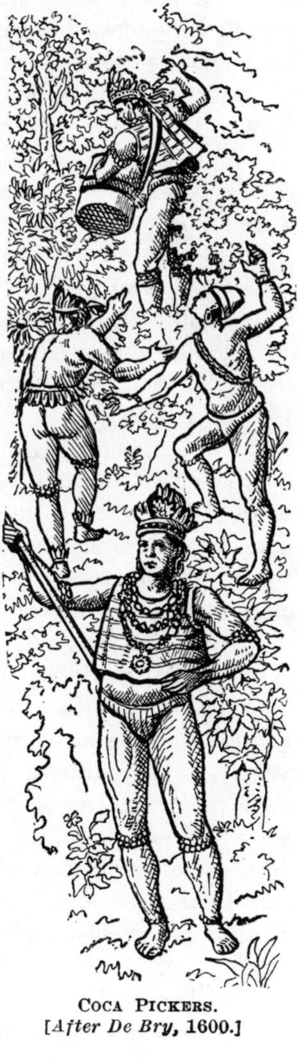

COCA PICKERS.
[*After De Bry,* 1600.]

These facts of travellers and naturalists have been elaborated by the historians, and Prescott, in his story of the *Conquest of Peru*, and Helps, in the *Spanish Conquest in America,* have embodied the salient points regarding the efficacy of Coca, or *Erythroxylum Peruvianum,* as the former as well as Miller terms it. Mr. Prescott had voluminous manuscripts at his disposal in the compilation of his famous work, with ample opportunity to verify statements. He particularly alludes to the assertion of Poeppig as to the injurious influence of Coca, of which he says: "Strange that such baneful properties should not be the subject of more frequent comment by other writers! I do not remember to have seen them even adverted to."[36]

A scientist who rendered particularly valuable service in the interest of cinchona was the English

[35] Weddell; 1853. [36] Prescott; *Note;* Vol. I, p. 143; 1848.

botanist, Richard Spruce, whose name is associated with one variety of Coca. He went to South America in 1849, and for ten years devoted himself to a study of the flora along the Amazon and tributary streams. His researches were varied and extensive, particularly in mosses and the *Hepaticæ*. Among his collections were examples of twenty or more native languages, while the botanical specimens numbered thousands of species, examples of which have enriched the herbarium at Kew. Dr. Spruce remarked the dependence for support which the Indians of the Rio Negro placed in the constant chewing of a certain variety of Coca. The powdered leaves were mixed with tapioca and the ashes of *imbauba—cecropia peltata*—as a *llipta*. With a chew of this in his cheek, he said, the Indian would travel two or three days without food or without a desire to sleep.

Though many expeditions had been made through Peru in behalf of other powers, it was not until 1854 that the United States government sent an exploratory expedition under Lieutenants Gibbon and Herndon in search of the source of the Amazon. Many facts pertaining to the customs of the Indians, and the use of Coca in the districts these officials travelled, are embodied in their entertaining narrative report to Congress. Herndon, while in the valley of Chinchao, where the cultivation of Coca commences in the northern montaña—between the central and eastern Cordilleras—mentions a visit to Señor Martius at his *hacienda* of Cucheros. The Señor told him this *quebrada* produced seven hundred *cargas*, or mule loads of two hundred and sixty pounds each, yearly. The value of such a crop at Huanuco, estimated at three dollars the *arroba* of twenty-five pounds, would make the gross yield $21,840, which, requiring seven hundred mules for transportation at a rate of $4 apiece, would reduce the earnings to about $19,000, though many of the small farms in the neighborhood then sold their Coca on the spot for two dollars the *arroba*.[37]

At Tarma the expedition separated, Herndon to follow the head waters of the Amazon, while Gibbon was to seek the

[37] Herndon and Gibbon; Vol. I, p. 129, *et seq.*; 1853.

source of the Madre de Dios—or, as it is termed in Quichua, *Amaru Mayu,* or snake river—and explore the Bolivian tributaries. The route led Gibbon to Cuzco, where he had opportunity to observe the industry about the royal city among cocals which had been plantations ever since the time of the Incas. As a rule Coca is grown in a small way by farmers who till their own land, but in a frontier settlement was seen a cocal which gave employment to a hundred laborers.[38]

There is a legend of the naming of the southern tributary of the Amazon by Padre Revello. The savage Chunchos, who are much feared in this region, at one time made a raid upon a neighboring settlement, killed the Christianized Indians, and destroyed their little church, throwing the sacred images into the stream. These were carried to the *Amaru Mayu,* where they rested upon a rock and afforded a suggestive hint for christening these waters, "Madre de Dios," by which name they have since been known. The most inveterate *coqueros* consider the Coca grown on the tributaries of the Madre de Dios, in Peru, to be superior to that produced along the waters of the Beni, in Bolivia. These two streams have their origin near to each other, between the gold washings of Tipuani and Caravaya, but a separating ridge of mountains causes the Madre de Dios to flow directly into the Amazon, while the Beni goes to the Madeira River.

The markets of La Paz are well supplied with fruits and vegetables from Yungas[39] on the Beni, and at one time nearly five hundred thousand baskets of Coca of seventy pounds each were annually produced there.

Of the wages paid to Coca cultivators who are unfortunate enough to be compelled to farm for others, it is related that the superintendent of a cocal below the valley of Cochabamba in Bolivia, received his shelter, scant cotton clothing, and fifteen dollars a year, a pittance sadly reduced by tithes to the Church.[40] Yet this man was not happy! He longed for the gay days in his native town of Socaba, where he might

[38] Herndon and Gibbon; Vol. II, pp. 46-47; 1854.
[39] *Yuncu* in Quichua implies a tropical valley, and Yungas is its Spanish corruption.
[40] Herndon and Gibbon; Vol. II, p. 185; 1854.

indulge in an occasional cup of *chicha* instead of impersonating "the man with the hoe" all day long in the Coca patch.

An epoch in the introduction of Coca to the medical men of Europe was marked by the *prize essay* of Dr. Paolo Mantegazza, published at Milan on his return after a residence in Peru, where he had been engaged in practice. He refers to the employment of Coca not only as a medicine but also as an article of food, a use not confined to the rich, like luxuries usually, but which, on the contrary, is prevalent among the working Indians, who enjoy Coca as a nutriment and restorative. So that a laborer in contracting for work bargains not only for the money which he shall receive but the amount of Coca which shall be furnished him.

"The child and the feeble old man seize with eagerness the leaves of the wonderful herb, and find in it indemnification for all suffering and misery."[41]

Contemporary with these writings was the labor of Mr. Clements Markham, who visited Peru in 1859, for the purpose of collecting specimens of cinchona to establish its cultivation in India. This gentleman is a scholar of South American literature, and has rendered available to English readers the knowledge of the doings of the Spanish conquerors through translations of their early writings. His intimate study of Incan customs and the affairs of modern Peru, enables authoritative statements.

Of Coca he says: "Its properties are to enable a greater amount of fatigue to be borne with less nourishment, and to prevent the occurrence of difficulty in respiration in ascending steep mountain sides. Tea made from the leaves has much the taste of green tea, and if taken at night is much more effective in keeping people awake. Applied externally, Coca moderates the rheumatic pains caused by cold, and cures headaches. When used to excess, it is like everything else, prejudicial to the health, yet of all the narcotics used by man Coca is the least injurious and the most soothing and invigorating. I chewed Coca, not constantly, but frequently, from the day of my departure from Sandia, and besides the agree-

[41] Mantegazza; 1859.

able soothing feeling it produced, I found that I could endure long abstinence from food with less inconvenience than I should otherwise have felt, and it enabled me to ascend precipitous mountain sides with a feeling of lightness and elasticity and without losing breath. This latter quality ought to recommend its use to members of the Alpine Club, and to walking tourists in general. To the Peruvian Indian Coca is a solace which is easily procured, which affords great enjoyment and which has a most beneficial effect. The shepherd watching his flock has no other nourishment."[42]

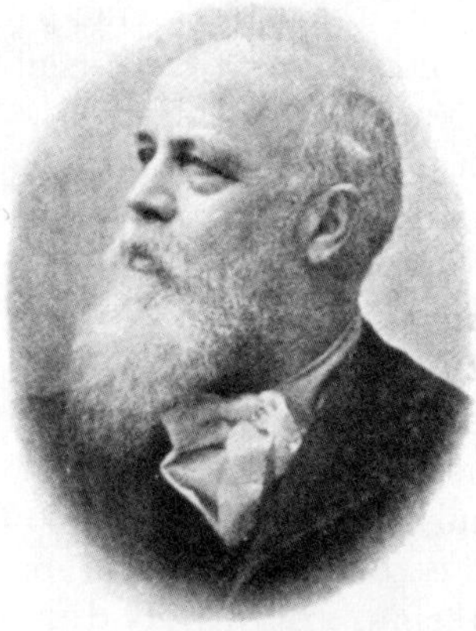

ANGELO MARIANI.

But just as the mass of Peruvian manuscript in Spanish and native Quichua was of little utility to the working world until rendered so by the practical hand of the translator, so the wonderful qualities of Coca remained locked as a scientific mystery unsolvable by the multitude, until it was finally released from its enchanted spell as through some magic touch of a modern Merlin.

It has been said that a man is created for some especial work, and this seems happily applied in the present instance. Angelo Mariani was born in Bastia, the largest city of Corsica, where a foundation for scientific training through an ancestry of physicians and chemists preceded him. But better than ancestry is the work that a man does which shall live after him. Reared in an atmosphere where chemical possibilities were daily thoughts—while united with these was a love for books, and allied art and antiquities—it seemed but natural that he should experiment on the then much talked of Coca of the Incas, an ideal of endurance, interest in

[42] Markham; p. 152 *et seq.;* 1862.

which the tales of travellers and scientists from Cieza to Mantegazza had only intensified. The problem of the elixir of life, so baffling to philosophers since long before the days of Hermes Trismegistus, which many now believed was pent up in Coca—seemed capable of as definite solution as is possible through human intervention. Commencing investigation with the unmistakable evidence regarding the properties of Coca, it was sought to present these in a positive and available form, which fluid and solid extracts, or the volatile herb, had not uniformly preserved. Experimentation led to combining several varieties of leaf, setting aside those which contained chiefly the bitter principle—since known to be cocaine—and selecting those which contained the aromatic alkaloids. An extract of these blended leaves embodied in a wholesome wine, was found to represent the peculiar virtue of Coca as so much prized by the native users.

There is no secret other than method claimed in the process which has made the name of its inventor synonymous with that of Coca, though I heard an anecdote related of this gentleman—who personally scrutinizes every detail of manufacture, that: "after everything else is done he goes around and drops something else in." Whether this be so or not, it is certain that the preparations of Coca manufactured by Mariani are entirely different in aroma and action from other Coca preparations which I have examined. These latter have not the agreeable flavor of Coca, but the fluid extracts are usually bitter and the wines have a peculiar birch-like taste comparable with the smell of an imitation Russia leather. That this "musty cellar flavor," as it is technically termed, is due to the quality of Coca leaf was evidenced by a preparation of wine made for me in Paris in the fall of 1898, from choice leaves direct from the Caravaya district, which, however, were rich in cocaine.

It seems appropriate in a history of Coca that I should say something of the personality of one whose life work has been devoted to rendering the "divine herb" popular. It may be said that Coca is the hobby of Mariani. It is his recreation, his relaxation and constant source of pleasure, wholly removed from sordid commercial interests. At Neuilly, on the Seine, Paris, France, where his laboratory is located, his study is tastefully arranged with rich tapestries and carvings, in which the exquisite designs possible from conventionalizing the Coca leaf and flower are so artistically used as the motif of decoration that they are not obtrusive but must be pointed out in order to be recognized. Here he has extensive conservatories, which are filled with thousands of Coca plants of various species, among which he takes the greatest delight in experimenting upon peculiarities of growth and cultivation. From this collection specimen plants have been freely distributed to botanical gardens in all parts of the world.

As I had difficulty in preserving appropriate examples of the Peruvian shrub for my study, ten choice Coca plants were sent to me from Neuilly, and these, for proper care and preservation, I presented to the New York Botanical Garden, while still being permitted to continue my experiments upon them. In addition to this courtesy, I have been the recipient of numerous favors from M. Mariani, who has generously accorded me details upon the subject of research not readily obtainable elsewhere, and who literally extended the resources of his vast establishment to the furtherance of my investigation. Aside from papers in current journals Mariani wrote a monograph upon Coca and its therapeutic application, a translation of which by Mr. J. N. Jaros, of this city, has been the most available authority for the English reader.[43]

I am convinced no more happy realization can occur to this savant than the knowledge that his efforts to render Coca popular and available have met with a spontaneous approval from representative personages in various parts of the world. Entirely aside from any personal interest, a voluminous testimony has literally showered in from those whose motive and sincerity must be accepted as an unquestionable regard for recognized merit. Eminent artists and sculptors have painted and chiseled some dainty examples which serve to typify their esteem for a modern elixir vitæ. Roty, President of the *Academie des Beaux Arts,* and probably the most eminent liv-

[43] Mariani; 1888.

ing medalist, has executed a presentation medal of appreciation. Famous musical composers, such as Gounod, Faure, Ambrose Thomas, Massenet, and many others have sung their hosannas in unique bars of manuscript melody. Poets and writers without number have versed the qualities of the Coca leaf and the present happy idealization of its powers. Royalty has set upon it the meritorious seal of patronage, and the modern Church, more liberal than its edicts of long ago, has welcomed its use. Only recently Pope Leo XIII sent a golden medal of his ecclesiastical approval, for it is said that for years His Holiness has been supported in his ascetic retirement by a preparation of Mariani's Coca, of which a flask constantly worn is, like the widow's cruse, never empty.

So numerous have been these expressions from eminent characters of the day, that it has been possible to compile from them a cyclopedia of contemporary biography which has already reached several large octavo volumes. A brief outline of each notable is given, with an etched portrait, and often accompanied by a sketch showing some known forte of the individual. Where these are artists their impromptu illustrations display a happy humor associated with their characteristic touch. The resultant compilations, exquisitely printed and bound as an *edition de luxe,* are much sought by bibliophiles. A short time since, while the Princess of Battenberg was on a visit at Nice, she was presented with one of these copies, and in acknowledging the courtesy suggested that her mother, the Queen of England, would be delighted to have one for her private library. In fulfillment of such a hint, which was accepted as an imperial command, two sets, especially illuminated by Atalaya, were forwarded to Her Majesty, who wrote that she considered them among the finest specimens in her collection.

With this first advance in securing the properties of the leaf in convenient form for use, came the important re-

---

Description of Mariani's Coca Garden on opposite page.

1. The Salon, in Conventional Coca Designs by Courboin. 2. A Corner of the Coca Conservatory. 3. Garden Looking toward Conservatory. 4. Plastic Leather Modeling by Saint André. 5. Conventional Binding by Meunier. 6. Coca Nymph by Rivière. 7. In the Palm House.

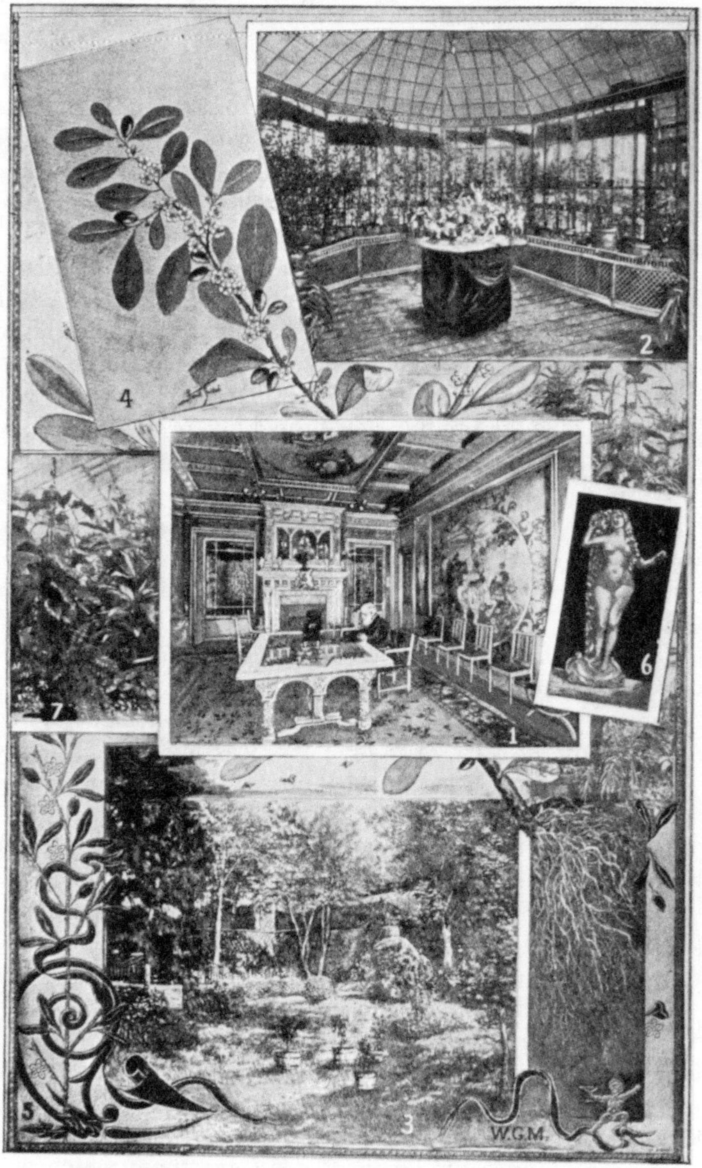

MARIANI'S COCA GARDEN, NEUILLY ON THE SEINE, PARIS, FRANCE.
[For description see opposite page.]

searches of Niemann upon the alkaloids of the Coca leaf. The work of this investigator was speedily followed by a host of ardent experimenters, as is recounted in the chapter which relates some of the chemical problems involved in Coca. The more pronounced advantages, however, which were to benefit all humanity, were not immediately utilized, and for nearly a generation cocaine was regarded as but an expensive curiosity of the laboratory.

In 1884 the attention of the scientific world was suddenly concentrated on the remarkable possibilities of the Coca leaf through the discoveries of Dr. Carl Koller, on the application of cocaine to the surgery of the eye. Manufacturing chemists turned their attention to the parent plant, for there was a desire to make the product now brought so prominently into great demand as to be held at exorbitant prices. An incident will serve to illustrate its rarity at that time. I was then on the staff of physicians at the hospitals of the almshouse, Blackwell's Island, and through a former interest as a pharmacist in the study of Coca, was desirous of obtaining some of the new alkaloid. Upon requisition a supply of about a drachm of a two per cent. solution of cocaine was sent for use in a service of some two thousand patients.

Among my classmates, in the medical department of the University of the City of New York, was my friend Henry H. Rusby, then regarded as a botanist of great promise, and at present Professor of Materia Medica of that university and of the New York College of Pharmacy. Immediately after his graduation he went to South America on a botanical expedition for Parke, Davis & Co., and they forwarded instructions to him to devote sufficient time to study Coca in its native home.[44] The result of his research is full of interest as showing the similarity between modern customs of Coca cultivation, as compared with the descriptions of the early Spanish historians. These investigations were chiefly carried out in the district of Coroico, of the Yungas of Bolivia. This botanist was the first to clearly show that: "the best quality of Coca leaves, to a manufacturing chemist, means those which will

[44] *Person. com.;* Parke, Davis & Co.; March, 1898.

yield the largest percentage of crystallizable cocaine, while the same leaf might be considered for domestic consumption as representing one of the lower grades." For, as he has explained: "The Indian selects a Coca rich in the aromatic and sweet alkaloids instead of the bitter leaf in which cocaine is predominant."[45] Since 1885, most of the writings and the experiments of physiologists upon Coca seem to have been based upon the idea of a single active principle which should represent the potency of the leaf. As is clearly indicated in the history which has been traced through nearly four centuries, this is a false supposition. The qualities of Coca are not fully represented by any one of its alkaloids thus far isolated.

[45] Rusby; *person. com.*; 1898.

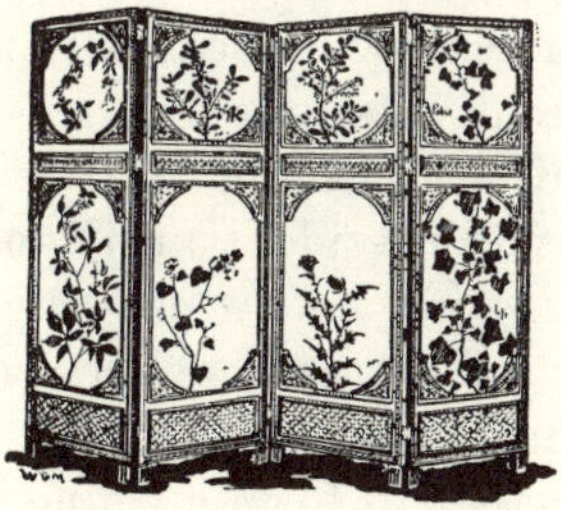

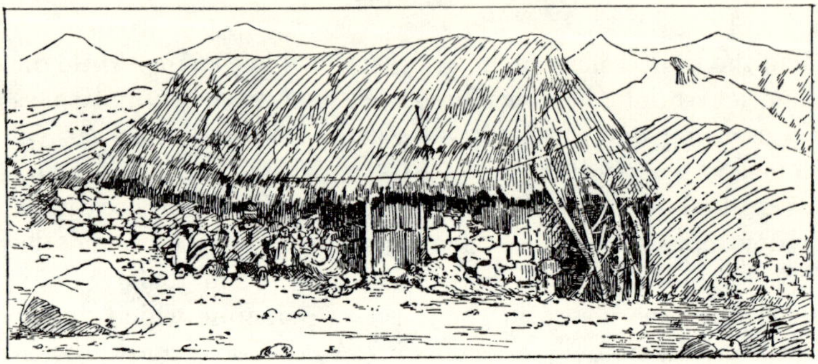

CHAPTER VII.

THE PRESENT INDIANS OF PERU.

> "Three Leaves supply for six days' march afford.
> The *Quitoita* with this Provision stor'd
> Can pass the vast and cloudy Andes o'er."
>
> —*Cowley.*

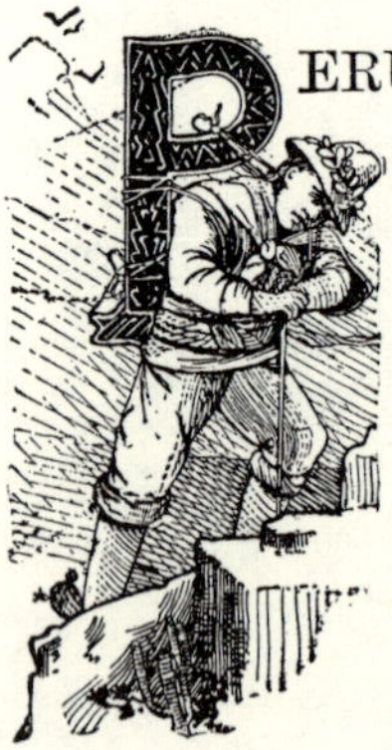

PERU is divided into nineteen departments, which are similar to our States. At the head of government is a president, the chief executive, whose term of office is four years, and who cannot be re-elected nor elected as vice-president until an equal period has elapsed. There are two vice-presidents, and affairs are in charge of ministers representing the several departments meeting together to form a council, the functions of which are similar to our Congress. Each department is under the head of a prefect, and is sub-divided into provinces under sub-prefects, while these are divided into districts each in charge of a *curaca*—governor—under whom are the alcaldes, who look after the best interest of—themselves—the governor and lesser villagers.

The alcaldes, who are commonly Indians, belong to a class of very consequential chaps, exceedingly proud of their position. They carry a staff of office, a sort of long walking stick, with a large copper head and copper ferrules around the stick, which indicate their years of service. Every alcalde has a half dozen or more henchmen under him; these each carry a staff of office and collect the Indians when necessary for any designated labor, to which all are obliged to go when assigned, at a pay agreed upon by the governor, an individual who not only arranges the terms, but often pockets the fees as well.

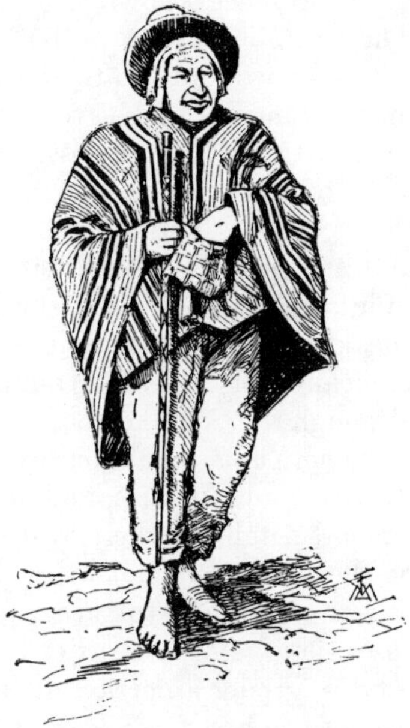

ANDEAN ALCALDE.
[*From a Photograph.*]

The present people of Peru comprise foreigners, creoles who are native born, Indians, *mestizos* who are part Indian, negroes, mulattos, and *zambos* —part Indian and part negro. The upper class is mainly of pure Spanish blood, and, as indicated by their names, their ancestry represented every part of Spain. Some of the Indians are of Incan stock, from which the native pride always endeavors to trace an ancient lineage. Indians are often spoken of collectively, but in Peru there are several types under this designation, each of which is wholly distinct from the other in feature, color and characteristics. Like the absolute variation of climate which this land displays in accordance with locality, so the Peruvian Indians vary with their environment, but the real difference is dependent upon heredity. There are the *Cholas* of the coast, and the *Serranos* —or *Indios de la Sierra*—or *Cholas de la Sierra,* living in the mountains. These are both civilized and more or less educated; then there are the savage Indians—*Indios silvestros*, literally wood Indians—located east of the Andes, upon tributaries of the Amazon. The term *Chunchos* or *Antis* usually covers all of this latter class, although there are many small tribes with differing names and customs. The savage Indians are very much feared, having resisted all efforts to civilize them, being "no Christianos," as the Andeans say of them. They are not very often seen, but occasionally make their presence known near the banks of some of the rivers. They wander about perfectly naked through the forests by tracks known only to themselves, armed with bow and arrows made from the tough wood of the *chonta* palm. They make their attacks just at dawn, and come like the wind, no one knows from whence, leaving only their depredations to mark their course. The women of these people do their hard work, and are probably representatives of the original type of the fabulous stories of the fierce Amazonian fighters. When speaking of the Andean it is the Indian of the mountains that is meant, for the coast Indians do not go into the mountains, although the Serrano goes to the coast.

The Cholas are a happy and contented lot. They gather in little communities, and are usually busy, either in working a small patch for their own necessities or else laboring in one of the many *haciendas,* in the cultivation of cotton, grapes, olives, or some of the other products of the valleys. In some cases they become a sort of half serf-like tenantry of the larger estates, giving a portion of their time and work for the privilege of a house, for it seems but natural to them that they shall always be subservient to a master. As a class they are kindly and gentle, not exactly lazy, for they are always busy at something, but listless and without ambition, while their wants are easily satisfied. Maize and potatoes in varied form, with some few vegetables and fruits, constitute their commoner articles of food, though they are not averse to a liberal dietary when occasion permits, and will relish a meal of fowl, beef, mutton, goat, or even their favorite guinea pig. Frugal as their methods of living may be, the same spirit of hospitality cultivated in Incan times is still spontaneous between themselves and towards those whites whom they like, though in this latter case it is always with the humility of a servant to his master.

The Indians delight to participate in the numerous festivals, which are everywhere frequent among them, for throughout Peru there are more *fiestas* than working days; and upon these occasions not only the villages, but even the larger cities, put on gala array, and there is an abandonment of all cares for the present jollity. The festival which precedes Easter Sunday is always particularly grand, when fun and revelry runs riot, and one is unusually fortunate who is not showered with flour or sprinkled with scented water from one of the numerous *chisquetas,* a trick in which the ladies seem to take particular delight. On these gala days there are booths established just for the occasion, where all the holiday folk dine, for like the coming of a country circus in one of our smaller towns, the festivities make the women too busy to waste time on household duties. These people have a numerous lot of peculiar dishes very highly seasoned, which are offered at these times. Perhaps it may be the tough goat served in a savory *seco*—or stew with rice and sweet potatoes, or the more crisp *chicharones*—the pieces of pork separated from the fat in rendering lard, or *salchichones*—which are what we should denominate sausages, or *tamales*—a sort of highly seasoned meat dumpling made from pork and chicken, with an outer paste of ground maize, and steamed in wrappings of maize leaves. Then there is the stew of beef in a *salsa picante,* seasoned hotly with *aji,* or the more tempting *churasco*—a fried steak prepared with onions and served with an egg, suited as an appetizing breakfast for a hungry man anywhere. In many of their dishes they use *achote*, from which *annotta* is made, imparting an apparent warmth in color, which an unstinting use of *aji,* the native red pepper, manifests in reality. There are numerous indigenous species of this pepper, which is used throughout Peru in everything eatable. They are sweet, strong and far superior to anything of the kind in our markets. Then there is the delicious *dulces,* a sort of guava jelly-like preserve of native fruits, so sweet that the eating provokes a thirst for water, which suggests the dietetic maxim: "*Tomar dulce, para beber agua.*"[1]

[1] Take sweets in order to drink water.

On all festal occasions alcoholic beverages in numerous forms are not forgotten, and *capitas,* or offerings of drink, are gratuitous. The Indian followers of Bacchus often drink themselves into one continuous drunk, that ends only with their own incapacity for obtaining more liquor; and these poor fellows are killing themselves from an unrestricted use of alcoholics; it matters not so much as to the method as to the quantity, either raw alcohol or *chicha.* This latter, which is made from corn, has been the celestial drink of the country since the time of the Incas, when it was known as *acca.* To witness its brewing would scarcely excite a profound thirst in the traveller from more enlightened parts. Usually chicha is made in a primitive way by old women, who chew the bruised maize kernels, the mass being ejected into a vat, when it is boiled with water, and then subjected to fermentation. Notwithstanding this loathsome means of preparation, it has been asserted that the resultant product is superior to that made from the more prosaic method of grinding the maize in a mill, which is viewed by the natives as an innovation, yet probably the bulk of manufacture of this liquor is now made in this more civilized way. The product is a preparation of varying strength, all the way from sour water to a strongly spirituous liquor. It is sometimes termed Peruvian beer, but is really neither wine nor beer; possibly resembling more closely the Russian *kwiss,* a sort of cider sometimes made from bread. Some chicha is sparkling, and the different regions in which it is prepared vie with each other in its manufacture by adding little extra delicacies to it, such as chicken, which may increase the local repute. In the primitive method of making this drink, where the corn is chewed, there is, of course, a probability that the ptyalin of the saliva has some very de-

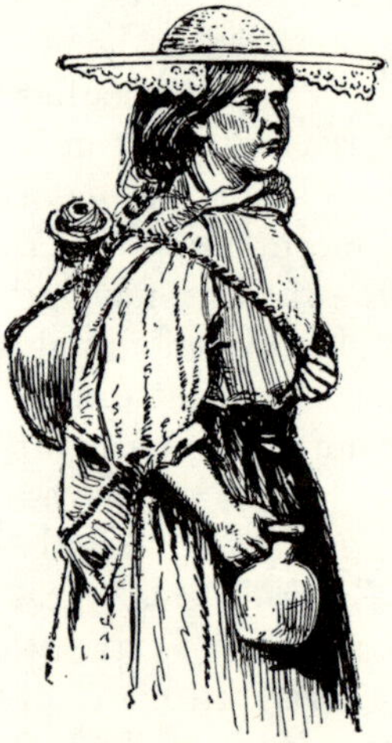

A Chicha Seller.
[*From a Photograph.*]

cided influence in regulating the flavor through its malting action on the grain, which would be absent in the more improved process. In one case the result might yield a product more nearly resembling beer; in the other a more pronounced spirit resembling whiskey.

Chicha was the royal drink of the Incas, and though not considered sacred as was Coca, which was always carried about the person of the nobles, their doings were often sealed with a royal bumper. Thus, when Pizarro established Manco on the throne, the ceremonies for his coronation were studiously observed. The young prince kept the prescribed fasts and vigils, and on the appointed day the nobles and people, with the whole Spanish soldiery, assembled in the great square at Cuzco to witness the concluding ceremony, which was sanctified by offerings of Coca made by the high priest, and completed by pledging the Spanish commander in a golden goblet of sparkling chicha.

The laboring class of the Peruvian coast is chiefly comprised of negroes, many of whom are descendants of the slaves imported during the first years of the Conquest, when it was found that the Indians were not adapted to successfully cultivate the then newly introduced sugar, cotton and grapes. There are also a number of Chinese laborers who, first brought here in 1849, were continued to cheaply supplant the negro slaves, who had since been made free, and these Chinamen have fallen into a sort of contract slavery from which they cannot seem to escape. There are many German settlements throughout Peru, together with some French, Italian and Portuguese, and many of the larger industries of the country are furthered by capital from England and by the enterprise of the United States.

Lima, eight and a half miles from the sea, at an altitude of four hundred and forty-eight feet, is situated in a fertile sloping delta. The city has over one hundred thousand inhabitants, a cosmopolitan place, with many and diverse interests, and with social qualities manifested through numerous clubs and scientific societies. The sanitary condition of the city is excellent; there is a good water supply and well constructed sewers, which are flushed from the river, and modern improvements, such as gas, electric lights and telephones, have been introduced everywhere, and there are several miles of street railways. The churches are numerous, and the imposing cathedral is filled with relics; among these there lies in the crypt the embalmed remains of Francisco Pizarro. The society of the capital is brilliant and exclusive, the beauty of the Limaian ladies being proverbial, while much to the chagrin of the traveller in search of the fanciful, they are clothed similarly to the better classes in any civilized community, their gowns being even rigorously patterned after the latest Parisian models. What an element of disappointment it is to go thousands of miles from home and find a continuance of the same customs which are conventional! And yet in this picturesque land there is sufficient that is unique even among the habits of the better class; for though the *saya y manto* of earlier days has been cast aside, the ladies commonly wear a lace fichu thrown over the head and shoulders, which lends charm to a graceful carriage. There are two medical schools in Lima—the College of San Toribio and La Academia Libre de Medicina. Foreign physicians have little repute unless they have been educated in France. The capital is well advanced in the sciences, indeed, education maintains a very high standard in every department, and the growing element often displays a cleverness akin to precocity. Lima has one of the best appointed general hospitals outside of Europe. It occupies an entire square, and the original cost was $1,000,000. Twelve wards, each bearing the name of a saint, radiate from a great central garden which extends between the several wards. There are two public gardens, one devoted to botany, the other to the study of botany and zoology.

Throughout Peru the morals of the people are good. The Indians are punctilious in the observance of conventionalities in accordance with their point of view. Few of them are legally married, for a religious ceremony would be too ex-

---

DESCRIPTION OF VIEWS OF LIMA, PLATE I., ON OPPOSITE PAGE.

1. General View and Cathedral. 2. The Port of Callao. 3. Calle Mercaderes. 4. Plaza de Armas. 5. San Augustin. 6. Santo Domingo. 7. San Francisco.

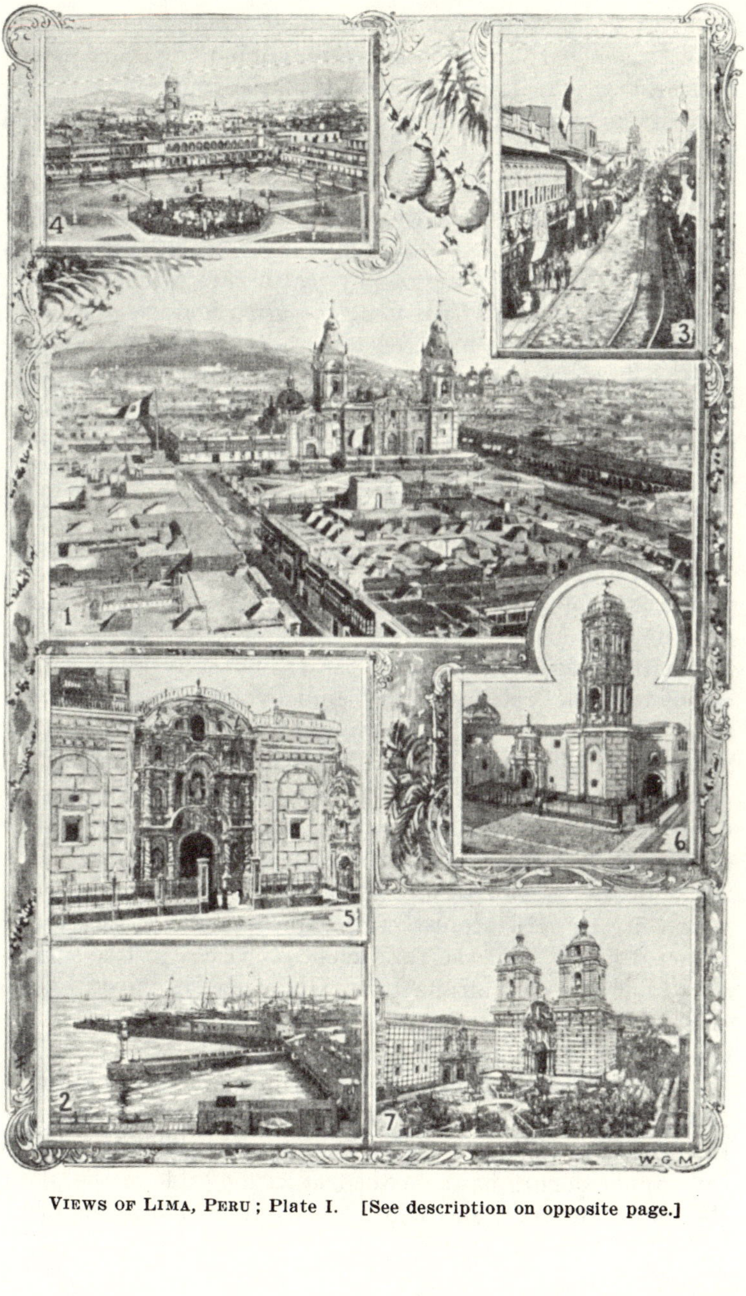

VIEWS OF LIMA, PERU; Plate I. [See description on opposite page.]

pensive; yet prostitution, as we understand it, is unknown among them. Here, as in all warm climates, Nature brings her children to maturity very early, and at fourteen or fifteen years some of these Indian girls are quite pretty, with the actual large gazelle-like eyes so often quoted, perfect teeth, glossy black hair, and with the blush of the rose stealing through a thin dark skin, while their figures, voluptuous, yet chastely molded and graceful, display a wealth of charms which only the awakening of physical nature teaches them is distinctive. At one of the many *fiestas* a maiden may meet some man who shows preference for her and who later manifests his love through small presents and slight attentions, but wooings are brief in this poetic land of the sun; the parents are consulted as a matter of course, just as during the old Incan days. If they give their consent to a union, all well and good, but should they oppose it the would-be husband takes his bride-elect to his home, where she is recognized as his wife, and from thenceforth his dominion over her is supreme, and she will continue faithful to her lord and master.

The Catholic religion is the state worship of Peru, which the Indians accept kindly, for they are greatly interested in ceremonies, and religion with them is often only the outward and visible sign without the inward spiritual grace. They celebrate all the feasts of the Church, and their offspring are now named after every saint in the calendar, instead of after natural objects, as was the custom in Incan days. They know their children must be baptized, while confession seems essential, and the sign of the cross appears to them a ceremonial which must guard against every danger. A candle burned before a saint brings the fulfillment of wishes just as sure as a scapular will ward off the devil. They live in the consciousness that the good see heaven and the bad are burned, active consummations, which seem practical to them.

The chief cities of Peru cannot be outrivaled for churches, for one cannot look out of a window in any important town of that country without seeing several, while every village that can support a *cura* has a "cathedral" at one side of the plaza, the importance of which is out of all proportion to the place, and from which bells may be heard in discordant clanging through almost every hour. Since the days of the conquerors the missionary work of the Catholics has been so persistently and aggressively effectual that the ecclesiastics still continue a ruling power which it may not always be well to ignore, even though they may not manifest this power through a personal goodness. Some of these spiritual instructors neither display the abstemiousness nor that rigid celibacy which was so markedly characteristic of the Incan priesthood, and often the village *padre* is father to more sins of commission than to those of omission. There is almost a constant succession of church festivals, and ceremonial processions are very common in the streets. Whenever the bishop passes in holy array he is preceded by a bearer of a staff of bells, the jingling of which is a signal for every one within sight to kneel, a subservience which is rigidly enforced by the police. At times bearers go about with little boxes with a glass front, under which is a picture or image of some saint which has been blessed by the Church. In the bottom of the box is a drawer filled with little cotton balls attached to bits of string. The glass is kissed as a salutation to the image, which is regarded with great veneration, but the full benefit from this respect does not become effectual unless *largess* be given to the carrier, in which case one of the cotton balls is given in return, and these little tufts are commonly worn on festal occasions. At some of the principal festivals of the Church small altars are erected in front of private houses, and the religious procession passes from one to another of these places with appropriate ceremony. At Christmas time there is usually open house everywhere, and it is customary to display a miniature scene of the manger at Bethlehem, which is set out with plaster figures or even simple toys, or perhaps among the very poor with merely playing cards. All are welcome on these occasions to the good cheer offered.

The Serranos are considered direct descendants of the Incan race. They are commonly referred to by writers as "Quichua," a term not applied to them at all in Peru, but only to their language. These Indians of the mountains have been

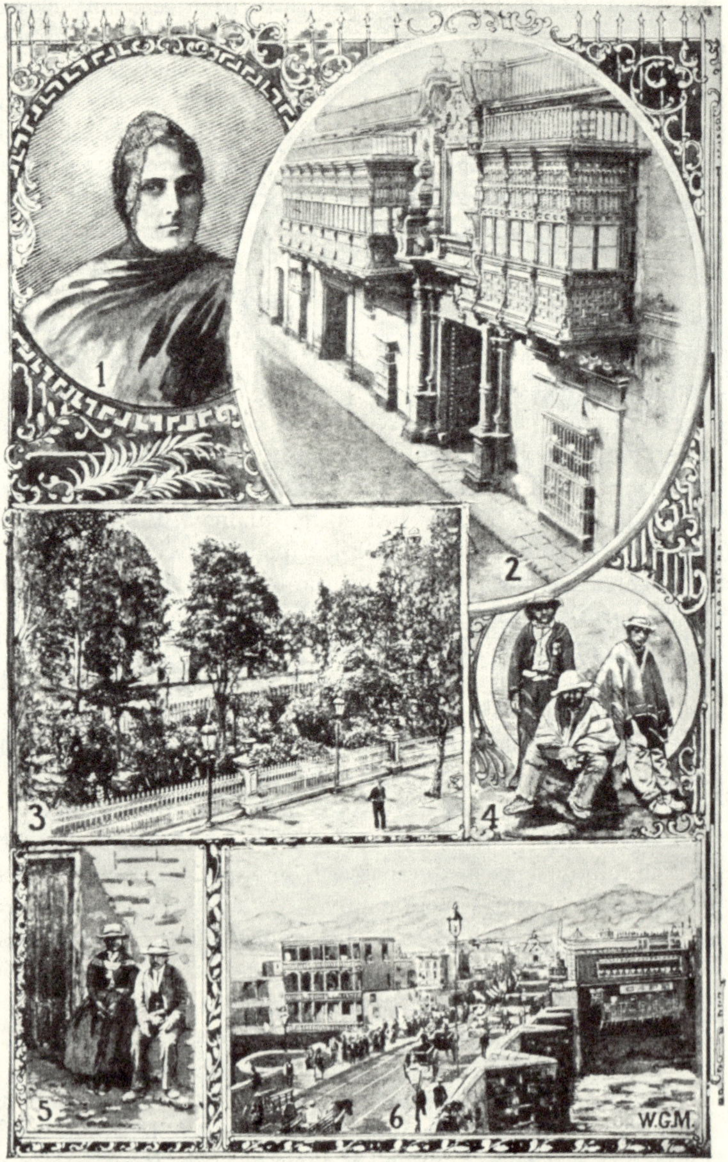

VIEWS OF LIMA, PERU; Plate II. [See description on opposite page.]

so much influenced through environment and the heredity of oppression that, while their customs have changed but little since the days of the Incan dynasty, the race has sadly deteriorated. If we consider the present Andeans as descendants of the lower order of the early empire, then it is doubtless they are still much as Garcilasso wrote some fifty years after the Conquest: "The common people, as they are a poor, miserable lot, do not aspire to things higher than those to which they have been accustomed." The Indians are naturally reticent, and can only be drawn into conversation when they become attached to a person, but once enlisted they would prefer working for nothing to receiving good wages from a stranger. They are very respectful, and subservience is inborn, while their usual expression depicts a profound despair, as though of the hopelessness of the condition of their race; yet, on being drawn into conversation, they often prove good talkers. During the time of the Incas it was said that no one was permitted to enter the presence of the sovereign, or, indeed, to enter the royal city, unless bearing a burden as a token of his humility,[2] and to this day the poor Indian realizes that he is so essentially a burden bearer that if met on the road without a pack he seems to feel it is absolutely necessary that he should apologize, or make some explanation for his want of a load; and even though he should not be questioned, he will tell you, "I am going on an errand; that is why I have no *ccepi*."*

These Serranos live in adobe huts which are built from blocks made of chopped straw and clay, molded in a box possibly a foot square, and dried in the sun, the blocks being set and plastered with wet clay. The huts are thatched with the long ychu grass, and usually have but one low door and no window or chimney. The Incan costume was prohibited after the Conquest, and now the common dress of the men is a short-skirted baize coat, which they prefer either of blue or green, with a red vest and black breeches open at the knee, or com-

[2] Salcamayhua. * *Ccepi*—burden, Quichua.

DESCRIPTION OF VIEWS OF LIMA, PLATE II., ON OPPOSITE PAGE.

1. Type of Limeños Beauty. 2. Old Spanish Balcony. 3. Plaza of Santa Ana. 4. Chola Types. 5. Chola Types. 6. Bajada del Puente.

monly two pair of trousers which are well turned up. This usual costume may be supplemented by a poncho, and an additional poncho worn over the shoulders serves to carry packages. Their legs and feet are usually bare, though at times they wear knitted woolen stockings and sandals. For a head covering the usual slouch felt hat is worn, under which the Indians of some of the Eastern provinces wear a knitted skull cap with long side pieces, which are either tied under the chin or left flying. This cap often serves as a convenient hand bag for any small parcel they wish to carry. In other provinces the Indians wear a *montero*, or velvet hat, having a broad brim, covered with cloth and ornamented with tinsel lace

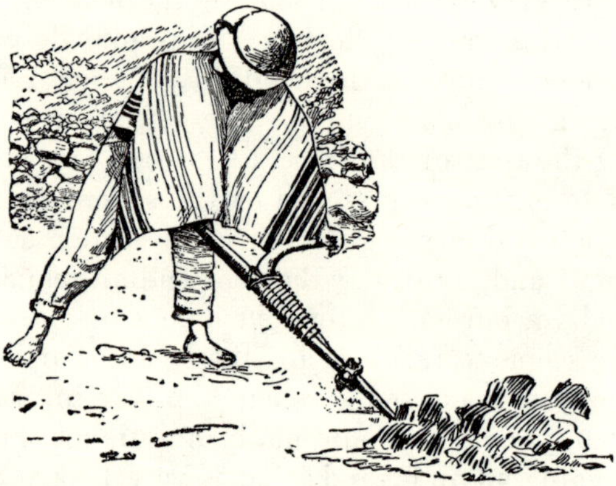

ANDEAN PLOW OR REJKA. [*From a Photograph.*]
See description on page 145.

and colored ribbons. This same style of covering is used by the women, while in some localities they wear an embroidered cloth lying flat on the head and hanging down behind, after the manner of Swiss peasant women. The men wear their hair long except in the front, where it is cut off short, while the women commonly braid theirs into two long strands plaited with wool, which hang down the back. The same little bags known as *chuspas* for carrying Coca leaves, which formed a portion of the vestment of the ancient sovereigns and nobles, are still carried as a constant part of the accoutrement of the present Indians. The women wear bright-colored skirts reaching a little below the knees, and a mantle, or *lliclla,* which is secured over the breast by a large pin, with a head resembling the bowl of a spoon, known as a *topus.* Some of these, in wrought silver, are very pretty and similar in design to patterns which have been found in Incan tombs.

The Indians commonly sing while at their work, and some of their love songs, or *haravis,* that have been continued since the days of the Incas, express very pretty sentiments. Here, for example, is a verse of such a song, descriptive of a lover's return after an absence of many months, which suggests the elfin god in his travels has not neglected the Andeans:

> "At length, my dove! I have returned
> From far distant lands
> With my heart steeped in love;
> O, my dove! come to my arms."

The following verse, which is one of four from a chorus in the drama of Ollantay, is still chanted by the Indians on their long journeys, or at harvest time. It is addressed to the little bird called *tuya,* which commonly eats the corn in the fields, the refrain presumably being an imitation of the bird's call:

> "O, bird, forbear to eat
> The crops of my princess;
> Do not thus rob
> The maize which is her food.
> Tuyallay, Tuyallay."

The Indian mother often quiets her babe to sleep with some plaintive lullaby descriptive of the trials and subjections into which their race has been forced. The following is often heard through the Department of Ayacucho, being a literal translation without rhythm or meter, merely to show the sentiment:

> "My mother begot me, amidst rain and mist,
> To weep like the rain, and be drifted like the clouds.
> You were born in the cradle of sorrow,
> Says my mother, as she gives me the breast;
> She weeps as she wraps me around.
> The rain and mists attacked me
> When I went to meet my lover;

Seeking through the whole world,
I should not meet my equal in misery.
Accursed be my birthday;
Accursed be the night I was born,
From this time forever and ever."[3]

It must not be considered, however, that the Indians are profoundly melancholy, for they are jovial, and even addicted to a keen wit when they feel sufficiently acquainted to talk freely.

Although the language of Peru is Spanish, which is generally spoken by all classes along the coast and through the larger cities, the Serranos continue the Quichua, the ancient language of the Incas, which the conquerors termed "*La lengua general.*" This remains to-day the most widely spread of all South American languages, being spoken not only by the descendants of the Incas, but by many of the Spanish through the interior. The priests of the large cities at certain seasons preach their sermons in this language, while in the Indian villages it is used altogether.

The name Quichua was first applied to that language by Friar Domingo de San Tomas, the first doctor who was graduated at the University of Lima, in his grammar printed at Valladolid, in 1560. The derivation of the word has been traced to a combination of the Indian terms, *quehuasca,* twisted, and *ychu,* straw, literally twisted straw, possibly suggested from the predominance of straw throughout the mountains, and its use by the Indians for every conceivable thing. It is a unique tongue, there being none other found in any part of the globe of which it is even supposed to be a dialect. It lacks our letters b, d, f, g, j, v, w, x and z, the plural being generally formed by adding *cuna,* and the sentence concluding with the verb.[4] Quichua is spoken pure in Cuzco, but elsewhere is so much corrupted through local dialects that what is spoken in one province might not be understood in another. The Bolivian Indians, who resemble those of Peru, originally formed the Collas, one of the early tribes of the

[3] These songs are from Mr. Markham's translations of the Quichua in his work on Cuzco.
[4] Ludewig; *Lit. of Am. Aborig. Lang.*

ancient empire. Their language, known as Aymara, is built upon the same general lines. Humboldt called Quichua "agglutinative," because of the formation of new words by adding particles as affixes to the root, as in some of the Asiatic tongues. A peculiar method of conjugation, which the Jesuits termed "verbal transition," consists in incorporating the accusative—if a pronoun, as well as the nominative—into the verb. Thus, "I love you," or "he loves me," becomes one instead of three words, as *"munayqui,"* or *"munahuanmi."* Perhaps one of the most peculiar features of this tongue is that a man uses a different form of expression from that employed by a woman when speaking of the same person. Thus:

A brother, speaking of his sister, says *panay*.
A sister, speaking of her sister, says *ñañay*.
A sister, speaking of her brother, says *huanquey*.
A brother, speaking of his brother, says *llocsimasiy*.
A father, speaking of his son, says *churiy*.
A mother, speaking of her son, says *ccarihuahuay*.
A father, speaking of his daughter, says *ususiv*.
A mother, speaking of her daughter, says *huarmihuahuay*.

There is also a difference whether the male or the female speaking is related to the side of the father or to that of the mother of the one addressed. In this manner entire sentences are often expressed by one word, very suggestive of some of those German words running across an entire page, which Mark Twain has humorously termed "alphabetical processions."[5]

The Quichua numerals admit of any combination. These are:

1. *Huc.*	6. *Zocta.*
2. *Yzcay.*	7. *Canchiz.*
3. *Quimza.*	8. *Pussac.*
4. *Ttahua.*	9. *Yzcun.*
5. *Pichca.*	10. *Chunca.*

At a period during the vice-royalty it was proposed by the Viceroy, Don Augustin de Jauregui, as one means of remov-

[5] *Innocents Abroad;* p. 611.

ing discontent and furthering complete subjugation, that Quichua should be prohibited, and the Indians compelled to speak Spanish. This was found wholly impracticable, and instead of rooting out the language it was determined—just as had also proved the better policy when it was suggested to exterminate Coca—to improve and cultivate it. Numerous grammars were written, and the language was taught in the colleges, where it has been continued by regularly appointed professors ever since the first chair of Quichua was occupied by Don Juan de Balboa in the University of Lima.

The Incas did not have an alphabet, nor any mode of writing, so that their words, first written phonetically by the Jesuit missionaries, often show many variations in spelling. Garcilasso de la Vega mentions certain hieroglyphics used by the wise men of Cuzco, and Montesinos, who is not always the best authority, declared that in the early ages the use of letters was known among the Incan people, but had been lost during the reign of Yupanqui. A European missionary found among the Panos Indians, on the banks of the Ucayali, a manuscript written on paper made of plantain leaves containing hieroglyphics and separate characters, which was said to be a history of their ancestors. Rivero and Von Tschudi described hieroglyphics cut upon rocks near Arequipa, and also in Hiaytara, and the Province of Castro-Vireyna, and others on the coast near Huara, and there are very many such specimens found over a wide area.

Now that we have formed some acquaintance with the country, with the people and with the Indians, we can better appreciate a trip over the mountains, best done with pack and train, in order to study local customs; for while the modern means of transit may be more comfortable, it offers little opportunity for either scientific study or even a leisurely view of Nature's bounties here presented on every hand. Before we can commence such a journey, there are many details which have to be arranged. *Peons,* or laborers, are to be secured to care for the baggage, and a *piara,* or train of mules, with the *arriero,* or driver, must be engaged to bear the necessary traps of travel. To get these, application must be made to the governor, who notifies the alcalde, and his henchmen round up both mules and men.

It is always difficult, and unless one has considerable influence almost impossible, to secure the necessary mules for transportation. The cost of hire varies with the district from seventy-five cents a day upward, and mules are commonly engaged with the driver, or *arriero*, to travel only their accustomed beat. Hence arrangements must be made for a period of time which will presumably cover this journey of usually about a hundred miles. The drivers push on to consummate this trip speedily, and stragglers must be left behind.

The proper equipment for the road is a heavy box saddle of wood covered with pigskin, with deep knee pads. This affair, which weighs about fifteen pounds, is fastened with two girths to prevent slipping either over the head or tail. With this is worn the pillion—or saddle rug of wool, or silk, spun into a thick fringe-like fur, lined and faced with leather, which serves the traveller as a bed during the journey. Some of the finest of these are worth several hundred dollars. Across this is slung the *alforjas*—or saddle bags, woven from cotton in gaudy colors. In these are carried the clothing and whatever is required for immediate use. The food, which must be so concentrated that it shall take up but little space, usually consists of parched corn, cheese, chocolate, spirits and Coca extract. With this is carried an alcohol lamp, with sufficient fuel to last for about five days. The bridle is of finely braided rawhide, ornamented with silver rings and buckles galore, and the reins terminate in a long lash—*chicote,* which serves as a whip. The stirrups are heavy boxes cut from a single piece of wood, ornamented with carving and silver filigree. These are made heavy for the purpose of protecting the feet from crushing in the narrow passes, while they also serve to shed the rain. Spurs with immense rowels are worn often so heavy that they must be supported by a rest attached to the heel; their rhythmic jangle makes music for the mule and serves to warn a traveller coming from the opposite direction, for in the stillness of the mountain they can be heard for more than a mile. The armament consists of a revolver, worn conveniently, and a carbine carried at the side, for highwaymen who are not Indians, but *mestizo* outcasts, are a possible feature of the lonesome mountain paths. The wraps are a heavy woolen poncho, or a padded overcoat, and heavy woolen gloves with thickly woven wristlets, which serve to prevent the wind from blowing up the sleeves.

For protection against rain a rubber poncho is carried. This is an oblong sheet of heavy rubber cloth with a hole in the centre, through which the head is thrust, the folds serving to

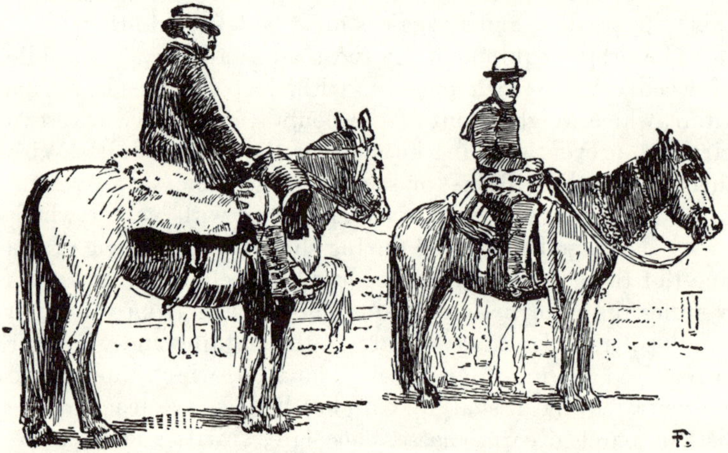

READY FOR THE START. [*From a Photograph.*]
The figure on the left is Captain Zalinski, who invented the dynamite gun.

protect not only the rider, but the flanks of his mount. Double suits of underclothing, paper vests, and fur-lined boots or "arctics," are additional luxuries which serve to keep the traveller warm in the higher altitudes. At night a leather sleeping bag is used, and wrapped in blankets and buttoned up in this bag a bed on barren rocks, sometimes softened by the fleecy snow, seems a luxury. The baggage is commonly carried in small boxes—twenty-two by thirty-two inches—such as are used by the English army officers. When packed these weigh about eighty pounds; one or even two of these may be carried on a mule. They are tin-lined, and the edge is set with rubber to make a water-tight joint, so that they may be completely submerged without the contents getting wet. Sole leather, which would seem to be appropriate for such packages, mildews immediately when wet, and is not suited for travelling over these mountains.

But all of this preparation is only preliminary and in no way assures the probability of an early start, for having engaged and even paid in advance for the service, it will be necessary to keep a close watch over the individual members of the proposed train in order to keep it intact up to the period of starting. It has been suggested that the proper way to set out on such a journey is to harness and load the baggage mules, mount the riding mules, and after a few turns around the square dismount and unpack and—wait patiently until to-morrow to start. *Mañana!*—to-morrow. Everything is put off until to-morrow, after that usual deliberative Spanish habit, which was quickly adopted by the Indians. If you should tell these people you intend to leave in the morning at sunrise it would be very remarkable if, trusted to themselves, they appeared before noon, while before that time even, unless a very close guard has been kept over the train, either mules or men may be missing. When the period for departure actually arrives the Indians throw Coca in the air, just as did the Incan priests of old, to propitiate the gods of the mountains, who, presumably, do not wish their domains invaded; and when by this a successful trip is assured, these people continue faithful and persistent, and thoroughly trustworthy.

From the coast the ascent is usually made through some ravine, which at the outset may be thickly populated and filled with profuse vegetation. Passing through a succession of deserts and fertile valleys the ascent is at first so gradual that four days' journey only reaches an altitude of some eight hundred feet. But from the plain the mountains rise suddenly, and when the climb of the western cordillera really begins the path is through grand valleys with walls towering for thousands of feet on either side. Perhaps fifteen miles would be the average day's journey, and it is quite impossible to make more than thirty miles. The Indians take little account of distance or time; they stop when they get tired, and they estimate everything by the period that a chew of Coca will last. A *cocada*—as it is termed—is equivalent to about three-quarters of a league, or about forty minutes.[6] The path is often shaded by willow trees, and sometimes even darkened by overhanging foliage, while the road may be obstructed with droves of laden llamas or mule trains. The mules used resemble the same sturdy animals that grow in the blue grass region of our own country, though of smaller build. They have great endurance, are remarkably sure-footed, and are usually docile, although at times they may manifest their customary obstinacy by an endeavor to rub off their load against a side hill, or to lie down just at some unpropitious time. While the *arriero* may ride, his accompanying Indians seem to prefer to go afoot, travelling quite as rapidly as the mules do, and aided by an occasional *acullico*—chew of Coca, they retain a freshness and vigor for endurance that is phenomenal. They will jog along all day under a burning sun up these rugged mountain steeps, and will be just as ready to travel at night, which is the time often selected, to avoid the intense heat. In the ascent of the western cordillera, which is not timbered, there is no vegetation, but there is no absence of coloration, for the sterile rocks are of all tints, and here and there is a profusion of wild flowers, especially heliotrope. In places the narrow pathway, just sufficient for the *machos,* or mules, in single file, winds around some *cuesta,* or hill, at the base of some immense cliff, where the walls tower above for thousands of feet, while below there is a yawning gulf into which it momentarily seems both rider and mule must be hurled. But one becomes accustomed to these dizzy heights after a time, and the grandeur of the scenery is sufficient to so engross the imagination that peril is unthought.

The Indians that are met are always busy, not only loaded with the customary burden, but with both hands actively employed as well, usually in spinning or knitting. They run along at a sort of dog trot, and seemingly never tire, the men often carrying enormous loads of barley or wheat which completely hide them from view, while the women, never with-

[6] Herndon; Vol. I; p. 146; 1853; also Raimondi; 1874.

out the customary baby, borne in a *ccepi* on their back, from which the little round head wobbles about as if it might drop off, drive the *burro* with a miscellaneous load of potatoes, corn, fruit, or mutton, intended for the market. The *serranos* are the reverse of the hospitable and vivacious people of the lowlands. They are commonly poor and view all travellers with suspicion. Their huts are dirty and uninviting, and usually crowded in one apartment are chickens, children, dogs, cats, guinea pigs and vermin, affording little room for guests. They cannot be counted upon to grant any favors, and even when letters are brought from the alcalde they must be emphasized with threats. Even when bound for market the Indian will not part with any of his stores while en route. If he is seen to have anything in his load which you absolutely need, he will not sell it at any price, and is inconvincible through argument, so that the only method of acquiring necessities is to help one's self and pay what is considered proper afterwards. During this enforced sale just sufficient annoyance may be displayed to prompt another chew of Coca, but there is never any complaint, and he accepts what is offered as though thoroughly well pleased at the bargain. This same peculiarity prevails everywhere and may have been developed through the custom of the Incan purveyor to the sovereign appropriating such articles as he chose for his lord, a procedure which the invaders did not hesitate to continue. In any case the Indian has grown to feel that his superiors will help themselves to what they want regardless of any personal expression he may manifest, and thinking perhaps with the followers of Mohammed—"Whatever is, is right," saves himself unnecessary worry. The natural reserve of the Serrano extends to an actual disinclination to grant the slightest hospitality even in their homes, and as a traveller approaches a hut he may often be challenged by *manam cancha*—"we have nothing," even before having expressed a desire for anything, and in some instances before the dwellers have taken the trouble to see who approaches. It seems then that one is compelled to be aggressive in order to reap those latent benefits and blessings which otherwise might not be applied to advantage.

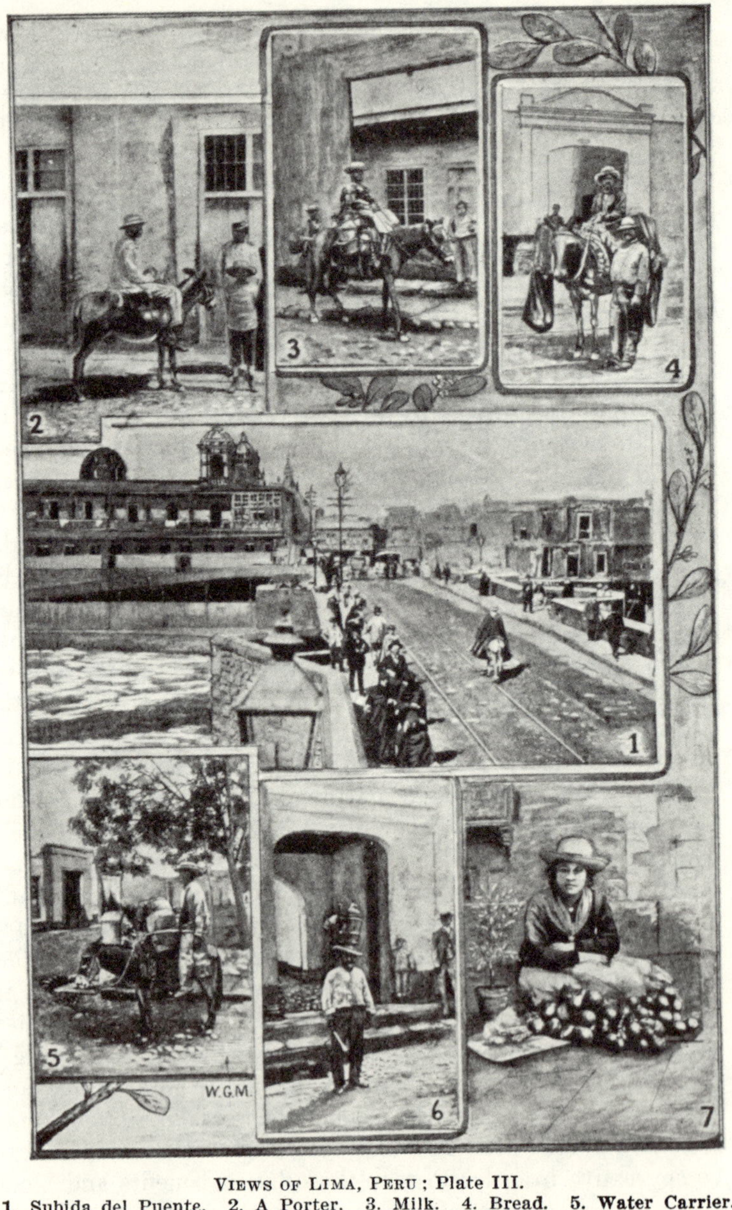

VIEWS OF LIMA, PERU; Plate III.
1. Subida del Puente. 2. A Porter. 3. Milk. 4. Bread. 5. Water Carrier. 6. Ice Cream. 7. Fruit Seller.

As a higher elevation is reached the air becomes cold, and the snow-capped mountains in the distance are seen through the clear atmosphere that seems to bring them very near. As night approaches, an encampment is made in the open air, usually by preference, because of the numerous insects which infest every habitation. These are particularly annoying to travellers, though the natives do not seem to mind them, and, in fact, the Indians often relish them. As one means of protection against the multiplicity of these pests, Nature has placed here a large, black bug, about an inch and a half long, heavy bodied, with an ant-like waist, and with transparent wings. The natives call it *amigo del hombre*—the "friend of man," on account of its killing and burying all poisonous insects. At times it may be absolutely necessary to take refuge in one of the *tambos,* or shelter houses, where protection may be found from the cold winds, now often filled with snow and hail. Here the traveller, wrapped in heavy woolens and fleecy poncho, supplemented by rugs or a sleeping bag of vicuña skins, may barely succeed in keeping himself warm by the physical exertion of shivering, while his Indians, scantily clad, squat together outside upon the frozen ground in some sheltered nook, where they apparently rest comfortably in a sweet slumber that is uninfluenced by the elements. The Indian squats on every occasion, rarely sitting on a chair. It is very much as Gilbert's song of the Admiral in *Pinafore* says: "This is his customary attitude," for he not only squats to sit, but he takes his sleep in this way, and even does much of his work in this same pose, while his dead body is buried in the same position. It is amusing to see the deliberation with which these people cut grain with a small sickle; they do this squatting, grasping a handful of grain it is carefully cut and carefully laid down. The Indian women squat in the market place when offering their wares for sale, while at their weaving they get still lower and lie prostrate. It has been suggested that this position is assumed as a means of keeping warm, but they never are known to display any annoyance from the cold, and are seemingly as oblivious to the elements as to the pangs of hunger, a relief they attribute to having propitiated the genii of the mountains through their constant use of Coca. At any rate, they are sustained by Coca in their travels, and it affords them not only *callpa*—or force, but warmth and comfort during the still hours of the coldest night in the high altitudes. And it is still here, so still that one may actually feel the awe of utter loneliness, a stillness which, in the reverberations of the slightest sound, lends a profundity to the echo.

Speaking of echoes suggests the weird and the ghostly. These Andeans are full of superstition, but amidst such crags and peaks in the darkness and stillness of the night, with only the occasional cry of some bird, it doesn't require an exalted imagination to think of spooks and hobgoblins. But it is not only at night that the Indian is full of dread, for there is a constant possibility that some enemy may cast a sort of *ojo*—or evil eye, upon him or upon his belongings, while, if he escape this terror, there is yet a dread that *chucaque*—another mysterious spell, may be thrust upon him. *Chucaque,* they say, is as though a man were made "to feel cheap," and as it is often manifest by severe cramp, it not unnaturally does make one feel humiliated. These conditions are only promptly to be relieved by some *curadora,* an old woman who understands the secret, when, by means of a poultice of mustard and tobacco, aided by certain cabalistic signs, the evil influence is driven out. Similar superstitious beliefs are entwined throughout all the customs of these people. The Indians live to a good old age on the mountains, a fact which has been set down to the long-continued use of Coca as a promoter of vigor and endurance. At any rate eighty, ninety and a hundred years is not at all uncommon here, even though life is commenced at so early an age that *mestizo* girls may be mothers at ten.

The Indians in the mountains have an intuitive knowledge of physical conditions. They can tell you with unerring accuracy in the morning, under a clear sky, just what hour of the day it will rain, and yet they seem to have no idea of time or distance. If you ask an Indian how far it is to a certain place he will reply: "*Mucha questa*"—"much up hill," or "just a little way." They measure their journeying as they do the extent of their labor, by the amount of Coca it is necessary to consume to reach a given place or perform a certain task.

The Indians chew Coca just as they do everything else, very deliberately and systematically. The mouthful of leaves taken at each time is termed *acullico,* or *chique,* which is as carefully predetermined as would the skilled housewife apportion the leaves of some choice *bohea* intended for an individual drawing. In preparing the chew the leaf is held base in between the two thumbs, parallel to the midrib, the soft part of the leaf being stripped off and put in the mouth. From the constant presence of this quid through many years the cheek on the side in which it is usually held presents a swollen appearance known as *piccho.* It is an error to suppose that the Indian journeys along and plucks the Coca from bushes by the wayside to chew, for the leaf must be carefully picked, dried and cured, and, just as tobacco or tea or coffee has to undergo certain processes before ready for consumption, so the full property of the Coca leaf is only developed after a proper preparation. Usually carried in the *chuspa,* or *huallqui,* with the leaves, or fastened to it outside, is a little flask or bottle made from a gourd and called *iscupuru.*[7] The word is not Quichua, but belongs to the dialect of the *Chinchay-suyus* along the banks of the Marañon. The Spanish authors termed it *popóro.*[8] In this gourd is carried a lime-like substance made from the ashes left after burning certain plants or by burning shells or limestone.[9] This, which they term *llipta,*[10] or *llucta,*[11] is intermixed with the leaves when chewing by applying it to those in the mouth with a short stick dipped into the gourd from time to time. After this application the lime left on the stick is wiped about the head of the gourd in an abstracted way, leaving a deposit of lime which increases with time, for the Indian never parts with his *popóro.* M. Gaugnet presented M. Mariani with a *popóro,* brought from Colombia, a cast of which in my possession well represents this formation.

[7] *Iscu,* lime; *puru,* gourd. [8] Oviedo wrote it *baperoñ;* Vol. II; p. 286; 1556.
[9] Herndon; Vol. I, p. 132, 1853. [10] Von Tschudi; 1840. [11] Paz Soldan; 1862

The operation of chewing is termed in Bolivia and Southern Peru *acullicar,*[12] while in the North it is called *chacchar.*[13] The *llipta* is made in different localities from various substances; in the South from the ashes of the algarroba,[14] the fruit of which has an immense reputation as an aphrodisiac, the mass being held together with boiled potatoes, while in the North quicklime is used, and in some of the montaña regions ashes of the *musa*[15] root or that of the common cereus are employed. The ashes of the burnt stalk of the quinoa plant, *chenopodium quinua,* mixed with a little lime, is the ordinary

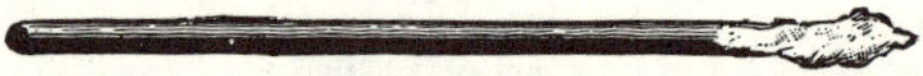

STICK FOR EXTRACTING LLIPTA FROM THE POPÓRO.

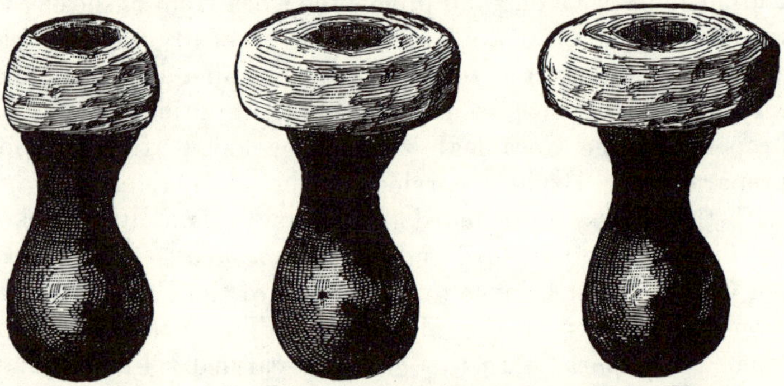

1. YOUTH. 2. MIDDLE AGE. 3. OLD MAN.

POPÓRO OR GOURD IN WHICH LLIPTA IS CARRIED, SHOWING INCRUSTATIONS AT VARIOUS AGES. [*Mariani.*]

preparation. In Caravaya the *llipta* is made in little cone-like lumps;[16] in other places it is found in flat dried cakes, which are scratched into a powder with a stick as it is required for use. Tschudi mentions the use of sugar with the leaves, but this must have been a European innovation which was supposedly an improvement, but not warranted by local customs. In Brazil, Coca—or *ypadú* as there termed, is powdered and mixed with the ash of *Cecropia palmata* leaves.[17]

[12] [13] [15] Von Tschudi; 1840. [14] Paz Soldan; 1862. [16] Markham; 1862.
[17] Schlechtendal; 1834.

LOCAL TERMS IN COCA USAGE.

People.	*The pouch for carrying Coca.*	*Gourd for alkali.*	*Gourd for tobacco and alkali.*	*Alkali used with Coca.*	*Alkali if with tobacco.*	*Stick to apply alkali.*	*To use Coca.*	*A chew of Coca.*
Businka.....	yóbru-mósi[1]..	yumbúro[2]... yóbru[1].......	....	impúsi (c),..	....	sôkáne (g).....	....	....
Chibcha.....	....	....	....	anńa (d)[9]...	....	....	bchuscua[2].....	....
Colombian.	....	....	duamosi..... yuamosi.....	mambi[5]......	duámba[2].... yuabíre[1].....	....	....	....
Guajiro......	kartáure.......	jurú[1]	....	guarépo (e)[3] guaréto	....	sutánia[2].......	....	taguará[3]...
Guamaca...	....	dumbúro[1]... dumburú[2]...	....	....	....	shugúna[1]......	dumburujái[2]	....
Habitos.....	....	....	....	manbi[6]......	ambiro.....	....	....	....
Köggaba....	sugaméi (a)[2].	súgui[2]	....	núgui (f).....	....	zugkálla (h)[2]	zugzahíñ[2].....	....
Quichua....	chuspa........ huallqui.......	iscupuru(b)	....	llipta[4]....... tocera........ llucta[7]....... yechta[10].....	....	....	coquero........ chacchar...... acullicar.......	acullico ... chique.....
Spanish.....	....	popóro........ baperoń......	....	....	....	....	poporear.......	....

(a) *Sugui*, gourd; *gama*, little sack. (b) *Iscu*, lime; *puru*, gourd. (c) *Buzi*, luminous. (d) *Anná*, bluish lime. (e) *Uretá*, white. (f) *Ñugui*, lime. (g) *So*, gourd; *kan*, wood. (h) *Sugui*, gourd; *kalli*, stick.

[1]Isaacs. [2]Celedon. [3]Simons. [4]Von Tschudi. [5]Ulloa. [6]Delano. [7]Paz Soldan. [8]Oviedo. [9]Uricoechea. [10]Probably phonetic.

Ernst has traced the derivation of a number of the terms which are applied to the use of Coca among the Colombian Indians. These have been built up from the name of the gourd used to carry the lime or from the little sack in which the leaves are carried, which is always worn by the Indian. Thus the Chibchas term the alkali *anńa,* which signifies a bluish lime.[18]

Dr. Monardes speaks of the use of tobacco combined with Coca and says of the Indians: "When they will make themselves to be out of judgment they mingle with the Coca the leaves of the tobacco, at which they totter and go as though they were out of their witts, or if they were drunk, which is a thing that doth give them great contentment to be in that sorte."[19] Tobacco is still mixed with Coca by some of the Colombian Indians, but it is doubtful if such a mixture alone would produce the effect described. The hallucinations and narcotic action attributed by early writers to Coca are largely confusional from imperfect facts. Some of the Indians gather the leaves of a plant they term *huaca* or *huacacachu.* It is a running vine with a large obvate leaf, pale green above and purple beneath, growing in the montaña only upon ground where there has previously been a habitation; for what is now an apparent virgin forest it is thought may three or four hundred years ago have been thickly inhabited. No scientific facts are known regarding this leaf as far as I could learn after submitting specimens of it to several of our leading botanists. The Indians term so many things *huaca*—which is a name they apply to anything they consider sacred—that it is very difficult to determine simply from the name. Von Tschudi probably refers to this leaf in what he describes as *bovachero,* or *datura sanguinea.* Several writers refer to the use of this leaf as a remedy for snake bite and against inflammations. A liquor is prepared from the leaves which the Indians term *tonga,* the drinking of which, they believe, will put them in communication with their ancestors, and from its strong narcotic action perhaps it may. Tschudi describes the symptoms observed in the case of an Indian who had taken

[18] Uricoechea; 1871. [19] Clusius, *trans.*, 1601.

some of this narcotic. He fell into a heavy stupor, his eyes vacantly fixed on the ground, his mouth convulsively closed and his nostrils dilated. In the course of a quarter of an hour his eyes began to roll, foam issued from his mouth, and his body was agitated with frightful convulsions. After these violent symptoms had passed off a profound sleep followed of several hours' duration, and when the subject recovered he related the particulars of his visit with his forefathers. Because of this superstitious property the natives termed *huaca* "the grave plant."

The Indians have fixed places along the road where they rest and replace their chews of Coca. Usually it is in some spot sheltered from the wind; and if near one of these retreats, they will hurry until reaching there, where they may drop exhausted, and after resting for a few moments will begin to prepare the leaves for mastication. In about ten minutes they are *armado*—as it is termed, or fully prepared to continue their journey. The distance an Indian will carry his *ccepi*—or load, of about a hundred pounds, under stimulus of one chew of Coca is spoken of as a *cocada,* just as we might say a certain number of miles. It is really a matter of time rather than distance, the first influence being felt within ten minutes, and the effect lasting for about three-quarters of an hour, during which time three kilometres on level ground, or two kilometres going up hill, will usually be covered.[20] Although the roads are marked out with league stones, the exact number of miles these represent is a varying quantity, and travellers soon fall into the local habit of computing distance by the *cocada* as more exact.

These *ccepiris*—or burden bearers, which is the Quichua term or *cargaderos*—as they are termed on the coast, commonly travel six to eight *cocadas* a day without any other food excepting the Coca leaf used in the manner as indicated. It is not at all unusual—as related by numerous travellers—for a messenger to cover a hundred leagues afoot with no other sustenance than Coca. The old traditional *chasqui,* or courier, who has been continued since the time of the Incas, is still

[20] Raimondi: 1874: also Herndon: I: p. 146, 1853.

given messages to carry on foot rather than by horse or mule. He always carries a pack, which is fastened on his back and to his head also, leaving both arms free; and where the road is so steep that he cannot walk he will scramble along on all fours very rapidly. When the Indians come to their resting place they throw off their burdens and squat down, and the traveller might just as well decide to rest here as to attempt to go on. All persuasion would be just as useless to induce a resting Indian to proceed as it would be in the case of their favorite beast of burden, the llama, which is as unalterable of purpose as is his master.

The amount of Coca that is used by an Indian in a day varies from one to two handfuls, which is equivalent to one or two ounces. The leaves are not weighed out, but are apportioned to each man in accordance with the amount of work that is to be done. As an extensive operator in Peru expressed it to me, "the more work the more Coca," while conversely, the more Coca the more work they are capable of doing. If the placid calm of an Indian is ever ruffled, it is only manifest through his taking an extra chew.

Away up in the cold and barren regions of the mountains wood and brush are too scarce to supply fuel, so the dried droppings of the llama are used instead; and as no one ever thinks of having a fire in this region merely for the purpose of keeping warm, this fuel is only used for cooking and necessity soon corrects any over-fastidiousness in the epicure. One of the remarkable peculiarities of the llama is that the beast deposits this mountain fuel always in the same places; a whole herd will go to one fixed spot, and so greatly lessen the labor of gathering the dung. In some of the particularly dangerous passes in the mountains there are rude crosses erected, which have been set up by the missionaries to mark the piles of sacred stones of the early Incan period. These stone piles are often far removed from loose stones, which must be carried for a long distance in anticipation of adding to the heap. As the Indian makes his offering he also expects all travellers as they pass to make a like obeisance to the god of the mountain, expressive of gratitude for a journey that has been safe thus far, and imploring a favorable continuance. Often these places are decorated with little trinkets, which are hung upon the arms of the cross or thrown upon the pile of stones. Any object that has been closely attached to the person is offered; sometimes this may be even so simple as a hair from the eyebrow, but commonly the cud of Coca is thrown against the rocks, the Indian bowing three times and exclaiming—"*Apachicta,*" which is an abbreviation of the term *Apachicta-much-*

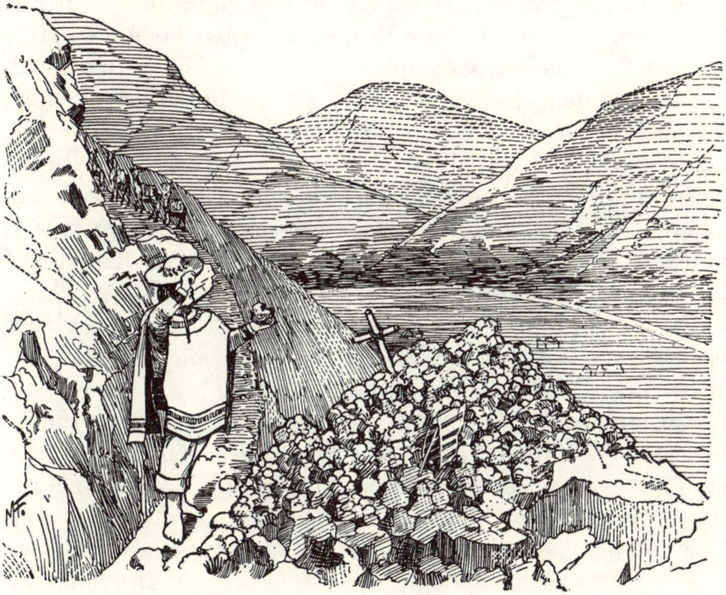

ANDEAN STONE HEAP TO PACHACAMAC.

hani,[21] "I worship at this heap," or "I give thanks to him who has given me strength to endure thus far." The offering is made to *Apachic,* or *Pachacamac,* of whom the stone pile is an emblem. It is a curious fact that diametrically opposite on the globe, in that portion of Chinese Tartary where the priests are called *Lamas,* offerings are made by the natives to similar stone piles which are there termed *obos.*

Arduous as may be the task of the cargo bearer, the severest trial the Indian is subject to is mining. They commence

[21] Rivero; 1854.

this labor as boys of eight and spend the greater part of their lives in the mines. These places are wet and cold, and the work is very hard. In getting out the ore the workers must use a thirty-pound hammer with one hand, while the carriers are obliged to bear burdens of about one hundred and fifty pounds up the steep ascent of the shaft to the surface. This mining is continuous, being carried on by two gangs of men, one of which goes on duty at seven at night, working until five in the morning, when, after a rest of two hours they continue until seven at night, and are then relieved by the other party. Some of the silver mines employ thousands of operatives, both men and women, the men working in the mine and the women breaking and sorting the ore which is brought to the surface. Unless there is at least twenty per cent. of silver in the ore it is cast aside; and these women are so expert that as they break the stones into small pieces they determine instantly how it shall be sorted. A similar cleverness is shown on the part of the Indians who select the Coca or cinchona plants. They will walk rapidly through a nursery and determine at a glance the value of individual plants or of the whole field without apparent hesitation. The Indians do not always select mining through choice, but are almost driven to it through the influence of the authorities. They have a dreadful fear of temporal powers and dare not disobey, even though their inclinations might suggest that they were born agriculturists. But these people have no inclinations; they have always been taught to do as commanded. It is suggestive of an instance I once met with when a physician, in reprimanding his colored servant, asked him why he did a certain thing, to which the poor fellow started to explain by "I thought." "Thought!" said the doctor—"there you go thinking again; you have no right to think!" And so it is with these poor Indians; they can have no opinion, they have no right to think.

The Incas did a prodigious amount of work in their mining efforts, which, even if primitive, were forcible and effective. A system of waterway, similar to the extensive aqueducts of the coast, was made use of to conduct these operations, and several of these canals still exist, some many miles long. They are from three to five feet wide, and five to eight feet deep; in places cut through the solid rock, and in others, when over a porous soil, they are lined with sandstone. Numerous smaller ones were extended from the main canal, generally ending in reservoirs, from which sluice gates might be opened to permit the pent-up volume of waters to suddenly rush down a hill, carrying with it hundreds of tons of golden gravel. At the same time other streams were run along the base of the cliffs, undermining them, and by this ancient method of hydraulic mining, continued through centuries, whole mountains have been washed away. At Alpacata, in the upper part of Aporoma, at an elevation of seven thousand five hundred and fifty feet, is still to be found one of these old canals, together with the huge tanks for storing water, in a fair state of preservation.

An engineer, extensively interested in mining interests, who spends several months of each year in Peru, has described to me the peculiar methods followed by the Indians, who sometimes conduct their gold washings in the streams to their own profit. Selecting a part of some river bed that is left without water during the dry season, the Indian paves it with large sloping stones, forming a series of riffles. When the freshets of the rainy season cause the stream to rise and overflow these paved spots, any gold carried down is caught between the stones and is gathered during the following dry season. The annual returns from such farms are almost exactly the same each year, so that the Indian may count with as great accuracy on the yield of gold from his several mining *chacras* as he would upon the products of his corn or Coca fields. This primitive form of mining is still carried on to a limited extent, and these gold farms are handed down from father to son as regular property. The Indians appear to have an intuitive and very accurate knowledge of the relative richness of the various streams, but their natural reticence makes it extremely difficult to gain this information from them.

Prior to the Conquest the only domestic animals of the Incans was their household pet, the *cuè*—or guinea pig, and the llama, their beast of burden. The wool from these latter, together with that from the immense flocks of native sheep, which have been guarded and preserved through centuries, has continued an important source of Peruvian wealth. The llama, alpaca, vicuña and guanaco, all somewhat resemble each other. The first two are not found wild at all, but have been developed through long, patient effort from the wild species. Though in no way related to the camel of the Old World, the appearance of the llama is suggestive of both that beast and the sheep. They have the long neck and camel-like appearance of the head, with a sheep-like body and long legs, with feet peculiarly adapted for rough mountain travel, cushioned beneath, and having a claw-like hoof above. The guanaco—commonly termed the Peruvian sheep, lives in small herds, and like sheep places implicit obedience in a leader. If deprived of this guardianship they become bewildered and are easily hunted. They are wonderfully sure-footed on rocky heights, and are also good swimmers, taking voluntarily to the water; and they have even been known to drink the briny waters of salt springs. The vicuña is a smaller animal, living near the region of perpetual snow. It bears some resemblance in habits to the chamois, being extremely active and so timid as to have resisted all efforts at domestication. They travel in herds of ten to fifteen females, with one male, who is the leader, ever on the alert, and who, upon approaching danger, gives a peculiar whistle or cry somewhat resembling that of a wild turkey, when the herd is off like a flash. The short silken fur of this animal is nearly uniformly brown, or tinged with yellow on the back, shading into gray on the belly, and is highly prized. It is from this wool and from that of the alpaca that the Incan robes and the fine Coca pouches carried by the sovereigns were woven, llama wool being more coarse and only used for rougher fabrics.

The use of the llama as a beast of burden by the early Peruvians was continued by the Spanish, and these animals still form an important means of transporting the wealth of the interior country across the mountains. They travel for immense distances by short stages, going, like the camel, long periods without water, while their sustenance is cropped by the wayside from the coarse blades of *ychu* grass, which appears to be their natural food, for they will not thrive where it does not grow. The llama will carry from eighty to one hundred pounds for about ten miles a day, but soon becomes exhausted, and not only requires rest, but in its peculiar way, demands it, so that double the number bearing the packs must be taken in train to admit of shifting the burdens frequently to avoid delay. This animal is an example of what can be done by coaxing rather than driving, for if overburdened or forced to travel beyond its ability the beast will sit down and absolutely refuse to budge, an obstinacy from which neither force nor blows will persuade it, but only excites a retaliation manifested by spitting an acrid saliva which, mixed with chewed cud, is extremely offensive, and is supposed to raise blisters wherever it touches the skin, but which in any case renders the person upon whom it falls an unenviable object. The Indians treat these beasts very kindly, talk to them, encourage them, and so get them to do their work. A drove of llamas bearing their cargo of Coca over the mountains is an imposing sight. The leader, chosen for his height—usually about six feet, has commonly his head decorated with tufts of colored woolen fringe hung with little bells, and his pointed ears, large, restless eyes and quivering lip make a very pretty picture. (*See page* 140.)

When the llamas are met by other travellers in some narrow defile the leader passes up or down the cliff and is followed by his train, scrambling over places that would not be attempted by a mule. The alpaca—the most beautiful of all the native animals, is in size a more refined modeling of the llama; it is probably merely a domesticated variety of the wild guanaco. Its color is commonly black, often variegated with brown and white, while the wool is long, silky and very valuable. At one year's growth the fleece is one foot long, and ten to twelve pounds may be taken from one animal. The fine fancy tapestries of the Incas were woven from this wool, specimens of which, found in some of the ancient tombs, will to-day rival any of the most exquisite weaves of other countries in texture as well as in picturesque design and brilliancy of coloring. The extreme docility and kindness of the Andeans is nowhere better shown than by their care for their animals. As one writer has very clearly shown, "it is probable that no other people could have successfully domesticated so stubborn an animal as the llama so as to use it as a beast of burden, and constant watchfulness and attention have alone enabled the Indians to rear their flocks of alpacas, which need assistance in almost every function of nature and to produce the large annual outturn of wool."

Smallpox has played havoc in the villages of the Andes. It is prevalent all over Peru and all along the Amazonian valley, and through the interior one meets with many faces showing the ravages of the disease. That the disease is here ancient is evidenced by many examples of Incan pottery which depict it. The Indians do not take kindly to vaccination, and will not willingly submit to it, though in the cities it is compulsory.

That giant vulture, the condor, which is probably the fabulous roc of the stories of our childhood, is at home in the highest and coldest peaks of the Andes, where the most daring and experienced climbers are unable to reach their young or find the two eggs which they commonly lay upon some lofty ledge. The general color of the bird is a grayish black, of variable depth of glossiness in different individuals, the adult male being distinguished by the amount of white upon the feathers and a downy white collar about the neck. There are many exaggerated stories told of the power of the condor and of its attacks upon the native animals, but it prefers carrion to the living, or even to the flesh of those recently killed, and enjoys, unrestricted, the advantages of the barrenness of its lofty home, being seldom seen below the line of perpetual snow. While this bird is large and powerful, it hardly equals in strength the mighty roc, which carried poor Sindbad, the sailor, from the island on which he had been deserted by his companions. One claw of that bird, Sindbad said, was "as big as the trunk of a large tree," while "its egg was one hundred and fifty feet in circumference." The full spread of the condor's wings rarely exceeds fourteen feet, and the bird is so clumsy and stupid as to afford favorite sport for the Indian boys, who often cleverly lasso them.

As one travels up the mountains the glaring rays of the sun, bursting through some gorge, are so dazzling, especially when falling upon the new-laid snow, as to occasion much inconvenience. *Surumpe*—as this snow blindness is termed, is a very common affection of the Indians, which the traveller must guard against by wearing protecting goggles. Added to this disability is the *zoroche,* or mountain sickness, induced by the rarefied atmosphere of the high altitudes. This often comes on suddenly without any premonitory symptom; at times it may be wholly absent, or it may be manifest all the way from a nervous irritability or uncomfortable fullness in the head and palpitating heart to complete prostration, suggestive of collapse. At times travellers may drop from the saddle from sheer muscular weakness, and Squier relates having drawn off his glove to go to the assistance of one of his party who had thus fallen, when they were at an altitude of 14,750 feet, and being surprised to see blood oozing from the pores of his own hand. Upon reaching his companion he found him nearly senseless, with blood trickling from his mouth, ears, nostrils and the corners of his eye. Copious vomiting followed, the condition being relieved by the application of the usual restoratives. It is very unusual that such serious symptoms are shown, and *zoroche,* like seasickness, does not often excite even sympathy, while, like *mal de mer,* often after one has experienced a first attack, they may never be troubled again, or they may be similarly affected upon every occasion when going into high altitudes. It is remarkable how utterly prostrated one will feel under the influence of *zoroche,* the most speedy relief from which is to lie flat and perfectly still until sufficiently recovered to continue the journey. The slightest movement seems to be a difficulty, and just as the poor seasick victim, at first afraid he will die, becomes finally so physically demoralized through his suffering that he is afraid he will not die, so the subject of mountain sickness in its severity prays to be left alone to what seems his inevitable and immediate end. Rest and a judicious use of Coca, now best taken as an elixir or wine, acts so magically as to soon change all this, and the sufferer lives to enjoy the bounties which Nature has in store in brighter, smiling scenes beyond.

Even the animals suffer from an impossibility of taking in sufficient stimulus in the thin air of high altitudes, and the owners of the mules often slit the nostrils of their beasts—when they have not already been cut through from thistle eating—so as to remove even the slightest impediment to deep breathing. It is not known that the mules have been induced to feed upon Coca leaves, as the horses of the far East are sustained by opium, but their suffering is supposedly relieved by the odor of garlic; and the *arriero,* ever mindful of the welfare of his charge, attempts to relieve the trembling and panting beasts by rubbing over the foreheads of these animals an ointment made of tallow, garlic and wild marjoram. Some of the Indians have peculiar ideas about this disability, which they call *veta*—or vein, because they believe it is occasioned by a vein of metal in the mountains diffusing around some poisonous influence and so contaminating the atmosphere. But whatever his interpretation as to the cause may be, the Indian knows from experience that if Coca will not wholly prevent, it will speedily relieve this annoyance; and its use for this purpose is mentioned in all the historical accounts of the Andeans. All travellers who have written of their journeys over these mountains, speak in praise of this particular property of Coca. Dr. Benjamin F. Gibbs, U. S. N., in his report on Coca to the United States Government, attributes this great virtue to the direct action of Coca in stimulating the cardiac muscular fibre, thus assisting the natural force of the heart to make its greatest effort to pass the summit of the Andes.[22]

One of the frequent disabilities for both man and beast travelling in the mountain is *empacho,* or indigestion, probably induced not only by irregularity in eating, but by improper and insufficient food, as well as imperfect oxygenation. Against this condition Coca exerts an influence by the increase of respiratory power, as well as increased capacity in the

22 *Sanitary and Medical Report, U. S. N., 1873-4;* Washington, 1875.

heart, holding at the same time hunger and thirst in abeyance, for it not only does not impair appetite in the least, but increases it; and when opportunity offers, the Indian who has gone for days without food will dispose of a meal with a deliberation and fixedness of purpose that is astonishing. Dr. Weddell, in speaking of this property of Coca in sustaining the strength without food, particularly refers to this fact, and says that it did not impair the appetites of the Indians who accompanied him in his travels and who chewed the leaf incessantly, yet who, in the evening, at the completion of their labors, always ate ravenously of a quantity sufficient to compensate fully for any omissions since the previous meal.

Through these long mountain journeys, where it is necessary to carry the food supply, the Indians use the indigenous potato—*papa,* as they term it, which is found throughout Peru in great variety, and which they prepare for their use by numerous ways of preservation of drying and freezing. *Chuno* is made by soaking the common potato in water for several days and then pressing out the moisture and freezing the pulp, while *Chochoca* is another frozen preparation, and both of these have long proved so serviceable in the journeys on the Andes that Rivero suggested such a form of preparation might be desirable to add to the supplies of the army and navy. *Oca* is a species of potato of a purple color; it is a favorite article of diet from which *caya,* another preserved variety, is made. *Mashua* is made from *oca* by rotting it until it is so offensive that no palate but that of an Indian accustomed to such dainties could tolerate it. *Macas* is a potato tuber which when boiled looks and tastes like turnips. The Indians expose it in the frost and sun for a number of days, and then dry it indoors and prepare a sort of syrup from it which smells very offensive, but is said to be a stimulant to reproduction. On the mountains there grows a yellow potato—the *amarillo,* which is far superior to anything similar found in our markets; it will only grow at a certain elevation and has resisted all efforts of cultivation elsewhere by degenerating, after the first crop, into the common variety. Preserved meats are carried in the mountains as *charqui*—or jerked beef, which is the whole carcass of a sheep, dried in cold air; but alcohol is neyer forgotten on these trips, and the Indian will drink it straight, if it is given to him; for although his reliance is upon Coca as of necessity for the force and endurance it gives, he loves alcohol for its own sake. It is as was once expressed to me by a plethoric individual of our own clime, "I don't drink because I need it, doctor, but because I like the taste of it." The application that alcohol is a spur or whip to urge on over some immediate emergency, while Coca is an imparter of continuous force, is well illustrated by a story told of some Indians to whom whiskey had been given, and upon being asked an opinion as to its influence, one fellow replied: "Coca helps a man to live, but whiskey makes him row a boat."[23] This is an empirical application which has been fully determined by physiological fact, which establishes an alcoholic preparation of Coca—such as Coca wine—as an ideal tonic-stimulant, possessing not only immediate but lasting effects.

In looking through the log book of an Andean traveller with reference to the burdens carried by the Indians, I remarked that the packs for the party were chiefly made up of Coca, preserved foods and sugar alcohol, the first and last being predominant. The food supply in travelling over the mountains is one of the most serious problems, and at best the preserved foods are not very inviting, while it requires a good appetite and vigorous imagination to enjoy the compact portion of dried compounds, offered as an available ration. A gentleman recently returned from a trip across the Andes expressed himself of the belief that people commonly eat too much, and that during his sojourn there he had been forced, through sheer necessity, to be abstemious in eating, and for days at a time had lived upon Coca because it was the only thing convenient in the supplies at hand, but as a result he felt not only more strong, but younger.

The Indians carry a pack of from eighty to one hundred pounds, the amount of burden for both men and mules being regulated by law in the several districts, being less on the Eastern Andes than on the western cordillera, while the pay is the

[23] Rusby; *person. com.*; 1898.

same. The wages of these carriers is sixteen cents of our money a day, yet these people work on amidst all inclemency of weather, through shifting seasons from increased altitude, willing and contented, with a *cusi-simirac,* or happy smile, so long as *callpa,* or force, be sustained with the essential Coca.

In the villages of the Sierra there is found an abundant supply of native fruits in great variety. Some of these are very luscious, and one soon acquires a liking for them, which may remain a happy remembrance throughout life. Among these are the *chirimoya*—a heart-shaped fruit, from two to five inches in diameter, growing on a tree—*amonacherimolia*—fifteen to twenty feet in height, which requires a number of years to bring it to perfection. The fruit is a brownish green, externally covered with small knobs and scales, with fine black lines like a network spread over it. The pulp is a creamy white, containing a number of dark brown seeds arranged about a central core, the taste of which has been referred to as "spiritualized strawberries and cream," and it is comparable, with nothing else. *Palta*—sometimes called *aguacate*—the alligator pear, which is also seen in our markets, is the fruit of *Persea,* or *gatissima*—a tall, slender tree, fifty feet or more in height. The fruit is pear-shaped, having a tough rind containing a pulp which seems to melt upon the tongue like marrow, it is eaten with pepper and salt, or dressed like a salad. Then there is *granadilla*—the fruit of *tassiflora quadrangularis,* a hard, thick-skinned, egg-shaped fruit, with a grayish, gelatinous pulp of an agreeable sub-acid taste, which, with hosts of others, must all be novel to the traveller who first visits Peru. These, together with bananas, oranges, water melons, peaches, apples, grapes, cherries, figs and dates, comprise a tempting variety to select from.

Heavy clothing is always necessary in the elevated towns, the accustomed overcoat being replaced by the native poncho, a sort of blanket-like garment woven of llama wool, with a hole cut in the centre, through which one sticks the head, allowing the softly woven fabric to fall closely over the figure. It is commonly worn, not only by the natives, but by travellers, and is very light, fleecy and warm. With this the town folk of some provinces wear a white sombrero on week days, which is changed for black on Sundays, while the ladies don expensive silks, with fancy shawls and elaborate lace mantuas, with which they drape the head after the manner of the Limaian ladies in a style far more picturesque than would be the conventional bonnet.

Here in brief is an attempt to show some of the surroundings which the Andean of to-day is subjected to. These Indians represent the remains of the plodding masses of that once mighty nation of the Incas, whose customs and traditions have descended to them. The "divine plant," once so far beyond the privilege of this plebeian class, is now theirs through right of inheritance, and they have adapted the sacred Coca to their present necessities. That we may more readily understand what those necessities are which have continued this use through so many centuries, we should study these Indians at their labors, when it will be shown—as it long ago became apparent to the Spaniards—that Coca chewing among them is not a mere idle practice, but that Providence has truly granted them in this ancient plant a possibility for their survival despite the hardships of a peculiar environment.

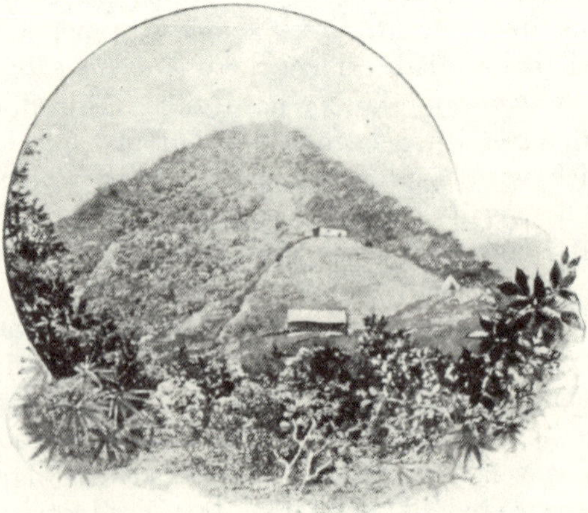

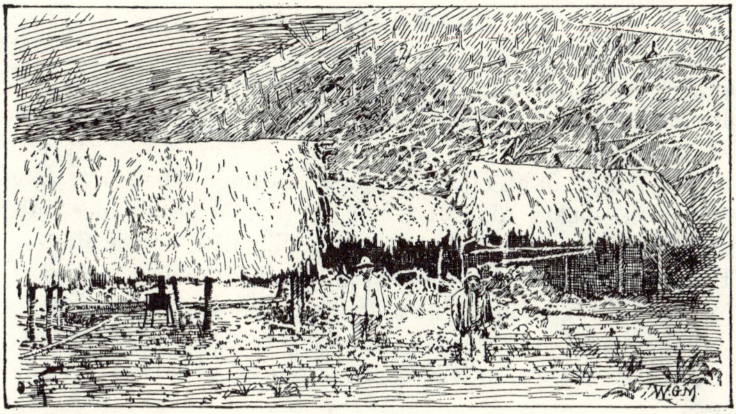

CHAPTER VIII.

THE BOTANY OF COCA.

"There is a Grecian fable that says a child had shown Æsculapius a plant that would cure all ills; Coca is that plant."
—Henri Houssaye, French *Académicien*.

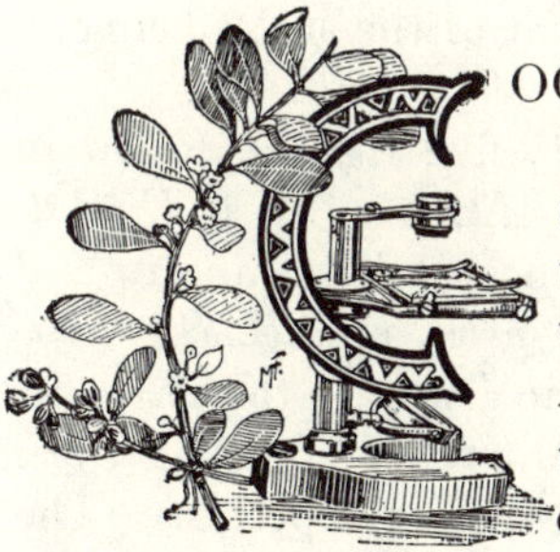

COCA—the "divine plant" of the Incas, belongs to the family of the *Erythroxylaceæ*, which is broadly distributed throughout the tropical world. There are two genera, the *Erythroxylon* and *Aneulophus*.[1] Of the former there are at least a hundred species, the majority of which are found in South America; in tropical Asia there are six, in Africa five or more, and two in Northern Australia. The characteristics of the entire family are similar, while several peculiarities are predominant, among which are the nerve markings of the leaf, the tongue-like appendage of the petals of the flower, and the early obliteration of a certain number of the original compartments

[1] Reiche, Engler und Prantl; Vol. III; (4); 1897.

of the fruit, two or three of these aborting even while in flower, leaving an indication of their former presence only by minute openings.

Peyritsch, in an elaborate classification of the genus *Erythroxylon,* makes four divisions of this in accordance with the size of the leaf and certain peculiarities of the flower.[2] The first division describes seven species growing in Brazil, Northern Mexico and Cuba, of which the leaves are up to a thumb's length, the flowers occurring from one to six in the axils of the bracts, or scales, the styles being at least in part free.

The second division enumerates twenty-eight species, among them several employed for economic uses, *E. anguifugum*, Mart., *E. squamatum*, Swaitz, and *E. areolatum*, Jacq., together with *E. Coca,* Lam., which is by far the most important of the entire family. The plants of this species are scattered through Peru, Colombia, Guiana, Panama—*E. Panamaense,* Turez, Mexico—*E. Mexicanum,* HBK., Colombia—*E. cassinioides,* Pl. *et* Lind, and *E. rigidulum,* DC. In this division the leaves are commonly longer than the thumb, though less than a finger's length. The flowers occur from three to ten in clusters, the arrangement of the styles being as in the first division.

The third division embraces thirty-five species, found in Peru, Guiana, Colombia and Brazil. Among this is *E. Pulchrum,* St. Hil., growing in the province of Rio Janeiro and locally known as *subrayil* or *arco de pipa*, and *E. Spruceanum*, Peyr., growing in Panuré to Rio Uaupés, the *E. suberosum,* St. Hil., and *E. tortuosum,* Mart. The *Mama Coca* of Martius is also classed here as a distinct species. The leaves of this class are of a finger's length or over. The styles of the pistil are joined up to their stigmas.

In the fourth division there are twelve species, the leaves of all of which are from a span to a foot or more long. In the entire classification eighty-two species are described.

Many of the species of *Erythroxylon* are employed for economic uses. *E. anguifugum* is used in Brazil as a remedy

[2] Martius; 1878.

against snake bite. *E. campestre* is employed in the same country as a purgative. The bark of *E. suberosum,* and also of *E. tortuosum,* yields a brownish red dye. The former is termed in Brazil *gallinha choca* and *mercurio do campo.*[3]

E. areolatum is a native of the northern parts of South America and Jamaica, in the latter place being known as red wood, or iron wood, and some excellent timber is derived from

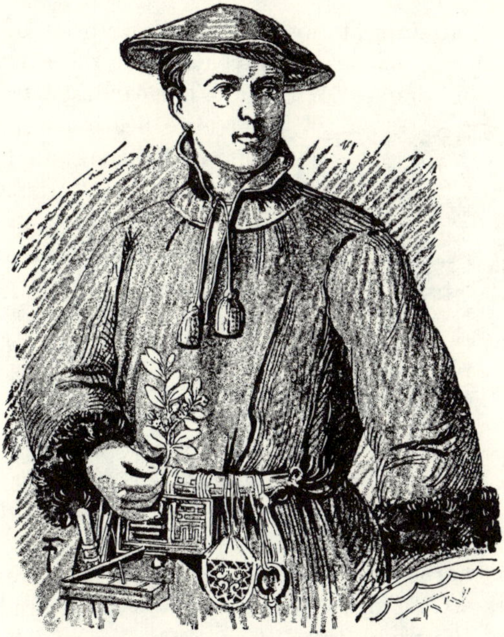

THE BOTANIST LINNÆUS IN EARLY LIFE.

this species. It is a small tree from fifteen to eighteen feet in height, with a trunk from five to six inches in diameter, growing in the lowlands. The twigs and leaves of this species are said to be refrigerant and when mixed with *benne* oil form a refreshing liniment, while the bark is also a tonic and the sub-acid of its fruit is purgative and diuretic. The wood of *E. hypericifolium* is the *Bois d'huile* of the Isle of France. *E. monogynum* is a native of the East Indies, where it is

[3] Lindley; 1853.

known under the native name of *gadara.* Its wood is fragrant and takes a beautiful polish, being considered as a sort of bastard sandal. An empyreumatic oil is derived from it, which is used in preserving the wood of the native boats. The important properties of Coca have directed attention to the plants of these several species of the *Erythroxylon* family in the hope that their leaves might contain a similar series of alkaloids.

The first attempt at any technical description of Coca was that made by Monardes some years after the early publications upon the conquest of Peru. The earliest purely botanical classification appears to be that of Plukenet, in 1692. He describes the "Mamacoca," or the "Mother of Coca," as the deified name used among the Peruvians.[4] About a generation later Antoine de Jussieu described the specimens which he had received from his brother Joseph while he was with the expedition of La Condamine. Jussieu placed Coca in the family of the *Malpighiaceæ* of the genus *Sethia* because of certain characteristics of the leaf and the three-compartment fruit. Cavanilles, who drew his account and his illustrations of the plant from these examples, which were preserved in the herbarium of the Museum of Natural History at Paris, also followed this classification.

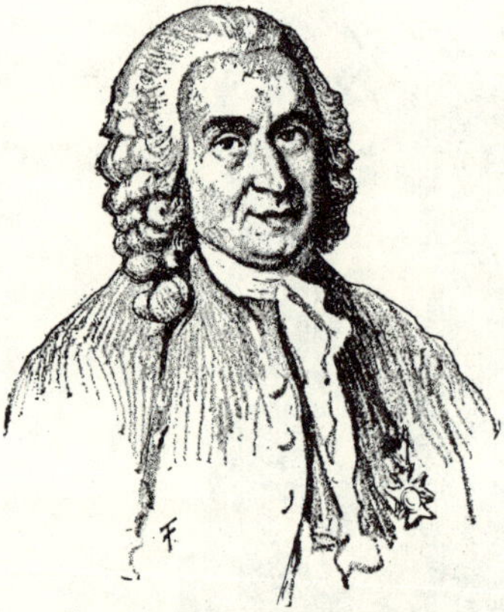

CARL VON LINNE. [*Linnæus.*]

Dr. Browne in 1756, in his *Natural History of Jamaica,* included Coca among the plants of that region and placed it in the family *Erythroxylum,* deriving this generic name from the red color of the wood of some local species.[5] About this same time Linnæus placed Coca in the family of the *Erythroxyleæ* of the genus *Erythroxylon,* and subsequently this classification was followed by Antoine Laurent de Jussieu, a nephew

[4] Plukenetii; *mantissa* 25; 1692. [5] Patrick Browne; p. 278; 1756.

of Joseph, who changed the classification from *Malpighiads* because of certain characteristics of the Coca flower.

The observation was made by the poet Goethe in his "Metamorphosis of Plants," that the flower was merely a reproduction of the modified plant leaf, just as the stem, trunk, stalk or root is shaped to satisfy particular requirements, all originating from the germinal embryo in the seed. Because it determines the perpetuation of the plant, botanists regard the flower as an important organ in the consideration of any classification.

The *Erythroxylons* differ from the *Malpighiads* by their flowers growing from amongst small imbricated scales, having no glands on the calyx, capitate stigmas, and having the ovules united superiorly. Lamarck has followed the classification of Antoine Laurent de Jussieu, and this has since been regarded by the majority of authorities as classic. Eichler and Martius have continued the description of the early Jussieu, while Ballieu, Planchon, and Bentham and Hooker, because of the frequent occurrence of a five-compartment fruit, have placed Coca with the *Linaceæ*—the flax family, and have assigned it as number thirty-four of the division of that order. Commers has placed Coca in the genus *Venelia* and *Roelana,* and Spreng associates it with the *Steudelia,* while Humboldt, Bonpland and Kunth class it with *Sethia,* of which Jussieu formed a genus.

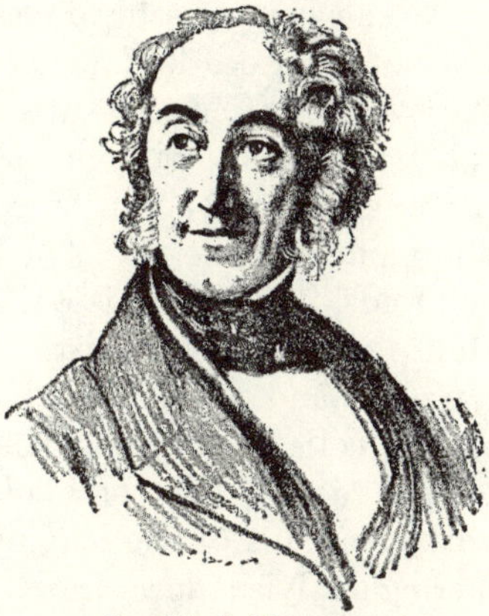

SIR W. J. HOOKER.

One of the most marked characteristics of the Coca leaf is the areolated portion bounded by two longitudinal elliptical lines curving toward the midrib. These lines are commonly more conspicuous on the under surface of the leaf. The areolated portion is slightly concave, and of a deeper color than the rest of the leaf, probably from a closer venation. This peculiarity is not confined to the *Erythroxlon Coca.* It is marked in *E. areolatum,* and it furnishes a character for the section *Areolata* of de Candolle's *Prodromus,* Vol. I, p. 575, in which five specimens are included. In many other species, where there are no demarking lines, the leaves are sometimes marked by similar bud pleatings or have a peculiar color bounding the area. In his early account of this species Browne described the leaf as: "Marked with two slender longitudinal lines upon the back which were the utmost limits of that part of the leaf which was exposed while it lay in a folded state."

Some botanists have considered the characteristic lateral lines of the Coca leaf as nerves. Martius was of the opinion these result from pressure of the margin of the leaf as it is rolled toward the midrib while in the bud, the pinching of the tissue causing the substance of the leaf to be raised, resembling a delicate nerve. The lines have been designated as "tissue folds,"[6] but there is no fold in either the epidermis or substance of the leaf. Histologically the lines are formed by a narrow band of elongated cells, which resemble the collenchyma cells of the neighboring epidermis,[7] and these doubtless serve to stiffen the blade. The lines have no connection with the veins of the leaf and in transmitted light seem like mere ghostly shadows which vanish under closer search.

Many observers have supposed they had found the original locality of wild Coca. Alcide d'Orbigny describes in his travels, having entered a valley covered with what he supposed to be the wild Coca shrub, but thinking he might be mistaken, he showed the plant to his mule driver, who was the proprietor of a cocal in Yungas, and he pronounced it undoubtedly Coca and gathered a quantity of the leaves.[8] It has been asserted that wild Coca may be found in the province of Cochero,[9] and one of the former governors of Oran, in the province of Salta, on the northern borders of the Argentine Republic, claims to have found wild Coca of excellent quality in the forests of that district.[10] Poeppig also described having found wild specimens, known by the natives as Mama

[6] Hananseck; 1885. [7] Schrenk; 1887. [8] D'Orbigny; 1830. [9] Peyritsch; 1878.
[10] Villafane; 1857.

Coca, in the Cerro San Cristobal, near the Huallaga, some miles below Huanuco. These examples closely resemble the shrubs of cultivated Coca collected by Martius in the neighborhood of Ega, Brazil, near the borders of the Amazon, and correspond to the wild specimens commonly found throughout Peru.

In Colombia Humboldt, Bonpland and Kunth described *Erythroxylon Hondense* as the possible type of the originally cultivated Coca shrub, but there is a difference between the leaves of *E. Coca* and *E. Hondense* in the arrangement of their nervures, from which Pyrame de Candolle considers them as entirely distinct species. Andre speaks of Coca in the valley of the river Cauca as in abundance in both the wild and half-wild state, but an excellent authority denies that Coca is found wild in Colombia.[11]

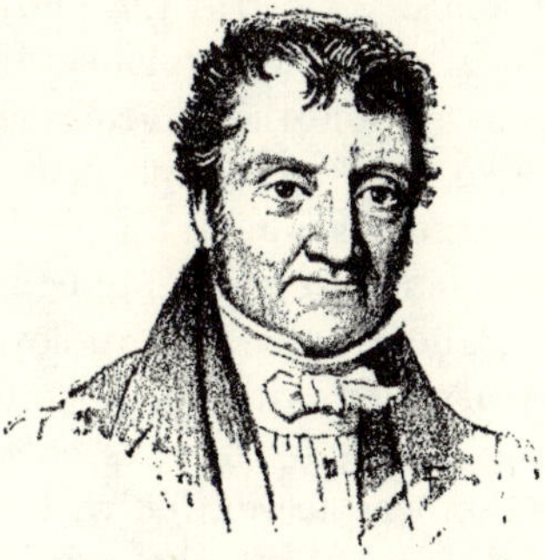

AIMÉ BONPLAND.

The exact locality where Coca is indigenous in a wild state has, however, never been determined. Though there are many Coca plants growing throughout the montaña outside of cultivation, it is presumed that these are examples where the seeds of the plant have either been unintentionally scattered or else are the remains of some neglected plantation where might have flourished a vigorous cocal under the Spanish reign. There are evidences of these scattered shrubs throughout the entire region where Coca will grow, but there is no historical data to base a conclusion that these represent wild plants of any distinct original variety, while the weight of testimony indicates that they are examples of the traditional plant which have escaped from cultivation.

Although the heart of the habitat of Coca is in the Peruvian montaña from 7° S., north for some ten degrees, the shrubs are found scattered along the entire eastern curve of

[11] Triana and Planchon; p. 338; 1862.

the Andes, from the Straits of Magellan to the borders of the Caribbean Sea, in the moist and warm slopes of the mountains, at an elevation from 1,500 to 5,000 and even 6,000 feet, being cultivated at a higher altitude through Bolivia than in Peru. Throughout this extent there are to be seen large plantations and many smaller patches where Coca is raised in a small way by Indians who come three or four times a year to look after their crop. In some localities, through many miles, these cocals cover the sides of the mountains for thousands of feet. During the Incan period the centre of this industry was about the royal city of Cuzco, and at present the provinces of Caravaya and of Sandia, east of Cuzco, are the site of the finest variety of Peruvian grown Coca. In this same region there grows coffee, cacao, cascarilla, potatoes, maize, the sugar cane, bananas, peaches, oranges, paltas, and a host of luscious fruits and many valuable dyes and woods.

There are still important Coca regions about Cuzco, and at Paucartambo and in several Indian towns along the Huanuco valley, situated in the very heart of the northern montaña and noted for its coffee plantations. At one time this region was accredited with supplying Coca for all Peru, which probably meant the mining centres of Huancavelica—formerly more prominent than at present—and Cerro de Pasco, where the mines are still extensively worked. There are fine cocals at Mayro, on the Zuzu River, and at Pozuso—which are German colonies; at the latter place is located the laboratory of Kitz, one of the largest manufacturers of crude cocaine, whose product supplies some of the important German chemical houses. Still further to the northwest—in Colombia, there are a number of small plantations along the valley of Yupa, at the foot of the chain of mountains which separates the province of Santa Marta de Maracaibo, at the mouth of the Magdalena River. Eastward from the montaña Coca is cultivated near many of the tributaries of the Amazon, and through some portions of Brazil, where it is known as *ypadú* (*E. Pulchrum,* St. Hil.). The Amazonian plant is not only modified in appearance,[12] but the alkaloidal yield is inferior.[13]

[12] Poeppig; 1835. [13] Parke, Davis & Co.; *person. com.;* 1898.

The temperature in which Coca is grown must be equable, of about 18° C. (64.4° F.). If the mean exceeds 20° C. (68° F.), the plant loses strength and the leaf assumes a dryness which always indicates that it is grown in too warm a situation, and though the leaves may be more prolific, they have not the delicate aroma of choice Coca. It is for the purpose of securing uniform temperature and appropriate drainage that Coca by preference is grown at an altitude above the intense heat of the valleys, and where it is virtually one season throughout the year, the only change being between the hot sun or the profuse rains of the tropical montaña. As the temperature lowers with increase of altitude, when too great a height is reached the shrub is less thrifty and develops a small leaf of little market value, while as only one harvest is possible the expense of cultivation is too great to prove profitable. Even close to the equator, in the higher elevations, there is always danger from frost, and for this reason some of the cocals about Huanuco have at times suffered serious loss. All attempts at Coca cultivation on a profitable scale near to Lima have failed not only because of the absence of rain, but because the season's changing is unsuited.

A peculiar earth is required for the most favorable cultivation of Coca, one rich in mineral matter, yet free from limestone, which is so detrimental that even when it is in the substratum of a vegetable soil the shrub grown over it will be stunted and the foliage scanty. While the young Coca plants may thrive best in a light, porous soil, such as that in the warmer valleys, the full grown shrub yields a better quality of leaf when grown in clay. The red clay, common in the tropical Andes, is formed by a union of organic acids with the inorganic bases of alkaline earths, and oxides—chiefly of iron—which in a soluble form are brought to the surface by capillarity. These elements enter the Coca shrub in solution through its multiple fibrous root, which looks like a veritable wig. The delicate filaments are extended in every direction to drink in moisture, and as these root-hairs enter the interspaces of the soil, the particles of which are covered with a film of water, absorption readily takes place. The clay soil of the montaña affords this property in a high degree, while the hillside cultivation admits of an appropriate drainage of

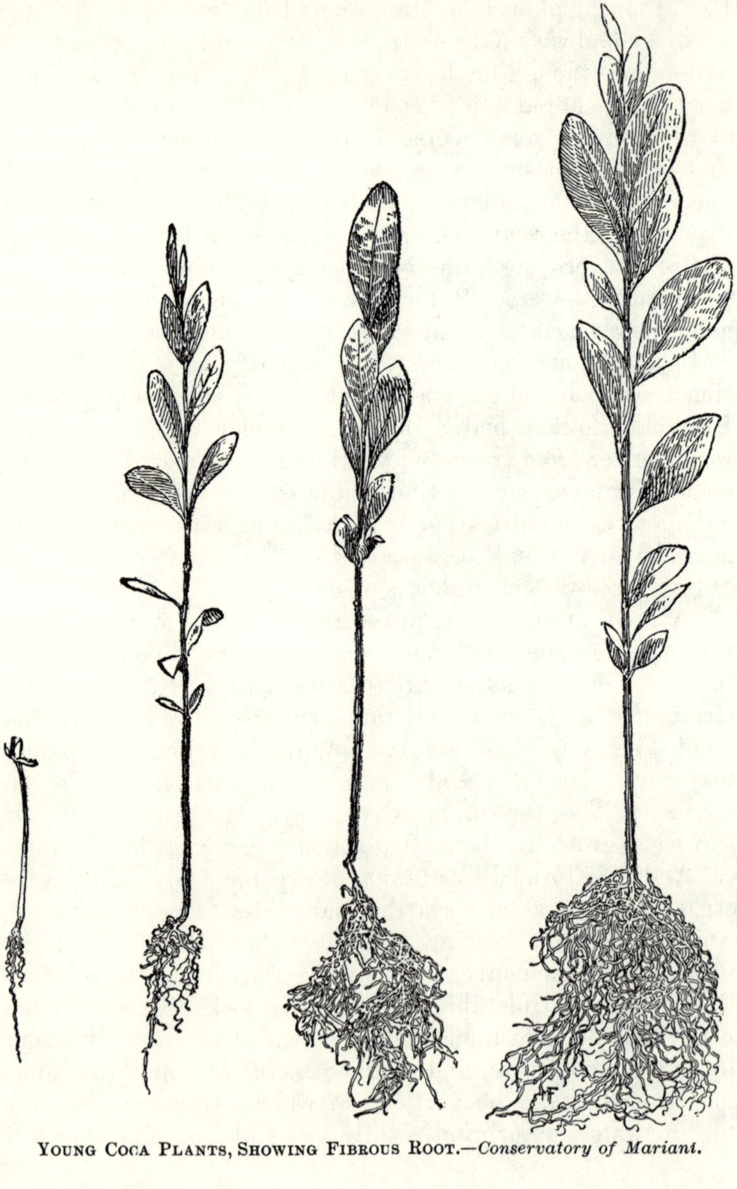

YOUNG COCA PLANTS, SHOWING FIBROUS ROOT.—*Conservatory of Mariani.*

the interspaces without which the delicate root would soon be rotted. As the water is absorbed from the soil, a flow by capillarity takes place to that point, and so the Coca root will drain a considerable space.

It is possible a metallic soil may have some marked influence on the yield of alkaloid. At Phara, where the best Coca leaves are grown, the adjacent mountains are formed of at least two per cent. of arsenical pyrites, a fact which is noteworthy because this is the only place in Peru where the soil is of such a nature. Most of the soil of the Andean hills where the best Coca is grown, originates in the decay of the pyritiferous schists, which form the chief geological feature of the surrounding mountains. This, commonly mixed with organic matter and salts from the decaying vegetation, or that of the trees burned to make a clearing, affords what might be termed a virgin earth—*terre franche ou normale*—which requires no addition of manures for invigoration. In the conservatory it has been found, after careful experimentation, that a mixture of leaf mould and sand—*terre de bruyère,* forms the best artificial soil for the Coca plant.[14]

Aside from an appropriate soil that is well drained, there is another important element to the best growth of Coca, and that is a humid atmosphere. Indeed, in the heart of the montaña it is either hazy or drizzling during some portion of the day throughout the year, the intense glare of the tropical sun being usually masked by banks of fog, so that it would seem that one living here is dwelling in the clouds. At night the atmosphere is loaded with moisture and the temperature may be a little lower than during the day, though there is usually but a trifling variation day after day.

The natural life of the Coca shrub exceeds the average life of man, yet new Cocals are being frequently set out to replace those plants destroyed through accident or carelessness. The young plants are usually started in a nursery, or *almaciga,* from seeds planted during the rainy season, or these may be propagated from cuttings. In the conservatory slips may be successfully grown if care is taken to retain sufficient moist-

[14] Mariani; *person. com.;* 1899.

ure about the young plant by covering it with a bell glass.[15] The birds are great lovers of Coca seeds, and when these are lightly sown on the surface of the nursery it is necessary to cover the beds at night with cloths to guard against "picking and stealing." Before sowing the seeds are sometimes germinated by keeping them in a heap three or four inches high and watering them until they sprout. They are then carefully picked apart and planted,[16] either in hills or the seeds are simply sown on the surface of the ground, "and from that they take them up and set them in other places into earth that is well labored and tilled and made convenient to set them in."[17] There is commonly over the beds of the nursery a thatched roof—*huasichi,* which serves as a protection to the tender growing shoots from the beating rain or melting fierceness of the occasional sun. The first spears are seen in a fortnight, and the plants are carefully nourished during six months, or perhaps even a year until they become strong enough to be transplanted to the field.

As a rule, all plants that are forty or fifty centimetres high (16 to 20 inches) may be set out, being "placed in rows as we might plant peas or beans."[18] In some cases they are set in little walled beds, termed *aspi,* a foot square, care being taken that the roots shall penetrate straight into the ground. Each of these holes is set about with stones to prevent the surrounding earth from falling, while yet admitting a free access of air about the roots. In such a bed three or four seedlings may be planted to grow up together, a method which is the outgrowth of laziness, as the shrubs will flourish better when set out singly. Usually the plants are arranged in rows, termed *uachas,* which are separated by little walls of earth—*umachas,* at the base of which the plants are set. In some districts the bottle gourd, maize, or even coffee, is sown between these rows, so as to afford a shield for the delicate shoots against sun or rain. At first the young plants are weeded—*mazi* as it is termed—frequently, and in an appropriate region there is no need for artificial watering; but the Coca plant loves mois-

[15] Mariani; *person. com.;* 1899. [16] Rusby; *person. com.;* 1898.
[17] [18] Monardes; 1580.

ture, and forty days under irrigation will cover naked shrubs with new leaves, but the quality is not equal to those grown by natural means.[19]

In from eighteen months to two years the first harvest, or *mitta,* which literally means time or season—is commenced. The leaves are considered mature when they have begun to assume a faint yellow tint, or better—when their softness is giving place to a tendency to crack or break off when bent, usually about eight days before the leaf would fall naturally. This ripe Coca leaf is termed by the Indians *cacha.*

The Coca shrub, growing out of immediate cultivation, will sometimes attain a height of about twelve feet, but for the convenience of picking, cultivated plants are kept down to less than half that height by pruning—*huriar* or *ccuspar*—at the time of harvesting, by picking off the upper twigs, which increases the lateral spread of the shrub. The first harvest—or rather preliminary picking, is known as *quita calzón,* from the Spanish *quitar*—to take away, and *calzón*—breeches. As the name indicates, it is really more of a trimming than what might be termed a harvest, and the leaves gathered at this time have less flavor than those of the regular *mittas.* Each of the harvests is designated by name—which may vary according to the district. The first regular one in the spring—*mitta de marzo,* yields the most abundantly. Then, at the end of June, there is commonly a scanty crop known as the *mitta de San Juan*—the harvest of the festival of St. John—while a third, following in October or November, is the *mitta de Todos Santos*—the harvest of all saints.

Usually the shrubs are weeded only after each harvest, and there seems to be a prejudice against doing this at other times, though if the cocals are kept clear the harvest may be anticipated by more than a fortnight.[20] Garcilasso tells how an avaricious planter, by diligence in cultivating his Coca, got rid of two-thirds of his annual tithes in the first harvest.

Picking exerts a beneficial influence on the shrub, which otherwise would not flourish so well. The gathering—*palla*—is still done by women and children—*palladores* as they are

[19] Weddell; 1853. [20] Garcilasso; Hakluyt; 1871.

termed—just as was the custom during the time of the Incas, though the Colombians will not permit women to take part in the Coca cultivation at any time. Many writers have spoken of the extreme care with which the leaves are picked or pinched from the shrub, one by one; but to a casual observer the gathering seems to be done far more carelessly. The collector squats down in front of the shrub, and taking a branch strips the leaves off with both hands by a dexterous movement, while avoiding injury to the tender twigs. The pickers must be skilled in their work, for not only a certain knack, but some little force is requisite, as is shown by the wounds occasioned to even the hard skin of the hand of those who are accustomed to the task.

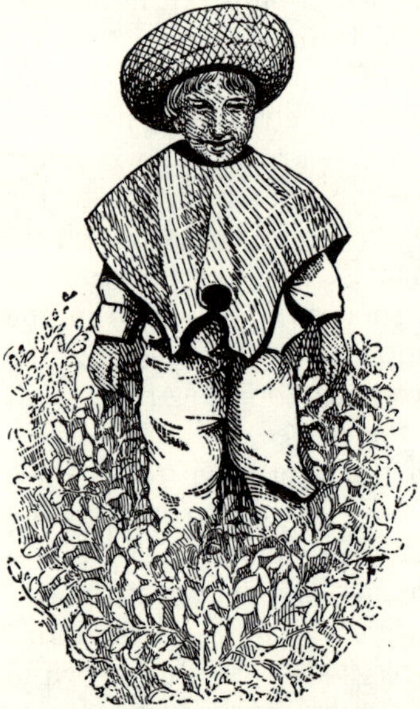

A Little Coca Picker —*Brettes.*

The leaves are collected in a poncho or in an apron of coarse wool, from which the green leaves — termed *matu* — are emptied into larger sacks—*materos,* in which they are conveyed to the drying shed—*matucancha.* Four or five expert pickers in a good cocal can gather a *cesta*—equivalent to a bale of twenty--five pounds, in a day. Harvesting is never commenced except when the weather is dry, for rain would immediately spoil the leaves after they have been picked, rendering them black in color and unsalable, a condition which the Indians term *Coca goñupa,* or *yana Coca.*

Coca when gathered is stored temporarily in sheds—*matuhuarsi,* which open into closed courts, the *cachi,* or *matupampa,* and the contents of these warehouses indicate the prosperity of the master of the cocal.[21] In the drying yards of

[21] Gosse; 1861.

these places the leaves are spread in thin layers two or three inches deep, either upon a slate pavement—*pizarra,* or simply distributed upon a hard piece of clear ground of the *casa de hacienda.* The closest guardianship must now be maintained over the leaves during the process of drying, and on the slightest indication of rain they are swept under cover by the attendants with the greatest rapidity. Drying may be completed within six hours in good weather, and when properly dried under such favorable conditions, the leaf is termed *Coca del dia* and commands the highest price. A well cured mature Coca leaf is olive green, pliable, clean, smooth and slightly glossy, while those which are old or are dried more slowly assume a brownish green and are less desirable. After drying, the leaves are thrown in a heap, where they remain about three days while undergoing a sort of sweating process. When this commences the leaf is crisp, but sweating renders it soft and pliable. After sweating the leaves are again sun dried for a half hour or so, and are then ready for packing. If the green leaves cannot be immediately dried, they may be preserved for a few days if care be taken not to keep them in heaps, which would induce a secondary sweating or decomposition and give rise to a musty odor, termed *Coca ccaspada,* which clings even to the preparations made from such leaves.

The refinement of curing maintains a certain amount of moisture in the leaf, together with the peculiar Coca aroma, and it is exact discernment in this process which preserves the delicacy of flavor. When drying has been so prolonged as to render the leaf brittle and without aroma, the quality of Coca is destroyed. It has been suggested that an improvement might be made in drying through the use of sheds, where the leaves could be exposed in layers to an artificial heat, and a current of dry air, after the manner of the *secaderos* used in Cuba for drying coffee. But whether because of an unwillingness to adopt new methods, or because of some peculiar influence of the atmosphere imparted to the leaf in the native way of drying, all attempts to employ artificial methods have proved unsatisfactory.

The exquisite little creamy white flower of Coca is seen in

the fields of the cocals after each harvest, the flowering continuing for about two weeks. The Coca plants which were presented to the New York Botanical Garden have continued to blossom at irregular intervals throughout the year, while

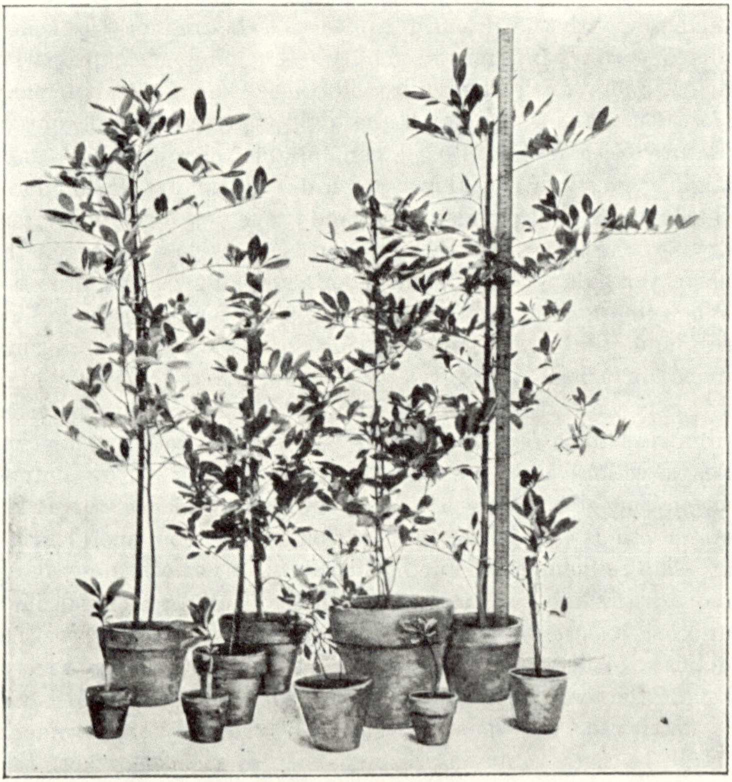

TEN COCA PLANTS RECEIVED FROM PARIS, FRANCE, SEPTEMBER, 1898.
[*From a Photograph.*]
The upright rule on the right is one metre high. These plants, presented to the New York Botanical Garden, have in two years fully doubled in size.

M. Mariani told me that the shrubs grown in his conservatories flower in October. The blossoms are very delicate and the petals quickly fall.

When the fruit has formed it changes color in ripening,

through all the hues from a delicate greenish yellow to a deep scarlet vermilion, and upon the same shrub there may be a number of such colorations to be seen at one time. Monardes, writing centuries ago, said: "The fruit is in the form of a grape, and as the fruit of the myrtle is reddish when it is ripening, and about of the same dimensions—when attaining its highest maturity becoming darker black." I was going to say that the fruit resembles the smallest of oval cranberries, both in color and in shape, for I at one time found some little cranberries which appeared so much like the Coca fruit as to seem almost identical; but all cranberries are not alike, and there has already been too much confusion in hasty comparison, so I shall reserve my description for the more technical details. The fruit is gathered while yet scarlet during the March harvest, but if it is permitted to remain on the bush it becomes dark brown or black and shrivels to the irregular lobing of the contained nut.

In selecting the seeds care is taken to cast aside all fruit that is decayed, the balance being thrown into water, and those which are light enough to float are rejected as indicating they have been attacked by insects. The balance are then rotted in a damp, shaded place, to extract the seed, which is washed and sun dried. When it is desired to preserve these any length of time the fruit is exposed to the hot sun, which dries the fleshy portion into a protective coating. But the seeds do not keep well. In Peru perhaps they will retain germinating power for about fifteen days, while those from plants grown in the conservatory must be planted fresh, when still red, for if allowed to dry they become useless.[22]

With every detail to cultivation which tradition has inspired, the Coca crop is not always secure, for the cocals are subject to the attacks of several pests, which, while a constant source of annoyance may at times seriously damage the shrubs. Below an altitude of four thousand feet there is the *ulo,* a little butterfly, which during a dry spell deposits its eggs, and as the grubs develop they devour the younger leaves. In the older cocals an insect called *mougna* sometimes intro-

[22] Mariani; *person. com.;* 1899.

duces itself into the trunk of the shrub and occasions its withering. M. Grandidier speaks of a disease termed *cupa,* or *cuchupa,* in the valley of the Santa Marta, which has destroyed an entire crop within eight days. From an attack of this not only the immediate leaf is rendered small and bitter, but during the following year the shrub remains unproductive, and a gall-like excrescence is developed termed *sarna mocllo*—seeds of gall. Some cultivators at the first indication of this disease prune the affected twigs and so succeed in raising a new crop by the next harvest.

The ant, *cuqui*, which is a great pest through all the montaña, is a dangerous evil to the Coca plant. It not only cuts the roots, but disintegrates the bark and destroys the leaves, and in a single night may ruin an entire plantation. In fact, the sagacity of the traditional ant is outdone by these pests. Some of them are capable of carrying a kernel of corn, and an army of them will run off with a bag of corn in a night, kernel by kernel, making a distinct trail in the line of their depredations. They build their nests of leaves, twigs and earth, and even construct an underground system of channels to supply their hillocks with water. It is extremely difficult to keep them out of a cocal, as they will burrow under the deepest ditches, and the only method of being free from them is to destroy their hills wherever they are found. Another enemy to the shrub is a long bluish earthworm, which eats the roots and so occasions the death of the plant. Then a peculiar fungus, known as *taja,* forms at times on the tender twigs, occasioned by injury or from poor nutrition. Aside from these pests, there are a number of weeds which are particularly injurious to Coca, among which are the *Panicum platicaule, P. scandens, P. decumbens, Pannisetum Peruvianum, Drimaria,* and *Pteris arachnoidea.*[23] These plants grow rapidly and take so much nourishment from the soil as to destroy the nutrition of the Coca shrub. For a similar reason the planting of anything between the rows is now abandoned.

There grows on the trunks and branches of the older Coca shrubs various species of lichens, termed *lacco,* which, while

[23] Poeppig; 1836.

not known to be detrimental, may even have a marked influence on the alkaloidal yield of the leaf. Two very pretty specimens in the herbarium of Columbia University show the *Parmelia* and *Usnea*. These formed part of a collection

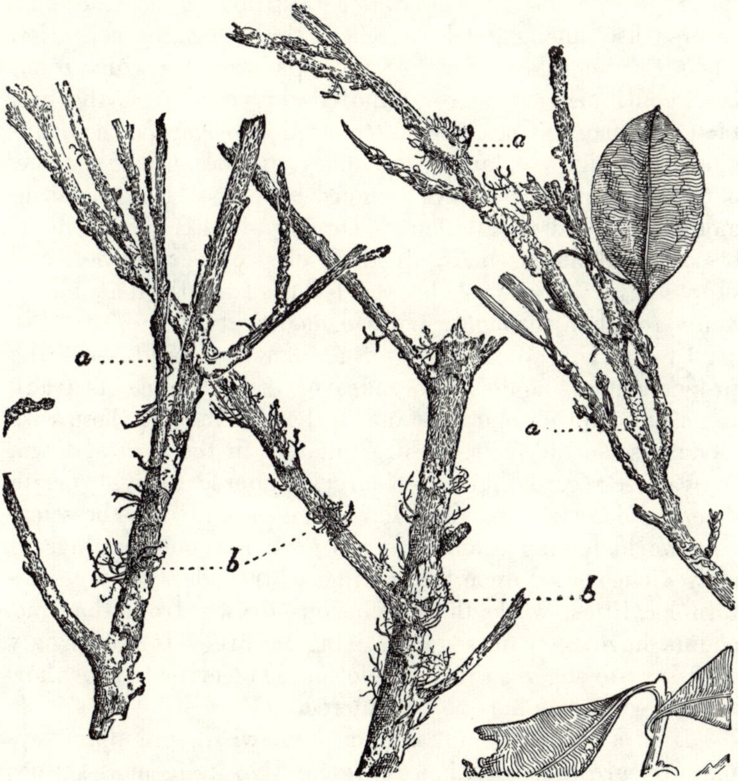

LACCO OR LICHENS ON SPECIMENS OF COCA.
From the Herbarium of Columbia University. *Drawn from Nature.*
a, a, a, Species of *Parmelia; b, b, Usnea Barbata.*

made by Miguel Bang, during 1890, in the Province of Yungas, Bolivia, from a cocal at an altitude of 6,000 feet.[24]

In describing any plant it is the ideal of botanists to base their studies upon an example growing under natural conditions. It is inferred that cultivation causes a variability which may occasion considerable alteration from the original

[24] Distributed by Drs. Britton and Rusby.

type. Considering the centuries elapsed during which we have any historical references to the use of Coca among the Peruvians, it is remarkable to note how uniformly the characteristics of the plant are continued. Even at the period of the Spanish invasion there was a tradition which traced its revered use among the Incans back through many centuries, when it was employed for the precise purposes for which it has been continued. Yet for hundreds of years after the first facts concerning Coca were introduced into Europe the available knowledge was largely legendary, and because of the phenomenal properties always assigned to its use Coca was commonly regarded as fabulous. During all this period, however, the plant has maintained its classic peculiarities, and supposed variations probably result more from the demands of commerce than through a natural modification.

In studying the history of a plant it would seem the proper course should be to endeavor to first trace its traditional description and uses and to then harmonize these with modern scientific facts. Unfortunately in the case of Coca, the earlier records have been largely ignored through prejudice, the descriptions which have been presented to the scientific world having often been the arbitrary outcroppings of convenience based upon the writings of travellers through certain localities, while the conclusions drawn from these accounts have been of a generalizing nature. It seems only necessary to suggest this possible source of error to show how readily confusion may be engendered.

It is always difficult to determine whether a plant, apparently growing wild, is a representative indigenous species which has existed from an early period or has been introduced from some distant locality. The scattering of seeds, by the winds, or birds, as well as by other unconscious means, may be one source of distribution of a plant through a wide region, though as a rule the abode of each species may be regarded as nearly constant. One of the strongest evidences of the an-

DESCRIPTIONS OF CLASSIC EXAMPLES OF COCA, ON OPPOSITE PAGE.

1. E. Coca of Commerce. 2. E. Coca, Bonpland; (Cuzco). 3. E. Coca, Weddle; (Bolivia). 4. E. Coca, Poeppig; (Peru). 5. E. Coca, Triana; (New Granada). 6. E. Coca, Triana; (New Granada). 7. E. Coca, Hondense, Kunth; (New Granada).

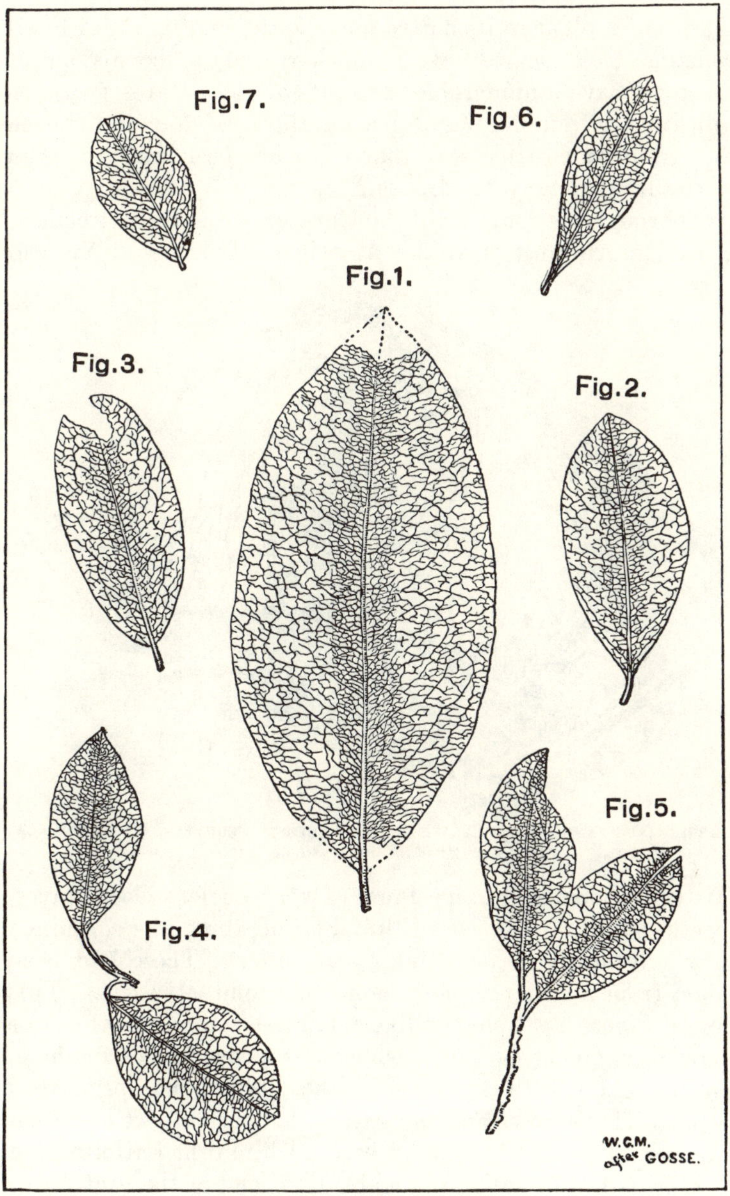

CLASSIC EXAMPLES OF COCA.
[See description on opposite page.]

tiquity of a plant in its native home is the finding of its fossil remains. While we have no such record in the history of Coca, we have innumerable examples of Coca leaves found in relics and with mummies of great antiquity, which indicate in the strongest possible way that Coca has been indigenous to Peru through many hundreds of years.

Through the courtesy of the Curator of the Department of Peruvian Antiquities at the American Museum of Natural

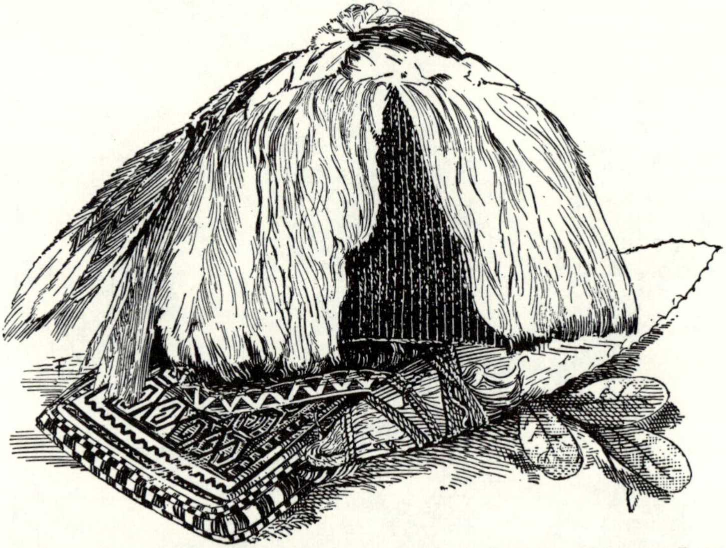

FEATHER CAP AND FLINT KNIFE FROM ANCIENT PERUVIAN MUMMY PACK.
American Museum of Natural History.

History, I obtained a specimen of very ancient Coca leaves, together with a little bag of llipta, all of which was contained in a chuspa of the ordinary Incan order. These had been taken from a mummy pack found in a tomb at Arica. This mummy wore a cap shaped like a Turkish fez, woven of coarse wool in unique design, over which was a covering of feathers, surmounted with a green tassel-like feather, máking a very imposing head dress and indicating that the subject had been a person of rank. One hand bore a white flint knife, with a handle made by binding cloth about one end of the flint.

In the pack with the mummy, which had every evidence of

extreme antiquity, was a papal bull dated 1571. Allowing some twenty years for this document to have found its way to Peru, this would make the mummy over three hundred years old. That this was so, may be inferred from the fact that no other European object was found in the pack, everything being of an aboriginal order before the influence of the Conquest had been manifest. The leaves were dry and very brittle and of a light brownish color. The llipta was in soft yellow lumps. A reproduction of these leaves proves them to be of the variety which we to-day understand as Truxillo or Peruvian Coca. They vary in size from a half inch in length to pieces showing a probable length of some three inches. They all plainly show the peculiar characteristic markings of Coca, the lateral lines being well made out. Unfortunately this mummy pack had been treated with antiseptics before it was opened, which rendered it impossible to note the taste of the leaves, and there was not sufficient of them to attempt an assay. By a comparison of the plate with the accompanying one of recent Coca leaves it will be seen that there is no material difference, and certainly no ground to presume that the classic Coca of Peru is extinct or modified. (*Page 250-251.*)

In a choice collection of leaves from the district of Caravaya I have found every variety of leaf present, the pronounced obovate, the long narrow leaf, the leaf with the little point extending as though a continuation of the inner leaf, and the distinctly lanceolate, so that it is quite probable that more than one variety of Coca is grown in one plantation.

The Coca which comes to the markets of the commercial world is broadly grouped in two varieties, the Bolivian or Huanuco and the Peruvian or Truxillo variety, the characteristic difference between the two varieties being that the Bolivian leaf is thick, dark green colored above and yellowish beneath, while the Peruvian leaf is smaller, more delicate, lighter color and grayish beneath. Manufacturers of cocaine use practically nothing except the Bolivian or Huanuco Coca, which contains the highest percentage of cocaine and the least quantity of associate alkaloids, which cocaine manufacturers have regarded as "objectionable" because they will not crystal-

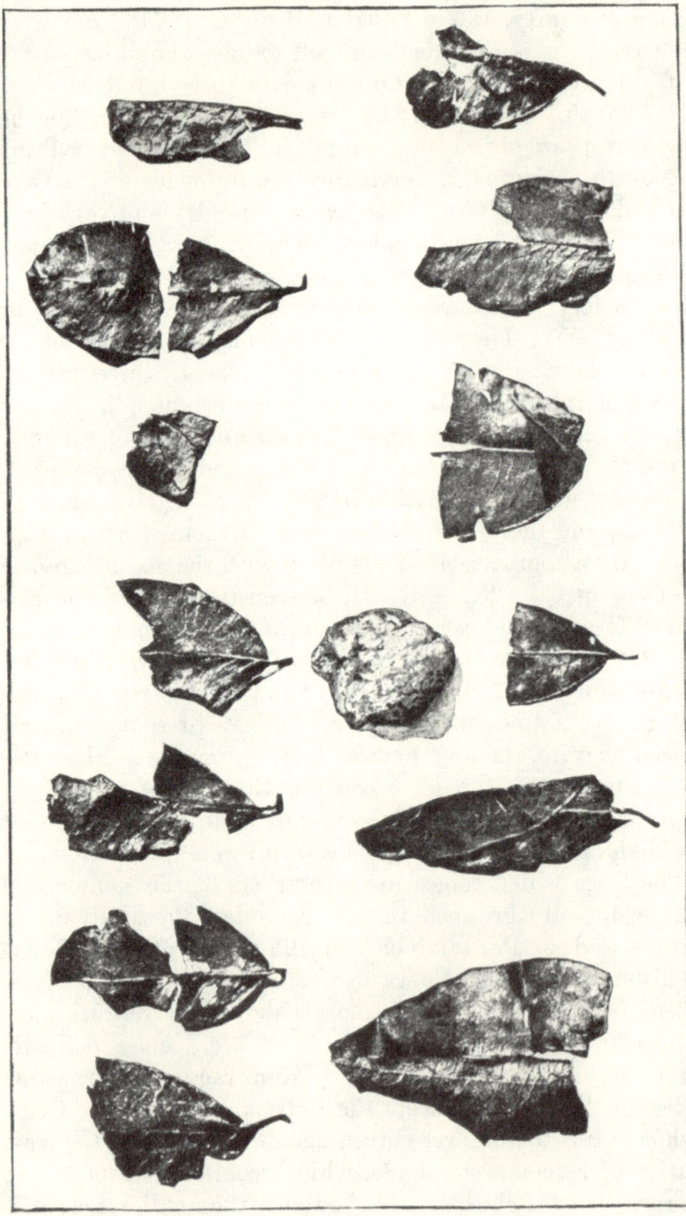

TYPICAL COCA OF THE INCAS. [*From a Photograph.*]
These leaves were taken from a mummy pack found at Arica, Peru, and presumed to be at least three hundred years old. The substance in the centre of the illustration is a lump of *llipta.* [Compare with type of Modern Coca on opposite page.]

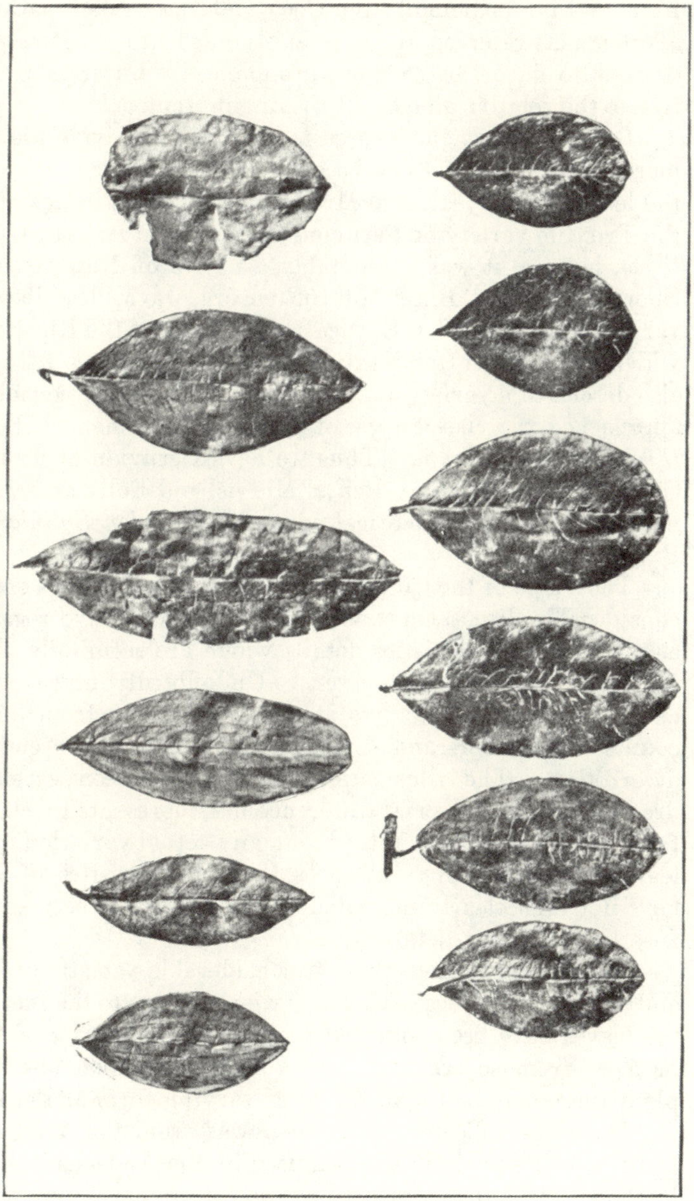

TYPE OF MODERN COCA.

These leaves were selected from a bale of choice Coca sent the author from Caravaya, Peru. Note their various shapes and sizes and similarity to the ancient leaves on opposite page.

lize. While medicinally the Coca yielding a combination of alkaloids is preferred, the two varieties of leaf are entirely distinct as to flavor, being more pronouncedly bitter in proportion to the relative amount of cocaine present.

Botanists have endeavored to still further divide the commercial varieties of Coca because of certain peculiarities of the leaf. Some years ago Mr. Morris, of Kew, in describing the Truxillo variety of Peruvian Coca, named it *Novo Granatense,* because it was presumably a native of New Grenada. Shortly after Dr. Burck, of Buitenzorg, Java, described the variety collected by Dr. Spruce on the banks of the Rio Negro, which he named after its discoverer, *E. Spruceanum.* He also described a variety of Huanuco Coca which he considered approached the classic type of Lamarck, and named it *Erythroxylon Bolivianum.* Thus we have Peruvian or Truxillo Coca, variety *Novo Granatense,* Morris, and Bolivian or Huanuco Coca, which is identical with *Erythroxylon Bolivianum,* Burck.

The shape of the Coca leaf is a question which has excited considerable discussion among botanists, who have regarded as striking characteristics details which are seemingly unimportant to the casual observer. Undoubtedly much of the early confusion in attempts at classifying Coca from the accounts of travellers and writers has arisen from unscientific description. The illustrations have often been carelessly drawn, and this pictorial difference has represented technical faults of the illustrator rather than any actual variation of the leaf itself. In many instances the characteristics of Coca have not been clearly indicated. The result has been to confuse those seeking details.

As a matter of fact, there is considerable variation in size and shape of the Coca leaf, a variation not due to the fact that the leaves have been collected from several varieties of Coca or even from several different shrubs, but upon one Coca plant there may be found leaves of varying form and size.

The Coca collected by Jussieu was from the Yungas of Bolivia, while the bulk of Coca used by the Andeans is grown in Peru. It is the plant used by these Indians, the properties of which have been exalted from the time of the Incas, to which all the traditions of Coca are attached, and really one would be more justified in saying that the specimens sent by Jussieu from Bolivia were a modification of the historical Incan plant than to say that the Peruvian grown species is a

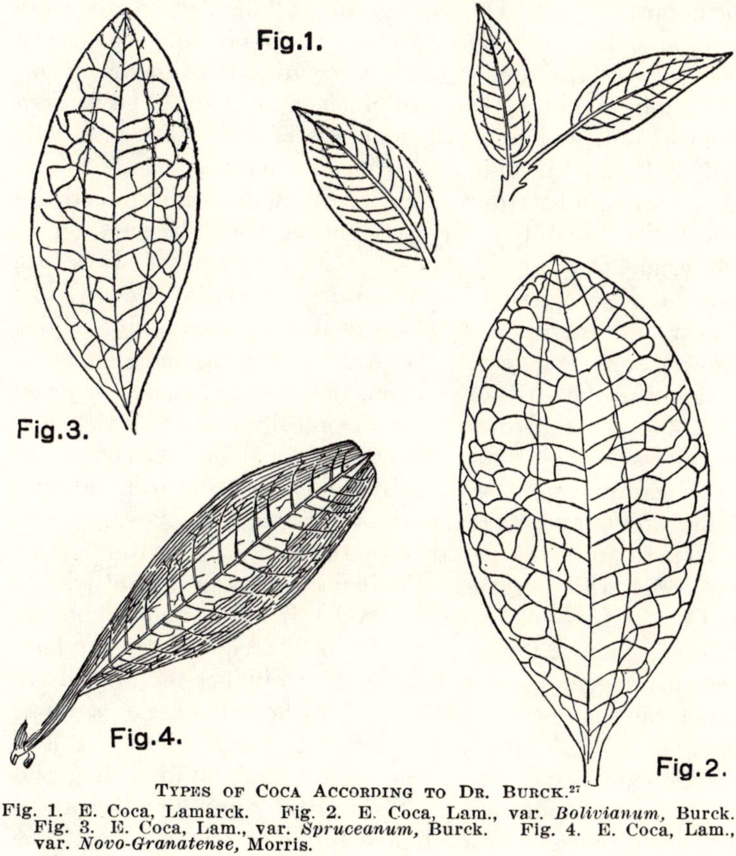

TYPES OF COCA ACCORDING TO DR. BURCK.[27]
Fig. 1. E. Coca, Lamarck. Fig. 2. E. Coca, Lam., var. *Bolivianum,* Burck. Fig. 3. E. Coca, Lam., var. *Spruceanum,* Burck. Fig. 4. E. Coca, Lam., var. *Novo-Granatense,* Morris.

variation. The Indians prefer Peruvian Coca, and but for the importance to Bolivian Coca through cocaine less of the latter variety would be grown. Any attempt to describe Coca as a whole from any one variety, it will be seen, must be confusional, Bolivian Coca being rich in cocaine, while Peruvian

[27] Burck; 1892.

Coca is richer in aromatic alkaloids. This variation is still maintained in the plants grown artificially at Paris and in the East.

Plants and seeds of several varieties of Coca have been distributed to the botanical gardens of the English colonies at Demerara, Ceylon, Darjeeling, and Alipore, where they are cultivated in a commercial way and where they have been carefully studied under the new conditions of environment. Having in mind the history of cinchona, which had been taken from its native home in the montaña of Peru and so successfully cultivated in the East, it seems a natural inference that Coca may also be grown scientifically under similar facilities where the possibility for distribution would be superior to the crude Andean methods. Certain parts of Java are particularly suggestive of the Coca region of Peru. The country is traversed by two chains of mountains which are volcanic, and, as in the Andean region, the vegetation varies with the altitude. From the seaboard to an elevation of 2,000 feet the growth is of a tropical nature, and rice, cotton and spices abound. Above this to 4,500 feet coffee, tea and sugar are raised, while still higher, to 7,500 feet, only the plants of a temperate region can be grown.

There are many details essential in the cultivation of tea and coffee which suggest similar necessities in the cultivation of Coca. In Ceylon the best coffee is grown from 3,000 to 4,500 feet above the sea, where rain is frequent and the temperature moderate, and, like Coca, the higher the altitude in which the shrub can be cultivated without frost, the better is the quality of the product. Although the yield may be less, the aromatic principles are more abundant and finer than that produced in the lowlands. Similar hilly ground where there is good drainage is best adapted for the growth of tea. The shrubs do not yield leaves fit for picking before the third year, the produce increasing yearly until the tenth year. The yield from the tea plant is about the same as that from Coca, but the young leaves of tea are usually gathered, while only the matured leaves of Coca are picked.

The climate, the environment, the method of cultivation

and even the uses all seem paralleled in tea, coffee and Coca, but the benefits of application are immensely in favor of Coca. Tea and coffee were introduced into Europe in the sixteenth century, about the period when we have the first historical record of Coca. They were not then popular beverages as now, and it was only after much prejudice had been overcome that they were considered necessary. As the properties of Coca become better appreciated there is every reason to suppose this substance will come into as general use in every household as a stimulant—rendering a clear head instead of the hot and congested one so apt to follow the use of coffee or tea—Coca does not impair the stomach, while it possesses the added advantage of freeing the circulation from impurities instead of, like tea and coffee, adding additional waste products to the blood stream, as has been suggested by Morton[25] and by Haig.[26]

The Coca leaf affords a most exquisite subject for histological study. Viewed in transverse section, the flattened cells of the upper epidermis are large, oblong and of irregular shape; their outer walls are thicker than the walls between the cells and give the surface of the leaf a wavy outline. Beneath this protective layer is a single row of upright cells—the palisade tissue—which are filled with chlorophyl granules. These cells have very thin walls and they are compactly set together, diverging only at their lower edge, where the underlying spongy tissue is less compact. Here and there may be found cells containing crystals of oxalate of lime. Immediately beneath the palisade row of cells are irregularly shaped and loosely united, affording many inter-cellular spaces except where the more compact tissue surrounds the fibro-vascular bundle, which constitutes the veins. The epidermal cells of the lower surface of the leaf are smaller and more uniform in size than those of the upper epidermis. The lateral walls of the cells are straight and their outer walls are much thicker at their central part than their marginal joinings, thus forming a papillary projection, which is characteristic. At intervals these cells are interrupted by the

[25] Morton, 1879. [26] Haig, 1897.

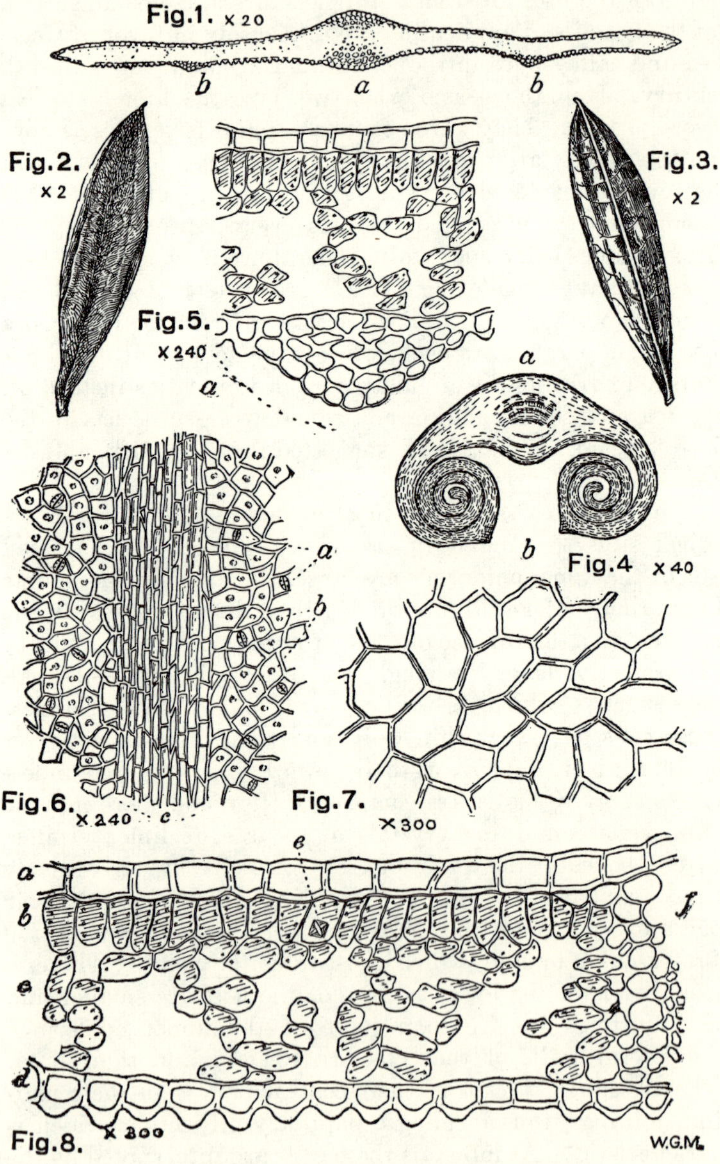

STRUCTURE OF THE COCA LEAF IN DETAIL—*Studies Drawn from Nature.*
[See description on opposite page.]

little breathing places or stomata, bounded on either side by modified epidermal cells that are not papillose.

A transverse section of the leaf in the bud shows that it is rolled from its margin toward the midrib in such a way that the lateral lines lie close together. When such a leaf is carefully opened the midrib may be seen to be of the same color as the leaf, pale green, and succulent, tapering from the petiole until it is lost in the upper third of the leaf, while from the tip there is a terminal projection, slightly hooked, one millimetre long and of a very much paler green than the rest of the leaf. The margin of the upper half of the leaf shows a slight wavy outline, probably due to the more rigid venation. The lateral curved lines are distinctly marked as projections on the under surface of the leaf, which is slightly concave from the midrib to the margin on either side.

The following is a résumé of the Coca shrub more in technical detail:

Erythroxylon Coca, as cultivated in the montaña of the Andes, grows upon a delicate shrub, which varies according to the altitude, locality and conditions of its culture. It is commonly kept by pruning to a height of from three to six feet for convenience of picking. Examples which are found growing out of cultivation are commonly seen ten or twelve feet high.

The root on which the Coca shrub is dependent to imbibe the nutrition for the plant forms a loose tuft or cluster of fibres, which end in fine hair-like rootlets.

The trunk is covered with a rough bark, commonly overgrown with various species of lichens—a complex colony of

---

DESCRIPTION OF STRUCTURE OF THE COCA LEAF, ON OPPOSITE PAGE.

Fig. 1. Transverse section of a young Coca leaf near the tip; *a*, midrib; *b*, *b*, lateral lines, prominent only on under surface. Fig. 2. Upper surface of an opening Coca leaf, showing manner of its unrolling. Fig. 3. Under surface of a similar leaf. Fig. 4. Transverse section of the lower half of a young Coca leaf, showing manner in which it is rolled; *a*, midrib; *b*, prominence of lateral lines. Fig. 5. Transverse section of Coca leaf through a lateral line, *a*. Fig. 6. Under epidermis of a Coca leaf along a lateral line; *a*, stomata or breathing places; *b*, papillose cells; *c*, cells of the lateral line. Fig. 7. Upper epidermis of the Coca leaf. Fig. 8. Transverse section of a Coca leaf near the midrib; *a*, epidermal cells of upper surface; *b*, single row of palisade cells, with contained chlorophyl granules; *c*, spongy tissue of body of leaf; *d*, epidermal cells of lower surface; *e*, crystal of oxalate of lime; *f*, region of the midrib.

algæ and fungi—which apparently find favorable growth from the nature of the plant and the surrounding moist atmosphere. The shrub branches sparingly and these are alternate, either opening straight out from the sides of the trunk or ascending slightly, at times a little forked and bearing scanty foliage, the entire arrangement being adapted to afford a large surface for light and air to favor the nutrition of the plant. The color of the twigs varies from the pale fern-like green of the scaly tips to a deeper apple green, and as the firmer stem is formed the color deepens through various tints of brown until the gray bark of the trunk is reached.

The leaves are arranged as the branches—alternate, and so placed that their upper surface looks toward the apex of the stem, while the lower surface is directed away from it—*dorsiventral* as it is termed. The shape of all varieties of the Coca leaf tends to oblong forms, narrowing at each end, in some examples gradually, in others more abruptly, the base of the leaf tapering into a short petiole or leaf stalk. Lamarck described the Coca leaf of Jussieu as "oval pointed." The leaf of Bolivian Coca is large, elliptical, oval, broader above its middle, while the Peruvian leaf is more narrow obovate, or lanceolate. The Brazilian, the Colombian and also the Javan Coca have each a smaller leaf than either of the preceding, tending to oval, broadest in the middle, from which it tapers to the apex above and to the base below. The margin of the leaf of all varieties is without notching—entire. The apex of some varieties is depressed at the extremity of the midrib—emarginate, and there is often a little soft hooked point, as though a continuation of the midrib—*mucronate*. This point

---

DESCRIPTION OF STRUCTURE OF COCA FLOWER, ON OPPOSITE PAGE.

Fig. 1. Flower bud, *a*, in axil of leaves showing the bracts, *b*. Fig. 2. Section of Coca flower showing the arrangement of its parts; *a*, the calyx; *b*, the petals; *c*, the stamens; *d*, ovary, and contained ovules, *e*. Fig. 3. The expanded flower. Fig. 4. Flower seen from below. Fig. 5. Flower seen from above. Fig. 6. Separate petal, showing tooth-like appendage, *a*. Fig. 7. Petal seen from above. Fig. 8. The tooth-like appendage of the petal seen from its attachment. Fig. 9. Flower stripped of petals; *a*, anthers of stamens *b*; *c*, styles and stigmas of pistil; *d*, ovary; *e*, cupule of stamens—the *urceolus stamineus* of Martius; *f*, calyx. Fig. 10. Pistil, with cupule and stamens removed. Fig. 11. Diagram of fertilization, [after Darwin]; *A*, long styled; *B*, short styled; *a*, legitimate union; *b*, *b*, illegitimate union.

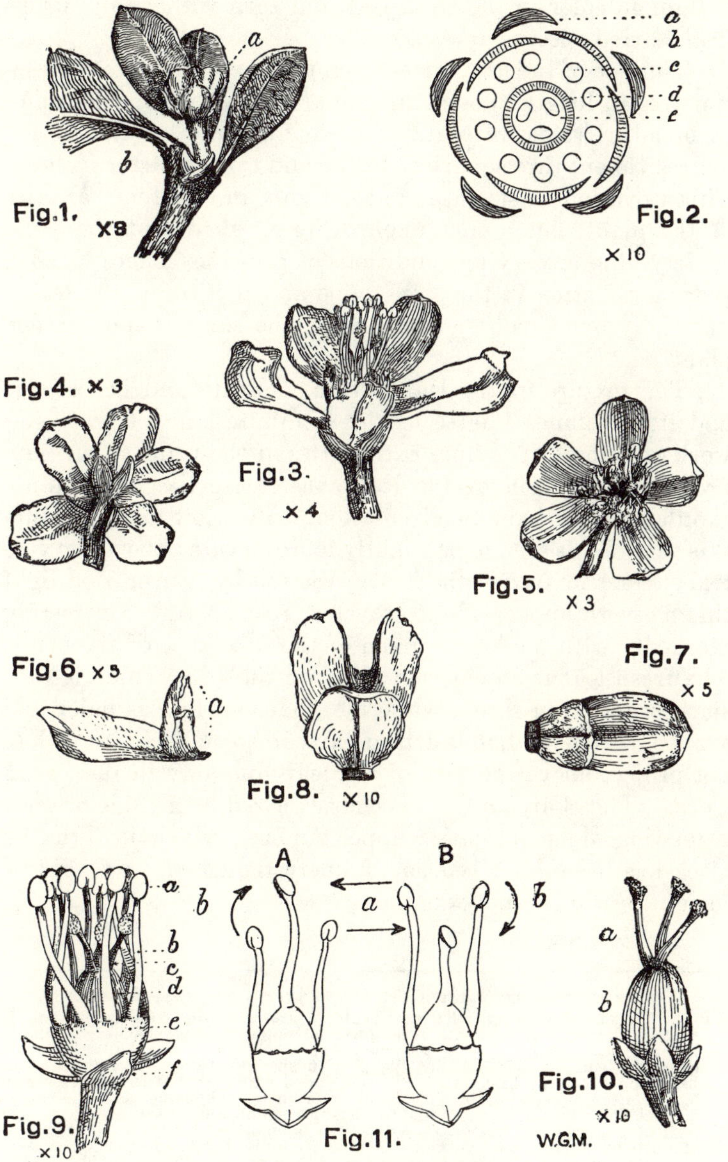

STRUCTURE OF THE COCA FLOWER IN DETAIL—*Studies Drawn from Nature.*
[See description on opposite page.]

is light in color in the fresh leaf, but soon withers and drops in the dried specimen.

The size of the leaf varies from two centimetres to ten centimetres in length (about three-quarters to four inches), and in breadth from two centimetres to four and one-half centimetres (about three-quarters to one and three-quarter inches). This variation in size is found not only in different varieties of the plant, but occurs upon different shrubs of the same variety, due to varying conditions of growth. There is, however, a variation in the size, shape and texture of the leaves upon any one shrub and even upon the same branch of one plant.

The texture of the leaf is thin, delicate and herbaceous and its substance intersected by a minute and intricate network of veins. The finer extremities of the veins as they approach the margin of the leaf anastomose like the minute capillaries of the animal circulation. By a low magnification this venation is seen to be slightly more elevated above the ventral surface or face of the leaf. Viewed by transmitted light this network appears light brown or rosy in tint, contrasting markedly with the bright green of the substance of the blade. The fresh leaf is an emerald green on the face, which is soft, smooth and even shiny, while the under surface is paler and grayish. The midrib is delicate and in some varieties it does not project above the face of the leaf—notably in the Javan Coca. The Bolivian Coca is characterized by a ridge or crest extending along its entire upper surface, which in Truxillo Coca has been described as obliquely truncate,[27] a feature I have not seen in any example.

[27] Schneider; 1898.

DESCRIPTION OF DETAILS OF COCA FRUIT, ON OPPOSITE PAGE.

Fig. 1. Tip of Coca spray, with ripe fruit, *a*, and growing stem with buds, *b*, with a young leaf and the triangular stipules at its base, *c*. Fig. 2. Dried fruit. Fig. 3. The six-lobed nut. Fig. 4. Longitudinal section through fruit; *a*, scarlet coat; *b*, pink fleshy substance; *c*, thin shell of nut; *d*, white starchy-albumen; *e*, suspended embryo; *f*, dried styles. Fig. 5. Transverse section of fruit, the references the same as in Fig. 4; *g*, two aborted ovules. Fig. 6. Embryo removed from seed; *a*, the radical; *b*, two cotyledons shown forced open at *c*. Fig. 7. *a*, Stamens of uniform length, seen from without the cupule, *b*, showing cells; *c*, relative size of pollen grains to anthers; *d*, pollen magnified 200 diameters. Fig. 8. *a*, Stamens of unequal length seen from within the cupule, *b*, showing attachment.

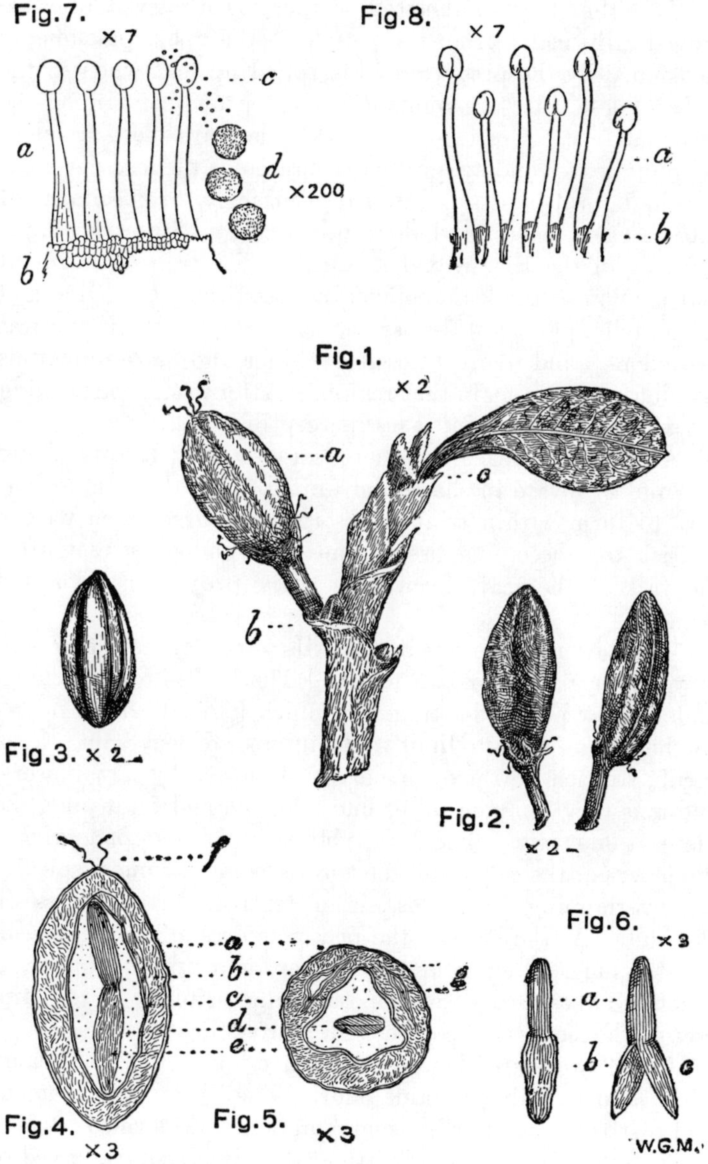

DETAILS OF THE COCA FRUIT AND SEED—*Studies Drawn from Nature.*
[See description on opposite page.]

To either side of the midrib there is a curved line, arranged elliptically from the petiole to the apex, presumably occasioned by the pressure of the rolled up leaf when in the bud. These lines are commonly more pronounced upon the lower surface. Gosse considers that they are more frequent in young leaves and are gradually effaced as the leaf develops, but the lateral lines are found in a majority of specimens of mature Coca leaves, and their presence constitutes a unique marking of the Erythroxylon family. By transmitted light that portion of the leaf included between the lateral line and the midrib appears of deeper shade, as though the tissue was more dense, and there is possibly a finer and more numerous division of the veins in that region. After prolonged soaking in water this deeper tint is less perceptible.

At the base of each leaf there is a pair of little appendages —stipules—ovate in shape and united along their inner borders to form a thin triangular organ, at first green with a whitish top, becoming brown and stiff, and persistent after the fall of the leaf, forming a scaly projection upon the branch.

The flower buds occur in the axils of the leaves, either solitary, or in groups of two to six. The bud is ovoid oblong, under a low power, looking very much like a bishop's mitre. As there is no definite limit to the number of leaves on a Coca shrub, so each new growth may be followed by new flowers, and it is very common to see bud, blossom and fruit upon the plant at one time. The floral plan is in five—*quincunxial*—the leaves of the calyx and the corolla being arranged spirally and overlapping like scales, either dextrorse or sinistrorse in the bud. At the base of the peduncle or stalk, about a centimetre long, which bears the flower, is a miniature leaf or bract. This is scaly, oval or triangular, similar to the stipules of the leaves, but shorter and more delicate.

The flowers are about a centimetre long, delicate, creamy white and exhaling a faint odor. They bear both stamens and pistils in the same blossom, and hence are termed perfect. Their outer circle of leaves—the calyx, is green, composed of five smooth, oval, triangular pointed, lobed sepals, united below and free above, the whole covered in some specimens with a delicate bloom—*glaucous.* That portion of the flower which is within the calyx—the corolla—is composed of five creamy leaves or petals, arranged above the sepals and alternate with them. The petals are of uniform shape, oval oblong, obtuse with a central nerve terminating in a little hooded point. Their upper surface is depressed longitudinally, which at the back shows as a keel. Their upper two-thirds is irregularly concave and the lower third is narrowed into a triangular groove or fold. Near the base inside is an ovoid wavy tooth, or claw-like appendage, half the length of the petal, and so attached that when the petals are united to form the corolla these processes present in the centre of the expanded flower as a little crown. The entire corolla soon falls, leaving the naked pistil.

The flower has ten slender stamens, the filaments of which are erect, pale yellowish green, either the length of the corolla or of alternate lengths, those opposite the petals being longer than those opposite the sepals. They are inserted below the pistil, coalescing on the inner side of a short membranaceous cupule—the *urceolus stamineus* of Martius, which surrounds the ovary and presents obtuse tooth-like projections outside and between the filaments. Upon each filament is attached by its base a small yellow oblong compartment or anther, which contains the pollen, the grains of which are granular and spheroidal, or smooth and oval similar to those of the lily.

The pistil has three irregular, divergent cylindrical, pale yellowish, green styles, which may be either longer or shorter than the stamens. Each bears a flattened cap of loose tissue—the stigma, to receive the pollen from the opening anthers. The ovary—with its contained ovules—fertilization of which generates the seeds of the plant, is situated above the calyx. It is obovate, pale yellowish green, smooth, with three compartments, from the summit of each of which is suspended an ovule, but before the ovary ripens to form the fruit two of its three compartments are obliterated.

When fresh the fruit is fleshy, mucilaginous, ovate, one to one and one-half centimetres long (three-eighths to five-eighths of an inch), smooth and having the remnants of the dried styles at its apex and the adherent calyx and cupule at its base. Its color, at first pale green, changes through varying tints to scarlet at maturity and is bluish black when dried, while its form shrivels to the irregular lobed shape of the contents. The seed, slightly shorter than the fruit, is pointed at each end, with six longitudinal lobes, smooth and of a pale flesh color. Its outer coat is very thin and the kernel, which completely fills the inner coat, is white, hard, albuminous and starchy. In this nutrient substance is suspended the straight green embryo or germ, half its length being the radical to form the root, while the balance composes the two flat cotyledons or seed leaves, and between these is the minute plumule, from which may develop the first shoot of the new Coca plant.

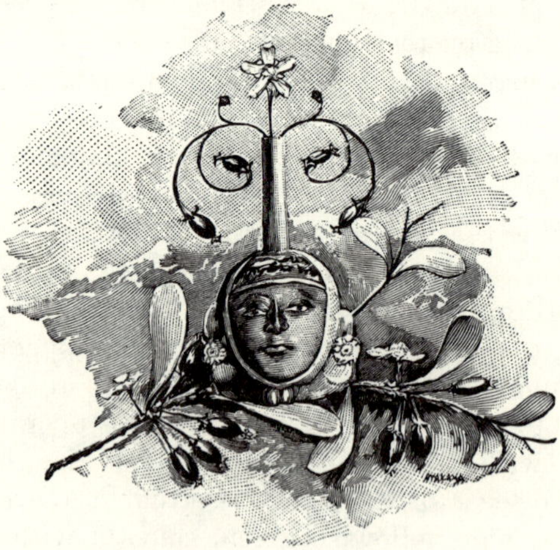

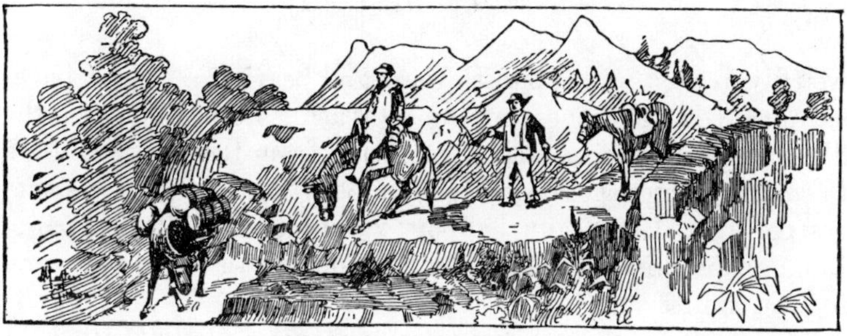

CHAPTER IX.

IN THE COCA REGION OF PERU.

"Of all the Plants that any Soil does bear,
This Tree in Fruits the richest does appear,
It bears the best, and bears them all the Year."
—*Cowley.*

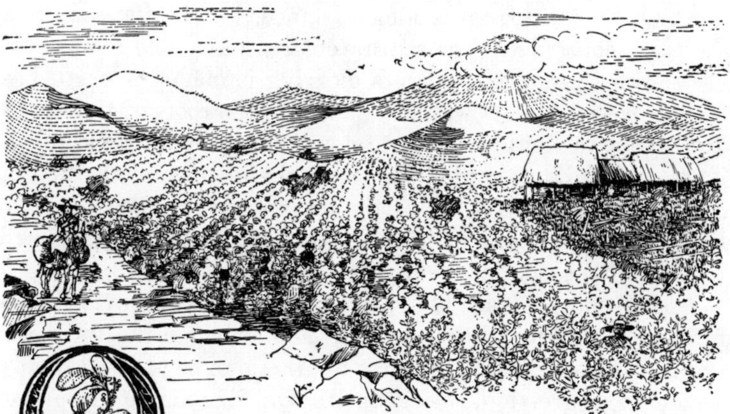

ON descending the slope of the Andes, from the bleak, barren heights of sierra to the eastern montaña, the soil at first thin gradually improves as the timber line is reached. What at first appears like the scrawly brush of the barren mountain is soon found to be the scraggy tops of a more favorable growth beneath. The trees now loom into full view, weirdly draped with Spanish moss and bearing a host of parasitic growths in witness of the increasing humidity. As the declivity is now more steep, transition from the colder heights to commencing vegetation seems to be with an abruptness suggestive of a descent by balloon, rather than Nature's panorama of the shifting seasons here set on end instead of traversing the country.

Everywhere there is a wealth of tropical plants, both wild and cultivated. The air is filled with the odor of sweet perfume from myriads of flowers, while here and there are sharply defined the clearings of the cocals, or Coca plantations, which commence at an altitude of about 5,000 feet. The whole scene presents a marked contrast to the former bleakness.

At times the mountains are surrounded by terraces, as though some giant stairway overgrown with an interlacing of tropical vegetation. In the utter barrenness of the western Cordillera terraces are built upon the bare rock with soil that must be brought from a long distance, but in the montaña these are constructed for a different reason. The mountains are so precipitous that when a clearing is made the earth has no longer the support which it had from the roots of trees, and during a rain would be washed away unless held by the walls. These are built around the sides of the mountain, the height of the wall and the width of the terrace varying according to the inclination of the hill, while retaining an appropriate soil in which the Coca bushes are set out.

Often these terrace beds are looked upon with envious eyes by some less industrious neighbor, and although the Indian is ordinarily honest and really too apathetic to be aroused to any serious transgression, the ease with which he may appropriate this desirable earth brought so ready to his uses may prove irresistible. The result is that the local tribunal has more occasion to settle the petty disputes arising from stealing a few bushels of dirt than for more serious offences.

The terraces—known as *andeneria*—are usually built along the base of some hill where the declivity may afford aid to the Indian in making a clearing and yet where the drainage

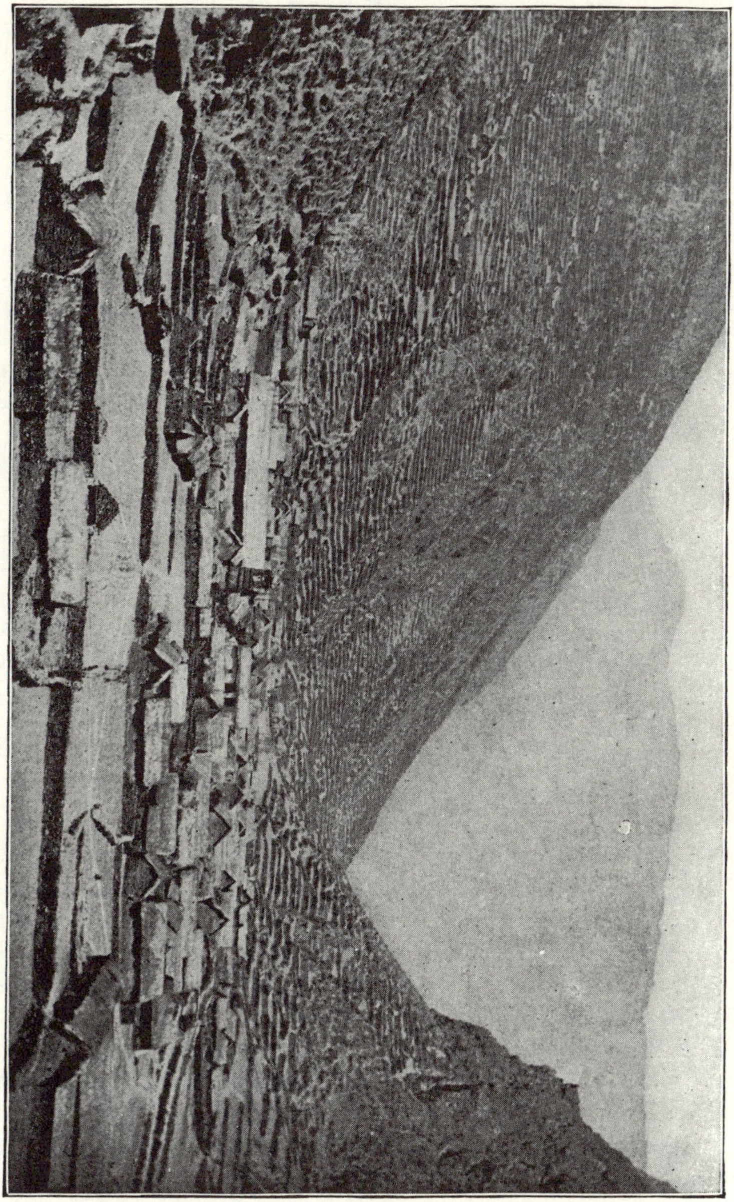

Incan Terraces at Cuyo-Cuyo, Peru ; Altitude, 7,000 Feet. See page 136. [*From a Photograph.*]

is suitable. On some slopes the inclination exceeds forty-five degrees, and the laborer is obliged to hold on with one hand while attending to cultivation with the other. There are many Coca plantations throughout Peru which are supposed to have existed for hundreds of years, and these choice locations are pointed to with reverential regard as having been continued from the days of the Incas.

The raising of Coca is the chief industry of certain districts of the montaña, and at one time the Peruvian government derived a considerable annual tax from it, but this is now only municipal, as at Huosa, where a tax of forty cents per quintal is imposed. In Bolivia the Coca traffic is said to be controlled by the State similar to the manner in which cinchona is regulated, the government reserving the right of purchase, a privilege commonly sold at auction to the highest bidder. Years ago Poeppig estimated the profit on a Coca plantation to be fully fifty per cent., and quite recently a prominent grower at Sandia said that a cocal would pay all expenses in two years if three crops could be obtained, while often there are four harvests.

Coca is cultivated in accordance with the same simple traditions which have been handed down from early Incan times, and there is still associated with it much of superstitious influence. Some Indians believe if a Coca bush be touched at its top by either man or beast the plant will surely die, while for a stranger to sleep near to a pile of drying leaves is considered dangerous. The Colombians say that no one should attempt to cultivate Coca who has not been favored with inherited talent in this direction, under the penalty of direful consequences, to say the least. Their women are not permitted to take any part in the several processes of the preparation of the leaf,[1] which is similar to a restriction against women at a certain period in some of the French vineyards.

Customs were so instilled in the laboring class of the Incas that the lapse of centuries has not changed them, and so the methods of cultivating Coca, described by Spanish writers immediately after the Conquest, may still be seen carried out

[1] Sievers; 1887.

with a minuteness of detail to-day. For just as Coca is indigenous to Peru, so too is the method of its cultivation, and each district has continued from generation to generation the traditions and processes of its predecessors, which, though varying in some trifle from those practiced in some other districts, are commonly similar throughout the Coca region.

During the time of the Incas the terrace method of growth was that generally pursued, for east of the Andes the montaña was thickly beset with unsubdued tribes of savages who resisted all attempts to infringe upon their territory. With the advent of the Spanish, and their recognition of the necessity for Coca in order to force the greatest endeavor from the Indian laborers in the mines, they pushed its cultivation further east and planted cocals in clearings made for that purpose. As these were abandoned for other localities more convenient to their interests, the surrounding savages who had been driven from this land were quick to return, and so what at one time was a luxuriant Coca plantation soon became covered through neglect with the prolific growths of the jungle and reverted into an apparently virgin forest.

So sudden may be the change here whenever cultivation is intermitted that it is difficult to appreciate its effect. The mighty trees of the forest are almost constantly falling, or are even pulled down by the parasitic vines with which they are encumbered, and once fallen they are immediately attacked and disintegrated by "a host of politic worms" and insects, which crumble them into humus, while above and about these fallen hulks there is soon entwined the unkempt network ot an impenetrable jungle. In some cases a tree may so fall as to span a stream and thus form a natural bridge, and such is the ordinary footpath over many a winding river.

Man does not walk through the montaña on the ground, unless paths have already been cut, but his way must be hewn with the machete, and then the walk is between an interlacing of vines and over the trunks of fallen trees, where progress at best is exceedingly slow and laborious. There is a wealth of everything, but it is of that wild, rugged and uncultivated nature which overpowers and even kills through a mere profusion. One may stand knee-deep in fuschias, geraniums, gentians and begonias, of a variety more choice than are commonly tenderly cultivated in more temperate climes, but which here are as great a nuisance as would be so many weeds where choicer growth is wished. Amidst an immensity of vegetation there are giant palms, tree-ferns, and an occasional cinchona towering far above one's head. Around are unnamed and innumerable dainty wax-like orchids, quite as common as is the hardy cactus of the bleak mountain heights, while butterflies, with the most gorgeous coloration, and of innumerable species, flutter like the fall of autumn leaves, but the beauty is lost in the annoyance of over-abundance.

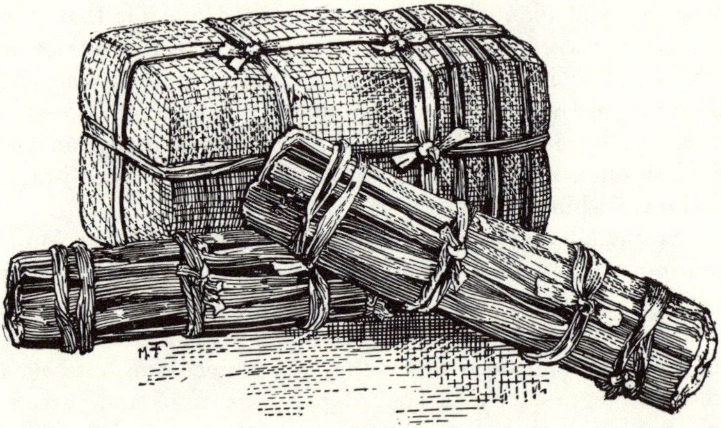

COCA PACKED FOR SHIPPING.

The surface under cultivation in the little *chacras,* or cocals where Coca is grown, is estimated by the *cato.* This is a piece of ground containing about nine hundred square meters or a little less than a quarter of an acre. Each Coca bush yields an average of four ounces of leaves, which dry out fully sixty per cent. Calculating the shrubs as set two by three feet apart, there would be upwards of seven thousand upon an acre of ground, or nearly eighteen hundred to a *cato.* A yield of four ounces from each bush would amount to four hundred and fifty pounds per *cato* at each harvest, and three harvests a year would yield an annual crop of thirteen hundred and fifty pounds of fresh leaves, or five hundred and forty pounds when cured and packed.

Usually the cocals are conducted by an Indian and his immediate family. When help is employed in harvesting the pickers are paid sixty cents of native money—at present equal to some twenty-nine cents of United States coin—for each thirty pounds of leaves picked. Adding to this an equal expense for cultivation, Coca under favorable conditions costs the planter less than three cents a pound at his cocal. When the product is exported the expense of transportation by mule or llama over the mountains to the sea must be considered in addition.

Coca is packed in a variety of ways, according to the district from which it is shipped. It is sometimes shaped by crude wooden presses into bales, or at times it is trodden into sacks—stamped Coca, though this is apt to break the leaf. In some districts the leaves are sprinkled with charcoal, to keep them moist. The bales are done up in huge banana leaves, bound with an outer wrapping of coarse woolen cloth known as *bayeta,* or *jerga;* these wrappings varying in color or quality in different localities. In Huanuco they are gray or black; in other provinces gray, white or brown. At times the sacking in which the bales are done up is woven in colored patterns. Such a package is termed a *cesta* and weighs from twenty-one to twenty-five pounds, the variation depending on the means adopted for transportation. Two *cestas* constitute a *tambor,* and in localities where Coca is conveyed on the backs of mules three *tambores* are united in one package, so that one hundred and fifty pounds may be carried each side of the animal, but where Coca is carried by llamas the *cesta* is smaller, because this beast can bear much less than half the burden of the mule.

Improperly packed leaves are liable to undergo secondary fermentation, and this not only deprives them of their essential qualities, but occasions the development of new ones which are undesirable, or, as the Indians term, *cholarse.* It has been presumed that it is at this time that objectionable alkaloids are formed as a result of decomposition. To avoid this it is desirable that the packages of Coca shall be in small bales.

For native consumption Coca is often packed in small lots sufficient to last one user about a month. Some of these packages are given various geometrical shapes and are covered with weavings of vari-colored wicker and cords so artistically, that the wrappings are sought as ornaments to hang in the houses after the Coca has been consumed.

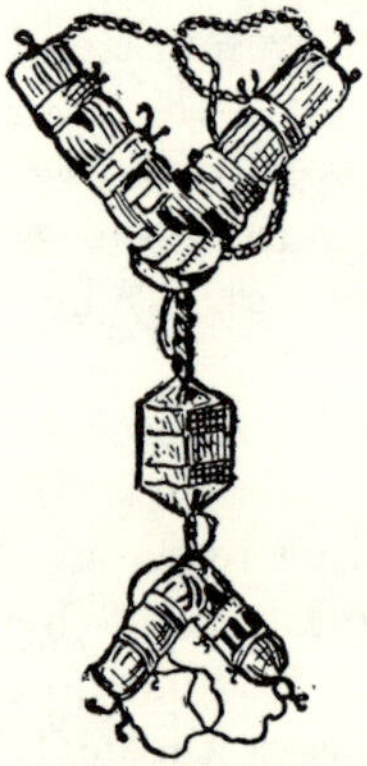

WOVEN PACKAGE OF COCA.

The chief places for the shipment of Coca are Salaverry—the port of Truxillo in the north, and Mollendo—the terminus of the railroad from the Titicaca region in the south.

There are two varieties of leaf coming to the North American market: the Huanuco—or large leaf, sometimes referred to as the Bolivian Coca, and the Truxillo—or narrow leaf, known as Peruvian Coca. In selecting a leaf the several manufacturers with whom I have corresponded have assured me that they base their choice upon the assay and yield of cocaine. For this reason the Huanuco leaf is the variety commonly found in the market, as it contains a larger amount of cocaine than the Truxillo leaf, which is considered less profitable because of its lower yield of this alkaloid. The native user, however, does not select the *hatun-yunca*—or large leaf Coca, his choice never being influenced by the amount of cocaine presumably present in the leaf chosen. Locally the distinction is made between *hajas dulces*—the sweet leaf, and *hajas amargas*—the bitter leaf, the amount of cocaine present occasioning the bitter quality, while a combination of aromatic principles renders the leaf of more desirable flavor. These principles, though commonly asserted to be exceedingly volatile, are still found in well preserved exported leaves.

The physiological accounts hitherto published of the action of Coca are often confusional because this distinction in the variety of leaf has not been considered, while many experimenters have contented themselves with enumerating the physiological effects of cocaine rather than that of Coca. In this connection Dr. Rusby says: "In my article* I took account of the Bolivian Coca only, which is practically the same as the Peruvian, or Huanuco variety, which is the one used for the manufacture of cocaine. As the leaves are found here in the dried state, their properties are, I believe, almost wholly due to the presence of cocaine, quite different from the properties of the fresh, or very recently dried leaves. There is another variety of Coca differing from the Huanuco variety, known as Truxillo leaves, the properties of which as found in this market differ from the Huanuco leaves, while more nearly resembling them in their fresh or recently dried state and as used in the Andes by the natives. You will thus see that all your labors in the direction of physiological research are likely to be fruitless, unless you will be able to ascertain in each case which variety of leaf was used by the one making the report. This I believe to be wholly impossible. Ninety-nine per cent. of our physicians scarcely know that there are two varieties, or at least that the varieties differ in any way medicinally. The endeavor has been to prevent physicians from learning facts concerning drugs. It is not likely that they can learn from the pharmacist which leaf he used at any particular time, for various reasons."[2] The biased effort, therefore, to misjudge preparations of Coca because they are not rich in cocaine is but an outgrowth of imperfect knowledge, for the unique quality of the Coca leaf is not solely dependent upon the presence of that alkaloid. It is as Dr. Squibb long since asserted from an intimate study of the qualities of Coca: "But as there is undoubtedly a value to Coca which is not measured by the yield of alkaloid, the proportion of alkaloid does not disprove the alleged inferiority."[3]

Thus it will be seen that the Coca leaf as used among the Indians of Peru is one thing, and the variety exported because

* *Coca at Home and Abroad.* [2] *Person. com.*; 1898. [3] *Ephemeris;* May, 1880.

of its large alkaloidal percentage of cocaine is wholly another matter. This is a distinction which any lover of tobacco will readily appreciate, for surely a fine cigar is never estimated by the amount of nicotine which it contains, nor is the flavor or quality of a delicate tea measured by its percentage of theine. We are beginning to learn Coca more intimately and even the more casual observer may soon realize that there is a very wide interim between Coca absolutely inert, as Dowdeswell long since would have had us believe: "With less vigor than a whiff of mountain air or a draught of spring water," and the extreme potency which the whole world now recognizes in the alkaloid cocaine.

As in all other details of this research, a variety of expression has been given as to the odor and appearance of the Coca leaf. Doubtless this diversity is due to whether new or old leaves have been examined, or whether the leaves have been suitably dried. Poeppig thought one of the constituents of the leaves was volatilized by drying, and it is known that the characteristic aroma of the leaf is lost when it is improperly kept. The aroma of Coca has been compared to that of about every other thing under the sun, and in one case is actually described as having an odor between hay and chocolate.[4] One can appreciate that it is exceedingly difficult to describe an odor, as the nearest approach to exactitude which may be made is by way of comparison. When it is realized how few people can accurately define the tone from a blending of colors, and when it is considered how much more subtle is the correct perception and interpretation of odors, the difficulty of accurate description may be well understood. Perfumy is an art in which there is a very wide range for expression, which is not only dependent upon the integrity of the observer's sense of perception, but influenced by the temperament of the describer. A freshly opened bale of properly dried and well preserved Coca has a peculiarly aromatic odor, faintly like vanilla or perhaps suggestive of a finely blended China tea, though more delicate. It has, however, a distinct aroma —the Coca odor *sui generis,* which once learned can always be

[4] Bentley and Trimen; 1880.

readily detected and must afford a means for immediate recognition of true Coca preparations as distinguished from

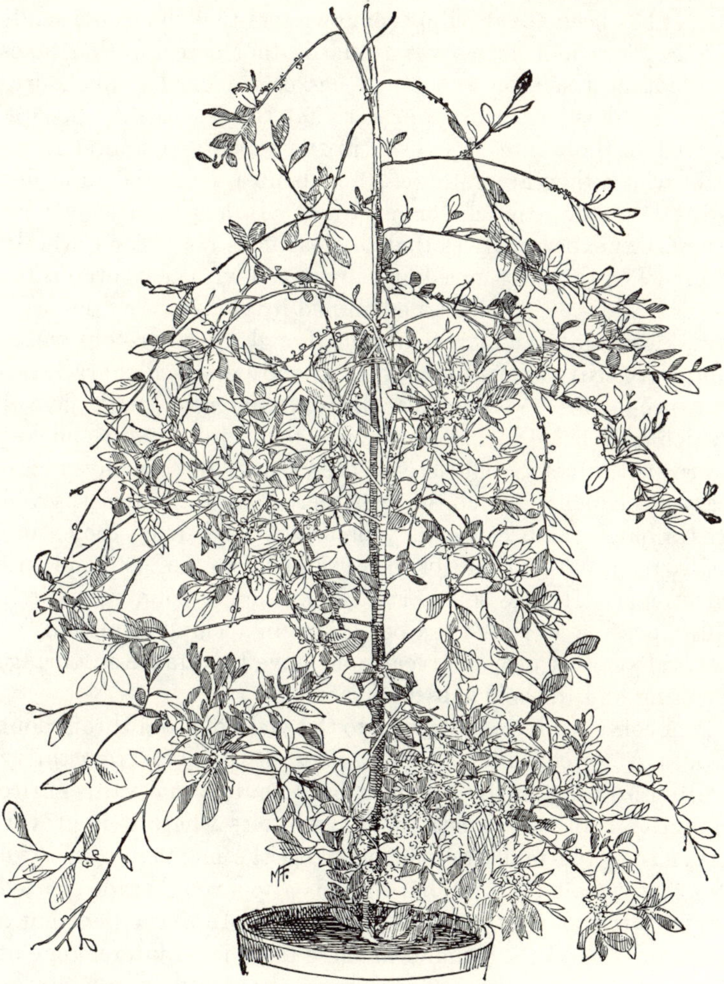

SHRUB OF PERUVIAN COCA. [*Conservatory of Mariani.*]

spurious combinations made with cocaine or from poor leaves. The Indians select the leaf from its characteristic odor alone, without necessitating even a tasting. This delicacy is only to be preserved by a proper drying and curing, to which end it is considered requisite that the layers of leaves in drying shall be so arranged that the exposure may be uniform to all parts.

It has been advanced by some writers that the constituents of the Coca leaf are so very volatile that deterioration takes place almost as soon as the leaf has been picked. The Peruvian Indians, however, consider that the leaves may be preserved in their integrity, even in the warm and humid localities where they are gathered, for about a year, and in cooler situations for a much longer time. It has been shown by numerous experimenters that the leaf does not become wholly inert when properly cured and preserved with care, even after several years. The leaves examined by Gosse were "the ordinary leaves of commerce, which, though three or four years old, were still greenish and spongy, and possessed characteristic properties." Shuttleworth experimented with leaves which had been in his possession for "eight years and yet were still intact." Christison used leaves for his physiological experiments which he considered were "at least seven years old," yet because they had been well dried they were still green, flat and unbroken, were bitter to the taste and full of aroma. It may be inferred from these accounts that it is quite possible to preserve Coca leaves in a sound condition for several years if proper precautions have been taken in curing, packing and in their subsequent care.

A conservative estimate as to the yield of Coca throughout South America under an average crop would be from thirty million to forty million pounds per annum, almost this entire quantity being consumed in the countries where it is grown. As a rule, the planters contract with the merchants in town for their whole product, but there is also a retail trade carried on with the country people. Every little Indian village has a fair to its patron saint, and at these there is an interchange of Coca, potatoes, maize and woolen cloths, which may again be sold at a considerable profit. There is possibly left for exportation from one million to one million five hundred thousand pounds of leaves, the value of which varies in accordance with the demand and facilities for transportation.

During the period of 1885-1886, when the newness of cocaine created such an exorbitant price for that alkaloid, Coca was held at thirty-five cents a pound on shipboard at Peruvian ports. Two years ago the leaves were quoted at seven cents a pound at Sandia, while at Asalaya, below Sandia, it was seven pesos and a half, and at Valle Grande, two days further in the montaña, it was four pesos the cesta—a peso being eighty Peruvian cents, at present equal to about thirty-six cents in United States coin. This would make the price of Coca about eleven cents and six cents respectively, varying with the district and subject to fluctuation according to the means of transit. The recent increase of demand for copper has so taxed the means for transportation that the llamas which were ordinarily used for carrying Coca leaves have been pressed into service for carrying copper ore, the result of which has been to advance the price of Coca on the Peruvian coast to twenty cents. Advices from Lima, dated January, 1900, stated that Coca leaves were then held there at twenty-four cents per pound in large lots.

With the recognition of a volatile principle in the Coca leaf, the proposition was made to solder the packages up in tins like China tea, but this has never been found practicable; in fact, it would be a serious problem to determine the arrangement for carrying such a package, as it should be recalled that the montaña is hundreds of miles from the coast, to which Coca can only be conveyed on the backs of mules or llamas in the most primitive way over rugged mountains and through lofty passes, where travel is exceedingly difficult.

Because of the annoyances of transportation, it has been supposed that the conveyance of Coca by water along the tributaries of the Amazon and down that great river to the sea might prove a more desirable means of transit, but the proposition is ideal rather than practical. In Northern Peru some advantage is taken of the Huallaga, but the mules compete with the Oroya railroad in the final stretch to Callao. Some years ago Dr. Squibb, through an interest that he endeavored to awaken in Mr. Wm. Brambeer, of Para, had a shipment of

Coca sent down the Amazon which turned out badly. Under the most favorable conditions it would take from twenty-eight to thirty days to reach the eastern port of the Amazon from the Coca region, while across the Andes the western coast may be reached in from ten to twelve days.

Perhaps more interest has been centered on the fertile region of the Amazonian valley than is invited by the cold and barren passes of the rugged Cordillera. From the eastern montaña, where the Amazon leaves the Andes under the name of the Marañon, it flows on over three thousand miles to the Atlantic from an elevation of some fifteen hundred feet, with a gradual fall of about six inches to the mile. As the river winds through the dense jungle of the tropics, it is met by numerous streams, all forming a water course of many millions of miles. When the Spaniards felt that they had conquered a country that was rich in gold and yet so soon had wasted these treasures, the more adventurous spirits, led by Gonzalo Pizarro, pushed on toward this mighty territory, passing down some of the tributary streams which have their source in the northern part of Peru. Although these expeditions did not result in the discovery of that fabulous city of El Dorado, the streets of which supposedly were paved with gold, these initial expeditions prompted a desire for further exploration into the interior in search of wealth. United to this was the desire of the Church to convert the savage Indians, a mission work which was furthered by the labors of the Franciscan monks.

Since these early times, the descent of the Amazon has prompted as many expeditions as has the discovery of the North Pole, while the stories of exploit, hardship and suffering have often been related with painful exactitude. During the vice-royalty of the Count of Chinchon, in the seventeenth century, the passage of the Amazon was made to and from Para through the river Napo. In 1835 Count Castelnau made a memorable trip through the Ucayali, and in 1852 Lieutenants Gibbon and Herndon, on behalf of the United States Government, explored the Ucayali and Huallaga, Mamore and Madeira rivers. An effort was to be made to find

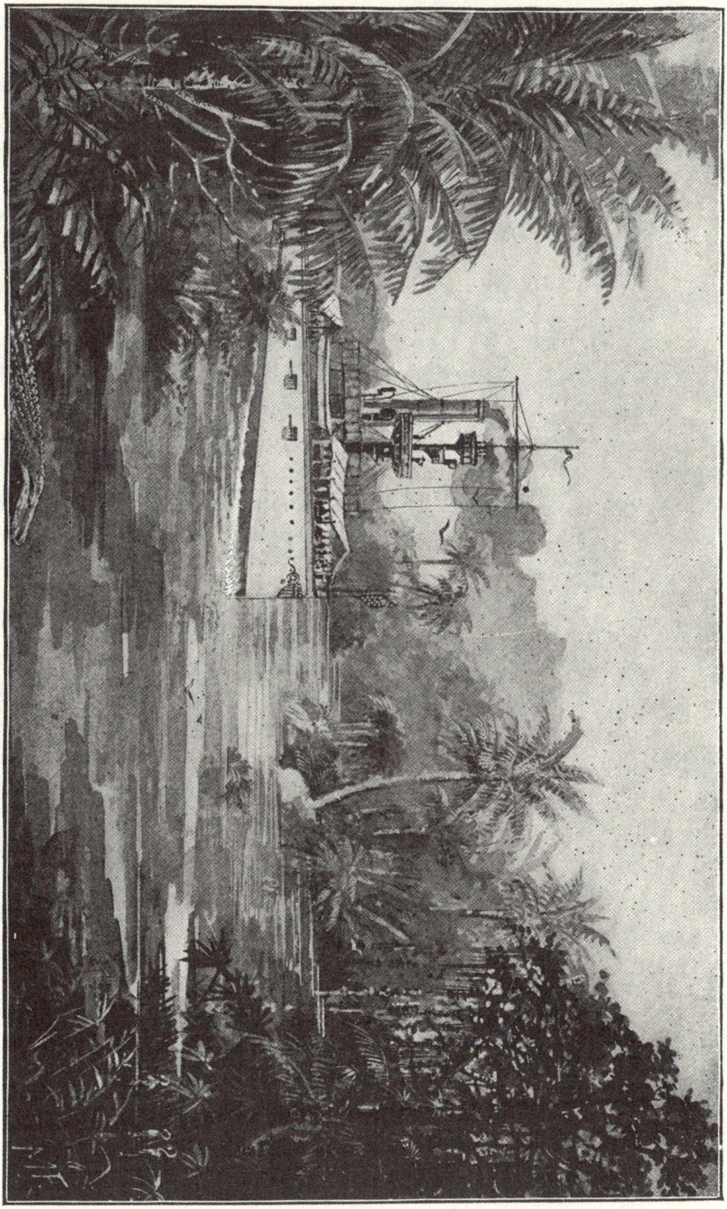

UNITED STATES GUNBOAT WILMINGTON DESCENDING THE AMAZON, MARCH, 1899.

some source of navigation between the numerous streams of the Eastern Andes through the Amazon to the Atlantic Ocean. The importance of this had been advocated as early as 1819 by Vincente Pazos, a citizen of Buenos Ayres, prompted through the introduction at that time of steam navigation into the United States.

The waters which go to form the Amazon are so filled with cataracts and treacherous rocks that for hundreds of miles they are unnavigable, while the severity of the tropical climate and the depredations of the Indians would seemingly retard exploration. But the greatest factor to overcome has been the persistent unwillingness of the Government of Brazil to permit extended surveys. It was not until 1867 that the Amazon was thrown open to the world, and steamers now ascend as far as Yurimaguas, on the Huallaga, close to the Eastern Andes, in the northern montaña, while the many tributary streams afford a source of commerce for numerous merchant vessels.

In March, 1899, the United States gunboat Wilmington, under Commander Todd, sailed from Para, ascending the Amazon and the Solimoens 2,300 miles to Iquitos, on the northwestern boundary of Peru. By this expedition the United States had the honor of entering the first man-of-war in Peru from the Atlantic, though the exploit came near creating unpleasant relations with Brazil, in consequence of the passage of the Amazon. Perhaps this was engendered through the suggestion of an article by Mr. Cecil Rhodes that destiny would impel the United States to acquire all of South America, a confirmation of which some over credulous natives saw in the presence of the vessel, which was presumably making surveys preparatory to annexing this tropical belt. Navigation through the entire extent of the Amazon is dependent upon the guidance of pilots, but so much feeling was created that pilots were refused to take the Wilmington back to Para, and the descent was completed under the guidance of charts made from surveys by the United States steamer Enterprise, in 1878, then commanded by Thomas O. Selfridge, now rear admiral, retired.

The Amazon has its source between the Peruvian Cordilleras from a number of streams which are supplied with the melting snow from the Andes. In its upper part it is called the Marañon as far as the frontier of Brazil, where it takes the name Solimoens as far as the river Negro. The Amazon has a length, following its curves, of nearly four thousand miles and is considered to be the largest, if not the longest, river in the world. Its depth varies from forty-two feet in the Marañon to three hundred and twelve feet at its mouth, where it is one hundred and eighty miles wide. Throughout its extent it is deep, even at the banks, which are without sloping shores. The water is muddy and still, though drifting logs and floating islands of grass and water plants indicate a current which runs about three miles an hour. The winding stream, in some places of a width of many miles, cuts through a dense forest, which ends abruptly at the water's edge. Here the trees shoot up to a great height before branching and are overhung with vines and creepers so as to present an almost solid wall, into which the passage seems at times directed.

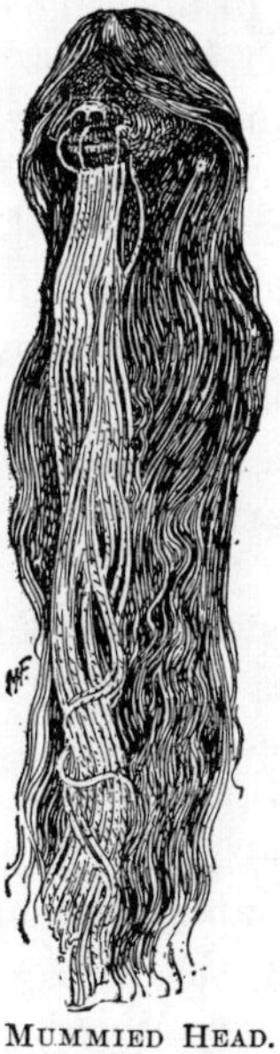

MUMMIED HEAD.
[*Tweddle Collection.*]

The tropical nature of the surroundings is well adapted to favor animal life, and the water is filled with strange fishes, alligators, turtles, anacondas and porpoises, while along the river banks there may be perhaps a few huts at every hundred miles, which are occupied by the rubber gatherers. Some of these huts are built on piles only elevated a few feet above the water, but the dwellers seem acclimated against the endemic fevers. The climate through the Amazon valley has but little variation, the chief fluctuation being from profuse rains to humid heat. The rainy season begins in September and continues until April, during which the river overflows its banks, and in the succeeding dry period it gradually recedes again, the difference between high and low water being as great as forty or fifty feet.

There are some savage tribes along the northern tributaries who have unique customs. Among these is a tribe of head hunters who preserve the heads of their enemies as trophies of their valor. The bones of the skull are crushed and removed and the head is then mummified to about a fourth of its natural size, while still retaining the features in reduced proportions and the long, straight black hair as in life. These little heads are not repulsive, but resemble an ebony carving more than the remains of something once human. Through the upper lip is put a fringe of string, each cord of which is said to indicate the number of enemies the warrior had overthrown.

While this immense river system must prove a great benefit in opening to the commerce of the world a vast territory rich in spices, food stuffs, cabinet woods, rubber, dyes and numerous drugs, yet it cannot render any material service to that section of country through which Coca is grown. Though some species of Erythroxylon are found along the Solimoens and the tributaries of the Amazon, the Coca producing regions of the montaña are still separated by long portages and hundreds of miles of canoe navigation, to say nothing of impassable cataracts and the uncertainty of such precarious travel.

Under the most favorable conditions the journey to the eastern coast may not be made in less than a month, while, as has already been stated, the trip over the Andes can be completed in from ten to twelve days. Yet there are those who are willing to accept the one hardship in place of the other and select the longer passage by preference to the arduous climbing through the great altitudes necessary in surmounting the passes of the Andes. This was recently shown by Señor Moises Ponce, a Peruvian gentleman of Iquitos, who, being desirous of going with his wife and four little boys to Truxillo, on the coast of Peru, preferred to go by boat to Para, thence by steamer to New York, and across the Isthmus of Panama and by steamer to Salaverry—a distance of nine thousand miles, rather than the more direct route over the Andes, which is less than four hundred miles. Indeed the officials journeying between Lima and Iquitos are allowed mileage by the government for this extended trip, though some more venturesome spirits cross the Andes by way of Caxamarca and so may make the journey in twenty-eight days.

Many fabulous tales have been told of the Amazonian region. Count Castelnau repeats with much earnestness a story of Father Ribeiro, a Carmelite, of a tribe of Indians seen on the banks of the Jurua with short tails, supposedly

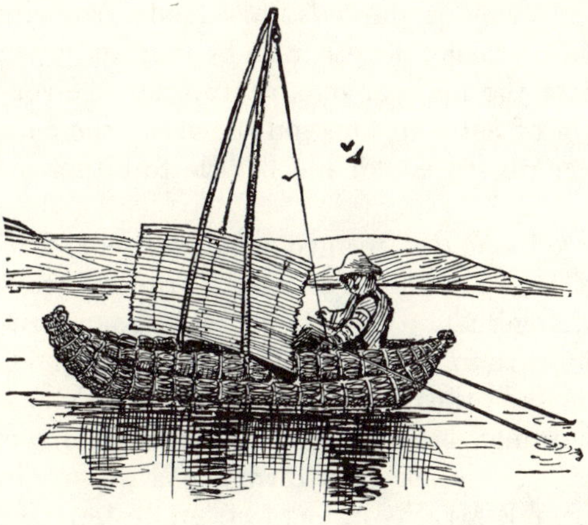

PERUVIAN BALSA, LAKE TITICACA. [*From a Photograph.*]

resulting from their literal union with one of the tribes of ancestral monkey. Many of the Amazonian streams are navigated by immense canoes, often forty feet long, which are made from a single log. These are conducted by a *puntero,* or bowman, who is the lookout, and poled or paddled by *bogas,* who stand up, one foot on the gunwale and one on the bottom of the canoe, and paddle it along, while the *popero* stands on a platform at the stern and steers.

The Incans were expert navigators in a peculiar form of boat known as the *balsa,* one of which it will be recalled Pizarro saw when he entered the Guayas River. These boats are still in use along the coast and on Lake Titicaca. They are constructed in a variety of ways; some of them resemble huge rafts, others are shaped like canoes. In the first instance they are made of trunks of the very light *balsa* trees, lashed together with cross-pieces. These primitive boats are often large enough to carry a number of passengers, who, together with the cargo, are placed on a small platform arranged above the deck as a protection from the water which constantly washes over the feet of the *balsero.* Some of these rafts are propelled under huge sails. Those on Lake Titicaca have sails which are made from the rushes growing near the lake. Other forms of the *balsa* are made from inflated seal skins, which are lashed together and connected by cross-pieces of wood, after the manner of a catamaran. Over this there is a platform of cane, at one end of which the *balsero* kneels and by alternate strokes of his paddle to either side propels his canoe.

The canoe-like *balsa,* termed *caballitos*—or "little horses," are made of conical bundles of rushes from ten to twelve feet long, bound together. Of course, these boats are not water tight, but they are unsinkable, riding easily on the huge waves of the Pacific, and they are so light that when borne inland by the swell they may be picked up and carried out of reach of the breakers. These boatmen form a floating, roving race, of whom my friend, Mr. Scott, has written designating them the "gypsies of the sea." They are seen everywhere along the coast, ready to carry the mail or venturesome passengers to and from the ships lying off shore. The traveller is often compelled to depend on this mode of conveyance on Peruvian waters, which, though absolutely safe, always awakens the gravest fears in the inexperienced voyager, who must maintain an equipoise for fear of momentary capsizing, while the motion is apt to excite an early oblation to Neptune.

The Indian arrow poison, *urary* or *curare,* which has been such a boon to experimental physiologists, is extensively prepared by the women of certain Indian tribes along the tributaries of the Amazon. It is not made from the venom of snakes, as is popularly supposed, though often venomous ants and scorpions are added to the pot in which it is concocted. It is commonly prepared from the juice of bruised stems and leaves of several varieties of *Strychnos* and *Apocynaceæ*, boiled and mixed with tobacco juice and capsicum, and thickened with the sticky milk of one of the *Euphorbiaceæ* to a hard mass. The first *curare* known to commerce was obtained from the Orinoco region.

There are now some eight or ten different varieties of this poison, of which that made by the *Macusi* Indians and the *curare* from Venezuela and Colombia, are considered the more powerful. It is a dark brown, pitch-like substance, usually kept in little earthen pots. The Indians spread it on the points of their arrows and on the tips of the little shafts of their blow tubes, termed by the natives *pucuna.* The result of the diffusion of *curare* into the blood is to occasion a torpor of the limbs, while the mind remains active until death follows from paralysis of respiration. The Indians shoot birds and monkeys which they wish to tame with darts tipped with a very weak *curare,* the influence of which soon wears away.

The blow guns are made of the long, straight wood of the *chonta* palm—of which bows, clubs and spears are also made. The guns are some eight feet long, tapering from two inches at the mouthpiece to half an inch at the extremity, shaped of two pieces in which a canal has been very smoothly polished, when the two pieces are bound together with twine and the whole covered with wax and resin. A sight, fitted to the top, made from an animal's tooth, and a couple of boar's teeth attached to each side of the mouth end, completes the implement. The darts, made from the central fibre of a species of palm leaf, are about a foot long and thin as a match; one end of this shaft is wrapped with a species of wild cotton, called *huimba,* and the other end is sharply pointed. The marksman uses this gun in a very unique way. Instead of stretching out one hand as a support, the tube is held to the mouth by grasping it close to the mouthpiece with both hands in a manner that requires considerable strength and much expertness to assure a correct aim. Yet the Indians kill small birds with their darts at thirty or forty paces. The outfit of a hunter consists of a gourd with a hole in it for carrying the *huimba,* with a joint of cane as a quiver for the darts.

In the depths of the forest there is at times heard the mournful cry of a bird which is known as *alma pérdida*—the lost soul. There is a legend that an Indian and his wife went from the village to work their little Coca farm, taking with them their infant. The woman, going to a spring to get water, gave the child in charge of her husband, but finding the spring dry, she went to look for another. The man, alarmed at the long absence of his wife, left the baby to go in search of her. When the couple returned they could not find the infant, and their agonized cries only provoked the wailing call of this bird, which, like the bewildered voice of their lost child, seemed to say: "Pa-pa, ma-ma," and the bird has since borne that name.[5]

There are an immense number of animals in the Amazonian region, among which are the ant eater, wild boar, armadillo, tapir, the boa-constrictor and numerous poisonous adders, to counteract the venom of which the Indians resort to various species of plants, among which is *anguifugum,* of the family of Erythroxylon and the *huaca* plant, mention of which has already been made. *Huaca* may be identical with the *guaco* described by Humboldt and Bonpland, of which several species are found in tropical South America belonging to the genera *Mikana* or *Aristolochia.*[6] The leaves are large, obvate, pale green above, the under side of an obscure purple hue with purple veins running through it, giving the leaf somewhat the appearance of mottled snake skin. The leaves grow singly, opposite on the stem, which is hard and ribbed and of a bluish color. The natives say no flower is ever seen. The Indians bruise the leaves to the consistence of a paste, which is made into small dried cakes and used as a remedy against snake poison.

When one is bitten by a snake one of these cakes is chewed until the bitter taste is gone. He is then bathed and the cud

[5] Herndon; Vol. I, p. 156; 1853. [6] *Journ. de Pharm.;* p. 99; 1867.

of chewed herb bound upon the wound. Stevenson was bitten in the hand by a coral snake, the bite of which is considered mortal if not immediately cured. There was a violent pain and burning in the wound and a sense of weight in the hand. He chewed *huaca* cake and the Indians squeezed the wound. In five minutes the pain abated and the bitter taste of the herb was gone. He then bathed in the river and was laid in his canoe, covered with ponchos and taken home, about four miles. During the time he was in the canoe he perspired profusely and more so after retiring. While the pain in his hand was much allayed, he felt general numbness and great debility, accompanied with nausea. He drank a glass of almond milk—*orchada,* slept for about an hour, but awoke feverish and for four days continued very ill. He felt much apprehension, but the natives assured him that after twenty-four hours had elapsed there was no danger, though for more than a fortnight he felt the effects.

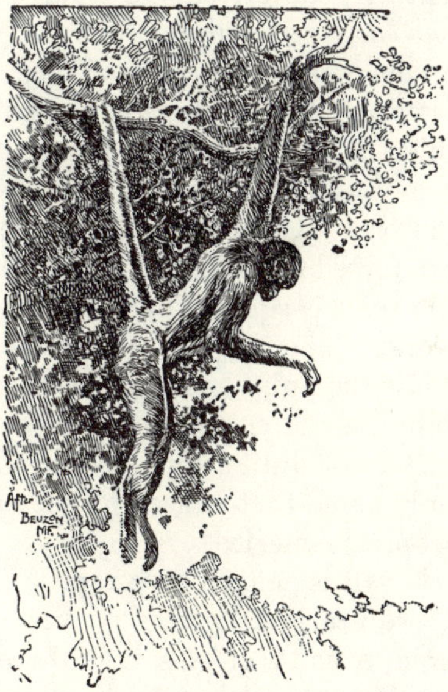

MAN'S PREHISTORIC STATE. [*Brettes.*]

Parrots and birds of beautiful plumage are very plentiful through the montaña and along the Amazon, while monkeys hanging by their tails continue an incessant chattering, as though asserting with their neighbors their representative right as descendants of man's prehistoric state. Yet the Indians, though not cannibals, are not averse to eating monkeys, while they also enjoy the armadillo, the peccary, agouti and tapir. Turtles are a common luxury, and in an emergency the savage Indian never hesitates to feed upon snakes, toads, lizards and the larvæ of insects.

Near the Orinoco there is a tribe of savages who feed upon a species of unctuous clay, a practice which, though probably the outgrowth of necessity, is not extremely rare throughout the Amazonian region. This clay, which is said to have a milky and not disagreeable taste, is a species of *marga,* or marl—*subpinguis tenax,* as it is called—which is found in veins of varying color. It is smooth and greasy, dissolving readily in the mouth, and is absorbed into the circulation.

The dietary of the Andean Indian, while chiefly of a starchy nature, is mixed with a fair supply of meat, principally mutton, with an occasional llama. The bread, or *farinah,* is generally made from the root of the mandioc—*jatropha manihot*—from which the juice is squeezed by a cleverly woven conical basket-work bag—*tapiti,* [*see page* 478] made from the coarse fibres of the palm. The bruised pulp of the tuber is placed in this bag and the whole suspended with a heavy weight attached to an eyelet woven in the lower end of the bag. Gradually this percolator elongates as the meshes are forced together, and so exerting a compression on the pulp the juice is squeezed out through the interstices of the wicker work. The starchy extractive of the juice yields tapioca, while the pulpy mass is dried into coarse granules and ground into flour from which a very palatable biscuit is made which tastes not unlike stale bread. This *farinah* is practically the only bread that is used by the natives through a vast region of tropical America.

Salt is held in high repute by the Indians. It is said that there are some places on the coast of Africa where, next to gold, a handful of salt is the most valuable. The Peruvian Indians travel hundreds of miles for their salt supply, but they have their pepper in the form of *aji* near at hand, and they use it in all their dishes quite as liberally as Spanish custom has taught them. Keller says that some of the Indians of Bolivia in chewing Coca unite with their llipta a bit of some species of red pepper.

The collection of rubber is one of the chief industries of the Amazonian valley. The tree from the sap of which rubber is made grows only in a region where its root may be annually submerged by floods. It is not the ordinary rubber plant of our conservatories, the sap of which is sometimes used to make a spurious rubber, but the *siphonia elastica*, which yields the *cahuchu* of the South American Indians that has proved so valuable in the arts. The rubber collectors live in the little elevated huts already described as along the Amazon, which are so constructed that in the time of flood they may be raised. During the dry season holes are chopped in the bark of the tree and from these tappings the milky sap exudes and is conducted by a trough made of bamboo into clay cups. The rubber is prepared by coagulating the sap on a wooden paddle over the smoke of the *urucury*. As it is gradually smoked the sap takes a greenish yellow tint, and the paddle is repeatedly dipped until by successive coagulated layers quite a thickness is obtained, when the *plancha* of rubber is cut on one side and removed to hang in the sun to dry, by which process it is gradually darkened to the condition in which we commonly see crude rubber.

One may not visit the montaña without hearing the various topics which have been mentioned here discussed, although the one of supreme interest in our research, and that which has excited the greatest comment of travellers, is the production and use of the Coca leaf, the technical details of which we may now consider.

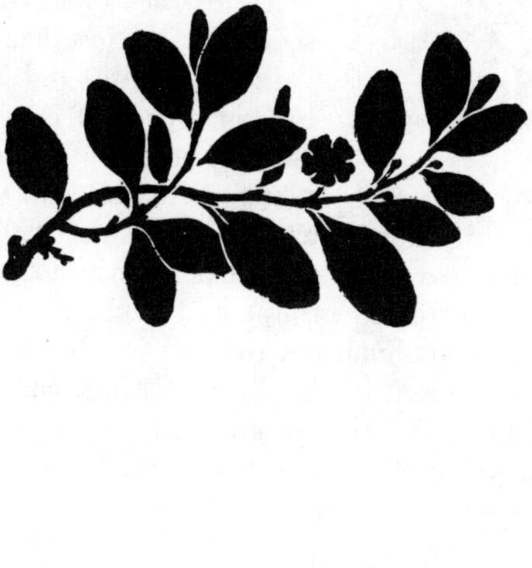

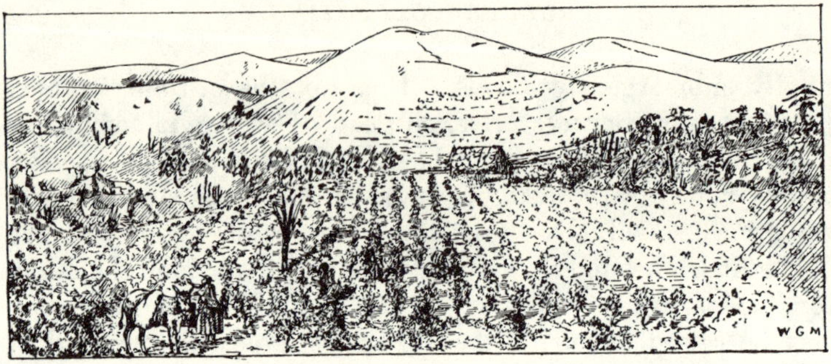

CHAPTER X.

THE PRODUCTS OF THE COCA LEAF.

"Nor *Coca* only useful art at Home,
A famous Merchandize thou art become;
A thousand *Paci* and *Vicugni* groan
Yearly beneath thy Loads, and for thy sake alone
The spacious World's to us by Commerce Known."

—*Cowley.*

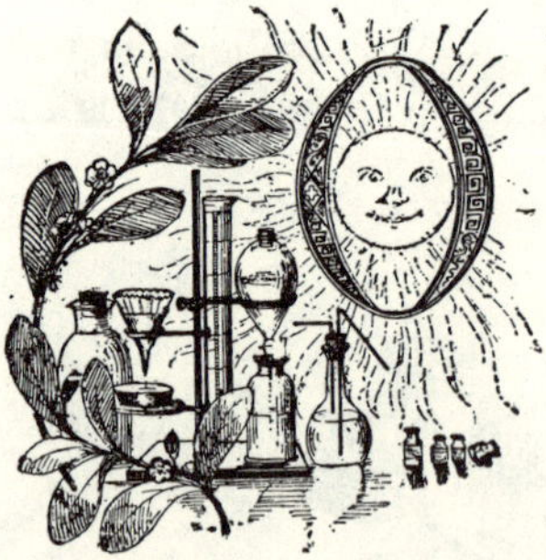

OF all the problems in the study of Coca the search for the force producing qualities of the leaf is the most profound. Science, ever alert to trace with exactitude the secrets of Nature, has struggled in vain to isolate and explain this hidden source of energy. But so cleverly are the atoms associated which go to build up the molecules of power in this marvelous leaf, that though the chemist through the delicacy of analysis has from time to time placed these atoms in differing groups and thus often given to the world some new combination, the one sought element of pent up endurance inherent in Coca has remained concealed. It is like the secret of life—though known to be broadly dependent upon certain principles which may readily be explained, the knowledge of the one essential element remains as great a secret as before research began.

Though all the accounts of travellers had directed attention to the peculiar qualities of Coca in sustaining strength, at the period when the first knowledge of this leaf reached Europe chemistry was not sufficiently advanced to admit of an exact analysis of plant life. Indeed, science met with little encouragement when the great powers were engrossed in political preferment, and it was not until the latter part of the eighteenth century that an impetus seemed given to research after Lavoisier had laid the foundation for modern chemistry. Though he lost his life on the guillotine through the whirligig of political fate during the French Revolution, just as he was at the height of his labors, a new interest was established and the work of the French chemists became active.

Humboldt was then making his extensive explorations through South America, collecting data which was to serve as a basis of research during many subsequent years. Cuvier, the anatomist, was advancing his theories on the classification of animals; Fraunhofer had established a means for studying the heavenly bodies through the spectrum, while chemical electricity had progressed from the experiments of Volta to the electro magnet of Ampère.

The method for expressing chemical equations, such as are now shown by those symbolic letters and figures which appear to the uninitiated as so many hieroglyphics, was not understood until Dalton, in 1808, had perfected his law of proportions. This was an important advance in chemical knowledge, for from it was built up the sign language which in a chemical formula expresses not only the symbol of each element, but tells the chemist the relative proportion of the combining atoms.

These fundamental facts are of interest as bearing upon the chemical history of the Coca leaf, while the combining nature of atoms has suggested an interesting theory that the physiological action of a chemical medicine is influenced by its molecular weight. This has been a matter of discussion among physiological chemists for years, and was suggested by

Blake as long ago as 1841 and since by Rabuteau. Thus an element of a fixed atomic weight may have special reference to the muscular system, while another of different weight may act upon the nervous tissue,[1] qualities which are fulfilled in the action of the several Coca bases.

Boerhaave may be said to have been the father of the present system of organic chemistry in the early part of the eighteenth century. So important were his teachings held that his works were translated into most modern languages. Although his attempts at analysis of living things attracted a wide interest, they could be in no manner exact, because the fundamental elements entering into the composition of all organic structure—carbon, hydrogen, oxygen and nitrogen—had not then been determined. Yet so skilled were his observations, even under limited opportunities, that many of his conclusions have not since been refuted in the light of improved methods. Perhaps the earliest hint upon alkaloids was that made by this scientist when he referred to the bitter principle in the juices from chewing Coca as yielding "vital strength" and a "veritable nutritive."[2]

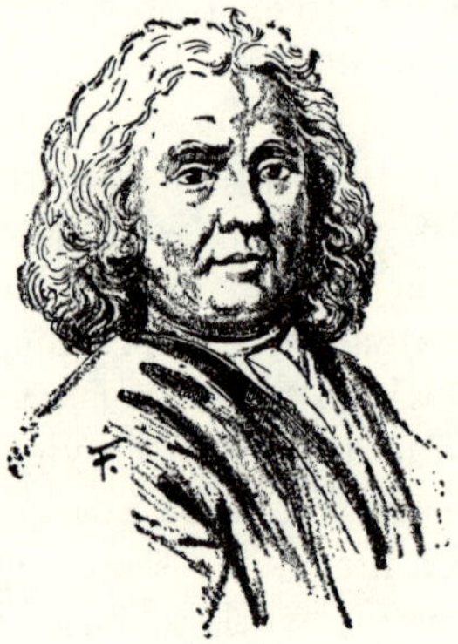

HERMANN BOERHAAVE.

It was reserved for Liebig some hundred years later to perfect the science of living structures, and to show there was not that exact separation between the chemistry of the organic and inorganic world that had previously been supposed. Following the teachings of this master mind, many compounds were constructed in the laboratory synthetically, and urea was thus produced in 1828 by Woehler, whose name is associated with the early investigators upon cocaine. Research upon the chemistry of organic bodies was now active. In England the work of Davy upon soils and crops, and the investigations of

[1] Brunton; p. 49; 1885. [2] Boerhaave; ¶68; 1708.

Darwin, unfolded in his theory of the origin of species, gave a new meaning to the study of organic life.

It was but a natural outcome of this spirit for research that turned the attention of explorers to South America, which had remained practically a new world since its discovery. Here were to be found innumerable strange plants indigenous to a country where everything was marvelous when viewed with the comparative light of the older world. In the height of this interest, the suggestive hints of naturalists and travellers were incentives to further the investigations of the European chemists. The writings of Cieza, Monardes, Acosta, Garcilasso and a host of others upon the wonderful qualities of the Coca leaf, stimulated a desire to solve its tradition of ages and prove its qualities by the test of science.

It is surprising to now look back over three centuries and recall these early authors, to consider under what conditions they wrote, and to read with what enthusiasm and exactness they gave expression to the knowledge they had gained from an observation of the novel customs about them. Thus the Jesuit father, Blas Valera, speaking of the hidden energy of Coca, wrote: "It may be gathered how powerful the *Cuca* is in its effect on the laborer, from the fact that the Indians who use it become stronger and much more satisfied and work all day without eating."[3]

It was not until after Coca had been botanically described by Jussieu, and classified by Lamarck, that its chemical investigation approached thoroughness. The researches of Bergmann and Black upon "fixed air"—as carbonic acid was then termed, the discovery of hydrogen by Cavendish, of nitrogen by Rutherford and of oxygen by Priestley, each following upon the other in quick succession in the latter half of the eighteenth century, displayed the great activity of chemistry at that period. Although no result was then arrived at in the investigations upon Coca, the spirit of the time was eminently toward exactitude, and this was displayed in many endeavors to trace to a chemical principle the potency of the Coca leaf.

Attention was very naturally directed to the method in

[3] Garcilasso; Vol. II, p. 371; 1871.

which Coca was used, and the *llipta* which was employed with the leaves in chewing was looked upon as having some decided influence. Dr. Unanue, who has written much concerning the customs of the Indians, was one of the first to suggest that possibly this alkaline addition to the leaf developed some new property to which the qualities of Coca might be attributed,[4] while Humboldt, as elsewhere referred to, through an error of observation considered this added lime as the supposed property of endurance.

Stevenson, in 1825, described the action of the *llipta* as altering the insipid taste of the leaves so as to render them sweet, and in 1827 Poeppig expressed the opinion that there was a volatile constituent in the Coca leaf which exposure to the air completely destroys.[5]

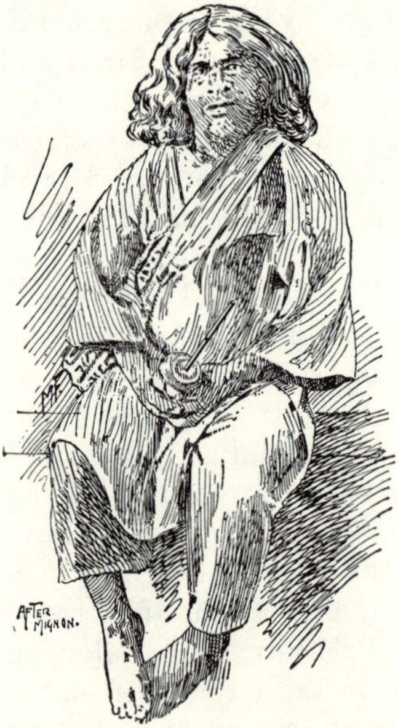

A COLOMBIAN INDIAN WITH HIS POPÓRO. [*Brettes.*]

Attention had now been directed to the isolation of alkaloids from plants, and during the first quarter of the nineteenth century several active principles were thus obtained and the possibility of tracing the hidden properties of Coca through analysis was suggested. Von Tschudi, when engaged in his extended explorations through Peru, became so impressed with the qualities of Coca that he advised Mr. Pizzi, Director of the Laboratory *Botica y Drogueria Boliviana*, at La Paz, to examine the leaves, which resulted in the discovery of a supposed alkaloid, but when on his return to Germany this body was shown to Woehler, it was found to be merely plaster of paris, the result of some careless manipulation.

[4] Unanue; 1794. [5] Gosse; p. 52; 1861.

Dr. Weddell, in 1850, after a prolonged personal experience in the Andes with the sustaining effects of Coca, pronounced it as yielding a stimulant action differing from that of all other excitants. This influence both he and other observers supposed might be due to the presence of theine, the active principle of tea, which had shortly before been discovered, and was then exciting considerable discussion. With this idea in view, Coca leaves were examined, and, though this substance was not found, there was obtained a peculiar body, soluble in alcohol, insoluble in ether, very bitter, and incapable of crystallization, and a tannin was obtained to which was attributed the virtues of Coca.[6]

About this same period there was found in the leaves a peculiar volatile resinous matter of powerful odor,[7] and two years later, from a distillation of the dry residue of an aqueous extract of Coca, an oily liquor of a smoky odor was separated together with a sublimate of small needle-like crystals, which was named "Erythroxyline,"[8] after the family of which Coca is a species.[9] So each new investigator made a little progress, and in 1857 positive results were very nearly reached through the following process: An extract of Coca was made with acidulated alcohol, the alcohol was expelled, and the solution rendered alkaline by carbonate of soda. Upon extracting this with ether, an oily body of alkaline reaction was obtained without bitter taste, which on application to the tongue produced a slight numbness. The reaction of platinum chloride yielded with the acid solution a yellowish precipitate, soluble in water. From a distillate of the leaves with alkali there was remarked a disagreeable, strongly ammoniacal odor.[10] Subsequently a peculiar bitter principle, extractive and chlorophyl, a substance presumed to be analogous to theine, and a salt of lime was found.[11]

These negative findings led some to assert that Coca was inert and its properties legendary, but more careful observation has shown the true difficulty was an inability to

[6] Wackenroder; July, 1853. [7] Johnston; 1853. [8] Gaedcke; 1855.
[9] It is claimed that Dr. S. R. Percy read a paper before the New York Academy of Medicine in November, 1857, upon an alkaloid of Coca which he had obtained and then independently named "Erythroxyline."
[10] Maclagan; 1857. [11] Stanislas Martin; 1859.

secure appropriately preserved leaves for examination. This was made evident through an essay upon Coca by an eminent Italian neurologist, from experiences while a resident of Peru, when a host of physiological evidence emphasized the powerful nature of Coca, wholly apart from any mere delusions of fancy or superstition.[12] The weight of facts presented proved sufficiently forcible not only to stimulate the waning spirit for scientific inquiry, but to awaken a widespread popular regard in what was now generally accepted as a plant of phenomenal nature.

In the height of this interest Dr. Scherzer, who accompanied the Austrian frigate Novara on the expedition to South America, opportunely brought home specimens of Coca leaves from Peru. These were sent to Professor Woehler of Gottingen for analysis, who entrusted their examination to his assistant, Dr. Albert Niemann, who is regarded as the discoverer of the alkaloid cocaine. Thus this chemist entered upon the investigation of Coca not in any mere accidental way, but with an understanding of the seriousness of his research and its probable importance.

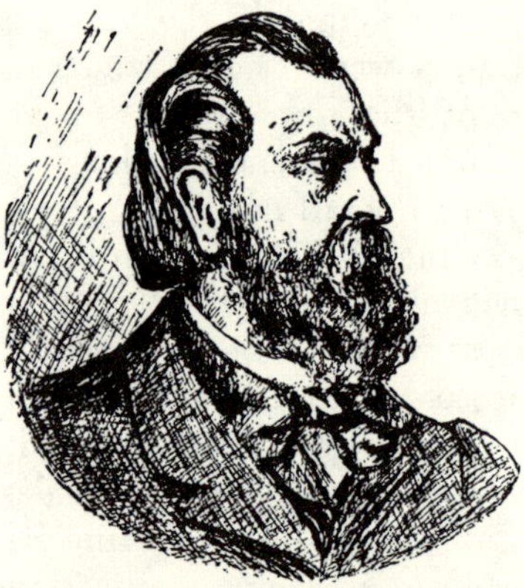

ALBERT NIEMANN.
[*From a Copper-plate Print at the Bibliothèque Nationale, Paris.*]

Niemann exhausted coarsely ground Coca leaves with eighty-five per cent. alcohol containing one-fiftieth of sulphuric acid; the percolate was treated with milk of lime and neutralized by sulphuric acid. The alcohol was then recovered by distillation, leaving a syrupy mass, from which resin was separated by water. The liquid then treated by carbonate of soda to precipitate alkaloid emitted an odor reminding of nicotine, and deposited a substance which was extracted by repeatedly shaking with ether, in which it was

[12] Mantegazza; 1859.

dissolved, and from which the ether was recovered by distillation. There was found an alkaloid present in proportion of about one-quarter of one per cent., which was named "*Cocaine*," after the parent plant, and the chemical formula $C_{32}H_{20}NO_8$, according to the old notation, was given it. Mechanically mixed with its crystals there was a yellowish brown matter of disagreeable narcotic odor, which could not be removed with animal charcoal or recrystallization, and was only separated by repeated washings with alcohol.

Pure cocaine, as described by this investigator, is in colorless transparent prisms, inodorous, soluble in seven hundred and four parts of water at 12° C. (53.6° F.), more readily soluble in alcohol, and freely so in ether. Its solutions have an alkaline reaction, a bitter taste, promote the flôw of saliva and leave a peculiar numbness, followed by a sense of cold when applied to the tongue. At 98° C. (208.4° F.) the crystals fuse and congeal again into a transparent mass, from which crystals gradually form. Heated above the fusing point, the body is discolored and decomposes, running up the sides of the vessel. When fused upon platinum the crystals burn with a bright flame, leaving a charcoal which burns with difficulty. The alkaloid is readily soluble in all dilute acids forming salts of a more bitter taste than the uncombined cocaine. It absorbs hydrochloric acid gas, fuses and congeals to a grayish white transparent mass which crystallizes after some days. The crystals from its solution are long, tender and radiating.

Besides cocaine, there was found in the alcoholic tincture precipitated by milk of lime a snowy white granular mass. This fused at 70° C. (158° F.), was slowly soluble in hot alcohol, more readily so in ether, and was not acted on by solutions of acids or alkalies. This substance was named *Coca wax* and given the empirical formula $C_{66}H_{66}O_4$.

Upon distilling one hundred grammes of leaves, a slightly turbid distillate was obtained, which when redistilled with chloride of sodium, yielded white globular masses lighter than water and having the peculiar tea-like odor of Coca.

In the dark red filtrate from which the cocaine had been

precipitated by carbonate of soda there was found after suitable treatment a *Coca tannic acid*, to which the formula $C_{14}H_{18}O_8$ has been given.[13] This latter result, it will be remembered, was as far as Wackenroder's investigations had gone in 1853.

The atomic weight of the amorphous compound determined from the double salt with chloride of gold, was found to equal 283, and when crystallized from hot water 280, or from alcohol 288. On heating this double salt benzoic acid was sublimed from it, which was recorded as the first observation of this nature from any known alkaloid.[14]

Following this research, the late Professor John M. Maisch of Philadelphia verified the several results. The small percentage of nitrogen announced in the original formula suggested that possibly cocaine was a decomposition compound, while the nicotine odor was thought to result from a nitrogenous body or another alkaloid. To determine this, the liquor and precipitate which had been obtained by carbonate of soda were distilled over a sand bath. A syrupy liquid was left, from which the alkaloid was separated by ether, while from the distillate was collected a resin-like mass of an acrid taste, having a narcotic odor, soon lost on exposure to a damp atmosphere, while the mass became acid and was now rendered easily soluble in water and alcohol. Whether or not this principle was nitrogenous this investigator left undecided.[15]

Continuing the same line of research as that of Niemann, and following the suggestions of Maisch, William Lossen[16] of Gottingen carried out an extended inquiry as to the nature of cocaine, and established its formula $C_{17}H_{21}NO_4$, in accordance with the new notation. In examining its composition he found by heating it with hydrochloric acid that it was split up into benzoic acid and another body, thereby confirming the observation which had been made concerning this sublimation from the double salt of chloride of gold and cocaine. This new base he named *"ecgonine,"* from ἔχγονος —son or descendant.

[13] Watts; 1889. [14] Niemann; 1860. [15] Maisch; 1861.
[16] Lossen; Juin, 1862.

The breaking down of cocaine was subsequently shown due to hydration, by saponifying it with baryta, and also with water alone. The first change being into benzoyl-ecgonine, followed by a sublimation of benzoic acid, while from the syrupy residue the ecgonine may be separated by repeated washings with alcohol and precipitation with ether. The crystals being only dried with great difficulty.

Ecgonine, $C_9H_{15}NO_3$, crystallizes over sulphuric acid in sheaves. It has a slight bitter-sweet taste, is readily soluble in water, less so in absolute alcohol, and insoluble in ether. Heated to 198°, it melts, decomposes and becomes brown. It forms salts with the acids, most of which crystallize with difficulty. With alkalies, it forms crystallizable combinations soluble in water and alcohol. In aqueous solutions the hydrochloride yields no precipitate with alkalies. Chloride of platinum in presence of much alcohol gives an orange yellow precipitate, chloride of mercury throwing down a yellow precipitate under the same conditions.

The unstable nature of cocaine in the presence of acids has suggested their avoidance in its preparation, plain water being considered preferable. In this process Coca leaves are digested several times at 140° to 176°, the infusions united, precipitated by acetate of lead, and filtered. The lead is removed by the addition of sulphate of soda, and the liquor concentrated in a water bath. Carbonate of soda is then added, and the whole shaken with ether to dissolve the alkaloid, when the ether may be recovered by distillation.

In his researches Lossen[17] also described the liquid alkaloid that had been hinted at by Gaedcke in 1855, and subsequently noticed by Niemann and Maisch, which, at the suggestion of Woehler,[18] who was associated in this investigation, was termed "*hygrine*," from *υγρος*—liquid, to which the formula $C_{12}H_{13}N$ was given. This was obtained by saturating the slightly alkaline mother liquor from which cocaine had been extracted with carbonate of soda and repeatedly washing with ether. Evaporation of the ethereal extract left a thick yellow oil of high boiling point with a strong alkaline reac-

[17] Lossen; CXXXII, 351; 1865. [18] Woehler und Lossen; CXXI, 372; 1860.

tion. Hygrine thus found is described as very volatile, distilling alone between 140° and 230° F. It is slightly soluble in water, and more readily so in alcohol, chloroform and ether, not in caustic soda, but readily in dilute hydrochloric acid. Its taste is burning and it has a peculiar odor similar to trimethylamine or quinoline. The oxalate and muriate are crystallizable, but very deliquescent.

With chloride of platinum, hygrine gives a flocculent amorphous precipitate which decomposes on heating. Bichloride of mercury gives an opalescence, due to the formation of minute oily drops.

Thus far there had been found in Coca leaves a crystallizable compound of unstable composition—cocaine; a second base which was only to be crystallized with difficulty—ecgonine; an intermediate compound—benzoyl-ecgonine; and an oily volatile liquid of peculiar odor—hygrine; together with Coca-tannic acid, and a wax-like body. Meantime, considerable was done in a physiological way in experimenting with the new alkaloids, though little decided progress was made during the following twenty years, until 1884, when the use of cocaine in local anæsthesia was announced. The importance of this application occasioned an increased activity of investigation regarding the Coca products. This interest tended to make our knowledge of the alkaloids more exact, as well as to enrich our understanding of those inherent sustaining properties of Coca which have for past ages excited wonder.

In the early days of the cocaine industry some manufacturers asserted that the several associate substances found in Coca leaves were decomposition products, developed by changes taking place in deteriorating leaves or arising during the process of obtaining the one alkaloid. The great demand for cocaine and the high price it commanded generated an apparent unwillingness on the part of manufacturers to admit the possible presence in Coca of any other principle than cocaine. Processes innumerable were devised to force the greatest yield of alkaloid from the leaves, and some of the earlier specimens of the salt placed upon the market were

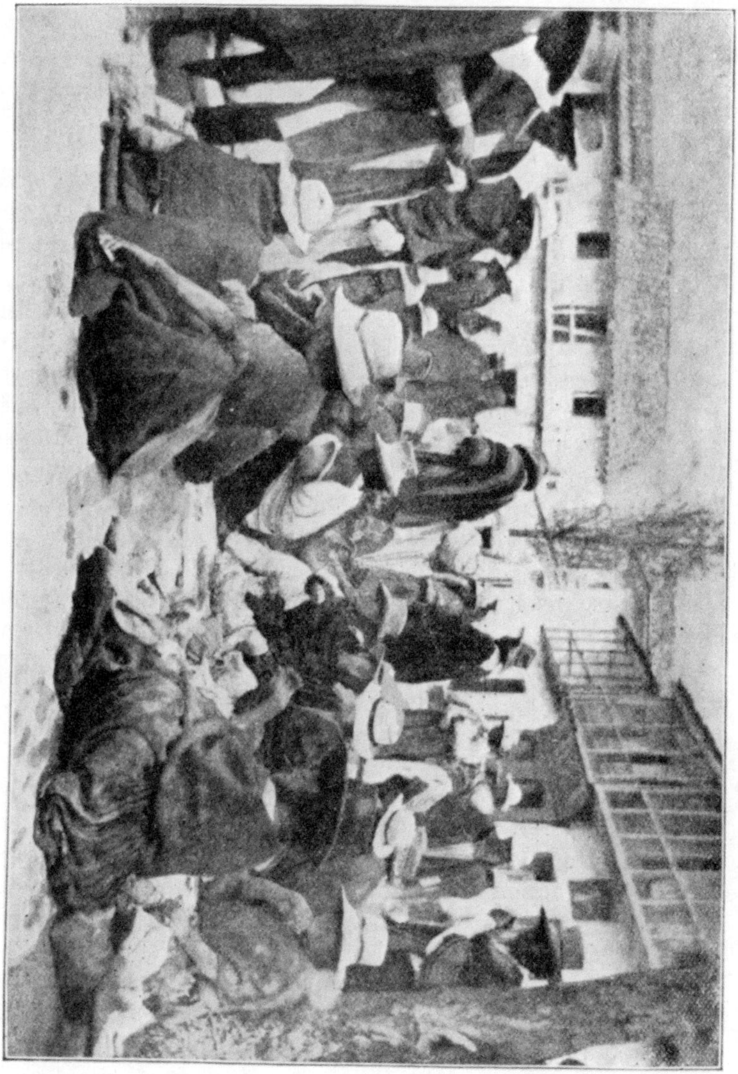

Selling Coca at Azangaro; Peru. [*From a Photograph.*]

more or less an uncertain mixture, dirty white in color and having a nicotine-like odor. This was defended as a peculiarity of the substance, the therapeutic action of which was asserted to be identical with cocaine, even though the appearance was not so elegant as the purer crystals. An endeavor to purify the salt by studying its sources of decomposition resulted in the separation of several important alkaloids.

The intermediate base *benzoyl-ecgonine*, $C_{16}H_{19}NO_4$, was described as a by-product of the manufacture of cocaine,[19] and it has been shown may be also obtained by the evaporation of cocaine solutions.[20] It has been prepared by heating cocaine with from ten to twenty parts of water in a sealed tube at 90° to 95° C., with occasional shaking until a clear solution is obtained. This is extracted with ether to remove all traces of undecomposed cocaine, and then concentrated on a water bath and crystallized over sulphuric acid. The crystals form as opaque prisms or needles, sparingly soluble in cold water, more readily so in hot water, acids, alkalies and alcohol, while insoluble in ether. It melts at 90° to 92° C., then solidifies, and again melts at about 192° C. The taste is bitter, its solutions are slightly acid, becoming neutral after recrystallization. The hydrochloride, at first of a syrupy consistency, forms tabular crystals which are freely soluble in absolute alcohol. Mayer's reagent produces a white, curdy precipitate; iodine in potassium iodide, a kermes brown precipitate; chloride of gold, a bright yellow precipitate, soluble in warm water and alcohol.

It will be recalled that Maclagan, Niemann and Maisch had each alluded to an uncrystallizable residue in their processes of extraction, and an effort was made to definitely determine its true quality. But just as cocaine was at first regarded as the only alkaloid, so this amorphous substance was studied as a whole instead of being regarded as a mixture of bases. Coca leaves, it was asserted, contained a crystallizable cocaine and an uncrystallizable cocaine. The latter product has been named *cocaicine*,[21] *cocainoidine*[22] and *cocamine*,[23] and is still the subject of investigation.

[19] W. Merck; 1885. [20] Paul; Oct. 17, 1885; March 27, 1886. [21] Bender; 1886. [22] Lyons. [23] Hesse.

The relative amount of this non-crystallizable body left in the mother liquor after the precipitation of cocaine varies greatly and is wholly dependent upon the kind of leaves used, or the processes to which they are subjected. The color of various specimens varies from dark yellow to dark brown, while the consistence is from that of a syrupy liquid to a sticky, tenacious solid, which, after spontaneous evaporation, may form short, fine crystals. The odor, while recalling nicotine, is more aromatic and less pungent; the taste bitter and aromatic. This body is of alkaline reaction, soluble in alcohol, ether, benzole, chloroform, petroleum ether, acetic acid, etc., and of varying solubility in water, according to its consistence. On gently heating it becomes quite fluid. It is very soluble in dilute acids, with which it forms non-crystalline salts, all of which dissolve readily in water. Dissolved in rectified spirit and treated with animal charcoal or acetate of lead, to precipitate the coloring matter, a pale yellow, sticky, non-crystalline body is obtained, which will not form crystals, even after standing for months. Solutions of the substance in alcohol, repeatedly precipitated by ammonia, yield a nearly white non-crystalline flocculent body, which is very hygroscopic, the original odor and taste remaining, no matter how often the purifying process is repeated.[24] Evaporated at gentle heat, the solutions darken, and if evaporated to dryness the substance becomes insoluble in water. The precipitation with permanganate of potash is brownish, which, on heating, yields an odor of bitter almonds; 5 c.c. of a solution 1-1000 reduces 20 to 40 drops of a permanganate solution of the same strength.

Professor Stockman, of Edinburgh, made an interesting study of these mixed bases, which he originally supposed to be a solution of ordinary crystalline cocaine in hygrine, basing his conclusions on the physiological action and chemical relations. As he stated, cocaine is extremely soluble in hygrine, and once solution has occurred it is practically impossible to separate the two bodies, as they are both soluble in the same menstrua and are both precipitated by the same reagents.

[24] Stockman; 1887.

This is also the case with the salts of these bodies, though not to the same extent, the presence of hygrine rendering any such samples of the salt hygroscopic, as well as imparting the peculiar nicotine-like odor of hygrine. Subsequent investigation, however, has convinced this physiologist that the substance he experimented with was cocamine dissolved in hygrine, together with some benzoyl-ecgonine.[25]

Thus it will be seen that the earlier conclusions regarding the Coca products were erroneous from imperfect knowledge. With the increasing usefulness of cocaine this confusion is a serious matter, because these mis-statements of the chemists and physiologists are often still quoted as authoritative. So positive were some of these earlier opinions that even after physiological proof showed the unmistakable presence of associate alkaloids with cocaine they were asserted, from interested motives, to be poisonous contaminations. In the face of this the result of physiological experimentation with the various Coca bases indicate that they are all more mild than cocaine, from which they differ markedly in physiological action. Dr. Bignon, Professor of Chemistry at the University of Lima, Peru, who from position and opportunities may be regarded as a competent authority upon Coca, long since asserted, when grouping the alkaloids of Coca in two classes, that the crystalline body is inodorous, while the non-crystalline has a peculiar odor and is weaker in action and less poisonous than the crystallizable cocaine.

The wholly different action of cocaine therapeutically from the Coca leaves of the Andean, or the more exact scientific preservations of Coca such as exhibited in the preparations of M. Mariani—which fully represents the action of recent Peruvian Coca, clearly indicates the presence of certain important principles in Coca, the properties of which are sufficiently distinct to markedly effect physiological action in a manner different from any one of its alkaloids. Happily we are now learning more definitely through research and experimentation, and these earlier errors are being corrected.

The diametrically opposite findings of investigators of

[25] Stockman; *person. com.*; 1899.

known repute indicate that these inharmonious conclusions were not wholly the result of carelessness nor prejudice. Just as Coca experimented with by one observer repeated the traditional influence, or in some other instance proved inert, so the chemists found the result of their labors at variance. Much of this confusion was cleared away when the botanists explained that there are several varieties of Coca. Those qualities which had formerly been attributed to superstitious belief, or which when reluctantly accepted as possibly present in an extremely fugitive form which was lost through volatility, were shown to be dependent upon the variety as much as upon the quality of the Coca leaf employed in the process of manufacture.

Cocamine, $C_{19}H_{23}NO_4$, was originally studied in the alkaloids obtained from the small leaf variety of Coca by Hesse.[26] It was regarded by Liebermann as identical with a base which he described as *γ-isatropyl-cocaine*, and afterward termed *α truxilline*, because supposedly found only in the Truxillo variety of Coca.[27]

The research leading to these conclusions provoked bitter controversy between these two investigators. It has since been determined that cocamine is of the same empirical composition as cocaine, though weaker in anæsthetic action. It is a natural product of several varieties of Coca, particularly of that grown in Java.[28] From hydrolysis by mineral acids cocamine yields *cocaic, iso-cocaic* and *homo-iso-cocaic* acids, while from its isomeride there is formed in a similar way *α-isotropic* or *β-truxillic* acid. Both cocaic and iso-cocaic acids yield cinnamic acid and other products on distillation. Subsequently a similar body was prepared synthetically from ecgonine and cinnamic anhydride, and named *cinnamyl-cocaine.*[29] It forms large colorless crystals, melts at 120°, is almost insoluble in water, and readily soluble in alcohol and ether. This body has been proved to occur naturally in Coca leaves from various sources,[30] being present in some specimens as high as 0.5 per cent.

Thus it will be seen there has been much discussion and

[26] Hesse; 1887. [27] Liebermann; XXI; 1888. [28] Hesse; Aug. 8, 1891.
[29] Giesel; 1889. [30] Paul and Cownley; XX, 166; 1889.

uncertainty upon the Coca products, particularly so as to those of an oily nature, originally designated as hygrine and the amorphous substances previously described under various titles.

It is the opinion of Hesse that hygrine is a product of decomposition of one of the Coca bases, and does not occur in fresh Coca leaves; in support of which he asserted that while dilute acid solutions of hygrine have a strongly marked blue florescence which is characteristic, this reaction is not shown when fresh leaves are first operated upon. But as this reaction develops gradually, he inferred that hygrine was formed by the decomposition of amorphous cocaine, from the solution of which it could be separated by ammonia and caustic soda as a colorless oil having the odor of quinoline. In fact, he considered the oil thus obtained a homologue of quinoline, possibly a tri-methyl-quinoline.

Another observer,[31] while experimenting with the alkaloids of Coca by means of their platinum salts, obtained an oily base, exceedingly bitter and differing in odor and solubility from that which had been described by Lossen, but which was presumably identical with the amorphous products, *cocaicine* and *cocainiodine*, and Hesse concluded there might really be two oily bases in amorphous cocaine, one found in the benzoyl compounds of the broad leaf variety and one in the cinnamyl compounds of the *Novo Granatense* variety, in both cases associated with *cocamine* and another base, which he named *cocrylamine*.[32] Liebermann, on the other hand, considers hygrine a combination of two liquid oxygenated bases which may be separated by fractional distillation. One—$C_8H_{15}NO$, an isomeride of tropine, with a boiling point 193° to 195°, the other, $C_{14}H_{24}N_2O$,[33] not distilling under ordinary pressure without decomposition, while still other experimenters from distilling barium ecgonate obtained a volatile oily liquid which strongly resembles hygrine.[34] Merck has shown this body yields, on decomposition, methylamine, from which it has been inferred that it is identical with tropine, and hence closely allied to atropine. With this fact in view it

[31] Howard; July 23, 1887. [32] Hesse; November, 1887.
[33] Liebermann; XXII; 1, 675; 1889. [34] Calmels and Gossin; 1885.

was presumed the dilating property of cocaine upon the pupil was due to hygrine, but this has been proved not to be the case.[35]

The assertion that hygrine is never present in Coca leaves, but is merely a decomposition product in the manufacture of cocaine, lends an added interest to the research of Dr. Rusby upon fresh Coca leaves made while he was at Bolivia. From repeated examinations he found a certain yield of alkaloids, while specimens of the same leaves sent to the United States yielded from treatment by the same process less than half the percentage of alkaloid that he had obtained. This prompted him to search for the possible source of error, and it was found that after all the cocaine was eliminated there was still a decided alkaloidal precipitate. From this it was concluded that: "native Coca leaves contain a body intimately associated with the cocaine and reacting to the same test, which almost wholly disappears from them in transit."[36]

This result indicates the presence in Coca leaves of some extremely volatile principle to which decided physiological properties are attached, which may also be obtained from suitably preserved leaves. When a preparation made from recent leaves in Bolivia was submitted to Professor Remsen, of Johns Hopkins University, his assistant reported that he found a bitter principle, and an oil, which presumably differed in no way from that found at the time of the examinations made in Bolivia. This is comparable with similar findings of those who have experimented with Coca, whether the leaves were recent and examined on the spot, or the examination had been made thousands of miles distant upon well preserved leaves. In each instance similar volatile alkaloids have been obtained, which have commonly been pronounced "decomposition products," yet, as these are always found by careful observers, it indicates they are the natural associate bases of Coca.

The conclusions are that crude cocaine is not merely a single alkaloid. As the yield of crystallizable cocaine from the crude alkaloid varies from fifty to seventy-five per cent., the

[35] Stockman; 1888. [36] Rusby; 1888.

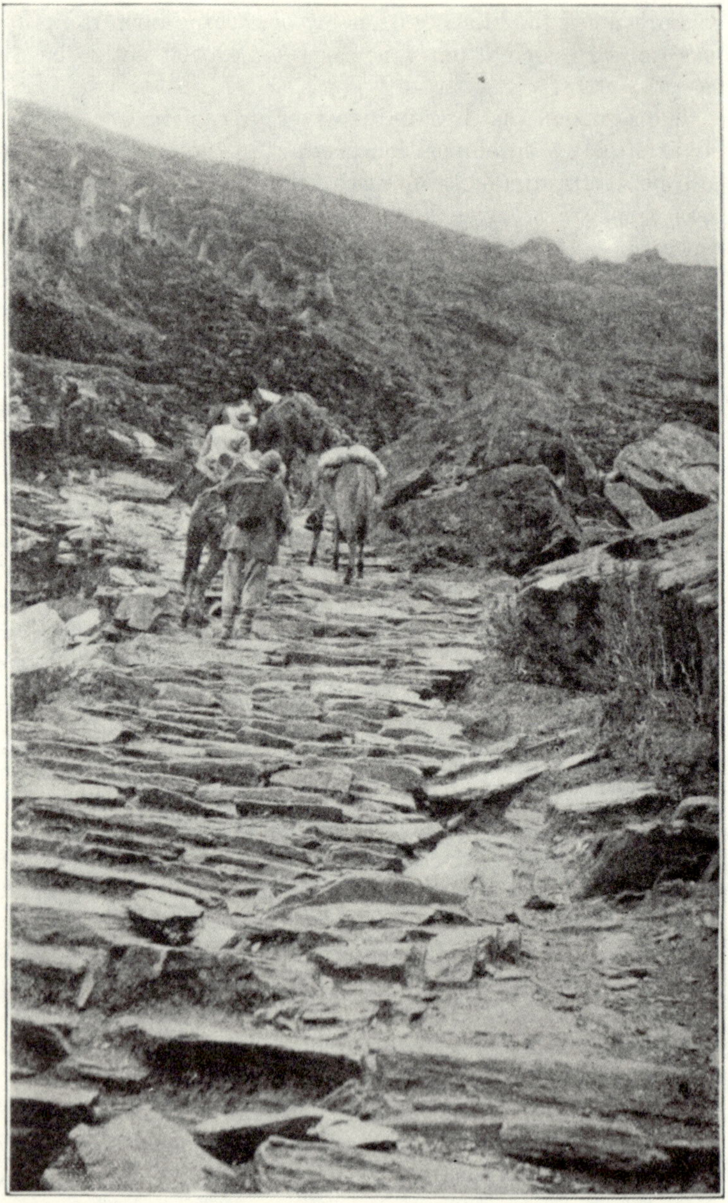

ROAD FROM THE COCA REGION OF PHARA; PERU. [*From a Photograph.*]

associate alkaloids, together with the impurities and contaminations of manufacture, must constitute the remaining twenty-five or fifty per cent. of the substance. Though our knowledge of these alkaloids is not yet exact, each of them has been found to possess certain chemical characteristics and sufficient physiological influence to prove a factor in the action of Coca. While these several Coca bases have been experimented with physiologically to a limited extent, they have never been individually applied to therapeutic uses. They have been regarded by the manufacturers of cocaine as simply so much waste from their yield of cocaine, and the attention of chemists has been directed to converting them by some synthetic process to what has been regarded as the pure alkaloid.

In the chemical constitution of cocaine there is a methyl, CH_3, and a benzoyl, $C_6H_5CO_2$, radical, either of which can be replaced by other acid radicals and so give rise to various homologues—or compounds of similar proportions. The methyl radical has been shown to be essential to the anæsthetic action, and its presence or absence in the chemical group constitutes a poisonous or non-poisonous Coca product.[37] By heating the Coca bases with alkyl iodides the corresponding esters are obtained. Thus *methyl-benzoyl-ecgonine*—cocaine; *ethyl-benzoyl-ecgonine*—homococaine; *methyl-cinnamyl-ecgonine*—cinnamyl-cocaine, etc., are formed. Acting upon this data, Merck, by heating benzoyl-ecgonine with a slight excess of methyl-iodide and a small quantity of methylic alcohol to 100° C., evaporating the excess of methyl-iodide and methylic alcohol, obtained a syrupy liquid containing cocaine hydriodate, from which an artificial cocaine was produced. In a similar way Skraup,[38] by heating benzoyl-ecgonine, sodium-methylate and methyl-iodide in a sealed tube, made a synthetic cocaine, although the yield was only about four per cent., while that of Merck[39] was nearly eighty per cent. of the theoretical quantity.

In following this process, but using ethyl iodide,[39] Merck obtained a new base, or homologue, *cocethyline,* or *homoco-*

[37] Crum-Brown and Fraser. [38] Skraup; 1885. [39] W. Merck; XVIII; 1885.

caine, with the formula $C_{18}H_{23}NO_4$, which crystallizes from ether in colorless, radiating prisms, and from alcohol in glossy prisms, which melt at 108°-109° C. The alkaloid is sparingly soluble in alkalies; chloride of gold gives a voluminous yellow precipitate, and chloride of mercury a white, pulverulent one, soluble in hot water. Falck has ascertained that cocethyline has an anæsthetic action similar to cocaine, though weaker.

In following a similar method, but employing propyl iodide and propyl alcohol, and again by the use of iso-butyl-iodide with its corresponding alcohol, *coc-propyline* and *coc-iso-butyline* have been respectively formed, both of which have a strong anæsthetic action, and, though chemically different, exhibit the same reactions as cocaine.

Ecgonine has been converted into a new base[40] by heating it for twenty-four hours with aqueous potash. This differs from ecgonine by being less soluble in absolute alcohol, in having a higher melting point, and in being dextro-rotary, and hence termed *dextro-ecgonine.* From this there has been prepared synthetically a *dextro-cocaine,* a colorless oil which solidifies and forms crystals on standing which are readily soluble in ether, alcohol, benzine and petroleum spirit. This body resembles cocaine, but its action is more fugitive.

From the ready conversion of the various Coca bases experimentally it was but a step to the building up of the associate bases into a synthetic salt of cocaine. This has given rise to a profitable industry, the process for which has been patented in Germany.[41] In this process the mixed bases are converted by hydrolysis to ecgonine, then to a solution of hydrochloride of that salt in methyl alcohol.[42] The hydrochloride of ecgonine methyl-ester is formed, and from this the salt is crystallized and heated over a water bath with benzoyl chloride, the homogenous mass being washed and separated from benzoic acid, and the cocaine precipitated with ammonia and crystallized from alcohol.

The proportion of alkaloids contained in Coca leaves is influenced by the method of the growth of the plant, and the

[40] Einhorn and Marquardt; XXIII; 1890. [41] Liebermann; XXI; 1889.
[42] Einhorn; XXI, 3335; 1888.

yield is dependent upon the manner of curing the leaves and their preservation. The percentage ranges from a mere trace to about one per cent. Bignon considers that well preserved leaves will yield fully as much as recent leaves, varying from nine to eleven grammes of the mixed alkaloids per kilogram, the latter being more than one per cent. Niemann obtained from his original process 0.25 per cent. of cocaine, while the present yield is more than double that. From a number of assays made during the last few years in the laboratory of an American manufacturer[43] the following percentages of alkaloid were obtained: 0.53, 0.51, 0.63, 0.63, 0.57, 0.60, 0.66, 0.55, 0.70, 0.70, 0.65, 0.67, 0.54, 0.70, 0.32, 0.42, 0.52, 0.85, 0.48, 1.3, 0.78, 0.70, 0.40, 0.63. This will serve as an index of the quantity of total alkaloid commonly found in the average leaf of good quality as it reaches North America.

In determining the amount of alkaloids present in a given specimen of Coca, it is essential that the selected leaves be finely powdered, and mixed with a suitable menstruum that will not cause undue annoyance from gummy and resinous matters while setting free the essential constituents. These are washed out of the solution by an appropriate solvent, dried and weighed, or estimated by using some reagent the equivalent values of which have been determined by experiment. Various alkalies, as lime, soda or magnesia, have been suggested for admixture with the leaves for the purpose of liberating the alkaloids, which are transformed to soluble salts by acidulated water and washed out with strong alcohol. The details of the production of the Coca alkaloids commercially are kept as a trade secret, but the broad methods of manufacture are all similar, as several will illustrate.

Dr. Squibb has suggested the following process for the preparation of cocaine on a small scale:

One hundred grammes of finely ground leaves are moistened with 100 c. c. of 7 per cent. solution of sodium carbonate, packed in a percolator, and sufficient kerosene added to make 700 c.c. of percolate. This is transferred to a separator, and 30 c.c. of 2 per cent. solution of hydrochloric acid added and

[43] Parke, Davis & Co.; *person. com.;* 1898.

shaken. After separation the watery solution is drawn off from below into a smaller separator, and this process is repeated three times, the alkaloid being in the smaller separator as an acid hydrochlorate. This is precipitated in ether with sodium carbonate, and evaporated at low heat with constant stirring and the product weighed.

Another process is to digest Coca leaves in a closed vessel at 70° C. for two hours with a very weak solution of caustic soda, and petroleum boiling between 200° to 250°. The mass is filtered, pressed while tepid, and the filtrate allowed to stand until the petroleum separates from the aqueous liquid. The former is then drawn off and neutralized with weak hydrochloric acid. The bulky precipitate of cocaine hydrochloride being recovered from the aqueous liquid by evaporation.[44]

Gunn made a series of tests to determine what relation the methods of extraction had to the alkaloidal yield, and concluded that the modified method of Lyons obtained the most alkaloids.[45] This is substantially as follows:

Shake 10 grammes of finely powdered leaves with 95 c.c. of petroleum benzin and add 5 c.c. of the following mixture: Absolute alcohol, 19 volumes; concentrated solution ammonia, 1 volume. Again shake for a few minutes, and set aside for twenty-four hours with occasional shaking. Decant rapidly 50 c.c. of the clear fluid, or, if it is not clear, filter it, washing the filter with benzin. Transfer to a separator containing 5 c.c. of water, to which has been added 6 to 8 drops of dilute sulphuric acid (1 to 5 by weight). Shake vigorously; when the fluids have separated draw the aqueous portion into a one ounce vial. Wash the contents of the separator with 2½ c.c. of acidulated water (1 drop of the dilute acid). Shake, draw off into the vial, and continue this two or three times, until a drop tested on a mirror with Mayer's reagent shows only faint turbidity. Add to the aqueous fluid 15 c.c. of benzin, shake, and when separation is complete, pour off the benzin. Add to the vial 15 c.c. of stronger ether, U. S. P., with sufficient ammonia to render the mixture decidedly alkaline. Shake, and when separation is complete, decant the ether carefully

[44] Pfeiffer; XI. [45] Gunn; 1896.

into a tared capsule. Wash the residue in the vial with two or three successive portions of fresh ether until the aqueous fluid is free from alkaloid, as shown by the test. Evaporate the ether over a water bath. Dry the alkaloid to constant weight, weigh, multiply the result expressed in decigrammes by two, which will present the percentage of crude cocaine.[46]

Instead of extracting the alkaloid from the acid aqueous solution a simple method adapted to use in the field may be followed, in which the alkaloid is estimated by titration with Mayer's reagent. An acid solution representing 5 grammes of the leaves should be made up to a volume of 15 c.c., and the reagent added as long as it continues to precipitate in the clear filtrate. In this way, with half strength solution, 3.5 c.c. reagent represents 0.2 per cent. of alkaloid.

Mayer's reagent, or the decinormal mercuric potassium iodide of the U. S. P., is prepared as follows: Mercuric chloride, 13.546 grammes, dissolved in 600 c.c. of water; potassium iodide, 49.8 grammes, dissolved in 190 c.c. of water; mix the two solutions and add sufficient water to make the whole measure, at 59° F., exactly 1000 c.c.

When Mayer's reagent is added drop by drop to an acid solution containing cocaine (1:200 to 1:600) there is at first produced a heavy white precipitate, which collects at once into curdy masses; a drop of solution should be examined on a mirror, and should not show more than slight turbidity when determining the final traces. Dr. Lyons suggests that after adding a certain quantity of the reagent it will be found that the filtered fluid which still gives a heavy precipitate with Mayer's reagent produces a precipitate also in a fresh solution of cocaine. It is thus evident that the precipitation is complete only when an excess of reagent is present in the fluid; and it is found advisable to correct the reading from the burette by substracting for each c.c. of fluid present at the end of the titration 0.085 c.c. (if the half strength reagent is used); the remainder multiplied by ten will give the quantity of alkaloid indicated in milligrammes. The best method of following the process is

[46] Lyons; *Manual*, p. 74; 1886.

to throw the fluid on a filter after each addition of reagent. Solutions of the alkaloid 1:400 appear to yield better results than solutions stronger or weaker than this.

One c.c. of Mayer's reagent will precipitate about 7.5 milligrammes of the mixed alkaloids from solutions in which alcohol is not present. As a rule the quantity of alkaloidal precipitate by this reagent is greater than the quantity of cocaine that can be extracted by washing out the alkaline solution with ether, so that in exact examinations a recourse to weighing is considered advisable. The dried precipitate weighed and multiplied by 0.406 will give about the amount of alkaloid present. With Mayer's reagent used in half strength the following values for the equivalent of the reagent are given:

Strength of cocaine solution.	1 c.c of Mayer's reagent (half strength) precipitates of cocaine.
1:200	0.0062
1:300	0.0066
1:400	0.0070
1:500	0.0074
1:600	0.0078

The following table may also be of service:

Quantity of Mayer's Reagent ($N\frac{1}{20}$) *Necessary to Precipitate a Given Quantity of Cocaine.*

Quantity of Cocaine.	Measure of Fluid Titrated.			
	5 c.c.	10 c.c.	15 c.c.	20 c.c.
.010	1.6	....	....	....
.020	2.7	3.1	....	....
.030	....	4.2	4.6	....
.040	....	5.3	5.7	6.2
.050	....	6.4	6.8	7.3
.060	....	....	7.9	8.4
.070	....	....	9.0	9.5
.080	....	....	....	10.6
.090	....	....	....	11.7
.100	....	....	....	12.8

Results higher or lower than those indicated are beyond the limits of the experiment and would call for repetition.[47]

The principal tests employed to determine the purity of

[47] Lyons; *Note;* 1886.

cocaine hydrochloride are the permanganate of potash and Maclagan's ammonia test. When one drop of a one per cent. solution of permanganate of potash is added to 5 c.c. of a two per cent. solution of hydrochloride of cocaine mixed with three drops of dilute sulphuric acid, it occasions a pink tint which should not entirely disappear within half an hour. When added to a stronger solution it occasions a precipitate of rhombic plates, which decompose on heating. If cinnamyl-cocaine be present the odor of bitter almonds is given off with the decomposition.

The Maclagan test is based upon the supposition that the amorphous alkaloids of Coca when set free by ammonia are separated as oily drops and so form a milky solution. It is employed by adding one or two drops of ammonia to a solution of cocaine, which is then vigorously stirred with a glass rod. If the salt is pure a formation of crystals will be deposited upon the rod and upon the side of the vessel within five minutes, while the solution will remain clear. If isatropyl-cocaine be present crystallization will not take place and the solution will become milky.

Considerable stress has been laid upon the value of this test for determining the purity of cocaine salts. Dr. Guenther[48] asserts that a perfectly pure cocaine will not show the Maclagan reaction, while if a small quantity of a new base which he described as *cocathylin,* with a melting point of 110° C., be present, the test will be pronounced. In endeavoring to show that this was an error, one of the largest manufacturers of cocaine in Germany worked up four thousand kilos of Coca leaves, and though they failed to find the new base which had been mentioned, they also proved that a pure cocaine will respond positively to the Maclagan test.[49] In support of this Paul and Cownley[50] have expressed the opinion that any cocaine which does not satisfy this test should not be regarded as sufficiently pure for pharmaceutical purposes, views which are also maintained by E. Merck.[51]

Of the various reagents that have been found delicate in

[48] Guenther; Feb. 2, 1899.
[49] Boehringer and Soehne; *person. com.;* Mannheim, Germany, 1899.
[50] Paul and Cownley; p. 587; 1898. [51] *Person. com.;* Darmstadt; July, 1899.

testing for cocaine Mayer's reagent will detect one part in one hundred thousand, while a solution of iodine in iodide of potash will determine one part in four hundred thousand, with a very faint yellow precipitate.

It has been shown by Gerrard that mydriatic alkaloids have a peculiar action with mercuric chloride, from the aqueous solution of which they precipitate mercuric oxide, the other natural alkaloids giving no precipitate at all, or at least not separating mercuric oxide. The late Professor Flücki-

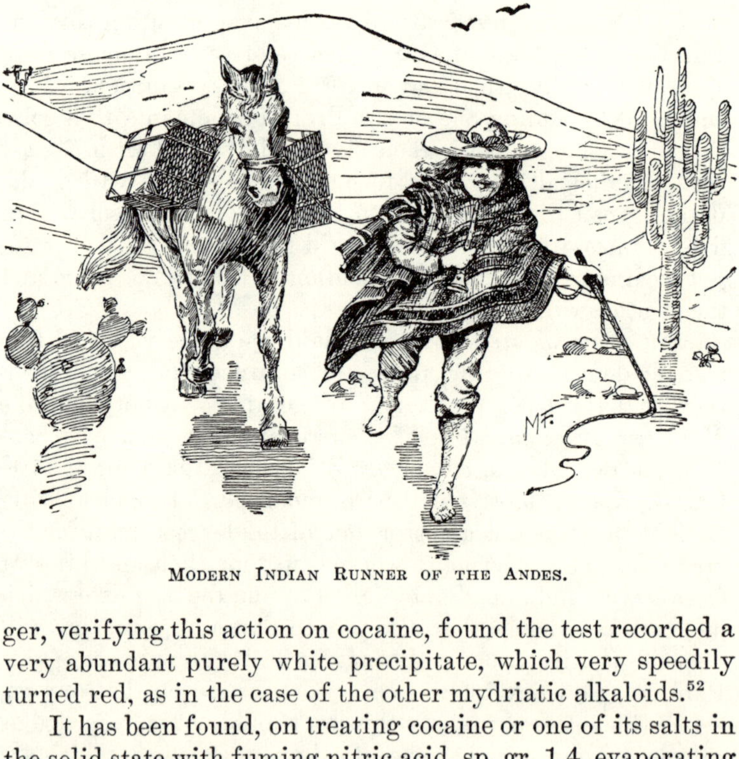

MODERN INDIAN RUNNER OF THE ANDES.

ger, verifying this action on cocaine, found the test recorded a very abundant purely white precipitate, which very speedily turned red, as in the case of the other mydriatic alkaloids.[52]

It has been found, on treating cocaine or one of its salts in the solid state with fuming nitric acid, sp. gr. 1.4, evaporating to dryness and treating with one or two drops of strong alcoholic solution of potash, there is given off on stirring this with a glass rod a distinct odor suggestive of peppermint.[53] This

[52] Flückiger; 1886. [53] F. da Silva; 1890.

odor test has been pronounced very delicate and is distinctive for cocaine, no other alkaloid having been found to yield a similar reaction.

There are several cocaine manufacturers in Peru. A few years ago there were five in Huanuco, one in the District of Mozon, one in Pozuso, two at Lima, one at Callao, at least two of which are run on an extensive scale. In 1894 the amount of the crude product manufactured in Peru and sent abroad for purification was four thousand seven hundred and sixteen kilos. A personal communication from Peru, dated January 15, 1900, states that the local manufacturers of cocaine are increasing their facilities and claim that they work with a better method than is followed elsewhere.

In 1890 Dr. Squibb called attention to the fact that crude cocaine was made so efficiently in Peru that it seemed highly probable that the importation of Coca leaves to this market was nearly at an end. This crude cocaine has a characteristic nicotine odor; it comes in a granular powder or in fragments of press cake, generally of a dull creamy white color, but rarely quite uniform throughout, the color ranging from dirty brownish white to very nearly white. Some of the fragments are horny, compact and hard, while others are softer and more porous. The following process has been given for determining the amount of cocaine present in the crude product:[54]

A small quantity being taken from a large number of lumps in the parcels, selected on account of their difference in appearance, the determination of moisture in the samples so selected is found by fusion at 91° C. The solubility of the samples in ether at a specific gravity .725 at 15.6° C., is then tested. The insoluble residue is thoroughly washed with ether, dried and weighed. The alkaloid dissolved by the ether is converted into oxalate, and the oxalate shaken out by water. The residue which is soluble in ether is then determined by evaporation of the ethereal solution. The aqueous solution of cocaine oxalate is rendered faintly alkaline by soda; the freed alkaloid shaken out with ether, and after spontaneous evaporation of the ether and complete drying of the crystals pro-

[54] Squibb; XXXVIII.

duced, the pure alkaloid is estimated. The usual yield of pure crystallizable alkaloid from this crude product varies from fifty to seventy-five per cent.

Crude cocaine when united with acids assumes an intense green color, due to the presence of benzoyl-ecgonine, while its characteristic chemical reaction is its property of splitting into benzoic acid and methyl alcohol.

Cocaine combines readily with acids to form salts, which are readily soluble in water and alcohol, though insoluble in ether. These salts, owing to their more ready solubility, have a more marked anæsthetic action on mucous surfaces than the pure alkaloid. There has been prepared benzoate, borate, citrate, hydrobromate, hydrochlorate, nitrate, oleate, oxalate, salicylate, sulphate, tartrate, etc.

According to the U. S. Pharmacopœia the following are the characteristics of cocaine hydrochlorate, the salt commonly employed: "Colorless, transparent crystals, or a white crystalline powder, without odor, of a saline, slightly bitter taste, and producing upon the tongue a tingling sensation, followed by numbness of some minutes' duration. Permanent in the air. Soluble at 15° C. (59° F.) in 0.48 part of water and in 3.5 parts of alcohol; very soluble in boiling water and in boiling alcohol; also soluble in 2,800 parts of ether or in 17 parts of chloroform. On heating a small quantity of the powdered salt for twenty minutes at a temperature of 100° C. (212° F.), it should not suffer any material loss (absence of water of crystallization). The prolonged application of heat to the salt or to its solution induces decomposition. At 193° C. (379.4° F.) the salt melts with partial sublimation, forming a light brownish yellow liquid. When ignited it is consumed without leaving a residue. The salt is neutral to litmus paper."

In reviewing the research of many workers it may be seen how each has closely approached, often with a mere hint or suggestion, results which later have been verified and described more in detail. Through this repetition many new facts have been made positive to us. Assertions have been strengthened or have been cast aside, and while the result has been to render a cocaine of purer quality, it has at the same time emphasized the immensity of our ignorance concerning the subtleties of alkaloidal formation.

More than all, these researches must impress the fact that similar changes to those which are possible in the laboratory of the chemist are also at work in Nature's laboratory, and that the therapeutic influence and efficiency of Coca, as of any remedy taken into the body, must be markedly affected by the transmutations of the organism.

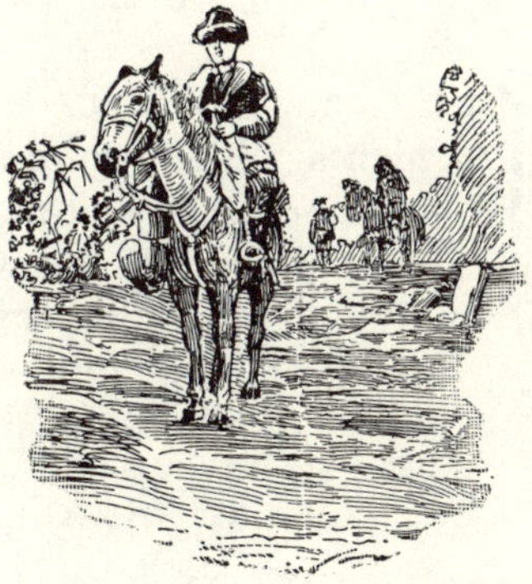

CHAPTER XI.

THE PRODUCTION OF ALKALOIDS IN PLANTS.

> **"Good wine makes good blood, good blood causeth good humors, good humors cause good thoughts, good thoughts bring forth good works, good works carry a man to Heaven; ergo good wine carrieth a man to Heaven."**
>
> **—J. Howell, *Familiar Letters*, Bk. II., liv.**

JUST how alkaloids are produced in plants, while a subject full of interest to the chemist and physiologist, is one upon which our knowledge is not yet very exact. But inasmuch as there exists an intimate association between plant physiology and that of animal life, there is also an ultimate comparison between those bodies which are considered as the excrementive principles of plants and similar waste products—which in some examples are closely allied chemically to these—that are cast out by the animal tissues.

The first separation of the active principle of a plant is attributed to a pharmacist of Eimbeck, in Hanover, named Sertürner, who about 1817 isolated from opium a basic substance to which he gave the name "morphium." This was rapidly followed by the discovery of strychnine and brucine, in 1818, and of quinine and cinchonine, by Pelletier and Caventou, in 1820, and later, in 1827, the volatile alkaloid conine was obtained from hemlock by Giseke, and by Geiger, while in the following year nicotine was described by Posselt and Reimann.

The plants yielding alkaloids are widely distributed throughout the vegetable kingdom, belonging chiefly to the botanical division of dicotyledons. These substances are not found in the familiar *Graminieæ* and *Labiatæ,* and are rarely obtained in plants of the extensive order of compositæ, and thus far in only one family of the monocotyledons—the *Colchiceæ.*[1] Alkaloids are nitrogenous carbon compounds, having basic properties, which are usually formed as the salts of organic acids. The greater number of them contain carbon, hydrogen, oxygen and nitrogen, though in a few cases oxygen is absent, and the resultant alkaloid is volatile, as nicotine, conine, sparteine, and some of the oily Coca bases.

Chemically, the vegetable alkaloids may be arranged in three groups, the first being derivatives of pyridine—as atropine and conine, the second derivatives of quinoline—as narcotine and cinchonine, the third those of the xanthin group—which are allied to urea, as caffeine. Nearly all the vegetable alkaloids belong to the first and second class, all of which contain nitrogen, and are probably formed by the action of ammonia, or amido compounds which are derived from ammonia, upon non-nitrogenous bodies.[2]

Pyridine—C_5H_5N, may be regarded as **a** benzin—C_6H_6, in which one CH group has been replaced by one of nitrogen. The pyridine bases, metameric with aniline and its homologues, are contained in coal-tar, naphtha, tobacco smoke, and many organic substances. Königs proposed confining the name alkaloid to plant derivatives of this origin. Quinoline—C_9H_7N, has the same relation to naphthalene—$C_{10}H_8$, that pyridine has to benzin; that is, it is derived by substituting one atom of nitrogen for one of the CH group in naphthalene.[3]

Originally an alkaloid was regarded merely as the active principle of the plant from which it was obtained, but as the number increased, and as allied substances were also found

[1] Thorpe; 1893. [2] Watts; 1889. [3] Allen: 1892.

in animal tissues which were often spoken of as alkaloids, the general term has become confusional when applied to these bodies without regard to their derivation. With the advance in organic chemistry, which has enabled the building up of compounds from coal-tar products in the laboratory to intimately resemble the true plant bases, it is often important to distinguish between those alkaloids which are natural and those which are of artificial production. Yet this very fact has indicated the correlation of all matter, and the investigations of the chemist and physiologist have happily progressed together, each furthering the research of the other.

It is not so many years ago that it was taught there was

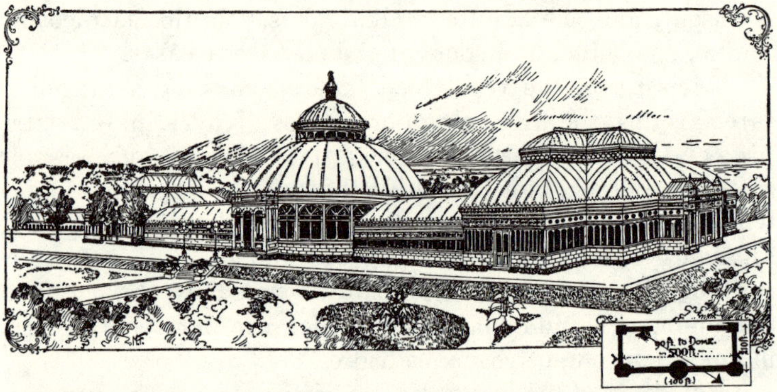

CONSERVATORIES OF NEW YORK BOTANICAL GARDEN AT BRONX PARK.

an abrupt difference between the chemistry of the inert and the living, while the several compounds that were described as cast out by living cells were supposed only capable of production by organized structures, but when Woehler manufactured urea synthetically, it was seen that this sharp distinction could no longer be true. Among organized bodies the association, and even interdependence, between the higher order of plants and animals is of course even far more striking. Long before the Christian Era Aristotle attempted to trace an absolute connection between all living things, and though it would seem that one might immediately pronounce to which class an organism belongs, it is really not so simple.

The lower forms of one so nearly approach the lower forms of the other order that biologists have often found extreme difficulty in determining a classification that shall be generally accepted by naturalists.

The old illustration as showing the distinction between plants and animals, that the former absorb carbonic acid and give off oxygen, while animals do just the reverse, is only partially true, for while it is a fact that animals give off carbonic acid, plants cannot live in the absence of oxygen, which is essential to furthering the processes of their metabolism. As another illustration, it was shown that plants have not the power of voluntary motion possessed by animals, but this assertion was shown to be wrong by numerous examples among the lower forms which are precisely the reverse. All individual cells must possess the power of motion, and some of the lower plant organisms actually move from place to place—indeed, locomotion is absolutely necessary to their existence.[4] On the other hand, some lower animal structures are permanently fixed, so that the older comparisons are not definite. Similar chemical changes take place in the cell structure of plants and animals. All must have motion incidental to growth, together with the functions of sleep, nutrition and irritability, which latter property is manifest by certain plants to a remarkable degree under the influence of such nitrogenous foods as raw meat, milk or albumen.[5]

As vegetable alkaloids are considered to be the excreta of plants, we cannot properly draw any conclusion concerning their probable formation without regarding the changes which are brought about in the life of the organism producing them. As these processes are intimately allied to changes which are undergone under similar conditions in the animal being, a review of the subject may not be wholly uninteresting, while it will enable us to more fully appreciate the possible action of the products of the Coca leaf when we come to consider the application of that interesting plant more directly in the human economy.

All organic structure is built up through a constant break-

[4] Darwin; 1880. [5] *Idem;* 1875.

ing down and rearrangement of simple chemical elements. In the case of plants, the compounds of the elements which have been admixed with the soil are carried in solution through the root to the most remote cells of the leaf. There these chemical bodies are converted into complex substances, which under suitable stimuli are built to form the tissues of the organism. These subtle changes take place only under the influence of that mighty alchemist, the sun.

It would seem that the Incas were not far wrong in regarding this great source of light and activity as at least the physical source of all power, for not only is plant life dependent upon the action of the sun, but the animal being is in turn dependent upon plant structure. Those compounds which have been so mysteriously molded into vegetable organisms must be torn apart and dissolved in order to set free the elements of which animal structure is composed. Here these elements are rearranged to the necessities of a higher organization, where they may continue a still more complex existence. This constant interchange is carried on through plants and animals—through animals and plants—each organism converting and reconverting, from age to age, the various elements appropriate to its own requirements. In the performance of these functional processes, each cell of the tissues creates for itself, as well as for surrounding bodies, that combination of energy which we call life. These changes are carried on without intermediary loss of matter—which we know is indestructible—regardless of the extent or method of the many conversions it may have undergone since creation, and shall continue to undergo until the end of time. So that it is theoretically, if not literally, possible that:—

"Imperious Cæsar, dead and turn'd to clay,
Might stop a hole to keep the wind away."

There are four principal elements of the sixty-seven or more known ones which may be regarded as the very basis of life. These are carbon, hydrogen, oxygen and nitrogen, and all organic changes take place in accordance with the varying proportions that these elements unite with each other. Carbon we are apt to carelessly regard as that coke-like substance made familiar to us through its employment in electricity, without stopping to recall its important relation to all organic tissue. It enters into the building of other cells than electric, for it is found, without exception, in every tissue of organic life. It seems difficult to understand how so apparently inert a substance can become intimately incorporated with living structures. Carbon, which as a product of combustion is everywhere diffused as carbonic acid, is carried as a gas and in solution to the plant and is absorbed by the roots and stomata of the leaves. Here under sunshine it is deposited for immediate use or to form emergency food for the tissues, while the oxygen is set free to again enter into the performance of those multiple chemical processes included in growth and decay. So important is the influence of carbon in all organic structures that Pflüger has advanced the theory that carbon united with nitrogen as cyanogen constituted the radical which formed the very nucleus of creation—of that molten chaos from which all existence sprung.

Nitrogen may be regarded, if not the source of all energy, certainly as the chemical creator of force, for it is absolutely necessary in all compounds from which power is to be derived. The changes due to oxygen are so much more spoken of that it would seem the importance of nitrogen is often disregarded. Though everywhere about us this element cannot, like oxygen, be readily forced into union, and plants cannot take in free nitrogen. But so essential is this subtle element to all organic energies through its formation of proteids and their decomposition, that it must be coaxed into suitable combinations by similar transmutations as those for the deposit of carbon—the activity of vegetable life under the stimulus of sunshine. Its combinations, however, are loose and maintained with difficulty, yet this very effort for constant freedom causes this to be the most important element of all chemical compounds in which it is associated. The property of nitrogen of escaping from union and liberating energy is made use of in the high explosives, and is also exhibited in the more subtle decompositions of decay, which owe their potency to the nitrogen contained in their ammonia.

Similar changes due to the influence of nitrogen are constantly going on in the processes of metabolism in all organic tissue. We have an instance of this when the carbohydrates of plants are converted into proteid structures, which, decomposing, again set free their nitrogen as excreta in the form of alkaloids. Again this property is shown in the human laboratory when the pent-up nitrogen in the Coca leaf is brought to bear upon the customary maize dietary of the Andean, and as a result the starchy elements are converted into the more complex molecule of the flesh-forming proteid.

With these four primary elements are mingled others, including sulphur, phosphorus, potassium, calcium, magnesium, iron, and the gaseous element chlorine, all of which may serve to nourish certain tissues of the organism to which they are carried in solution of various compounds. So while the several primary elements are essential to the structure of every organism, it is impossible for them to be utilized in the upbuilding of tissue until carried to the cell in fluid form. In the case of plant life, the elements are conveyed in such dilution of their salts that their presence is seemingly physically absent, while the fluids are apparently but simple water. This solution is taken up from the soil through the roots, yet the selection may not be only of such substances as are of positive nutritive value, but of other substances in solution, which may even be injurious.

That all living things are composed of cells has been known since Marcello Malpighi, Professor of Medicine in the University at Bologna, in 1670, first explained this arrangement of tissues coincident with an English botanist, Nehemiah Grew, who originally described the stomata—or little mouths of leaves. These two investigators, singularly enough, though working independently and many miles apart, each presented a paper before the Royal Society of London upon this subject on the same day. It seems remarkable, in view of the present regard for the importance of the cell doctrine, that this fact required nearly one hundred and seventy years for elaboration, for it did not receive final adoption until 1838, when it was accepted as the scientific basis of life.

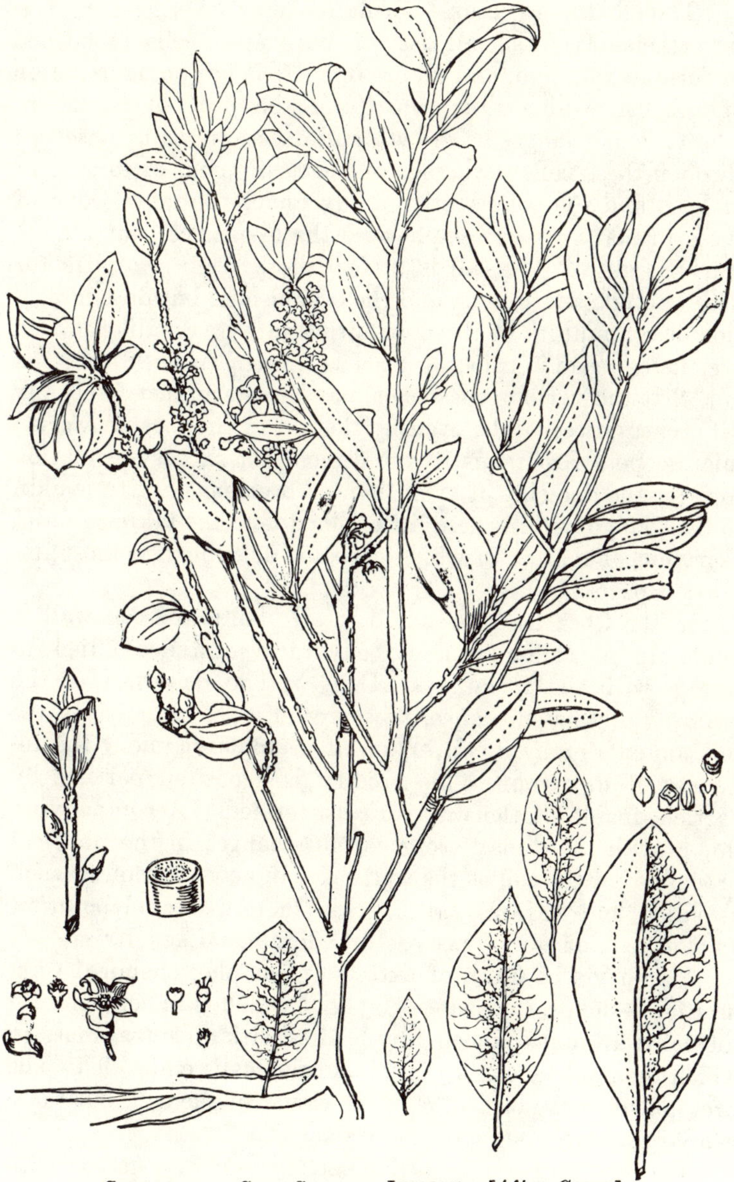

SPECIMEN OF COCA SENT BY JUSSIEU. [*After Gosse.*]
Herbarium, Museum of Natural History; Paris.

Though the structural formation may be different, it is nevertheless true that all tissue is built up of cells—modified in form or function, and all organic life is but an aggregation of the cell which thus constitutes the unit of existence. The various changes of growth and decay are to be observed through these cells—whether of bone, of wood, of muscle or of leaf, and the comparative study under the microscope of these primary tissues emphasizes the assurance that all the world is akin. The cell is in fact the beginning of life for both animals and plants, and the organism is but an aggregation or community of these primitive parts. So alike indeed are the embryonic cells, as Karl von Baer, in 1828, pointed out, that the various species cannot be determined from any differences discernible, even by the aid of the most powerful microscope. From this it would seem but an easy gradation to infer the doctrine of evolution. All change in life is akin to the change within these little cells due to the taking in and excretion of matter in which carbonic acid plays a most important part.

In the Coca leaf, as indeed in all plants, the cell wall is made up of cellulose, a carbohydrate substance allied to starch, with the formula $xC_6H_{10}O_5$. The material for the building of this substance, it is presumed, is secreted by the cell contents or by a conversion of protoplasm under the influence of nitrogen. This product is deposited particle by particle inside of the wall already formed. Accompanying this growth there may occur certain changes in the physical properties of the cell as the wall takes in new substances, such as silica and various salts, or as there is an elaboration and deposit of gum,[6] pectose and lignin. Each living cell contains a viscid fluid, of extremely complex chemical composition—the protoplasm—a layer of which is in contact with the cell wall and connected by bridles with a central mass in which the nucleus containing the nucleolus is embedded. The protoplasm does not fill the whole cavity of the cell, but there is a large space filled with the watery sap.

The sap carries in solution certain sugars, together with

[6] Frank; 1867.

glycogen and two varieties of glucose, and such organic acids and coloring matters as may already have been elaborated. Where metabolism is active, certain crystallizable nitrogenous bodies, as asparagin, leucin and tyrosin, with salts of potassium and sodium, are found, while in the vacuole there may be starch grains and some crystals of calcium oxalate. The protoplasm is chemically made up of proteids, of which two groups may be distinguished in plants. The first embracing the plastin, such as forms the frame work of the cell, and the second the peptones of the seeds, and the globulins found in the buds and in young shoots.[7] These proteids all consist of carbon, hydrogen, nitrogen, oxygen, and sulphur, while plastin also contains phosphorus. In active growing cells the proteids are present in a quantity, which gradually diminishes as the cell becomes older, leaving the plastin as the organized proteid wall of the cell, while the globulins and peptones remain unorganized. The whole constructive metabolism of the plant is toward the manufacture of this protoplasm, the chemical decomposition and conversion of which liberates the energy which continues cell life.

In certain cells of the plant associated with the protoplasm, and presumably of a similar chemical composition, are little corpuscles, which contain the chlorophyl constituting the green coloring matter of plants, a substance which from its chemical construction and physiological function may have some important influence on the alkaloid formation in the Coca leaf. In these bodies the chlorophyl is held in an oily medium, which exudes in viscid drops when the granules are treated with dilute acids or steam. Although no iron has been found in these bodies by analysis, it is known that chlorophyl cannot be developed without the presence of iron in the soil. Gautier, from an alcoholic extract, calculated the formula $C_{19}H_{22}N_2O_3$, and called attention to the similarity between this and that of bilirubin, $C_{16}H_{18}N_2O_3$—the primary pigment forming the golden red color of the human bile, which possibly may be allied to the red corpuscles of the blood. Chlorophyl, while commonly

[7] Reinke; 1881.

only formed under appropriate conditions of light and heat, may in some cases be produced in complete darkness, in a suitable temperature. Thus if a seed be made to germinate in the dark, the seedling will be not green, but pale yellow, and the plant is anæmic, or is termed etiolated, though corpuscles are present, which, under appropriate conditions, will give rise to chlorophyl.

It has been found that etiolated plants become green more readily in diffused light than in bright sunshine. The process of chlorophyl formation neither commences directly when an etiolated plant is exposed to light, nor ceases entirely when a green plant is placed in darkness, but the action continues through what has been termed photo-chemical induction. From experiments to determine the relative efficacy of different rays of the spectrum it has been found that in light of low intensity seedlings turn green more rapidly under yellow rays, next under green, then under red, and less rapidly under blue. In intense light the green formation is quicker under blue than under yellow, while under the latter condition decomposition is more rapid.

The function of chlorophyl is to break up carbonic acid, releasing oxygen, and converting the carbon into storage food for the tissues, the first visible stage of which constructive metabolism is the formation of starch. The activity of this property may be regarded as extremely powerful when it is considered that in order to reduce carbonic acid artificially it requires the extraordinary temperature of 1300° C. (2372° F.). In the leaf this action takes place under the influence of appropriate light and heat from the sun in the ordinary temperature of 10°-30° C. (50°-86° F.).[8] Plants which do not contain chlorophyl—as fungi—obtain their supply of carbon through more complex compounds in union with hydrogen.

Perhaps we are too apt to regard plants as chiefly cellulose—carbohydrates, and water, without considering the importance of their nitrogenous elements, for though these latter substances may be present in relatively small proportion,

[8] Curtis; p. 71; 1897.

they are as essential in the formation of plant tissue as in animal structures. The carbohydrates of plants include starch, sugars, gums, and inulin. The starch or an allied substance, as has been shown, being elaborated by the chlorophyl granules, or in those parts of the plant where these bodies do not exist, by special corpuscles in the protoplasm, termed *amyloplasts,* which closely resemble the chlorophyl bodies. In the first instance the change is more simple and under the influence of light, in the latter light is not directly essential and the process is more complex, the starch formation beginning with intermediate substances—as asparagin, or glucose, by conversion of the sugars in the cell sap.

Just as in the human organism, assimilation in plant tissue cannot take place except through solution, so the stored up starch is of no immediate service until it is rendered soluble. In other words, it must be prepared in a way analogous to the digestion of food in animal tissues. This is done by the action of certain ferments manufactured by the protoplasm. These do not directly enter into the upbuilding of tissue themselves, but induce the change in the substance upon which they act. Chiefly by a process of hydration, in which several molecules of water are added, the insoluble bodies are rendered soluble, and are so carried in solution to various portions of the plant. Here they are rearranged as insoluble starch, to serve as the common storage tissue for sustenance. Thus it will be seen how very similar are the processes of assimilation in plants and animals, a marked characteristic between both being that the same elementary chemical substances are necessary in the upbuilding of their tissues, and particularly that activity is absent where assimilable nitrogen is not present.

Several organic acids occur in plant cells, either free or combined, which are probably products of destructive metabolism, either from the oxidation of carbohydrates or from the decomposition of proteids. Liebig regarded the highly oxidized acids—especially oxalic, as being the first products of constructive metabolism, which, by gradual reduction, formed carbohydrates and fats, in support of which he re-

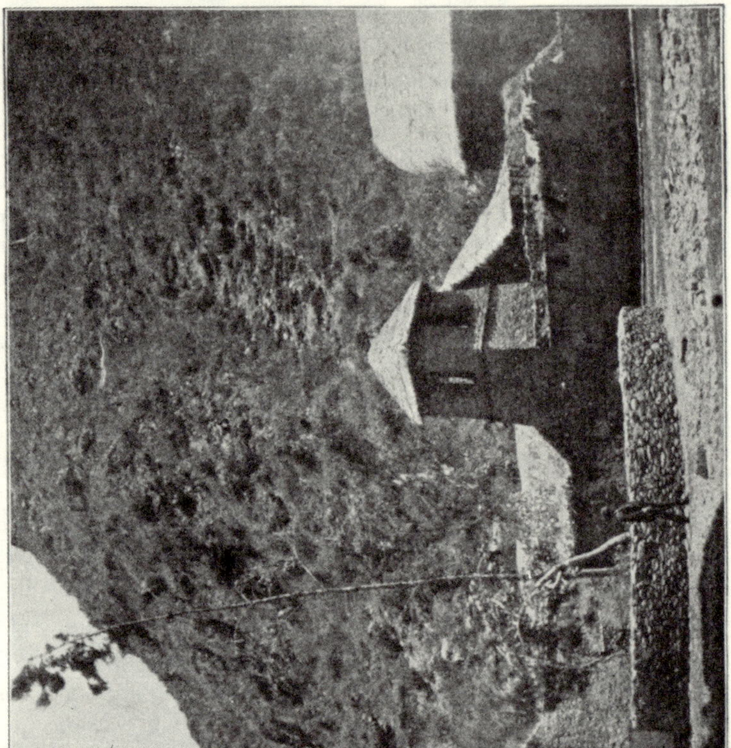

TOWN OF SANDIA, PERU, NEAR THE COCA REGION. [*From a Photograph.*]

ferred to the fact that as fruits ripen they become less sour, which he interpreted to mean that the acid is converted into sugar.[9] The probability, however, is that oxalic acid is the product of destructive metabolism, and is the final stage of excretion from which alkaloids are produced, while it is significant, when considering the Coca products, that acids may by decomposition be formed from proteid or may by oxidation be converted into other acids.

Oxalic acid is very commonly found in the leaf cells combined with potassium or calcium. It is present in the cells of the Coca leaf as little crystalline cubes or prisms. Malic acid, citric acid, and tartaric acid are familiar as the products of various fruits. Tannic acid is chiefly found as the astringent property of various barks. Often a variety of this acid is characteristic of the plant and associated with its alkaloid. This is the case with the tannic acid described by Niemann in his separation of cocaine, which is intimately related to the alkaloids of the Coca leaf, just as quinine is combined with quinic acid and morphine with meconic acid. It has been suggested that the yield of alkaloid from the Coca leaf is greater in the presence of a large proportion of tannic acid.

Tannin is formed in the destructive metabolism of the protoplasm, as a glucoside product intermediate between the carbohydrate and the purely aromatic bodies, such as benzoic and cinnamic acids, which are formed from the oxidative decomposition of the glucosides. In addition to these are found fatty oils, associated with the substances of the cell, and essential oils, to which the fragrance of the flower or plant is due, and which are secreted in special walled cells. The resins are found as crude resins, balsams—a mixture of resin and ethereal oil with an aromatic acid, and gum resins—a mixture of gum, resin and ethereal oil. The ethereal oils include a great number of substances with varying chemical composition, having no apparent constructive use to the tissues, but, like the alkaloids, regarded merely as waste. Some of these products serve by their unpleasant properties to repel animals and insects, while others serve to attract insects and

[9] Vines; p. 230; 1886.

thus contribute to the fertilization of the flower, so all these bodies may be of some relative use.

The proteids of the plant are supposed to be produced from some non-nitrogenous substance—possibly formic aldehyde—by a combination formed from the absorbed nitrates, sulphates and phosphates, in union with one of the organic acids, particularly oxalic. The change being from the less complex compound to a highly nitrogenous organic substance, termed an amide, which, with the non-nitrogenous substance and sulphur, unite to form the proteid. The amides are crystallizable nitrogenous substances, built up synthetically, or formed by the breaking down of certain compounds. They are similar to some of the final decomposition products found in the animal body. Belonging to this group of bodies is xanthin, which Kossel supposed to be directly derived from nuclein, from the nucleus of the plant cell. But in whatever manner the amides are formed, it is believed they are ultimately used in the construction of proteid, and although this substance is produced in all parts of the plant, it is found more abundant in the cells containing chlorophyl. Proteids are found to gradually increase from the roots toward the leaves, where they are most abundant. This would seem to indicate that the leaf is the especial organ in which proteid formation takes place, and it is in this portion of the Coca plant that the excreted alkaloids are found most abundantly.

According to Schützenberger, the proteid structures are composed of ureids, derivatives of carbamide, and Grimaux considers they are broken by hydrolysis into carbonic acid, ammoniac and amidic acids, thus placing them in near relation with uric acid, which also gives by hydrolysis, carbonic acid, ammoniac acid and glycocol. In animal tissues the last product of excrementition is carbamide—or uric acid, while the compounds from which proteids are formed in plants have been shown to be amides. It has been shown in the laboratory that the chemical products from the breaking down of proteids are also amides, with which carbonic acid and oxalic acid are nearly always formed. The presence of hippuric acid in the urine of herbivorous animals, the indol and the skatol found in the products of pancreatic digestion (Salkowski), together with the tyrosin nearly always present in the animal body, has led to the supposition that aromatic groups may also be constituents of the proteid molecule.[10]

All of this is of the greatest interest in the study of alkaloid production in connection with the fact, which has been proved, that when a plant does not receive nitrogen from outside it will not part with the amount of that element previously contained—in other words, the nitrogenous excreta will not be thrown off. Boussingault thought the higher plants flourished best when supplied with nitrogen in the form of nitrates, though Lehmann has found that many plants flourish better when supplied with ammonia salts than when supplied with nitrates, and this has been well marked in the case of the tobacco plant.

Nitric acid may be absorbed by a plant in the form of any of its salts which can diffuse into the tissues, the most common bases being soda, potash, lime, magnesia and ammonia. The formation of this acid, attendant upon the electric conditions of the atmosphere, may be one source of increase of vigor to the native soil of the Coca plant, where the entire region of the montaña is so subject to frequent electrical storms. Then Coca flourishes best in soils rich in humus, and various observers have remarked that nitrogen is best fixed in such a soil. An interesting point in connection with which is that the ammonia supplied to the soil by decomposition of nitrogenous substances is converted into nitrous, and this into nitric acid, by a process termed nitrification, occasioned by the presence of certain bacteria in the soil to which this property is attributed. Proof of this was determined by chloroforming a section of nitrifying earth and finding that the process on that area ceased.[11] The absorption of nitrogen by the Coca plant and the development of proteids is closely associated with the nitrogenous excreta from the plant, and the consequent production of alkaloids which we are attempting to trace.

The nitrogen of the soil, however induced, is transferred

[10] Kozlowski; 1899. [11] Schlösing and Muntz; 1879.

by oxidation into what has been termed the reduced nitrogen of amides,[12] which, in combination with carbohydrates, under appropriate conditions forms proteids, in which oxalic acid is an indirect product. Several observers consider the leaves as active in this process,[13] because the nitrogenous compounds are found to accumulate in the leaf until their full development, when they decrease. This is illustrated by the fact that in autumn, when new proteids are not necessary to matured leaves, it accumulates in the protoplasm, from which it is transferred to the stem, to be stored up as a food for the following season's growth.

It has been found that the nitrates, passing from the roots as calcium nitrate, are changed in the leaves by the chlorophyl in the presence of light with the production of calcium oxalate,[14] while nitric acid is set free, and conversely, in darkness the nitrates are permitted to accumulate. This change is influenced by the presence of oxalic acid, which, even in small quantities, is capable of decomposing the most dilute solutions of calcium nitrate.[15] The free nitric acid in combination with a carbohydrate forms the protein molecule, while setting free carbonic acid and water.

Cellulose, which we have seen is formed from protoplasm, is dependent upon the appropriate conversion of the nitrogenous proteid. When this formation is active, large amounts of carbohydrates are required to form anew the protein molecule of the protoplasm, and the nitrogenous element is utilized. When there is an insufficiency of carbohydrate material the relative amount of nitrogen increases because the conditions are not favorable for its utilization in the production of proteids, and this excess of nitrogen is converted into amides, which are stored up. When the carbohydrate supply to the plant is scanty in amount this reserve store of amides is consumed, just the same as the reserve fat would be consumed in the animal structure under similar conditions.[16]

The relation between the normal use of nitrogen in plants is analogous to its influence in animal structure, while the

[12] Kozlowski; 1899. [13] Sachs; 1862. [14] Schimper; 1888. [15] Emmerling; 1887.
[16] Schulze and Urich; 1875-1877; Kozlowski, p. 35, 1899.

final products in both cases are similar, the distinction being chiefly one in the method of chemical conversion and excretion due to the difference in organic function. Thus, although urea and uric acid are not formed in plants, the final products of both animals and plants are closely allied. We see this especially in the alkaloids caffeine and theobromine, which are almost identical with uric acid, so much so that Haig considers that a dose of caffeine is equivalent to introducing into the system an equal amount of uric acid.

There are numerous examples, not only in medicinal substances, but in the more familiar vegetables and fruits, which illustrate the possibilities of change due to cultivation. The Siberian rhododendron varies its properties from stimulant to a narcotic or cathartic, in accordance with its location of growth. Aconite, assafœtida, cinchona, digitalis, opium and rhubarb are all examples which show the influence of soil and cultivation.* Indeed similar effects are to be seen everywhere about us, certain characteristics being prominently brought forth by stimulating different parts of the organism, so that ultimately distinct varieties are constituted. The poisonous Persian almond has thus become the luscious peach. The starchy qualities of the potato are concentrated in its increased tuber, and certain poisonous mushrooms have become edible. The quality of the flour from wheat is influenced by locality and cultivation. The tomato, cabbage, celery, asparagus, are all familiar examples which emphasize the possibility of shaping nature's wild luxuriance to man's cultured necessity.

The chemical elements which are taken up by a plant vary considerably with the conditions of environment, and the influence of light in freeing acid in the leaf has been indicated. These conditions necessarily modify the constituents of the plant. When metabolism is effected certain changes take place in the tissues, with the formation of substances which may be undesirable to the plant, yet may be medicinally serviceable. Such a change occurs in the sprouts of potatoes stored in the dark, when the poisonous base *solania* is

* Paris; p. 72, *et seq.*; 1846.

formed, which under normal conditions of growth is not present in the plant. A familiar example of change due to environment is exhibited in the grape, which may contain a varying proportion of acid, sugar and salts in accordance with the soil, climate and conditions of its cultivation, nor are these variations merely slight, for they are sufficient to generate in the wine made from the fruit entirely different tastes and properties.

In view of these facts, it seems creditable to suppose that by suitable processes of cultivation the output of alkaloids may be influenced in plants, and such experiments have already been extensively carried out in connection with the production of quinine. When attention was directed to the scientific cultivation of cinchona in the East, it was remarked that when manured with highly nitrogenous compounds the yield of alkaloid was greatly increased. This is paralleled by the fact that when an animal consumes a large quantity of nitrogenous food the output of urea and uric acid is greater.

Alkaloids are regarded as waste products because they cannot enter into the constructive metabolism of the plant, though they are not directly excreted, but are stored away where they will not enter the circulation, and may be soon shed, as in the leaf or bark. Though, as indicating their possible utility, it has been shown experimentally that plants are capable of taking up nitrogenous compounds, such as urea, uric acid, leucin, tyrosin, or glycocol, when supplied to their roots. In some recent experiments carried out at the botanical laboratory of Columbia University, I found that plant metabolism was materially hastened under the stimulus of cocaine.

The influence of light in the formation of alkaloids has already been shown. Tropical plants which produce these substances in abundance in their native state often yield but small quantities when grown in hot houses, indicating that a too intense light is unfavorable, probably in stimulating a too rapid action of the chlorophyl, together with a decomposition of the organic acid. Some years ago the botanist, Dr. Louis Errera, of Brussels, found that the young leaves of certain plants yielded more abundant alkaloid than those that were mature. Following this suggestion, Dr. Greshoff is said to have found that young Coca leaves yield nearly double the amount of alkaloid over that contained in old leaves gathered at the same time. In tea plantations the youngest leaves are gathered, but it has always been customary to collect the mature leaves of the Coca plant, and these have usually been found to yield the greatest amount of alkaloid. The probability is that the amount of alkaloid present in the Coca leaf is not so much influenced by maturity as it is by the period of its gathering.

As regards the temperature at which growth progresses most favorably, Martins[17] has compared each plant to a ther-

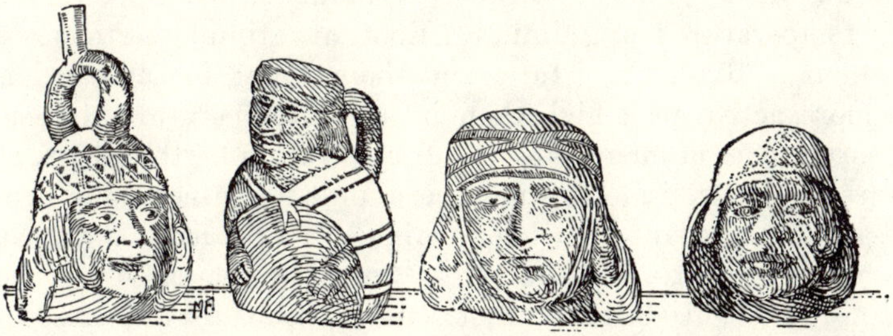

PERUVIAN PORTRAIT VASES. [*Tweddle Collection.*]

mometer, the zero point of which is the minimum temperature at which its life is possible. Thus, the Coca shrub in its native state will support a range from 18° C. (64.4° F.) to 30° C. (86° F.), an influence of temperature which is governed by the proportion of water contained in the plant. It has been found, from experiments of cultivation, that Coca will flourish in a temperature considerably higher than that which was originally supposed bearable, though the alkaloidal yield is less than that grown more temperately. The life process of any plant, however, may be exalted as the temperature rises above its zero point, though only continuing to rise until a certain height is reached, at which it ceases entirely. In the cold, plants may undergo a similar hibernation as do certain animals when metabolism is lessened,

[17] Martins; 1846.

though long-continued cold is fatal, and frost is always so absolutely to Coca. The influence of temperature on metabolism tends to alter the relations between the volume of carbonic acid given off and the amount of oxygen absorbed. Under a mean temperature these relations are equal, while in a lower temperature more oxygen is absorbed in proportion to the carbonic acid given off, and oxygen exhalation ceases entirely below a certain degree.

A relatively large proportion of water in a plant determines its susceptibility to climatic conditions. Thus freezing not only breaks the delicate parenchymatous tissues, but alters the chemical constitution of the cells, while too high a temperature may prove destructive through a coagulation of the albumen. The appearance of plants killed by high or low temperature being similar. Roots are stimulated to curve to their source of moisture, and their power for absorption is more active in a high than in a low temperature, but as absorption is influenced by the transpiration of the plant, it is less active in a moist atmosphere, unless the metabolic processes of the plant occasions a higher temperature than the surrounding air. Such activity would be increased by the heat of the soil about the roots, and is probably manifest in the Coca plant through the peculiar soil of the montaña.

The elevation at which a plant grows has an influence upon the absorption by the leaf. Thus it has been observed that while a slight increase in the carbonic acid gas contained in the air is favorable to growth, a considerable increase is prejudicial, while an increase or diminution of atmospheric pressure materially influences plant life. In some tropical countries Coca will grow at the level of the sea, provided there is an equable temperature and requisite humidity. Although in Peru Coca flourishes side by side with the best coffee, it will not thrive at the elevations where the coffee plant is commonly grown in either the East or West Indies. In Java, where experiments have been made in cultivating Coca, it has been stated that there is no perceptible difference in the alkaloidal yield due to the influence of elevation, while in the best cocals of Peru it is considered that the higher the altitude at which Coca can be grown the greater will be the alkaloidal yield. This is possibly effected by similar influences to that governing the aromatic properties developed in the coffee bean, which have been found more abundant when coffee is grown at an elevation, yet without danger of frost. This may be attributed to slower growth and a consequent deposit of nitrogenous principles instead of their being all consumed through a rapid metabolism.

It is therefore evident that as these several physical conditions have a marked bearing upon the life history of all plants, the more limited the range for any of these processes in any particular plant, the more it will be influenced. Thus in an altitude too high, the leaf of the Coca plant is smaller and only one harvest is possible within the year, while in the lower regions where the temperature exceeds 20° C. (68° F.) vegetation may be exuberant, but the quality of leaf is impaired. The electrical conditions of the atmosphere, it has been shown, have an important bearing upon the development of Coca, through the influence of the gases set free in the atmosphere and the possible slight increase of nitric acid carried to the soil.

It was thought by Martius that the mosses and lichens which are found upon the Coca shrubs were detrimental to the plant through favoring too great humidity. In the light of our knowledge on the development of alkaloids, however, it has seemed to me that here is an opportunity for very extended experimentation, as may be inferred from a reference to the alkaloidal production of cinchona. At first efforts were made to free the cinchona trees from the lichens and mosses which naturally formed upon them; but it was discovered accidentally that those portions of the trees which Nature had covered in this manner yielded an increased amount of alkaloid. When cinchona plantations were started in Java, experiments made upon the result of this discovery prompted a systematic covering of the trunks of the trees artificially with moss, which was bound about them to the height from which the bark would be stripped. At first very great pains was taken to collect just an appropriate kind of moss, which it was supposed from its association with the tree in its native home would be essential, but later experiments proved that any form of covering which protected the bark from light increased this alkaloidal yield. So that to-day this process, which is known as "mossing," is one of the most important in the cultivation and development of cinchona.

The chief interest of Coca to the commercial world has centered upon its possibilities in the production of the one alkaloid, cocaine, instead of a more general economic use of the leaf. Because of this, much confusion of terms has resulted, for chemists have designated the amount of alkaloids obtained from the leaf as cocaine, although they have qualified their statement by saying that a portion of this is uncrystallizable. Numerous experiments have been conducted to determine the relative yield of cocaine from the different varieties of Coca, and when uncrystallizable alkaloids have been found the leaf has been condemned for chemical uses. It will thus be appreciated how a great amount of error has been generated and continued. The Bolivian or Huanuco variety has been found to yield the largest percentage of crystallizable alkaloid, while the Peruvian or Truxillo variety, though yielding nearly as much total alkaloid, affords a less percentage that is crystallizable, the Bolivian Coca being set apart for the use of the chemists to the exclusion of the Peruvian variety, which is richest in aromatic principles and best suited for medicinal purposes. As a matter of fact, the Peruvian Coca is the plant sought for by the native users.

There is not only a difference in the yield of alkaloid from different varieties of Coca, but also a difference in the yield from plants of one variety from the same cocal, and it would seem possible by selection and propagation of the better plants to obtain a high percentage of alkaloid. At present there is no effort in the native home of Coca toward the production of alkaloid in the leaf through any artificial means. Regarding the quality of alkaloid that has been found in the different plants, the Peruvian variety has been found to contain equal proportions of crystallizable and uncrystallizable

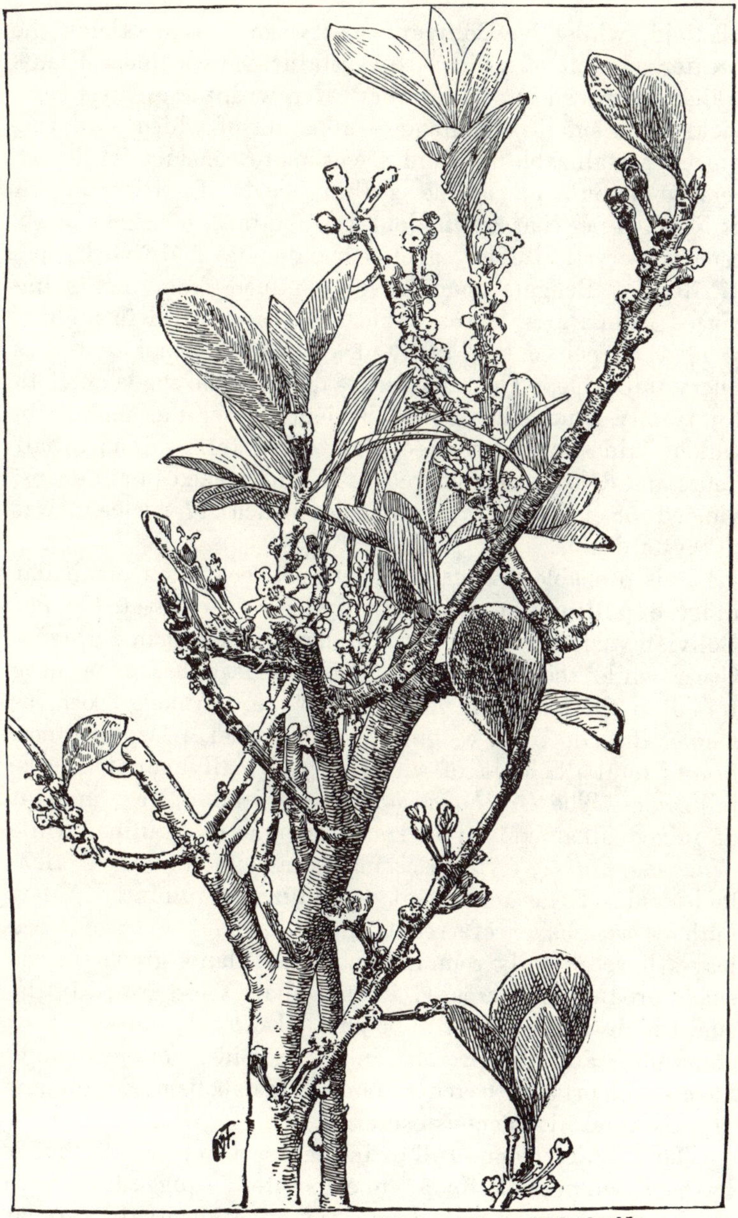

TYPE OF BOLIVIAN COCA. [*Conservatory of Mariani.*]

alkaloid, while the Bolivian variety contains alkaloids the greater amount of which are crystallizable cocaine. Plants which are grown in conservatory, even with the greatest care, yield but a small percentage of alkaloid, of which, however, the uncrystallizable alkaloid seems more constant while the relative amount of cocaine is diminished. In leaves grown at Kew .44 per cent. of alkaloid was obtained, of which .1 per cent. was crystallizable. From experiments of Mr. G. Peppe, of Renchi, Bengal, upon leaves obtained from plants imported from Paris, it was found that leaves dried in the sun yielded .53 per cent. of alkaloid, of which .23 per cent. was uncrystallizable. The same leaves dried in the shade on cloth for twenty hours, then rolled by hand, after the manner in which Chinese tea is treated, then cured for two and a half hours and dried over a charcoal fire and packed in close tins, yielded .58 per cent. of alkaloid, of which .17 per cent. was uncrystallizable.

It is probable that each variety of Coca has a particular range of altitude at which it may be best cultivated. The Bolivian variety is grown at a higher altitude than Peruvian Coca, while the Novo Granatense variety has even been found to thrive at the level of the sea. Among Coca, as among the *cinchona*, certain varieties yield a large proportion of total alkaloids, of which only a small amount is crystallizable. The *Cinchona succirubra* yields a large amount of mixed alkaloids, but a small amount of quinine, while *Cinchona Calisaya* yields a smaller amount of mixed alkaloids and a large amount of crystallizable quinine. A few authors who have referred to the alkaloidal yield of Coca leaves have casually remarked that the plants grown in the shade produce an increased amount above those grown in the sun, which would appear to be paralleled by the formation of chlorophyl and the production of proteids, both of which have so important a bearing upon the metabolism of the plant and the final nitrogenous excretion.

This subject is one full of interest, yet so intricate that it has not been possible for me to elaborate the suggestions here set forth in time to embody my investigation in the present writing, though I hope to present the result of my research at no very distant date. It would seem that sufficient has been shown, however, to indicate the possibility of modifying plant metabolism under appropriate conditions of culture so as to influence the development of the alkaloidal excreta. The comparisons between plant and animal life may have proved of sufficient interest to enlist attention to the higher physiology in which will be traced the action of Coca.

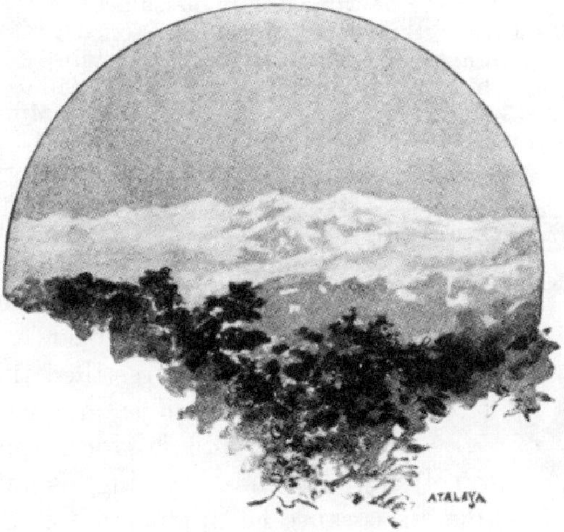

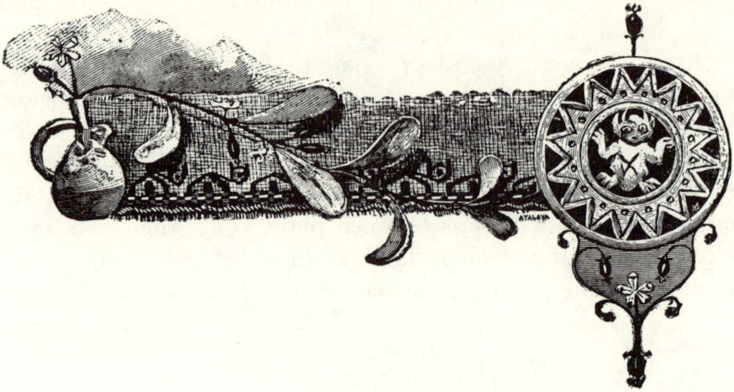

CHAPTER XII.

INFLUENCE OF COCA UPON MUSCULAR ENERGY.

*** * "Leaves of wond'rous nourishment,**
Whose Juice Succ'd in, and to the Stomach tak'n
Long Hunger and long Labour can sustain;
From which our faint and weary Bodies find
More Succor, more they cheer the drooping Mind,
Than can your *Bacchus* and your Ceres join'd."

—Cowley.

THERE has been no period since the command was given Adam in the Garden of Eden, when physical exertion was not essential to existence. The ancient philosophers instilled the doctrine that a sound mind is only possible in a sound body, and so Homer pictured the dejection of Achilles as eating his own heart in idleness because he might not fight. Idleness has ever been so recognized as a common precursor of discontent and melancholia, that when the children of Israel murmured against Pharaoh their tasks were wisely doubled to prevent retrospection. Occupation is not only essential to prosperity, but is morally and physically conducive to health and longevity and a rest is best attained not by total cessation, but by a change of employment. I believe it was Hammond who advised a wealthy neurasthenic to collect used corks, with the result that the patient became so interested in this unique occupation that his brooding was soon forgotten, while he became an expert in old stoppers.

With a popular regard for the benefits of appropriate exercise, the matter of athletics has been greatly overdone, and has often resulted in injury instead of the anticipated good. The early Greeks, who elaborated every form of gymnastics, only undertook the severe strain incidental to their games after a suitable preparatory period. They were encouraged to these performances—which were instituted in honor of the gods or deified heroes—through the idea that they were sacred, and in fulfillment of this the exercises always began with a sacrifice, and concluded in the same religious manner. In the period of Cæsar, a victory in the Olympic games was considered such a triumph that honors were not only extended to the victor, but to his relatives and even to his place of birth. There was, however, no impromptu emulation permitted in these contests, but those who desired to compete were obliged to submit themselves for preparatory practice at least ten months before the exercises began.

Wherever there is an incentive for supremacy, there is a possibility of overstrain, and Hippocrates cautioned the athletæ against the possible error of immoderate exercise. Galen foreshadowed the modern wear and tear theorists when he asserted:—"much exercise and weariness consumes the spirits and substances." Sustained and straining effort in any direction, whether it be mental or physical, cannot be continued without a following train of troubles. When any function of the body is put in action there is a chemical change within the tissues which gives rise to the energy set free, and before new power may be had the substance which affords this energy must be rebuilt. While this is true of all the tissues of the body, owing to the greater bulk of the muscular system the changes are apparently more active in this organism. Tire is recognized more speedily, while incessant activity often prevents an adequate opportunity for repair.

We have seen that the Incas, during the period when their young men were preparing for knighthood, devoted the greatest attention to athletic training. It was only when the young nobles had proved themselves worthy, by appro-

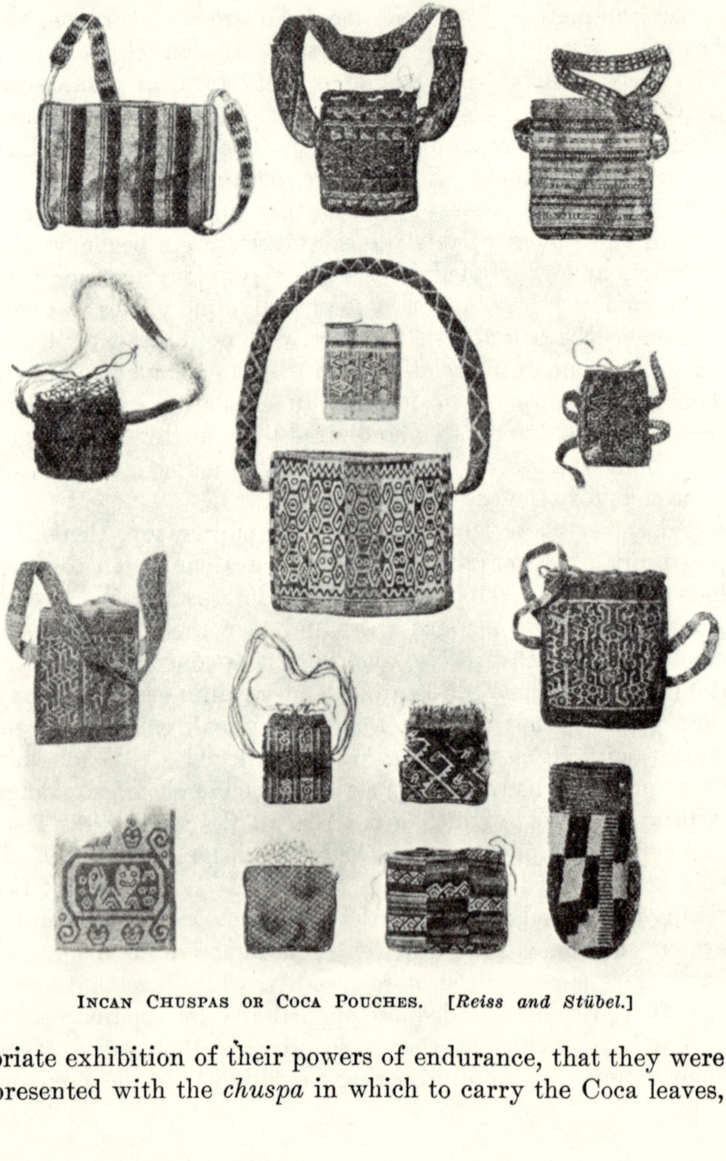

INCAN CHUSPAS OR COCA POUCHES. [*Reiss and Stübel.*]

priate exhibition of their powers of endurance, that they were presented with the *chuspa* in which to carry the Coca leaves, and the *popóro* to contain the lime to be employed in preparing the Coca for mastication. These decorations were thereafter worn through life as emblems of ennoblement, and buried with the mummied body, the Coca affording support on the journey to the unknown. The ancient philosophers were quite as ignorant of the exact changes which induced the transformation of energy displayed in muscular activity as were the Incas, or as are the modern Andeans regarding the true workings of Coca in its yield of force.

The muscular system comprises two varieties of muscles. One of these acts under mental influence, while the other acts independent of the will, while the heart—which is essentially a muscle—partakes of qualities in both of these varieties. The voluntary muscles are chiefly attached to the bony framework, and are concerned in bodily movements, while the involuntary muscles enter into the formation of the blood vessels, the lymphatics and the walls of various structures, as the air passages, the alimentary canal and other important organs, as well as forming parts of the skin and mucous membranes.

The framework muscles are supported by thin sheaths of tissue, which in their interior divide by numerous ramifications and separate the contained muscular substance into bundles. These are still further divided into little fibres, each ultimate fibre being enveloped with a close network of minute blood vessels. These vessels afford an ample means for bringing nutriment to the muscle substance, as well as for carrying away the waste products which are constantly being formed, even in the state commonly regarded as absolute rest. The importance of this hurrying stream of nutriment, and waste elimination to the muscular organism, may be inferred from the estimate that one-fourth of the entire blood of the body is contained in the muscles.

When the little muscle fibres are examined under the microscope, they are seen to be made up of alternating lines which appear as light and dark striations. The darker of these lines, when viewed in transverse section, is found composed of little polygonal compartments. Within these divisions is contained a semi-fluid material which has been demonstrated to be the contractile element of the muscle substance.

The ancients presumed the muscles acted by some pulling influence exerted through the nerves. Harmonious nerve action is essential to every movement, yet muscle substance has been shown to have an inherent property of contractility quite independent of nerve influence. The chief nerves controlling the movements of the muscular system have their origin in the brain and spinal cord. These each consist of fibres conveying sensation and fibres which control motion. These latter end in expansions on the surface of the muscle in intimate contact with the contractile element, the function of which it regulates through the reflex influence of the sensory nerves. In other words a stimulation of the sensory nerves excites the motor nerves to cause muscular activity.

Each fibre is not continuous through the entire length of muscle structure, but the tapering end of one fibre is united to the body of its neighbor by a cement-like substance to form a bundle which constitutes the muscle proper. These bundles taper, or are expanded, as the case may be, to a dense fibrous tissue for attachment to different portions of the movable framework of the body. When a muscle acts, each of its individual fibres shortens through some chemical influence of the contractile element. The combined action of the fibres exerts a pull toward either end of the muscle, which occasions movement of the less fixed portion of the framework to which the muscle is attached.

The involuntary muscles have not definite tendons like the voluntary muscles, and their microscopical structure is also different, their fibres being smaller and instead of being cross-striped they are marked longitudinally. In their arrangement the fibres are so interlaced that by their contraction they lessen the capacity of the vessels or organs in the walls of which they are located.

The property of contraction is inherent in the muscle itself, and continues even after its nerve supply has been cut off. For this experiment in the laboratory, curare is employed; this paralyzes the nerve filaments deep down in the

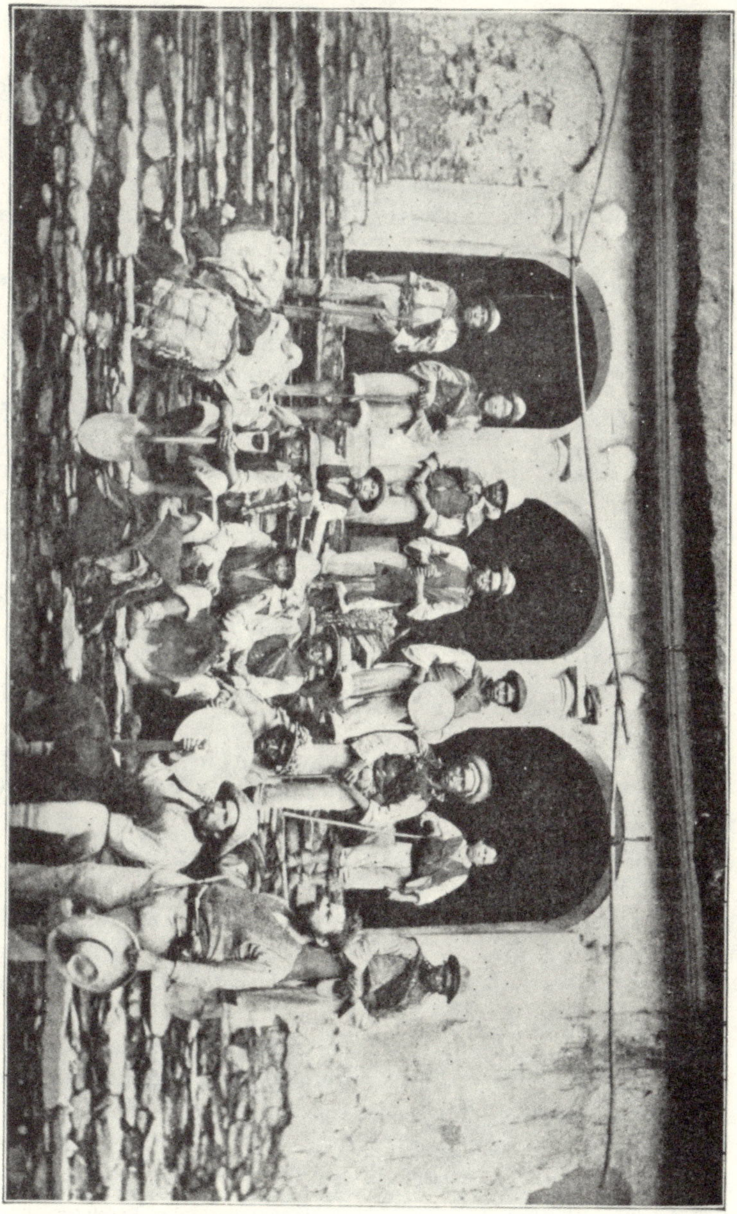

Andean Miners, on Church Steps at Phara, Peru. [*From a Photograph.*]

muscle substance yet leaves the muscle intact. Under these conditions though contraction will not be produced when the nerve is stimulated, movement will follow when stimulus is directly applied to the muscle substance. It is presumed that this inherent property is generated by some substance brought in the blood, which induces a chemical change in the contractile element and liberates the energy displayed as muscular movement. This change is influenced by temperature, and by the presence or absence of waste material in the muscle structure or in the circulation. Whatever this explosive substance may be, it is presumed to be built up in the muscle structure from some carbohydrate material—possibly glycogen—under the influence of a nitrogenous substance. For, as Foster has said: "The whole secret of life may almost be said to be wrapped up in the occult properties of certain nitrogen compounds."[1] Hermann named this hypothetical substance inogen.[2] During a muscle contraction it is inferred this carbohydrate splits into carbonic acid, sarcolactic acid and some nitrogenous material which may be myosin or a substance akin to it, the acids being carried off in the blood stream, while the proteid substance remains in the muscle to be again elaborated into the inogen energy yielding material. Helmholtz calculated that in the human body one-fifth the energy of the material consumed goes out as work, thus contrasting favorably with the steam engine, in which it hardly ever amounts to more than one-tenth.

According to the theory of Liebig the nitrogenous food is utilized in the building up of proteid tissues, and the non-nitrogenous food is exclusively devoted to heat producing purposes, being directly oxidized in the blood, while its excess is stored as fat. In accordance with this theory, muscular exercise increases the waste of muscle substance, while the wear and tear is estimated by the amount of urea excreted. Originally this idea was generally accepted, but was attacked from many sources when it was found that facts of subsequent research did not coincide. Troube suggested in opposition that muscle and nerve tissue is not destroyed by exercise, but

[1] Foster; p. 474; 1880. [2] Hermann; 1878. See also *Journal of Physiology*, I, p. 196, 1878.

that force is contributed to these tissues through the oxidation of non-nitrogenous substances of which the muscle and nerve were simply mediums of expression.

Following the idea of Liebig, that work results in wear and tear of the tissues, there should be an increased output of nitrogen during exertion, but many observers in trying to harmonize results with this view have found little increase of urea—which practically represents all the nitrogen passed out of the body—while a decided increase of urea is found from the consumption of nitrogenous foods. Among the more noted experiments which controverted the theory that the nitrogenous waste represented the relative expenditure of energy is that of Dr. Fick, Professor of Physiology, and Dr. Wislicenus, Professor of Chemistry, both of the University of Zurich.[3] They ascended the Faulhorn, two thousand metres high (6,561 feet) for the purpose of determining the resultant wear and tear upon the nitrogenous tissues from a known amount of exercise. To accurately determine this, they limited their diet to non-nitrogenous materials, taking starch, fat and a little sugar, with beer, wine and tea as beverages. For seventeen hours before the ascent they limited themselves to non-nitrogenous food, and their first examinations were made eleven hours before their start. The ascent was completed in eight hours, and after a rest of six hours they ate an ordinary meal, which included meat. The urine secreted was examined to estimate the nitrogen excreted for each hour's work, which showed the following results:

Nitrogen excreted per hour.
[Estimated in grammes.]

	FICK.	WISLICENUS.
Before work	0.63	0.61
Work	0.41	0.39
After work	0.40	0.40
Night	0.45	0.51

This indicates that the amount of nitrogen excreted was in relation to the food eaten and not to the work done, less

[3] Fick and Wislicenus; 1866.

relative nitrogen being passed in the "work" and "after work" periods when on a non-nitrogenous diet than during the period when nitrogenous food was eaten. The calculations were based on the amount of work which the oxidation of muscular substance containing fifteen per cent of nitrogen would produce as determined from the excreted urea. The result showed this inadequate to have enabled the experimenters to perform the task which they did, Fick's work exceeding the theoretical amount by one-half, while that done by Wislicenus was in excess by more than three-fourths the theoretical amount, without in either case considering the necessary work of the various vital processes. These facts led many experimenters to further investigation, and resulted in a decided reaction from Liebig's rigid theory, which had been accepted more literally than that physiologist intended. Instead of regarding the decomposition of proteids as the sole source of muscular energy, the carbohydrates were now looked upon as a formative element for generating force, because during muscular activity the glycogen stored in muscle disappears, to accumulate again during rest.

Pflüger, one of the most eminent of modern physiologists, in attempting to harmonize the theory of Liebig, experimented with a dog, which he kept upon an exclusive meat diet free from fat, and made him perform hard labor several times a day for weeks, during which the animal showed: "Very extraordinary strength and elasticity in all his movements."[4] In this experiment he wished to show that all the energy produced during hard work was from the transformation of proteid. To further show whether proteid simply was compensatory, he gave a mixed diet, and this led him to the conclusion that in a diet composed of proteid, carbohydrates and fats the quantity of the two latter substances destroyed in metabolism depends wholly upon the fact whether much or little proteid be fed. His conclusions are that: "In general the quantity of carbohydrates and fat that undergoes destruction is smaller the greater the income of proteid."[5] This may be regarded as the accepted view of modern physiologists

[4] Pflüger; L, p. 98; 1891. [5] *Idem;* LII; 1892; quoted by Verworn; 1899.

with this qualification, that proteids must be built up from carbohydrates under a nitrogenous stimulus, just as we have seen is the process in plant structure.

It has already been pointed out that the nitrogenous Coca has a direct bearing upon the structure of tissue through a possible quality of elaborating the carbohydrates of the protoplasm into proteids. Since the muscles form the largest bulk of tissues in the body in which chemical changes are constantly going on, it may be inferred how important is this upbuilding of the complex substance by which muscle activity is produced. The action of Coca on yeast as well as penicillium and other low organisms indicates its peculiar activity upon protoplasm. The experiments of Huxley and Martin[6] long since showed that penicillium can build itself up out of ammonium tartrate and inorganic salts, and can by a decomposition of itself give rise to fats and other bodies, and we have every reason, says Foster, to suppose this constructive power belongs naturally to all native protoplasm wherever found. At the same time we see, even in the case of penicillium, it is of advantage to offer to the protoplasm as food, substances which are on their way to become protoplasm, which thus saves the organism much constructive labor. "It is not unreasonable, even if opposed to established ideas, to suppose that the animal protoplasm is as constructive as the vegetable protoplasm, the difference between the two being that the former, unlike the latter, is as destructive as it is constructive, and therefore requires to be continually fed with ready constructed material."[7]

In further support of the influence of Coca upon the formation of proteid it may be again emphasized that the nitrogen found in the urea is not a measure of the proteid transformation of the body. This conclusion would be justified if it were known that all nitrogenous cleavage products of the proteid molecule without exception leave the body. But there is no ground for such belief. On the contrary, there is no fact known to contradict the idea that nitrogenous cleavage products of the proteid molecule can rebuild themselves syn-

[6] *Elementary Biology; Lesson V.* [7] Foster; p. 441; 1880.

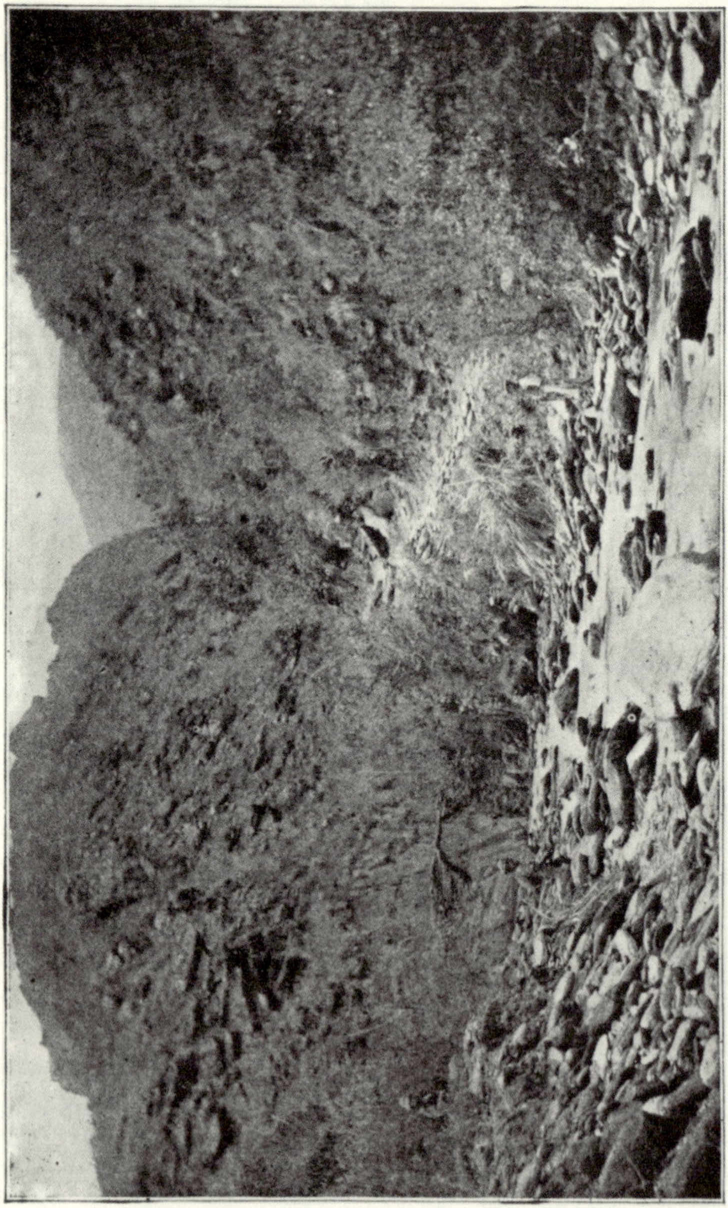

In the Montaña of Peru; The Puli-Puli River. [*From a Photograph.*]

thetically again into proteid with the aid of new non-nitrogenous groups of atoms. This latter possibility has been overlooked, and in consequence views have arisen, especially in relation to muscle metabolism, which though bearing the stamp of improbability have been accepted and handed down, but which recently have been criticised by Pflüger.[8]

Just where urea is manufactured in the organism is not definitely known. It is presumed that *kreatin, xanthin* and other nitrogenous extractives which are found in the circulation resulting from tissue activity may be converted either by the blood or by the epithelium of the kidneys, and discharged as urea. In certain kidney diseases it is known that these waste products are retained in the circulation, with consequent symptoms of poisoning. In addition to this it has been found that an increase of nitrogenous food rapidly augments this excretion, the products of intestinal digestion, the *leucin* and *tyrosin*, being carried to the liver and converted by the liver cells to urea, and this organ is considered at least the chief organ of urea formation.

It has been found that in functional derangements of the liver, when the normal urea formation is interfered with, there is imperfect oxidation of the products which should be eliminated as urea, and a deposit of lithates occurs in the urine as a signal of imperfect oxidation. This also may follow excessive exercise. In serious organic diseases the urea excretion may cease entirely, being replaced by the less oxidized *leucin* and *tyrosin*. M. Genevoix, from observations of his own and those of Charcot, Bouchardat and others, concludes that disorders of the liver which do not seriously implicate the secreting structure of that tissue increase the amount of urea excreted, while graver disorders diminish it very considerably.[9] A Belgian physician, Doctor Rommelaere, maintains that diagnosis of cancer of the stomach may be made when the urea excretion falls and continues below ten grammes a day for several consecutive days.[10]

The average excretion of urea is sixteen grains an hour,[11] the excretion fluctuating between thirteen and twenty-five

[8] Pflüger; L, p. 98; 1891; Verworn; p. 175; 1899. [9] Murchison; p. 598; 1885.
[10] Dujardin-Beaumetz; p. 233; 1886. [11] Haig; 1897.

grains, being greater soon after eating, and much less during the early morning hours. Uric acid, which is probably a less advanced form of oxidation, being present in the relation to urea as one to thirty-five, its relation to body weight being three and a half grains per pound; thus when urea excretion equals thirty-five grains for each ten pounds of body weight, there is commonly present one grain of uric acid. The effect of these waste products in the tissues is to so impede the functions of the cells as to occasion symptoms of depression and fatigue, whether this be manifested by irritability, drowsiness or profound muscular tire. There is a loading up —not necessarily within the cells of the tissues, but in the blood stream which supplies these—of excreta which vitiates the proper pabulum of the protoplasm, and a period of rest is absolutely necessary to enable the tissues to get rid of this matter before a healthful condition may be resumed.

All the symptoms of fatigue are due to the effort of the tissues at repair. There is an increase of respiration to bring the necessary increase of oxygen demanded, and accompanying this respiratory effort there is a frequency of the heart beat, while the body becomes cool because its heat is lessened through the evaporation of perspiration. In protracted fatigue there may be a rise of temperature due to irritation by the increased force of the blood stream, occasioning sleeplessness, while the digestive functions are interfered with because of the excessive demands of other organs on the blood stimulus.

In over exertion, where there is actual loss of proteid tissue, the effects of prostration and tire may not be experienced immediately, but only after several days. Similar symptoms to these accompany the infectious diseases when the blood is loaded with the products formed by invading bacteria. Again they are manifest when the organism is poisoned through toxic products of indigestion. These may be simply the products of proteid decomposition—*leucomaines* as they are termed, or they may be *ptomaines* produced by the activity of certain micro-organisms which affect the body through the toxic principles which they elaborate. Some of these are excessively poisonous in minute doses, and are chiefly developed in such articles of food as milk, ice cream, cheese, sausage and canned fish. It has been inferred that the muscles may also produce toxines which by their presence give rise to poisonous symptoms.[12]

From whatever source they may have been derived, waste products in the blood impede the action of all the tissues of the body. This influence is well shown in the laboratory upon a prepared muscle, the contractions being recorded by a series of curves upon a suitable machine. Following stimulation there is a short interval known as the latent period, and then contraction is indicated by a rising curve commencing rapidly and proceeding more slowly to a maximum height, and as the muscle returns to its normal condition there is a descending curve, at first sudden and then more gradual. After repeated shocks of stimulation these curves become less marked, until the contractions record almost a continuous line—a condition which is termed muscular tetanus.

Such tired muscle has a longer latent period than a fresh one, and a stronger stimulation is necessary to produce contractions equal to those at the beginning of experimentation. Bernard experimented with blue bottle flies—*musca vomitoria,* and found that the muscle of fatigued flies compared with that of flies at rest showed microscopical distinction, the contractile disks of the tired muscle being almost obliterated, while the capacity of such a muscle for taking a stain for microscopic examination evidenced an important difference over that of normal muscle, the whole contents of the segments staining uniformly, indicating that extraordinary exertion had used up the muscular substance more rapidly than it was repaired.

Ranke found that by washing out a fatigued muscle with common salt solution, though it added no new factor of energy, it freed the tissue from poisonous excreta and enabled it to again perform work. To confirm this a watery extract of fatigued muscle, when injected into fresh muscle, occasioned it to lose its working capacity.[13] Mosso has also shown

[12] Verworn; p. 468; 1899. [13] Ranke; 1865.

by experiments on the dog the presence of these fatigue substances. When the blood of a tired dog was injected into a dog which had been at rest all the phenomena of fatigue were manifest, but when the blood injected was from a normally resting dog no such symptoms were induced.[14] This physiologist has shown that in man small doses of cocaine remove the fatigue sense and raise muscular ability above normal.*

Dr. Alexander Haig, of London, attributes all the symptoms of depression and fatigue as due to the presence of uric acid in the blood, which he regards as the particular poison of the excreta. Uric acid, he claims, obstructs the capillaries throughout the entire body, the consequent deficient circulation preventing a proper metabolism by retarding the removal of waste products.

The relative excretion of waste is influenced not only by the routine of living, but by changes in the weather, tire being more easily produced in warm than in cold weather because of the increased elimination of acids by perspiration raising the alkalinity of the blood and permitting the passage of an excess of uric acid from the tissues into the blood. With this excess there is a diminished excretion of urea accompanied by the symptoms of fatigue. Exercise when excessive increases the formation of urea, which may at first be carried off in a free blood stream, but when the flow in the capillaries is diminished through the presence of uric acid in excess, the urea excretion is retarded and fatigue is manifest.

Cocaine, it is found, will free the blood of uric acid and abolish all the symptoms of fatigue both of mind and body, doing this by raising the acidity of the blood and so directly counteracting the effect of exercise by preventing the blood becoming a solvent for uric acid.[15] The effect of the pure blood is to produce a free circulation with increased metabolism in the muscles and nerve centres. When the blood is loaded with excreta the circulation is retarded and there is high blood pressure, which may ultimately result in dilatation of the heart.[16]

The long train of troubles which may follow retention of

[14] Mosso; 1891. * *Idem;* 1890. [15] Haig; p. 269; 1897. [16] Broadbent; p. 168.

waste have been found to be worse during the morning hours when the acid tide of the urine is lowest. These conditions are all relieved under the influence of Coca, a knowledge of which has been gleaned from its empirical use. As an instance of this, a lady suffering from a severe influenza accompanied with rheumatism, was induced to try a grog of Vin Mariani—as advocated by Dr. Cyrus Edson in the treatment of La Grippe,[17] and much to her surprise found that she was not only cured of her cold, but entirely relieved from the symptoms of her rheumatism as well, despite a preformed prejudice against Coca in any form. Acting upon this suggestive hint, I have found that alternate doses of Coca and the salicylates constitute an admirable treatment for rheumatism.

The influence of Coca in banishing the effects of extreme fatigue is well illustrated in an account of its use communicated to me by Dr. Frank L. James, Editor of the *National Druggist*, St. Louis. While a student at Munich he experimented with the use of Coca upon himself at the request of Professor Liebig, whose pupil he was. On one occasion, when exceedingly tired both physically and mentally, he was induced to try chewing Coca after the proper Peruvian fashion with a little *llipta*. Before commencing this experiment he was hungry, but too tired to eat and too hungry to sleep. In a few moments after beginning to chew hunger gave place to a sense of warmth in the stomach, while all physical weariness disappeared, though mentally he was still somewhat tired and disinclined to read or study, though this condition soon passed away, giving rise to an absolute eagerness to be at some sort of exercise. These sensations lasted altogether for probably three hours, gradually passing off after the first hour, leaving the subject none the worse for his experience and able to eat a hearty dinner the same evening.

Some years afterward, while practicing in the South, this gentleman returned from a thirty-six hours' ride so tired as to necessitate being helped off the horse and up-stairs to his room. While preparing for bed his eyes fell upon a package of Coca leaves which he had recently received by way of San

[17] Edson; p. 39; 1891.

Francisco, and the idea immediately occurred to him to repeat the experiment of his student days. In the course of a quarter of an hour—following the chewing of probably a drachm of Coca leaves—he felt so refreshed and recuperated that he was able to go out and visit patients about the town to whom he had previously sent word that he was too tired to call on them that night. In describing the result, Dr. James said: "I was not very hungry at the time before taking the Coca, but all sense of the necessity or of a desire for food vanished with the weariness."[18]

Professor Novy, of the University of Michigan, is referred to by one of his former classmates as having formed one of a group of experimenters upon the use of Coca leaves. The influence being tested during a walk of twenty-four miles, taken one afternoon without any other nourishment but water and Coca. Over four miles an hour was averaged, and although unaccustomed to such long walks or vigorous exercise, no special muscular fatigue was experienced by four of the party who chewed the leaves almost constantly during the journey. No change was noted in the urine and no depression was experienced the next day. One who did not chew Coca, but was addicted to alcohol and chewed tobacco constantly, was somewhat more fatigued than the others, and suffered considerably from soreness of the muscles on the following day.[19]

The experience of Sir Robert Christison, of Edinburgh, with the use of Coca upon himself and several of his students, is full of interest because of his extended experiments and the high rank of the investigator. Two of his students, unaccustomed to exercise during five months, walked some sixteen miles without having eaten any food since breakfast. On their return they each took two drachms of Coca made into an infusion, to which was added five grains of carbonate of soda, in imitation of the Peruvian method of adding an alkali. All sense of hunger and fatigue soon left, and after an hour's walk they returned to enjoy an excellent dinner, after which they felt alert during the evening, and their night's sleep was

[18] *Collective Investigation*, (924); 1898. [19] *Idem;* (586); 1898.

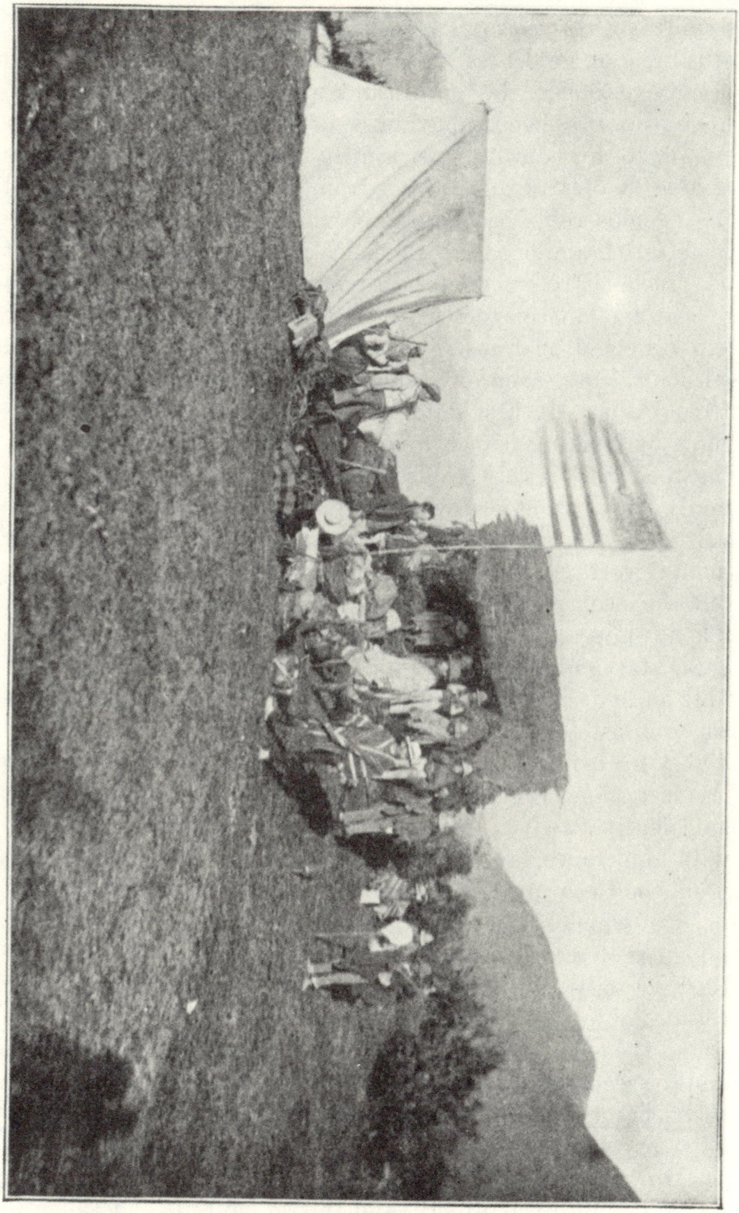

Camp of United States Explorers Between Phara and Aporoma, Peru. [*From a Photograph.*]

sound and refreshing. One of these students felt a slight sensation of giddiness after drinking the infusion, but the other experienced no unpleasant symptoms. Ten students, under similar conditions, walked varying distances, from twenty to thirty miles, over a hilly road. Two of these were unable to remark any effects from the use of Coca, several felt decided relief from fatigue, while four experienced complete relief, and one of these had walked thirty miles without any food. Professor Christison, though seventy-eight years of age and unaccustomed to vigorous exercise, subsequently experimented on himself by chewing Coca leaves, with and without *llipta,* some of which had been forwarded to him from Peru. He first determined the effect of profound fatigue by walking fifteen miles on two occasions without taking food or drink. On his return his pulse, which was normally sixty-two at rest, was one hundred and ten on his arrival home, and two hours later was ninety. He was unfit for mental work in the evening, though he slept soundly all night, but the next morning was not inclined for active exercise. Then, under similar conditions, he walked sixteen miles, in three stages of four, six, and six miles, with one interval of half an hour, and two intervals of an hour and a half. During the last forty-five minutes of his second rest he chewed eighty grains of Coca, reserving forty grains for use during the last stage, even swallowing some of the fibre. He felt sufficiently tired to look forward to the end of his journey with reluctance, and did not observe any particular effect from the Coca until he got out of doors and put on his usual pace, of which he said: "At once I was surprised to find that all sense of weariness had entirely fled and that I could proceed not only with ease, but even with elasticity. I got over the six miles in an hour and a half without difficulty, and found it easy when done to get up a four and a half mile pace and to ascend quickly two steps at a time to my dressing room, two floors up-stairs; in short, I had no sense of fatigue or any other uneasiness whatsoever."

During this walk he perspired profusely. On reaching home his pulse was ninety, and in two hours it had fallen to seventy-two, showing that the heart and circulation had been strengthened under the influence of Coca. The urine solids were the same as during the walk without Coca. In describing this walk, he said: "On arrival home before dinner, I felt neither hunger nor thirst, after complete abstinence from food and drink of every kind for nine hours, but upon dinner appearing in half an hour, ample justice was done to it." After a sound sleep through the night he woke refreshed and free from all sense of fatigue. An influence of Coca not anticipated was the relief of a tenderness of his eyes, which during some years had rendered continuous reading a painful effort. In another trial at mountain climbing, he ascended Ben Vorlich, on Loch Earn, 3,224 feet above the sea. The climb was along a rugged foot path, then through a short heather and deep grass, and the final dome of seven hundred feet rise was among blocks and slabs of mica-slate. The ascent was made in two and a half hours, the last three hundred feet requiring considerable determination.

His companions enjoyed a luncheon, but Sir Robert contented himself chewing two-thirds of a drachm of Coca, and after a rest of three-quarters of an hour was ready for the descent. Although this was looked forward to with no little distrust, he found upon rising that all fatigue was gone, and he journeyed with the same ease with which he had enjoyed mountain rambles in his youth. The experimenter was neither weary, hungry nor thirsty, and felt as though he could easily have walked four miles to his home. After a hearty dinner, followed by a busy evening, he slept soundly during the night and woke refreshed in the morning, ready for another day's exercise. During the trip he took neither food nor drink of any kind except chewing sixty grains of Coca leaves. Eight days after this experiment was repeated, using ninety grains of Coca. The weather had changed and the temperature was forty-four degrees at the top of the mountain and a chilly breeze provoked the desire to descend. While resting sixty grains of Coca was chewed. The descent was made without halt in an hour and a quarter, and followed by a walk of two miles over a level road to meet his carriage. He then felt slightly tired, because three hours had elapsed since he had chewed Coca.

In summing up his experience Professor Christison says: "I feel that without details the general results which may now be summarized would scarcely carry conviction with them. They are the following: The chewing of Coca not only removes extreme fatigue, but prevents it. Hunger and thirst are suspended, but eventually appetite and digestion are unaffected. No injury whatever is sustained at the time or subsequently in occasional trials." From sixty to ninety grains are sufficient for one trial, but some persons either require more or are constitutionally proof against the restorative action of Coca. From his observations there was no effect on the mental faculties except to prevent the dullness and drowsiness which follow great bodily fatigue.[20]

It is a matter of much interest to determine just what food is appropriate to generate muscle or to stimulate the tissues for work. As the capacity of an organ is in proportion to its bulk —under proper conditions—it seems essential that proteids should be eaten in order to create the muscle substances of which they form so great a part; but as has been repeatedly indicated, no one variety of food makes that same variety of tissue. All conversion in the body is due to a chemical change within the cell of the tissue; the food taken in is broken down by the digestive processes, and after assimilation is doled out according to the particular requirements of the individual parts of a normal organism.

The muscles are not set at work from the immediate intake of food, but are rendered capable for action by a chemical conversion of the material already stored up in the tissues, which is elaborated into energy as it may be required. It would seem as though this fact had not been carefully considered when calculating the effect of any diet upon muscular exertion during a brief period. The capacity of the body for work is due to the integrity of its tissue and the ability to draw suitable supplies from these stored substances. It is the ap-

[20] Christison; April 13, 1876; also *Pharmaceutical Journal and Transactions* (3); Vol. VI, p. 884.

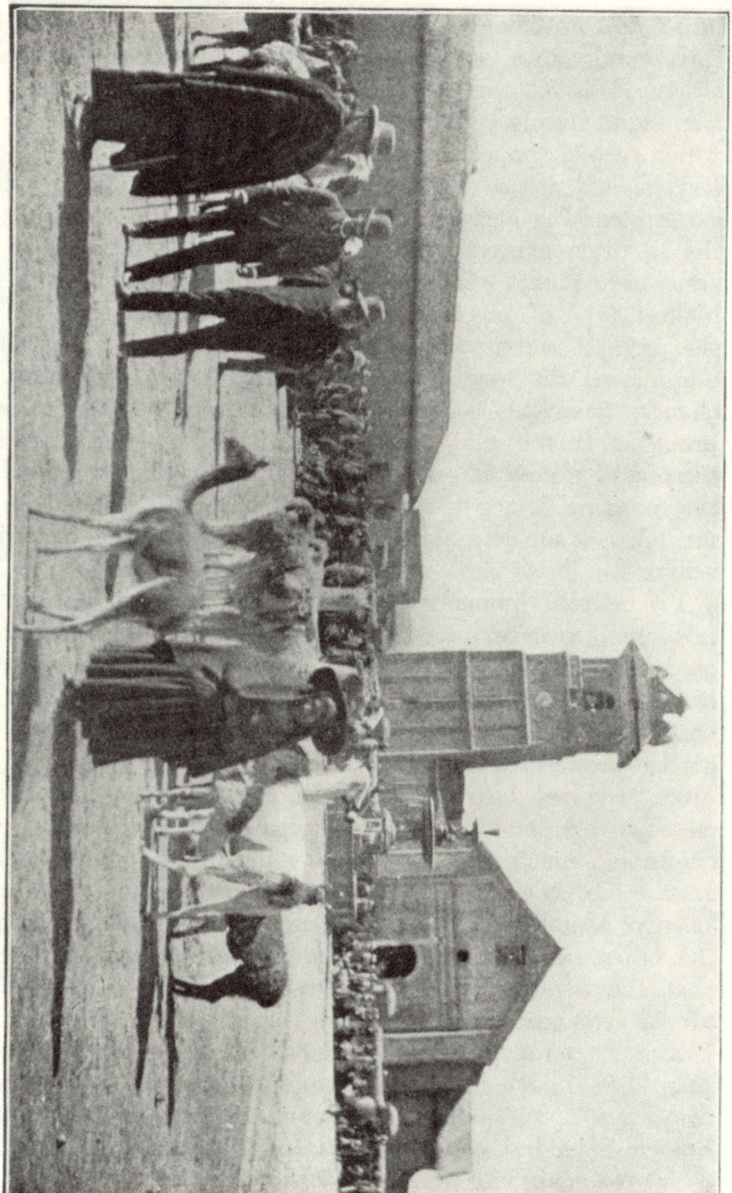

PLAZA AND CHURCH AT AZANGARO, PERU. ALTITUDE 15,000 FEET. [*From a Photograph.*]
The walls of the interior of the church are covered with sheets of gold.

propriate conversion of this stored-up material which constitutes energy in a capable being rather than a mere automatism. Without this power of conversion the human organism would simply be clogged up by an accumulation of fuel which would impede rather than create activity. The body should not be regarded as a machine constituted with certain working parts which are gradually worn out through the so often expressed "wear and tear." The facts long since have proved that life is a succession of deaths. The highest type of physical life is that which is capable of the greatest activity, creating useful energy and properly eliminating the waste matters resulting from the chemical changes from this conversion. Indeed, one of the gravest problems in the maintenance of a healthful activity is the one of excretion. To the retention of waste products in the blood or tissues a whole train of ills, both physical and mental, is unquestionably due, whether this poison be uric acid or not.

Preoccupied humanity seems constantly seeking some medicinal measure toward buoyancy and vigor rather than regarding the rational effects of appropriate eating and proper exercise. The success of many patent nostrums is chiefly based upon the fact of the necessity for elimination, and a good diuretic or laxative disguised as a panacea for all ills often produces the required result. As to the proper food essential to promote the greatest energy there have been many conflicting conclusions drawn from the known physiological facts. On the one side it has been asserted that all energy is induced from nitrogenous substances, while on the other side equally competent observers have asserted that the non-nitrogenous substances are alone used; yet all the evidence points to the fact that the constructive metabolism in animals is paralleled by similar processes in plant life, in which it has been shown that carbohydrates are built up into proteids, while these latter are also broken down into carbohydrates, and each of these may be converted again and again under the appropriate stimulus of the other substance. We know that starch, which is the representative of the carbohydrate class, is converted into glucose and carried to the liver to be stored up as the animal starch—glycogen—and as the various tissues of the body are called into activity this stored-up material is hurried to them in a soluble form to be utilized by the cell in the production of energy. When meat is eaten—which is the representative type of the nitrogenous class—its proteid material is changed into a soluble peptone, and this, carried to the liver, is converted into glycogen, which indicates, as has been proven by experiment, that either class of food substance is capable of maintaining the functions of the body so long as the chemical elements comprising the food taken be appropriate. While the meat eater and the vegetarian are each right, they are equally both wrong when advocating an exclusiveness in either dietary. The fact is, as will be shown in the chapter upon dietetics, it is purely an individual matter as to what particular food may be best. It all depends upon the body, or the machine—as you will—as to what substance each particular organism shall have the privilege of converting into energy.

While the body may be supported on either class of foodstuffs for a time, a man would surely starve as quick on a purely nitrogenous dietary as he would upon one purely non-nitrogenous. It will be recalled that the experiment of Fick and Wislicenus was conducted upon a food, the solid portion of which was carbohydrate, but with this tea was drunk as a beverage. Tea loaded with xanthin would afford sufficient of the nitrogenous element to convert the stored-up carbohydrates to action, but as Haig and Morton have both shown, tea contains so much of an equivalent to uric acid that it could not long be relied upon as an energy exciter, for while the tissue might be stimulated for a time, waste matter would soon be augmented in the blood. Coca, as we have seen, has the quality of freeing the blood from waste material, and yet possesses sufficient nitrogenous quality to convert the stored-up carbohydrates into tissue and energy. The Andeans are a race small of stature and of low muscular development. The average American or European could easily tire a native Indian in a day's travel, but while the former continuing on an ordinary diet would soon become stiff the Indian sustained by Coca remains fit and active, and is apparently fresh and ready after a hard day's jaunt. It seems probable that this condition is occasioned through the converting influence of the nitrogenous Coca acting upon the stored-up carbohydrates of the Andean's accustomed dietary. Thus while promoting metabolism and increasing energy the blood current is at the same time kept free.

The custom of the Andean to measure distances by the *cocada* has already been referred to; it is the length of time that the influence of a chew of Coca will carry him—equal to a period of some forty minutes—and during which he will cover nearly two miles on a level ground or a mile and a quarter up hill. Taking the suggestion from this a preparation of Coca made in Paris known as "Velo-Coca," is purposely intended for the use of bicyclists, a given dose of which is calculated to sustain the rider through forty kilometres—twenty-five miles. The advantage of Coca in long distance contests has long been known to certain professionals, who have endeavored to keep their use of this force sustainer a secret.[21]

Some years ago the members of the Toronto La Crosse Club experimented with Coca, and during the season when that club held the championship of the world Coca was used in all its important matches. The Toronto Club was composed of men accustomed to sedentary work, while some of the opposing players were sturdy men accustomed to out of door exercise. The games were all very severely contested, and some were played in the hottest weather of one summer; on one occasion the thermometer registered 110° F. in the sun. The more stalwart appearing men, however, were so far used up before the match was completed that they could hardly be encouraged to finish the concluding game, "while the Coca chewers were as elastic and apparently as free from fatigue as at the commencement of the play." At the beginning of the game each player was given from one drachm to a drachm and a half of leaves, and this amount, without lime or any other

[21] McLaumaille; 1875.

addition, was chewed in small portions during the game. The first influence experienced was a dryness of the throat, which, when relieved by gargling with water, was not again noticed, while a sense of invigoration and an increase of muscular force was soon experienced, and this continued through the game, so that fatigue was resisted. The pulse was increased in frequency and perspiration was excited, but no mental symptoms were induced excepting an exhilaration of spirits, which was not followed by any after effects.[22]

As has been shown, fatigue and its ills is occasioned by a diminution of the elements necessary to activity as well as to an excess of waste materials in the blood. This latter cause alone explains many problems dependent upon this condition which are commonly assigned to other causes. Under this hypothesis it is easy to appreciate not only the cause of muscle fatigue, but the irritability from nerve tire as well as the restlessness in wasting disease. When the tissues are not supplied with a blood stream that is pure and uncontaminated they cannot respond healthfully. A blood current already overburdened with waste can neither stimulate to activity nor carry off the burden of excreta.

The power of Coca to relieve the circulation, and so bring about a condition indicating a free blood stream, has been emphasized by a host of observers. Speaking of the action of but one of its alkaloids, Dr. Haig says: "Some have asserted that it is oblivion men seek for when they take opium, cocaine, etc., I believe this to be a great error. Give me an eternity of oblivion and I would exchange it for one hour with my cerebral circulation quite free from uric acid, and opium or cocaine will free it for me. When the blood stream is free the pulse tension is reduced, the rate is quickened, and the increased flow alters the mental condition as if by magic; ideas flash through the brain; everything is remembered."[23]

Hitherto the usual explanation that has been advanced as to the influence of Coca—when any influence has been accorded—has been its stimulant action upon the nerves. In view of the facts set forth in this research such a theory seems

[22] Shuttleworth; 1877. [23] Haig; p. 247, *et seq.*; 1897.

inadequate. I have endeavored to show by a succession of facts and many examples, that the sustaining influence of Coca in fatigue, as well as its curative power in so many diseased conditions, as to render it a seeming panacea, is largely due to a direct action upon the cells of the tissues, as well as through the property which Coca has of freeing the blood from waste. This influence may chiefly be upon the brain or upon the muscular structure, in accordance with the relative proportion of the associate principles present in the Coca leaf employed. Under this hypothesis, based upon physiological research as well as upon the theory of the formation of proteid in plants and in animals, Coca not only stimulates the cells to activity and so sets free energy, but may build up new tissue through exciting the protoplasm to appropriate conversion. Such an hypothesis is certainly plausible when we consider the action of amides and other nitrogenous elements in plant structure. This is again emphasized by its harmony with recent theories of Pflüger regarding the building up of proteid tissue in the animal organism. So much testimony points to this conclusion that in the entire absence of other scientific explanation this is certainly worthy of serious consideration. The facts of which will be more specifically elaborated in the chapter on physiology.

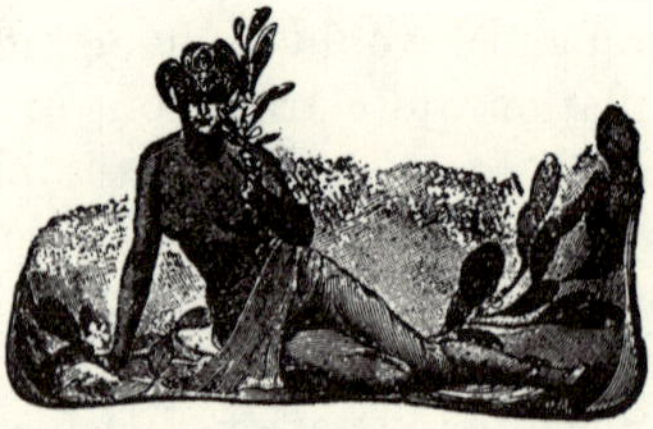

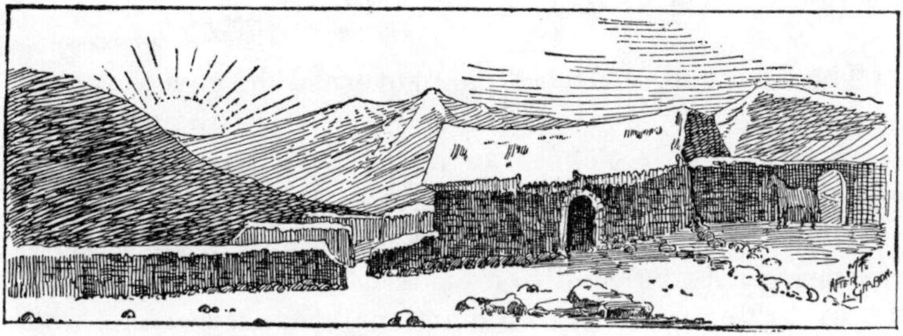

CHAPTER XIII.

ACTION OF COCA UPON THE NERVOUS SYSTEM.

"Man who man would be,
Must rule the empire of himself, in it
Must be supreme, establishing his throne
On vanquished will, quelling the anarchy
Of hopes and fears, being himself alone."
—Shelley, *Political Greatness.*

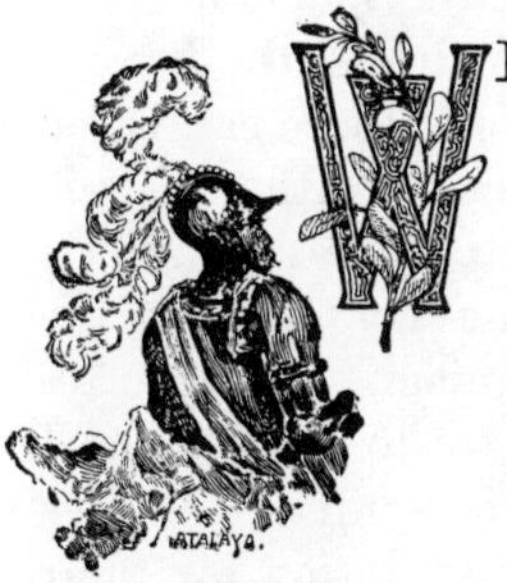

WE may presume an ideal condition of health, but there is no practical standard by which this can be gauged. Each individual organism presents a maximum and minimum range of vigor, between which the true balance must lie for that one being. The powers of the aboriginal Indian, while of a different quality, were not necessarily of a higher type than are those of the nervous worker of to-day, nor was the life of the former necessarily more natural because more active. We are creatures of the circumstances and environments in which cast. Each condition must be compared with its class. The possibilities of combating severe disease are vastly superior under the results of modern civilization. Man in every age must maintain a balance amidst the peculiar environment to which he is subjected, and the result of progress is to develop hygienic resources as well as keener susceptibilities.

The functions of the body are governed through the action of the nervous system involuntarily, whether the subject be asleep or awake, in sickness or in health. This action, however, may be influenced by the will either to depress or excite individual functions, so that their action may be modified or even perverted to a condition of disease. Dr. John Hunter, who was a victim to his own emotions, emphasized this when he wrote: "Every part of the body sympathizes with the mind, for whatever affects the mind, the body is affected in proportion."[1]

Among the annoyances incidental to a modern civilization are those troubles produced from a possible nervous perversion, engendered through overtaxing the powers mentally or physically in the modern whirl and bustle of a busy life. We all realize the effects of muscular fatigue, but few seem to appreciate the extreme tire which is possible to the nervous system of the purely sedentary worker. This may manifest itself in the mildest form as a mere irritability or restlessness, or more profoundly as peevishness and even despondency.

It is not as easy to demonstrate nerve tire in the laboratory as it is to show the fatigue of muscle, yet there can be no doubt that similar factors are at work to induce either. It is known that all the activity of the tissues, of whatever kind, is due to a chemical conversion of the substance contained in the minute cells which go to complete the organism. Fatigue results from the retention of products of waste in the blood which normally should be excreted. As a result the tissues are not properly nourished by a purified circulation for their work, and exhaustion is a consequence, whether the structure under this influence be muscle or nerve.

When we learn that Coca relieves muscular tire, mental depression or nervous fatigue, that it calms to refreshing sleep or stimulates to wakefulness and activity, that it allays hunger or induces appetite as the case may be, we can only harmonize such seemingly opposite applications through appreciating that this influence is extended to the tissues through the fluid which supplies them with nourishment. We

[1] Hunter; Vol. IV, p. 167; 1839.

have already seen that the blood is so speedily purified under the action of Coca that the circulation may at once return an appropriate pabulum to all the cells of the body and so may promote in them a normally healthful action.

The brain may be broadly considered as made up of cells and nerve fibres. The outer portion, which is termed the cortex, consists of many convolutions which through this arrangement affords a greater superficial area for the brain cells. These cells are located in layers over the surface, as well as arranged in groups at the base of the brain and in the medulla and spinal cord. The convolutions are merely rudimentary in animals and are poorly developed in the lower orders of the human race and in the uneducated. By intellectual development these are increased in a manner quite analogous to that in which muscle is increased by exercise. Gross bulk of brain substance does not necessarily indicate giant intellect, but merely the structure for such possible development.

The brain practically attains its greatest size in early childhood, at least this is the period of its most active increase, and remembering the law that the part of the body which is subject to the greatest physiological growth is most liable to disease, it will keep before us the fact that children are particularly susceptible to disorders of the brain and nervous system. In childhood the tendency should be to restrain these organs, which are already too alert, from an undue excitement.

From birth an education of the individual cells of this intellectual centre should be carefully conducted. A refinement of nerve tissue progressing by easy gradations until strength and power shall be secured. It is through this alone that man may be raised superior to the beast or savage. Not only present enjoyments but future comforts and realizations are so absolutely dependent upon this that even "Spiritual life can only reach the human form by and through the brain cell."[2]

Quite as important as the brain in maintaining mental stability is the action of the sympathetic nerve in controlling

[2] Wilson; 1899.

physical well being, while both brain and sympathetic nerve must act together to sustain the organism in true harmony. The sympathetic nerve runs on either side and in front of the spinal column as a double chain of little brains. From these centers not only the great organs are supplied, but also the coats of the blood vessels, through which association a controlling influence is maintained over the entire organism. Along its route these nerves are intimately connected with branch nerve fibres from the brain and spinal cord. Through groups of fibres sent to the heart, to the stomach and to the organs of the pelvis the functions of either one of these may be influenced in sympathy from the derangement of some other organ far distant, the workings of which are not directly associated, but the action of which is affected by a reflection of the troubles elsewhere. This reflex effect between distant parts of the body is analogous to the switching on of a branch telegraph loop to the main line to carry news to points with which it was not directly connected.

So intimate is the relation of this regulating nerve with the various functions of the body that it is possible for these to be seriously interfered with through action of the sympathetic on the blood vessels, by which the tension of their walls is altered and the circulation is accordingly hastened or retarded. Common examples of this effect are seen when the emotions are excited and occasion the capillary vessels to contract as in pallor, or, when these are suddenly dilated, to cause blushing. The idea that the emotions have their seat in the heart because of this influence of the blood vessels in occasioning an irregularity of its action has led to an erroneous and sentimental regard for that organ.

This intricate nervous development suggests the extreme importance of a well trained organization as a factor toward preventing that broad class of cases which are grouped under the generic title of neurasthenia. In this condition—rather than disease—a similar restlessness and over sensitiveness is present as in profound fatigue. In chronic illness the same symptoms are seen, but when these are complained of without any characteristic signs of disease the indications point to nerve irritability through imperfect elimination of tissue waste. If with this excess of waste materials in the blood there be associated a defective will, then the influence on the sympathetic nerve must be pronounced. Either cause may unbalance the circulation through the arterial system and so disarrange various functions of the body, while a low power of resistance intensifies the mental disability. It is remarkable that these sufferers are at first rarely treated appropriately, but are often impatiently urged to exert will power. While it is undoubtedly true, as so aptly phrased by Shakespeare: "There is no condition, be it good or ill, but thinking

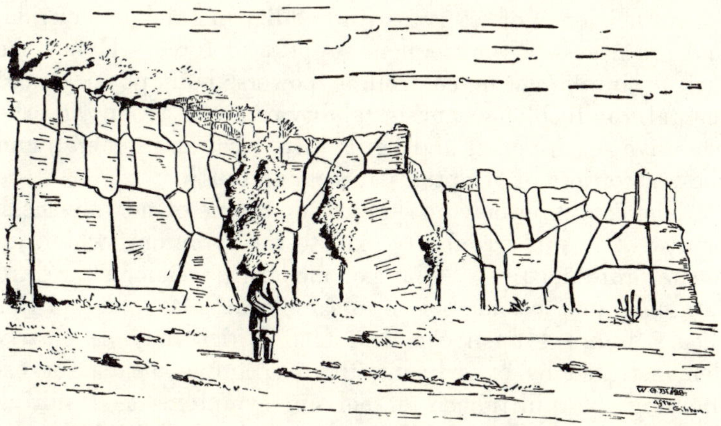

CYCLOPEAN WALL, FORTRESS OF SACSAHUAMAN, BACK OF CUZCO, PERU.

makes it so," will power must emanate from a primary store of bodily health.

The greatest factor, however, must be derived through the guidance of the emotions, particularly during the formative period of development. An early education of the will should form a basis for mental control. In this will be found a prominent factor in the production of future happiness, as well as a means of support in many a physical ailment, and even a source of contentment in hopeless disease. But as has already been indicated, the greatest benefit can only result from a healthful working of the entire organism. That there shall be a sound mind in a sound body is an old adage, and recently the great universities have appreciated this sufficiently to officially recognize physical training as an important part of a collegiate education.

Whether the title neurasthenia be scientifically correct for the peculiar train of symptoms which go to make up the complainings of the victims of over-nervous irritability, it has served since the classification of some thirty years ago to enable the acute medical examiner to group the particular sufferers from this morbid condition. As defined by Dr. Beard, neurasthenia is: "A chronic functional disease of the nervous system, the basis of which is the impoverishment of nervous force; deficiency of reserve, with liability to quick exhaustion, and the necessity for frequent supplies of force. Hence the lack of inhibitory or controlling powers, both physical and mental, the feebleness and instability of nerve action, and the excessive sensitiveness and irritability, local and general, and the vast variety of symptoms, direct and reflex."[3]

The condition may be summed up as one of nervelessness, or a weakness of irritability akin to the symptoms which indicate profound tire. A host of modern physiologists regard fatigue as due to some poison in the blood.[4] If we accept this theory founded upon chemical facts which may be clearly demonstrated by experiment, there is ample means for explaining the multiplicity of nervous symptoms as resulting from this cause alone. Waste matters in the circulation by clogging the capillaries prevent the venous blood from being appropriately purified. The nerve centers do not receive suitable stimulus for repair, and the increased irritability occasions an excessive waste which still further impedes the circulation. Functional changes must necessarily result in the heart, kidneys, liver and the brain from this continued irritation.

The subjective symptoms of neurasthenia are not so much engendered by a weakness of the nervous system, nor any lack of susceptibility of the nervous protoplasm to respond to irritation, as through excessive irritability, which renders the or-

[3] Beard; p. 36; 1886. [4] Foster; *Lancet*, Vol. I, p. 1457; 1893.

ganism over sensitive to normal and healthful stimulus. It is a condition which may be allied to the harp, so strung up as to permit the slightest breath to set its strings in a discordant hum. Often the subjects of this form of trouble are found among those who are in the prime of activity, in early adult life, when the various forces for the production of energy are being vigorously employed.

As it is that part of the body which is most active at any one period of life—particularly of growth—that is most liable to disease, so during the different epochs of pubescence, adolescence, and the early marital life in either sex, the symptoms of neurasthenia may be exhibited. These symptoms are particularly manifest when there has been at these periods a condition of overstrain, associated with mal-nutrition. Among all possible causes my experience has been that the genetic factor, through repeated explosive shocks upon the nervous system, is pre-eminent in the production of neurasthenic symptoms in those already overworked or suffering from imperfect nutrition.

Neurotics are prone to excesses as well as to extremes in any particular line. They are the class to which "habits" cling and "habit drugs" belong, and the apparent candor of their sufferings might often lead the sympathetic, unwary listener astray. In such subjects these habits and excesses should be regarded rather as symptoms than the underlying cause of the condition. If this fact were more generally thought upon we should hear less of those who have been wrecked by alcohol or opium. Indeed it is a fact that a perfectly healthy man rarely becomes a morphinist, cannabist, etc., but that such individuals are without exception neuropathic.[5]

The numerous symptoms which go to make up the condition of nervous prostration have only been made prominent through the push for supremacy, and even for maintenance, in the various specialisms of life. While the causes always have existed, modern civilization has greatly exaggerated them, and the present dwellers in cities are consequently emi-

[5] Tuke; Vol. II, p. 849; 1892.

nently of the nervous type. The sufferers are not all from one class, but are numbered among the high, the low, the rich and the poor, though the symptoms may be varied in accordance with the cultivation and environment of the patient. What the poor Andean Indian, working laboriously for days on scanty food, might regard as the ban of some "spirit of the mountain" cast upon him for presuming to invade some hallowed precinct and as a charm against which he chews the sacred Coca, the used up subject of protracted social functions considers in a different light. But the symptoms and conditions are similar, whether occasioned from over-indulgence and overwork, because of exalted ambition, or from enforced labor associated with hygienic errors.

The title neurasthenia has been made responsible for a multitude of evils, quite as bad as has that of "malaria" or "biliousness." While the group of subjective symptoms which Beard classed under this head has been expanded to embrace about every condition generated from nervous irritability, it remained for the classic guidance of Charcot to accentuate the importance of a certain few symptoms into what he styled "the stigma of neurasthenia," in an effort to combine these as an exact disease.

It is very different whether we consider this classic form or the commonly accepted type. On the one hand there may be mere nervous irritability, while on the other this is accentuated until it approaches the border line of psychical aberration. The more grave condition has been traced from a neurotic heredity or degeneracy, while the simpler application is made to embrace all forms of mental worry, from a mere nervous headache to some pronounced *phobia,* or dread. The two types, however, often intermingle on the threshold of some severe nervous affection, with hypochondriacal, epileptic or paralytic symptoms, or even insanity.

The popular idea of nervous debility held by the laity as well as by the general practitioner in medicine is not the serious disorder of the alienist any more nearly than is a "fit of the blues"—which, since the days of Burton's *Anatomy of Melancholy,* has been attributed to "biliousness"—is true melancholia. The two terms are used by the unknowing or the unthinking ones as interchangeable, the one being a simple temporary mental despondency, which may arise from any one of many causes, while the more serious ailment manifests this condition profoundly and characteristically all the time.

Charcot claimed that neurasthenia was entitled to a definite place in mental pathology, because the disease as witnessed by him maintains its identity under varying circumstances of origin. He believed the condition to be essentially distinct from hysteria, although it might be associated with that disease, and so present a complex hystero-neurasthenia—a combination which was also described by Beard. That is, the patient may exhibit only neurasthenic symptoms, or united with these the symptoms may be of positive hysteria.

Levillain[6] has, with many other authors, described two varieties of neurasthenia—that from heredity and the acquired. The two forms differ not only in their progress, but in their response to treatment. Among the peculiar train of symptoms commonly seen in this disorder are curious feelings of morbid fear or dread experienced by its subjects. This is similar to the hallucinations which the Germans term "*zwangsvorstellungen*" and "*zwangshandlungen,*" and which others have given a long list of terrible names. *Agoraphobia* is a dread of open spaces, *anthropophobia* is a fear of society, the antithesis of which is *monophobia*—the fear of being alone. Then there is *pantophobia,* a fear of everything, and a culmination which must be the last straw—*phobophobia,* a fear of being afraid. The French term this condition "*peurs maladies.*"[7] "*Folie de doute*" is the name given by Le Grande du Saulle to a condition of chronic uncertainty when there is a morbid doubt about everything.

Hereditary neurasthenia, it is asserted, may develop in those whose parents were distinctly nervous, even though the usual determining cause may not be present. Among predisposing causes, over-excitation including all forms of overstrain, whether sudden or gradual, is predominant, while the condition is not markedly influenced by alcohol or nar-

[6] Levillain; 1891. [7] Gélineau; 1894.

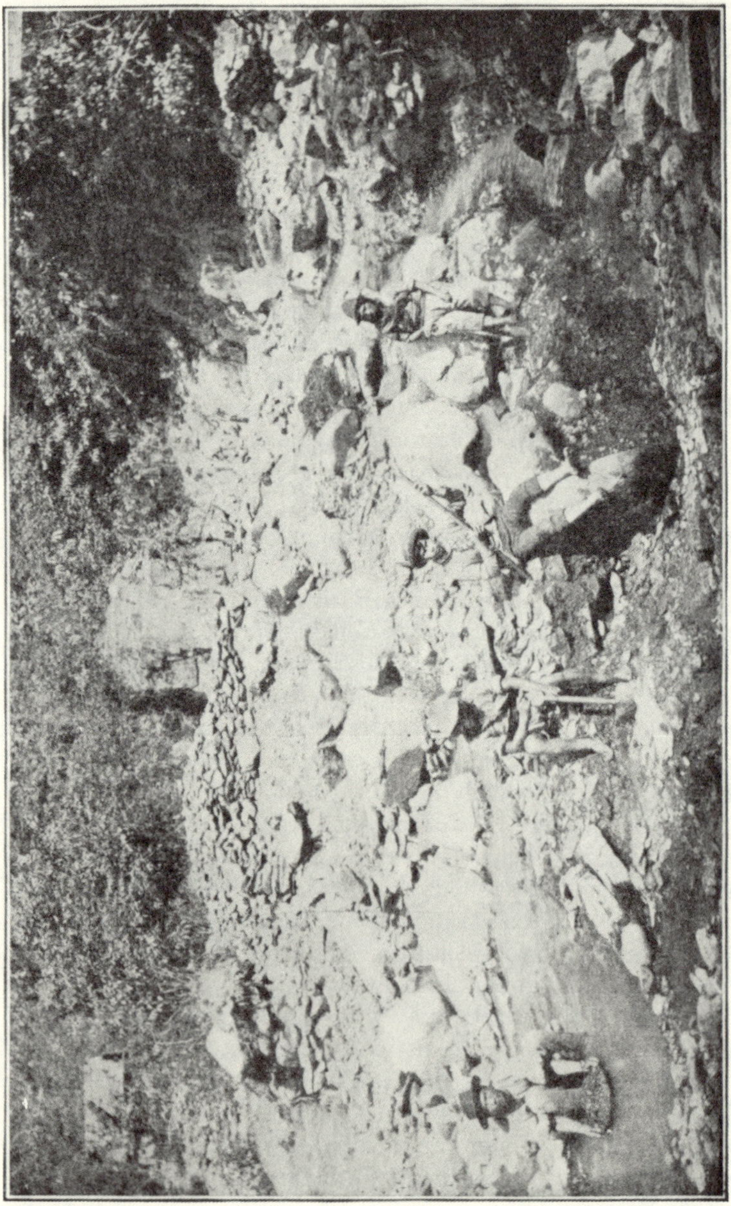

INDIANS WASHING GOLD FROM ANDEAN STREAM. [*From a Photograph.*]

cotics. The essential symptoms which Charcot described as the stigmata of the disease are: (1) Headache of a special kind; (2) Digestive troubles; (3) Incapacity for work; (4) Loss or diminution of sexual desire; (5) Muscular lassitude, marked by easily induced fatigue, and painful stiffness; (6) Spinal pain; (7) Insomnia; (8) Hypochondriacal views of life. Other symptoms which may appear are vertigo, cardialgia simulating angina pectoris, palpitation of the heart, feelings of faintness, and irritable pulse; but these may not be constant. The muscle weakness, with an indescribable irritability expressive of fatigue, Charcot considered so prominent a symptom that he reserved for it the term "*amyosthenia.*" The headache is of a peculiar character, suggestive of a weight or constriction over the back of the head or vertex, and sometimes over the whole cranium, described as the "neurasthenic helmet." In some cases this sense of pressure may be hemicranial. The insomnia, or troubled sleep, so annoying in pronounced cases, is a very important symptom. The backache may be limited to the sacral region, or to the neck, or may at times be in the coccyx, and is commonly aggravated by pressure. The digestive symptoms are of a general nervous type. With these there is incapacity for mental work, and particularly a lack of concentration of thought.

From the classic grouping it will be seen that it is often difficult to draw the line between actual organic nerve trouble and neurasthenia. Perhaps the usual type, as seen by the general practitioner, presents a nerve depression—an inability of the organism to speedily repair itself after some call for unusual strain, while the two most prominent factors of this condition are sleeplessness and mal-assimilation. Under such influences it is easy to understand that the symptoms presented may be manifest as cerebral, spinal, genital, chlorotic, vascular, cardiac, or gastric, while there may be an especial indication pointing toward the liver. It is quite plausible, as Boix has shown, to have a "nervous dyshepatia" as well as a nervous dyspepsia, due to defective innervation.

It should be understood that the vast array of symptoms which go to make up the condition known as neurasthenia are largely those of reflex irritation, an irritation which may arise from any part of the organism and be transmitted through the sympathetic, and acting chiefly upon the blood vessels through the vaso-motor nerves. It is because of this reflex nature of the symptoms that the condition is often confounded with other diseases, and the sufferer may go the round of the various specialists, and receive "local treatment" for conditions which are erroneously considered to be the chief cause of trouble. What the oculist regards as occasioned from eye strain the rhinologist may look for in the nose. If the patient be a woman, the gynæcologist locates the concentration of troubles in predominant functions. On the other hand, the genito-urinary expert has predetermined that in any nervous man the seat of ills is the prostate gland. It is, therefore, a very common occurrence to find that patients who are nervously irritable have become in themselves multiple specialists. Through constantly going the rounds in search of relief they become familiar with various local conditions, which may give rise to similar symptoms to those they suffer.

These subjects, as a class, are acute and quick; they belong to the clever people, and they are either all elation and prone to overdo or way down "in the blues." It is not surprising then that they soon become familiar with the various remedial efforts toward relieving their symptoms. They not only know in advance what their medical advisers may suggest, but are often prepared to offer a long series of protests against each particular effort toward aiding them to recover from their deplorable condition. If to such a patient, complaining of insomnia, the physician suggests sulphonal—that drug keeps them awake. Then ensues a hasty enumeration of the several hypnotics they have employed, while they recount wherein each had proved in their case an utter failure. If the symptoms complained of are pronouncedly about the head, they know all about refraction, astigmatism, and the cutting of eye muscles, or they have had their turbinated bodies taken out, or hypertrophied tissue removed from nose or throat, their ears inflated, or they have inhaled and been sprayed to an alarming extent. If by chance the stomach but manifests a twinge of protest, then that poor organ has been dieted and washed, both *gavage* and *lavage—ad nauseam.* Thus these patients are commonly treated through all the operative procedures until it is no wonder they should finally become nervous wrecks, ultimately going about from one resort to another, unable to find relief, unable even to find what they deem a competent trained nurse to cater to their imaginings, while a kindly disposed helpmate dances attendance upon their peevish whims.

Frequently these cases are subjects of plethoric prosperity, who, if not constitutionally weak, have had no education in self-control. They have spoiled themselves by fretting, and are being more rapidly ruined by petting; the very kindness and consideration that is bestowed upon them at home only adds fuel to their weakness. Often an entire change of environment affords the best condition for the treatment of such cases, such as the rest cure of Weir Mitchell, or one of the German watering establishments, where the regimen is rigid and exact. They must be coerced into recovery or else they will go through the balance of life a nuisance alike to themselves as well as to those who would wish to be their friends. Examples of this condition are legion, and the complainings are as multiple and varied as the ideas of man.

There are instances of self-control when sufferings are held in check while continuing at work. Some of the ablest men in the world's history have been those of weak nervous organization. "Wise judges are we of each other," says Bulwer. Often those whom we look upon as of indomitable will may suffer keenly from some seemingly trivial nervous symptom. A few years ago a prominent justice, who though outwardly was the very picture of health, assured me he suffered more keenly than the abject criminals brought before him, and was literally a coward from nervous dread. He came a long distance for consultation. Possibly it was a satisfaction to get out of his immediate environment and relate his sufferings to one who could listen patiently with a wish to guide him understandingly. Being a popular politician, he was often called upon to make speeches at the most inopportune times—for him, and he seriously proposed to give up a life position because he felt he could not stand the nervous strain.

This is but one example of many similar cases occurring among professional men, with mental faculties constantly at full tension. Whenever there is a lull in their work their thoughts revert to themselves, and the symptoms of an over tired nervous organism are magnified into some serious physical ailment. These are the cases that maintain the advertising quacks. They wish to be treated confidentially because they would not have their friends know for the world that they are ailing in any particular. They, who are seemingly so strong, would feel humiliated to recount a tale of personal weakness even to a medical man. It can readily be appreciated how necessary it is that a physician shall listen attentively to the story these patients tell, and advise with them openly and candidly as to the plan of treatment, which primarily must consist in some better means of living rather than a dependence upon medication alone. An interchange of confidence between patient and physician, while always advisable, is more necessary in these particular cases than in any other in the entire field of practice of medicine. There must be faith, and in this much I am an advocate of the faith cure. Indeed, faith is necessary in every walk of life. A chimney may blow off the roof, one may fall on a slippery pavement, a horse may run away, a bridge might fall, a boat might sink, and a hundred and one possibilities might occur to the nervously imaginative. Fear often becomes so exaggerated in the minds of these weak patients that they finally become too timid to attempt anything serious. Such a subject must be assured why and how he is to get well. I once had a patient who would be excited to an indescribable dread if, when walking in the street, he met a truck having any part of the load projecting, such as a chair leg or plank. To avoid it he felt compelled by some uncontrollable influence to turn off into a side street. In another case—a young man, could never go into the society of women, and actually avoided meeting them as much as possible in the street because of an expressed fear that he "must punch them." These were cases of simple neurasthenia, which appropriate hygienic measures, combined with the administration of Coca—a remedy which the homœopaths have long associated as a specific in cases of timidity and bashfulness—completely cured.

The numerous examples which Kraft-Ebing[8] relates of the "Jack the Ripper" order belong to this same class. The complainings of these patients should not be treated flippantly, for the subjects are earnest in their endeavor to find relief from a form of suffering which, while not actually painful, is profoundly humiliating and mentally agonizing. It can be well understood how readily such cases might adopt a drug habit in an unguided effort to find some means of relief.

There is a tendency in the human mind which is overweighted to seek support in unburdening a portion of trouble by recounting mental sufferings, whether of illness or not, to another. The celebrated actor, Mr. Frank Drew, related to me a curious example illustrating this, which occurred to him on a recent visit to England. He was dining alone in a restaurant, when a gentleman approached with the remark:

"I trust you will not mind if I take a seat at your table?"

"Not at all," replied the actor; "I shall enjoy company."

The two fell into a casual chat, which was resolved into the stranger telling a long and intricate story regarding a purely personal matter, of no interest to an outsider, yet which was patiently listened to without interruption to the end. Then, as though having unbosomed himself of a weight of woe, he arose, saying:

"You will excuse my having troubled you with this story, but really it has been a great source of comfort to me to have found some one to whom I could tell it. Knowing that we are absolute strangers, and shall never meet again, I have not hesitated to talk freely to you." On the assurance of a hearty sympathy, and that the secret should remain inviolate, they parted, neither expecting to ever see the other. But it so chanced, in the littleness of this world, that the following night brought them together again at a dinner party, where they were introduced under embarrassing recollections.

[8] Kraft-Ebing; 1892.

Not long since, a physician told me of an incident bearing upon this same tendency, which had occurred to him. One day at the close of his office hours he was preparing to leave for some outside work, when a lady was ushered into the consulting room, and instead of relating any physical ailment, entered into a long story of family history, which was listened to attentively, in expectation that it was to lead up to the real cause of her visit.

After this story was completed, the relator asked what she was indebted for the consultation, to which the physician, conscious of his hurry and delay, said in a perfunctory way: "Five dollars." "Five dollars! Why, I should think that was altogether too little for having taken up so much of your time." "Well, then, I will say ten dollars," said the doctor, treating the whole matter very much as a joke. But the sincerity was shown by the willingness with which the fee was extended with the query: "When shall I come again?" "Say in two weeks," said the consultant smilingly. "Two weeks! Hadn't I better see you in one week?" "Very well, make it one week." And so for several weeks in succession this patient returned and continued to revert to this same story, each time leaving well satisfied after having deposited the customary ten-dollar fee. A case of insanity! Oh, no, merely an over troubled mind which, without apparent physical ailing, had sought relief of mental worries from a physician, who undoubtedly prevented more serious trouble and effected a cure simply through being a good listener. While such instances are not rare in the routine of any practitioner, they seem almost incredible.

I was recently talking with a leading laryngologist, whose practice is in Philadelphia, upon this same line of thought, when he related an anecdote which had occurred in his own practice. He had gone to Paris for a short visit and had left instructions that his assistant would continue his practice. One day he was visited at his hotel in Paris by one of his Philadelphia patients, who, entering in the most casual way, said: "Doctor, I have a little trouble with my throat I would like to have you look at to-day." The physician, being really surprised to see his patient thus unexpectedly so far from home, asked him how long he had been in Paris and how long he proposed to remain, and was the more astonished at the reply: "Oh, I just ran over to have my throat treated, and shall take the steamer back to-morrow."

These examples, while in a measure indicating the smallness of the world, illustrate the fact that patients recognize and require the personal factor in the treatment of their troubles. An element of confidence is established, not necessarily in consequence of any superior preliminary qualifications on the part of the medical man, but because perhaps he has applied his knowledge understandingly.

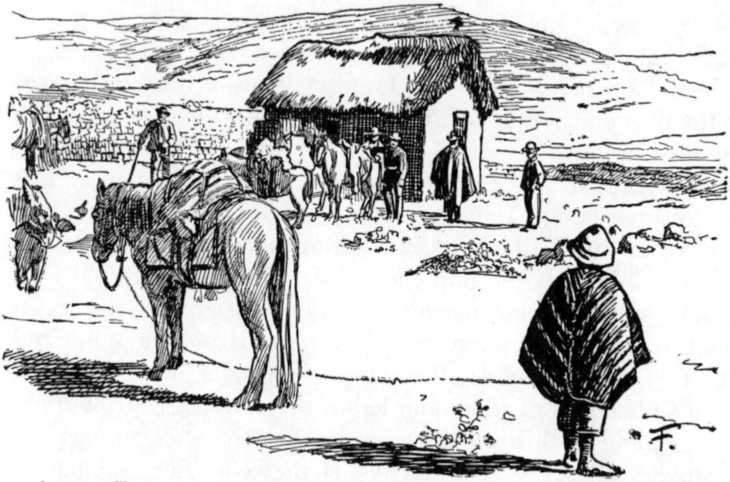

ANDEAN TAMBO AT ALTITUDE OF 13,500 FEET. [*From a Photograph.*]

Dr. Tuke[9] has written scientifically and very entertainingly regarding the subtle relations existing between mind and body—a subject which surely has a very important bearing upon the entire range of functional nervous troubles. The mind has an extraordinary influence, even in health, in causing disorders of imagination, sensation and also of organic functions. An outgrowth from this—a going off as it were on a tangent—leads to various beliefs in phenomena of a

[9] Tuke; 1884.

superstitious nature and forms a fertile field for the growth of unfortunate methods of treatment; unfortunate because disappointment must follow after the loss of valuable time in experimenting. In this connection I recall a remark made at an alumni dinner by the late Dr. John Hall in speaking of the so-called Christian science: "There is no Christianity in it, and it is not at all scientific."

It is a well-known fact to the physiologist that the mind may excite or depress the various nerve centres, and through these occasion functional changes in muscles or nerves. I hope it has been conclusively shown that this is the underlying factor occasioning many of the numerous subjective symptoms among that immense class known as neurasthenics. When the famous Dr. John Hunter's[10] attention was drawn to the phenomenon of animal magnetism—which was exciting the scientific world more than a century ago, he recognized the possible influence of expectancy upon the imagination, and in his lectures said: "I am confident that I can fix my attention to any part until I have a sensation in that part." It is because this possibility of the influence of the will is overlooked that greater success is not more commonly met with in the treatment of functional nerve troubles. Mr. Braid[11] emphasized this fact when he said: "The oftener patients are hypnotized from association of ideas and habit, the more susceptible they become, and in this way they are liable to be affected entirely through the imagination. Thus, if they consider or imagine there is something doing, although they do not see it, from which they are to be affected, they will become affected; but, on the contrary, the most expert hypnotist in the world may exert all his endeavors in vain if the party does not expect it, and mentally and bodily comply, and thus yield to it." A trite application of this thought is the example of the patient who felt "better" as soon as the clinical thermometer had been placed under his tongue.

In the answers received to my inquiry in this research regarding therapeutic application, fully one-half of those who went at all into detail advocated the use of Coca for cases of

[10] Hunter; 1839. [11] Braid; p. 32; 1843.

neurasthenia, and for the various symptoms of nerve and muscle depression grouped under that title. The whole train of ills resulting from debility, exhaustion, overwork, or overstrain of nerve or mind, recalls the early designation given to the classification of this long group of symptoms by some of the European physicians as "the American disease," the derangement of an overworked and overhurrying people. The general advocacy of Coca for this condition indicates that the causes which tend to produce such derangement are not only important problems to the general practitioner throughout our country, but must be predominant factors wherever there is an impulse to supremacy. It makes little difference under just what name the symptoms may be treated so long as the patient shall be relieved of suffering.

There is a general idea in the minds of the laity which, unhappily, is also shared by some physicians, that to name a disease is far more important than its treatment. I well recall, when attending lectures upon medicine, how eager the first year students were to make notes of the various remedies which each lecturer might advocate for different conditions. It is a difficult task to fill such a therapeutic notebook, but far more difficult to find an appropriate application for the prescriptions suggested. Diseases are of necessity broadly taught in types, and treatment is wholly a result of judgment on the part of the individual practitioner. When a physician has advanced far enough in his struggles in medicine to realize how few specifics there are, he surely broadens himself by cutting loose from the narrow channels of thought he had originally traced in his early student days.

Dr. E. G. Janeway, in a paper before the New York Academy of Medicine, refers to this tendency to treat the name of a disease rather than the condition in the following anecdote:

"Shortly after my entrance into the profession, a fellow interne at the hospital was stricken with a fever, the supposed cause of which was found in the condition of his urine, which contained blood, albumen and casts, and the name of his malady was at this time nephritis. He was given podophyllin to keep his bowels relaxed, and was made to take a hot bath each day. At the expiration of ten days of this treatment, an examination showed an eruption. The name of the disease was changed to typhus fever; the cathartics were discontinued, and in their stead whiskey was ordered. No marked change was noted in his condition to call for the change in the treatment; it was simply dependent upon the mental conception of the requirements of typhus fever then in vogue."[12]

Probably the majority of the laity regard therapy from the standpoint of specifics. If a proper diagnosis has been made, the medicine for that particular disease should be readily forthcoming. If a given prescription does not afford the relief as speedily as anticipated, the thought is suggested that possibly an error has been made in diagnosis, and—particularly in the larger cities, this leads to a "going the rounds" from one physician to another in search of one who will know "the right medicine." Then again the ill commonly want a remedy which they can continue for some particular disease, rather than for any immediate condition. This unfortunate state of affairs is largely the fault of the physician in not educating his patients.

While summering in a small country town in the western part of New York State, a hearty Irishman, a farmer, called at my office and asked for: "A somethin' for a kauld," emphasizing his necessity by a gurgling cough that seemed to rattle from his boots up. On my asking him to step into the consulting room that I might see just what his condition was by an examination, he replied in astonishment:

"Examined, is it! Sure I've lived here for the last twinty-foive years, and never yet was examined for a kaff or a kauld!" And he very indignantly left my office to seek some one who would supply him with the needful mixture, for it had been the custom of his usual consultant to give a mixture which might delight the heart of a veterinarian, with some such assurance as he patted a bottle of prodigious size, as: "What ye don't take now will do agen."

If the practice of medicine includes instructing the community as to the limitations of physic, and the necessity for

[12] Janeway; Vol. XII, p. 79.

appropriate methods of living, as well as writing prescriptions or dispensing medicines, it would seem that a physician should take pride in teaching his individual patients. It is only by some such method, that in the process of time people will become educated sufficiently to value a conscientious opinion that there is absolutely no trouble and no need for treatment, as of greater monetary worth than a piece of paper ordering something to take to assure a fee.

Again, I would impress that in no condition that the physician is called upon to treat is it more necessary to instruct the patient and endeavor to awaken a personal interest and inspire confidence than in the treatment of neurasthenia. These cases, as a class, are so prone to try all sorts of remedies, that they lapse into a condition where it seems as though remedial measures were almost of no avail. Any physician who tries to cure such a patient by the simple administration of medicine alone, or by any one unaided method of local treatment, will find that he has not only a very serious, but hopeless, time-consuming task to perform. Personally I have run the gamut of—I might say, about all methods that have been advocated, and have learned by repeated disappointment how difficult it is to employ one plan. Each case must be studied and treated independently.

From being an early admirer of Dr. Beard's work, I undertook to follow his procedures, not only in medication but in topical treatment. At one time I used electricity very largely and employed the static machine with considerable advantage in some cases. In view of our present knowledge, I hardly believe it will be presumed that this machine simply "strikes awe to the patient," nor that "they see the wheels go round and feel better." With a desire to know more profoundly the rationale for success in this direction, I sought to learn from the manufacturer of my machine—who had also made the instrument used by Dr. Beard, in just what manner he applied it. I was assured that the handles of his electrodes were made large and long, yet, in spite of this, were frequently being broken. When a suitable case presented, after describing the proposed method of treatment, the patient was asked

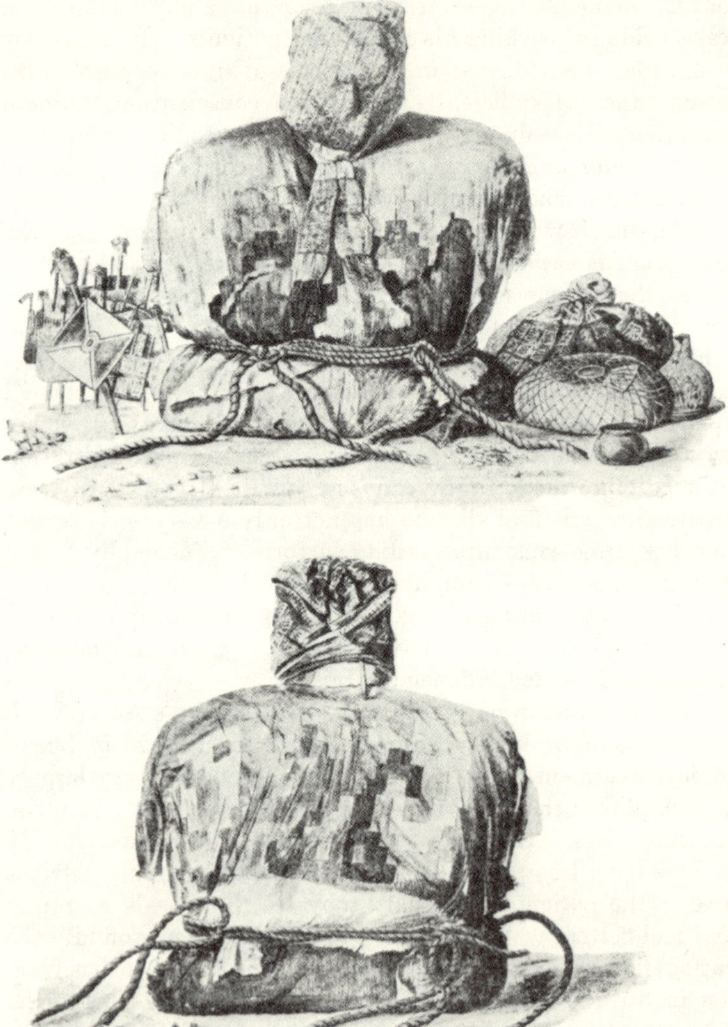

PERUVIAN FALSE HEAD MUMMY PACKS. [*Reiss and Stübel.*]

whether he wished to be cured immediately, or within a space of several months. As may be readily inferred, the majority of patients wished to be cured at once, and so treatment was commenced by a vigorous application of the electrode down the spine, in a manner which combined static sparks with massage in such vigorous blows as to account for the frequent breakage of handles. After this electric attack, the patient was usually quite resigned to accept treatment less severe, "even if it takes more time, doctor."

Here, then, was something of the personal not to be found in this author's works. A mild application of static electricity—that delightful aura—the gentle breeze of ozone which may be wafted from the wooden ball electrode is quite different from the more "magnetic method" described. And it was the method—the force perhaps, the personal magnetism at any rate which rendered the treatment successful.

Neurasthenia is a combination of many symptoms of very different nature; realizing this it is desirable to learn just what these symptoms may be, and whether they are pronouncedly mental or physical. An effort should be made, too, to learn something about the patient, as well as about the cause of complaint—about his work, ambition, hobbies and pleasures. Often these cases necessitate a gradual reparation of many functions before complete cure is to be hoped for, and this will necessitate time. Indeed, time alone with a case under appropriate guidance will work wonders. I usually advocate increasing the activity of the skin by a daily cold sponge bath, taken on rising. Patients quite commonly object to this—they "cannot stand the shock." But it is this very shock that is desirable when indicated. Judiciously used, the physician will find water one of the most useful measures in neurasthenic cases. Indeed, without being an advocate of any "pathy," I believe our friends, the hydropaths, certainly deserve much credit for popularizing so simple a remedy. I commonly advise, where there is any trouble with the digestive functions, the drinking of hot water after the method recommended by Dr. Salisbury and so ably advocated by Dr. Ephraim Cutter.

A glassful of water, as hot as can be borne, should be

slowly sipped while dressing. Where there is constipation the addition to this of a teaspoonful of Merck's dried sulphate of soda will bring the effects of the best of bitter waters of the German spas home. As to the action of this hot water drinking, I think it cannot be better explained than by repeating a conversation between two clergymen overheard while rummaging through the literary treasures of a book shop. One gentleman was extolling to the other, who was very deaf, the efficacy of drinking a glass of hot water before breakfast—not for deafness, however. To the subdued inquiry from the deaf gentleman as to how it worked, the other shouted: "Sort of washes out the insides," and perhaps this is as much as any of the advocates of this measure can say. It assists in dissolving and washing out the mucus from the stomach, and so prepares that organ for food after the prolonged stage of inactivity of the night.

A careful inquiry into the dietary of the patient and a proper regulation of that is always absolutely essential. Without any pet hobbies in this particular, I have often kept patients on an exclusive milk diet for months at a time, or again upon a diet of beef and hot water, at times associating with this a liberal supply of grapes. But fruit simply because it is fruit is a delusion as great as the brown bread of Dr. Graham—both should be taken guardedly and advisedly. I believe, with the late Dr. Fothergill, that usually sufferers from nervous troubles do not like fats, while at times they are great lovers of sweets, which by fermentation give an added discomfort. Physiology teaches us that the constituents of nerve cells are chiefly built up from fatty substances, and as the nerves will take from the other tissues it is very reasonable to understand that nervousness and mal-nutrition commonly go together.

Among these subjects the use of milk proves beneficial, because of the contained cream, which is the most easily digested of all fat. And when they will not, or imagine they cannot, drink milk, care should be taken that they shall be instructed how to use it. A patient confined to bed may put on flesh on an exclusive diet of two quarts of milk a day, but one that is up and about, engaged in mental or muscular labor, will require more than this amount.

Dr. Weir Mitchell[13] was an early advocate of absolute rest, enforced feeding, and passive exercise in these nervous cases, which is unquestionably the highest ideal treatment in certain forms of neurasthenia. But where the patient is not ill enough to be put to bed, or will not consent to undertake this ordeal, then the physician must endeavor as nearly as possible to imitate this method by regulating the diet, enforced feeding and massage. In the way of medication and as an adjunct to the food I know of no better remedy than Coca, preferably the original wine of Coca prepared by Mariani. In this the properties of Coca are appropriately preserved by some special method of manufacture, while the mild wine adds a temporary stimulation which is enhanced by the more permanent influence of the Coca.

Insomnia is very often an early, persistent and troublesome symptom to be combated. An exhaustion of the brain cells must be repaired just as are the cells of any of the other tissues, through rest and a healthful blood supply. Sleep is the natural rest for the brain, and without this sweet restorer there can be no recuperation from any nervous derangement. I disparage the use of the usual hypnotics and very rarely have recourse to them, except in an emergency—certainly not regularly in any one case. Yet our patients must sleep, and to establish the habit is going a long way toward ultimate cure. Coca, through its property of clearing the circulation, removes a source of irritation, and may ordinarily be relied upon to induce sleep. When more urgent measures are required the most magical benefit often follows the application of "wet pack." With a case of mania to treat, and with but one remedial measure to employ, I should rely by preference upon the wet pack. Admitting that at first it seems an almost suicidal undertaking to the patient and an alarming procedure to the patient's immediate family, who are anxiously looking on to see fair play, the result is all that could be hoped for. And it is for results that the physician's advice is asked.

[13] Mitchell; 1884.

To prepare a wet pack the bed is covered with a rubber sheet, and on this a blanket upon which is spread a sheet wrung out of cold water, say at 50° or 60° F. The patient is put naked on this wet sheet, which is quickly wrapped about and tucked in between the legs and arms, so that each limb and the trunk shall be separately enfolded. The underlying blanket is then wrapped about the wet sheet, a hot water bottle is put to the feet, and a cold towel applied to the head. In this condition the subject is permitted to remain from twenty minutes to one or two hours, according to indications. After the first annoyance of seeming imprisonment from the bindings the patient will not mind it any more than does an Indian papoose its wrappings, for pleasant sleep soon follows, or in any case there is a soothed and quieted condition. When the pack is taken off the subject is rubbed dry and tucked up snugly in a dry bed, quite prepared to enjoy a night's restful slumber.

There can be no greater mistake than to continue the use of bromides to allay nervous troubles without some other means added for strengthening the tissues. The bromides, as well as allaying peripheral irritation, always occasion marked depression. It was long since pointed out that Coca equalizes the various forces which constitute energy. A host of observers have remarked that Coca possesses the tranquilizing qualities of the bromides without the depressing effect,[14] and when it is considered necessary to give these salts this depression may be counteracted by Coca, which even dissipates the after effects of chloral, opium and alcohol.[15]

In the very nature of things, women are more commonly the sufferers from neurasthenia than are men, because as a rule women are less self-dependent. Formerly such a condition was termed hysteria, because it was supposedly only a disease of women, but since the group of symptoms which go to make up this condition have been more closely studied, they have been found quite as prevalent among men. It is only another instance of calling things by the wrong name. One who is diffident in society is often called nervous; a trem-

[14] Corning; p. 213; 1884. [15] *Idem;* p. 124; 1885.

bling old man is nervous; the timid child is nervous; the subject with a weak heart is nervous, as also is very probably the one whose stomach is distended with gas. We are apt to approach matters wrongly; as a result benefits are often lost. Drunkenness, for instance, has occasioned a fearful battle against alcohol, and millions of dollars had been spent to prove that alcohol caused people to be hopeless drunkards and wrecks, before it was learned that drunkenness may simply be a manifestation of a diseased nervous system, while alcohol is really a food often of timely benefit when rightly used.

Apropos of this thought, there comes to mind the instance of a recent interview of a professor in one of our leading colleges who, being interrogated as to his views regarding the researches of Professor Atwater of Wesleyan University on "The Nutritive Value of Alcohol," replied to the query whether he would class alcohol as a food: "If asked such a question by one of the laity I would reply no, but if asked by a scientist I must say yes." Unfortunately there is a tendency in some minds to jump at conclusions, and to this class the suggestion of food value seems to imply something which can take the place of beefsteak, while the facts of physiology clearly indicate the definition which I have formulated: *A food is any substance taken into the body which maintains integrity of the tissues and creates the energy we term life.* But this matter is more fully discussed in the chapter on dietetics.

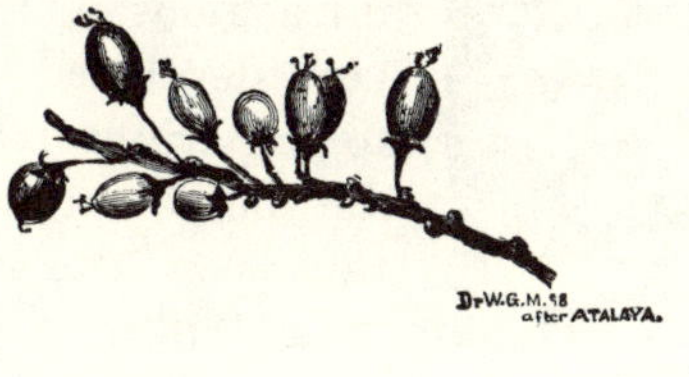

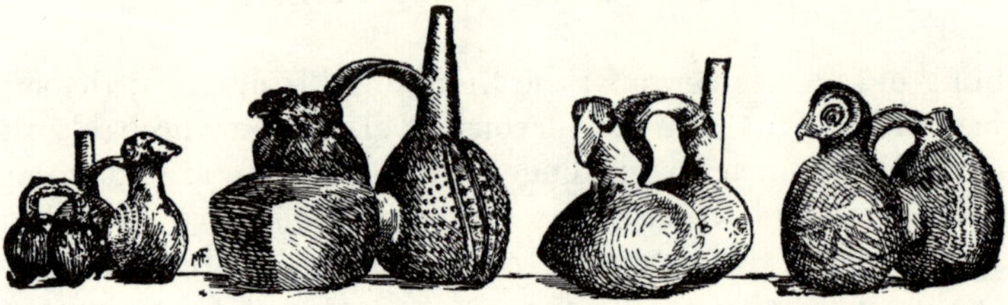

CHAPTER XIV.

THE PHYSIOLOGICAL ACTION OF COCA.

"Man's life, Sir, being
Too short, and then the way that leads unto
The knowledge of ourselves, so long and tedious,
Each minute should be precious."

—Fletcher, *The Elder Brother;* I, ii.

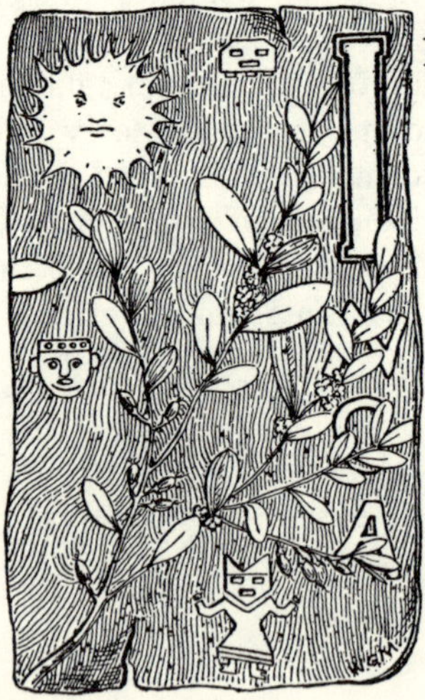

IN the study of any scientific problem the tales and traditions which associate it with an early race are always full of interest, for not infrequently there are hidden among simple and even homely usages suggestive hints. Influences which among a primitive people were regarded with superstitious awe, as of supposed miraculous origin, have often been developed by knowledge into important means. Many of the most useful inventions have thus been interpreted through the light of science. The amusing trifles of childhood's hour have become the absorbing powers of the present. Civilization has advanced by the adaption of primitive means. The history of applied science has shown this, and is paralleled in the art of medicine, which, while perhaps of slower growth, has evolved from primeval methods at first regarded as trivial and empirical, transformations of positive benefit.

If the history of any remedy be traced from its ancient uses it must be looked for amidst the fables and superstitions of the early people among whom it was associated. So closely allied has the practice of medicine been with the mysterious, that many still consider with Bacon, that: "Witches and impostors have always held a competition with physicians." There has ever been an association of caprice and prejudice in the application of any remedy. This is not merely due to an imperfect knowledge on the part of the physician, but to a false conception among the laity as to the action of medicines or of remedial measures. So when a prosaic real asserts itself over the false ideal, the result has often been an unfortunate scepticism. Science is but the outgrowth of truth, and truth must leave with the advance of time some record of its development.

Quinine came to us through the Incas, who had long been familiar with its uses before the advent of the Count of Chinchon, and although its introduction was clouded in mystery and prejudice, its application as a medicine has been none the less a benefit to millions of people. In the history of Coca, that shrub has been so intimately associated with the everyday customs of the simple people of its native land, that its actual merit remained uninvestigated for ages. For aside from the Spanish prejudice against its employment, the use of Coca was so general that any special effort to seriously study its true qualities seemed unnecessary.

There is a tendency in the human mind to jog along in beaten ruts of old familiar ways without questioning, and so we witness the shallowness of those who have grown up to blindly follow the methods of their predecessors, instead of shaping and adapting the suggestions of earlier times to modern requirements. The natural outgrowth from this spirit is a narrowness of mind which, while probably asserted to be conservatism, may often be regarded as merely ignorance. For example, one may have followed from childhood some certain religion, and yet know absolutely nothing of the doctrines advocated nor any individual reason for accepting them, yet would vigorously resent any innovation upon the customs that were so early grounded, although incapable of offering any plausible support for this narrowness of view. Such opposition is engendered of weakness, not of strength, it is not built upon true knowledge nor evolved from the logic of unbiased judgment. It is, as my preceptor, the famous anatomist, William Darling, would have said: "False and ridiculous—false because not founded upon fact, and ridiculous because contrary to reason."

Science does not advance a proposition which cannot be substantiated; hence the purest science is self-evident. It should be as clear and undisputable as Mark Twain would have the proof of Christian Science: "Capable of being read as well backwards as forwards, perpendicularly or sidewise, and bound to always come out the same."

There are relatively few physicians who can logically prove why they employ any certain method, yet these same practitioners would be quick to denounce any medicine used by others in a merely empirical way. The fact that the more familiar remedies are largely empirical has apparently not been recalled. The use of many modern medicines is a simple repetition of methods which have been continued from the traditions of antiquity. There are probably many who wield potent means who concern themselves little regarding the physiological action of opium or the salicylates, of iodide of potash, of quinine, or mercury, or a host of other drugs in everyday employment.

Even after having accepted a medicine for use the possibilities of its application are not always appreciated. Opium may be a laxative or an astringent, a stimulant or soporific, according to the method of its employment, nor are the whole benefits of the drug to be found in any one of its numerous alkaloids. A similar influence is more prominently manifest in the use of the various varieties of the Coca leaf, or even from the use of Coca of one variety in different preparations. Between such preparations and cocaine—which is commonly regarded as the sole active principle of Coca, the results are still more characteristic.

Linnæus considered that a medicine differed from a poison not so much in its nature as in its dose, and in this view food, medicine and poison may be considered as intimately allied to each other by indefinable gradations. A common example of this is illustrated in the use of certain condiments. Thus mustard, which, when applied in a small quantity to the food, gives a zest to the appetite, in a large dose acts as an irritant and provokes vomiting.

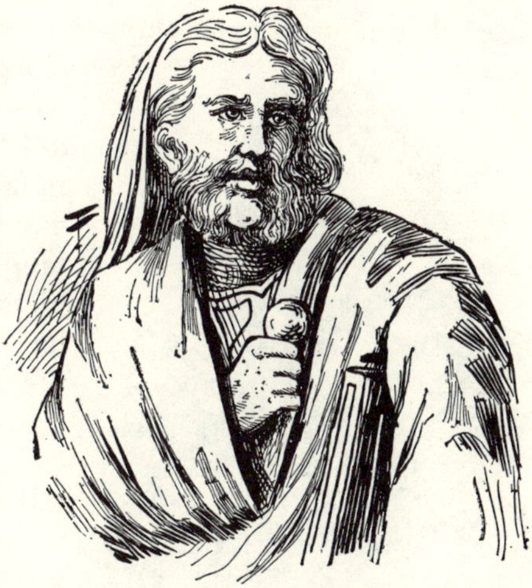

CLAUDIUS GALENUS.

It has been the aim of physiologists to learn the working of the human organism, and to trace through the tissues the influence of remedies in health as well as to understand their modified action in disease. The famous school of Alexandria, which flourished two centuries before Christ, may be regarded as giving the first inception to physiology, yet for centuries this science progressed only by slow stages. Herophilus and Erasistratus were permitted to practice vivisection upon criminals, an example which was followed by Fallopius. These experimenters did little more than examine the gross anatomy of parts, though Herophilus is considered to have been the first to describe the pulse. But there could be little done with the intricacies of physiology until minute anatomy was better understood.

Many of the early philosophers in medicine built theories which were blindly followed by their adherents, just as has been continued by their successors of the present. At the beginning of the Christian era Galen, following the doctrine of *pneuma*—which regarded life as a spirit, taught that the circulation was a sort of general respiration, the suction of air filling the vessels "with blood and spirits" and so causing the wave of pulse. He explained a multitude of qualities and varieties of the pulse, but his theories were so intermingled with superstition as to command little respect.

At the period when the Spanish were interested in the subject of conquests, anatomy and physiology was advancing along with the other sciences. Vesalius, who was physician to Charles the Fifth of Spain, in his researches pointed out many errors of Galen, and established the modern principles of anatomy, while Fallopius and Eustachius added the result of their investigations, and Porta and Kepler, following the earlier hints of Alhazen on refraction, laid a foundation for more perfect knowledge of the eye. The greatest impetus was given to physiology after Harvey made known his theory on the circulation of the blood, which he had built up from the researches of Bacon, the Spaniard Servetus, the Italian Columbus, the botanist Cæsalpinus, and other famous scholars of the school of Padua. This advance was supplemented by the work of Asellius on the lacteals, of Jean Pecquet on the chyle, of Rüdbeck on the lymph, and by the studies of Malpighi upon the capillaries and the process of oxygenation of the blood in the air cells. From this was gradually evolved our present knowledge regarding the assimilation and transference of food into nourishing blood.

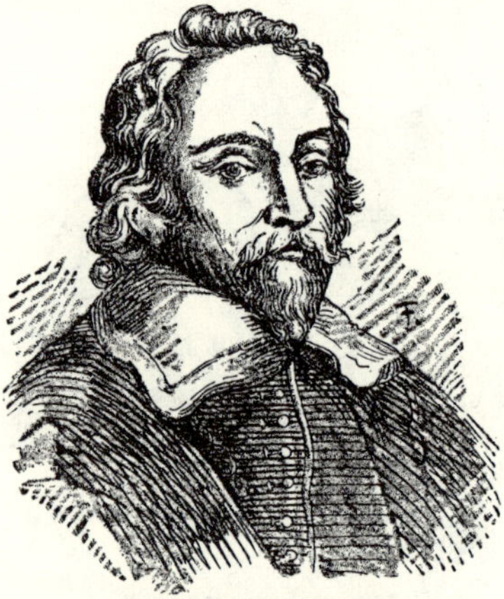

WILLIAM HARVEY.

Prior to this time it was not known how the tissues were constructed, nor what were the subtle processes of nourishment—aside from victuals. The science of physiology had only been dreamed of, and was slowly evolving from a belief in animal spirits and other vague controlling influences akin to the supernatural. The soul was regarded as the living force within the body, not only in stimulating the muscles to contract, but presiding over the secretions. Haller and John Hunter were the founders of comparative anatomy. The first was the originator of the doctrine of irritability, which he showed was not dependent upon the presence of the soul, and from this originated the experimentation which led to an understanding of the inherent contractile power of muscle when separated from its nerves.

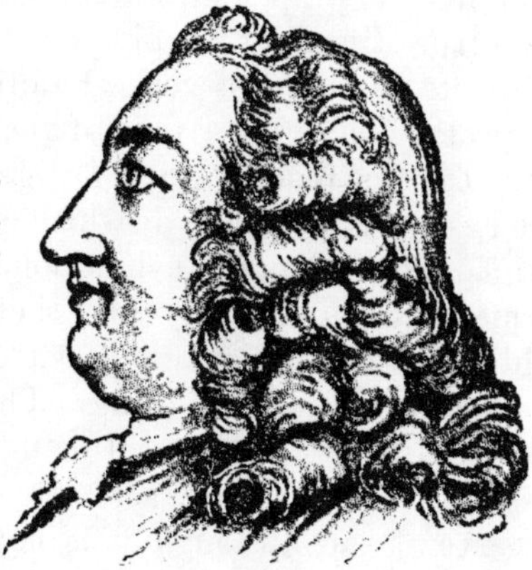

ALBERT HALLER.

Cullen, one of the greatest theorists in medicine, displayed an ingenious system of physiology. He supposed life to consist in an *excitement* of the nervous system, and especially of the brain, generating a *vital force* which diffused through the animal frame just as electricity prevails over nature. In addition to this force he inferred another which he termed *Vis Medicatrix Naturæ.* Through the interaction of both of these there must be maintained a balance to constitute health, while through their unequal activity the problem of disease was to be explained.[1] These teachings were modified by John Brown, who about the commencement of the nineteenth century was private secretary to Dr. Cullen. He taught that life is due to an excitability imparted to every man at his birth and that all disease must belong to either the *sthenic* or *asthenic* diathesis.

The misconception and confusion of the term stimulant originated from the teachings of those ancient philosophers who, in order to offer a physiological explanation for their theory of "vital force," established the supposition of an excitation of tissues from the irritation of stimulus, which they

[1] Cullen's *Physiology and Nosology;* Vol. I, p. 131.

presumed must necessarily be followed by depression. To this has been added a modern confusion through confounding stimulants with intoxicants, which is erroneous in fact. Quickly digested food is a stimulant, a cup of hot water slowly sipped may be a stimulant, and these or *any substance which increases natural action*—which is the true definition of stimulant—will not necessarily be followed by a period of depression corresponding to the previous sense of well being. Nor does a proper stimulant irritate to fretful excitement. The true stimulant simply rouses latent energies, which may be quite capable to work if only suitable impetus be given to promote activity. One of the most able writers upon this subject[2] has placed quickly digested and nutritious food at the head of stimulants, of which all other means can but be the faint reflex. Under such action, the pulse is given increased firmness without hurry and there is less feeling of fatigue, while a grateful warmth pervades the body, accompanied by a general sense of well being. These indeed are the physiological results of a good meal or may similarly follow from the use of Coca. These facts have been interpreted by many observers, and although it is not claimed that Coca replaces beefsteak, certainly it may in emergency act as a substitute for a more ample dietary, or may advantageously be used at other times to stimulate the assimilation and conversion of other food. It is the reconstructive action upon the tissues which forms one great benefit of the wide range of usefulness of Coca.

For more than three centuries the information that had come to the world in regard to Coca had been chiefly of a theoretical nature. The writings of travellers and of missionaries who were located in the sections of South America where Coca was used, had prepared the way for a scientific investigation of its properties as soon as there was a possibility of such work being done with exactitude. After the botanists had classified the plant, and chemists had begun to search for the hidden properties of its traditional action, the researches of the physiologists soon followed.

[2] Anstie; 1865.

In Europe the attention of the medical profession was directed to the action of Coca through a widely circulated paper by Dr. Mantegazza, who experimented upon himself, using the leaves both by chewing and in infusion. His description, while somewhat fanciful and full of imagination, fairly illustrates the physiological action of Coca, provided it is appreciated that observations made by an experimenter upon his own person are necessarily influenced by the temperament of the individual. He found from masticating a drachm of the dried leaves: "An aromatic taste in the mouth, an increased flow of saliva, and a feeling of comfort in the stomach, as though a frugal meal had been eaten with a good appetite." Following a second and a third dose there was a slight burning sensation in the mouth and pharynx with an increased pulse beat, while digestion seemed to be more active. Through the influence of Coca the entire muscular system is increased in strength with a feeling of agility and an impulse to exertion quite different from the exaltation following alcohol. While from the latter there may be increased activity, it will be of an irregular character, but Coca promotes a gradual augmenting of vigor with a desire to put this newly acquired strength in action. Mantegazza found that the intellectual sphere participates in the general exaltation produced by Coca, ideas flow with ease and regularity, the influence being quite different from that induced by alcohol and resembling in some degree that from small doses of opium. After drinking an infusion of four drachms of leaves he experienced a peculiar feeling as though isolated from the external world, with an irresistible inclination to exertion, which was per-

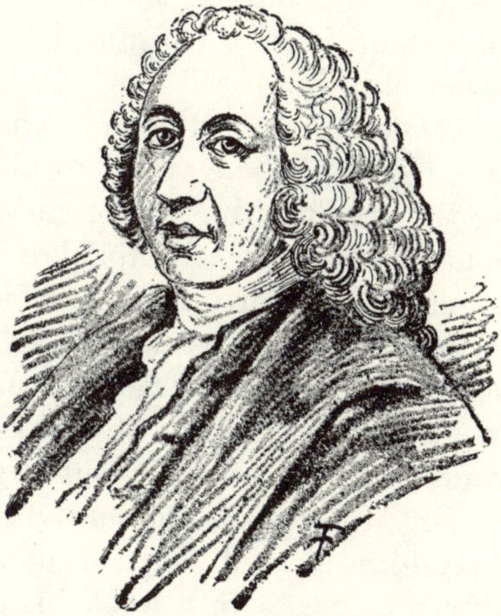

WILLIAM CULLEN.

formed with phenomenal ease, so that though in his normal condition he naturally avoided unnecessary exercise, he was now so agile as to jump upon the writing table, which he did without breaking the lamp or other objects upon it. Following this period of activity came a state of quietness accompanied by a feeling of intense comfort, consciousness being all the time perfectly clear. The experimenter took as much as eighteen drachms of leaves in one day, which is about the amount ordinarily consumed by the *Serrano* of the Andes. Under this increased dose the pulse was raised to one hundred and thirty-four, and when mental exhilaration was most intense he exclaimed to his colleagues who were watching the result of his investigation: "God is unjust because he has created man incapable to live forever happy."[3] And again: "I prefer a life of ten years with Coca to a life of a million centuries without Coca."[4] Following these experiments, during which he had abstained from any food but Coca for forty hours, he took a short sleep of three hours, from which he woke without any feeling of indisposition.

Dr. Mantegazza announced as a result of the studies made upon himself and verified upon other subjects that Coca, chewed or taken in a weak infusion, has a stimulating effect on the nerves of the stomach and facilitates digestion. That it increases the animal heat, and the frequency of the pulse and respiration. That it excites the nervous system in such a manner that the movements of the muscles are made with greater ease, after which it has a calming effect, while in large doses it may cause cerebral congestion and hallucinations. He asserted that: "The principal property of Coca, which is not to be found in any other remedy, consists in its exalting effect, calling out the power of the organism without leaving any sign of debility, in which respect Coca is one of the most powerful nervines and analeptics." From these conclusions he advocated the use of Coca in disorders of the alimentary tract, in debility following fevers, in anæmic conditions, in hysteria and hypochondriasis, even when the latter has increased to

[3] *"Iddio e ingiusto perche ho fatto l'nomo incapace di poter vivere sempre cocheando."*

[4] *"Io preferiseta una vitta di 10 anni con Coca che un di 1,000,000 secoli senza Coca."*

suicidal intent. He considered that Coca might be used with benefit in certain mental diseases where opium is commonly prescribed, and was convinced of its sedative effect in spinal irritation, idiopathic convulsions and nervous erethism, and suggested its use in the largest doses in cases of hydrophobia and tetanus.[5]

Some of the assertions of Mantegazza are directly opposed by our present knowledge of the action of Coca, particularly the observations as to its action on the heart and respiration. This is to be accounted for by the pronounced central action he observed, evidently prompted by a belief that the influence of Coca was primarily through the nervous system. It has been developed by more recent research that Coca has a direct action upon the muscular system. The action of Coca upon the heart is precisely as a regulator of that organ. If the heart's action is weak it is strengthened—if it is excessive the over-activity is toned down—if irregular the beat is made uniform. This indicates that Coca is a direct cardiac tonic. Let the heart be running riot in a palpitation from over-exertion and a teaspoonful of Mariani Thé—taken in a small cup of hot water—will speedily bring the heart's action to normal. This unique preparation of Coca is in the form of an agreeable fluid extract, said to represent in one part, two parts of the leaves, and presenting in concentrated form all the qualities of true Coca. It may be administered plain, or drunk as a tea with cream and sugar; in this latter form it has a taste resembling a rich English breakfast tea.

The especial influence of Coca upon the heart is alone sufficient to establish it as a remedy of phenomenal worth. Lieutenant Gibbs, U. S. N., from a personal experience with Coca in crossing the high passes of the Andes, considered the sustaining action of Coca in high altitudes due wholly to its enabling the heart muscle to perform the extra work then called forth.* Similar observations have been made by many travellers who have remarked the influence of Coca upon themselves. Recently Captain Zalinski, U. S. A.—who rendered the dynamite gun an effectual instrument of war—has been

[5] Mantegazza; 1859. * Gibbs; 1875.

experimenting upon a concentrated ration suitable for the army. In pursuing his studies under a severe test he submitted himself to the hardships of Andean travel, and through the high altitudes used Coca Thé and Coca Pâte prepared by Mariani, the timely use of which, he assured me, had supported his life through a serious ordeal.[6] Dr. Beverley Robinson, referring to the efficiency of heart tonics* has written: "Among well known cardiac tonics and stimulants for obtaining temporary good effects, at least, I know of no drug quite equal to Coca. Given in the form of wine or fluid extract, it does much, at times, to restore the heart muscle to its former tone." In this connection, Dr. Ephraim Cutter says: "Coca should be more used in heart failure from direct weakness, and in many cases might well replace the conventional digitalis which advances the treatment of heart disease no more than it was forty years ago."† Many physicians who have corresponded with me on the application of Coca have emphasized this influence from experiences in their practice. Coca is advocated to replace digitalis or to tone up the muscular structure of the heart after use of the latter, either employed alone or alternately with digitalis when that is considered essential.‡

The effect of Coca upon respiration is analogous to its action on the heart. It acts as a regulator, not increasing respiration, but giving force to the cycle—making inspiration deeper and expiration more complete.

The observations of Mantegazza were so soon followed by Niemann's researches upon cocaine, that the mistaken conception originated that the phenomenal activity of Coca had been discovered in that alkaloid, and subsequent physiological work was almost wholly carried out upon cocaine with the resultant neglect of the parent plant. The reports of many of the earlier experimenters, however, were so contradictory as to give rise to a suspicion whether cocaine had been used at all. But as the substance employed had been obtained from Coca leaves, and as the investigators were familiar with the methods

[6] Zalinski; *person. com.;* 1899. * Robinson, p. 238; 1867. † Cutter; 1898.
‡ See Heart, *Collective Investigation*, in Appendix.

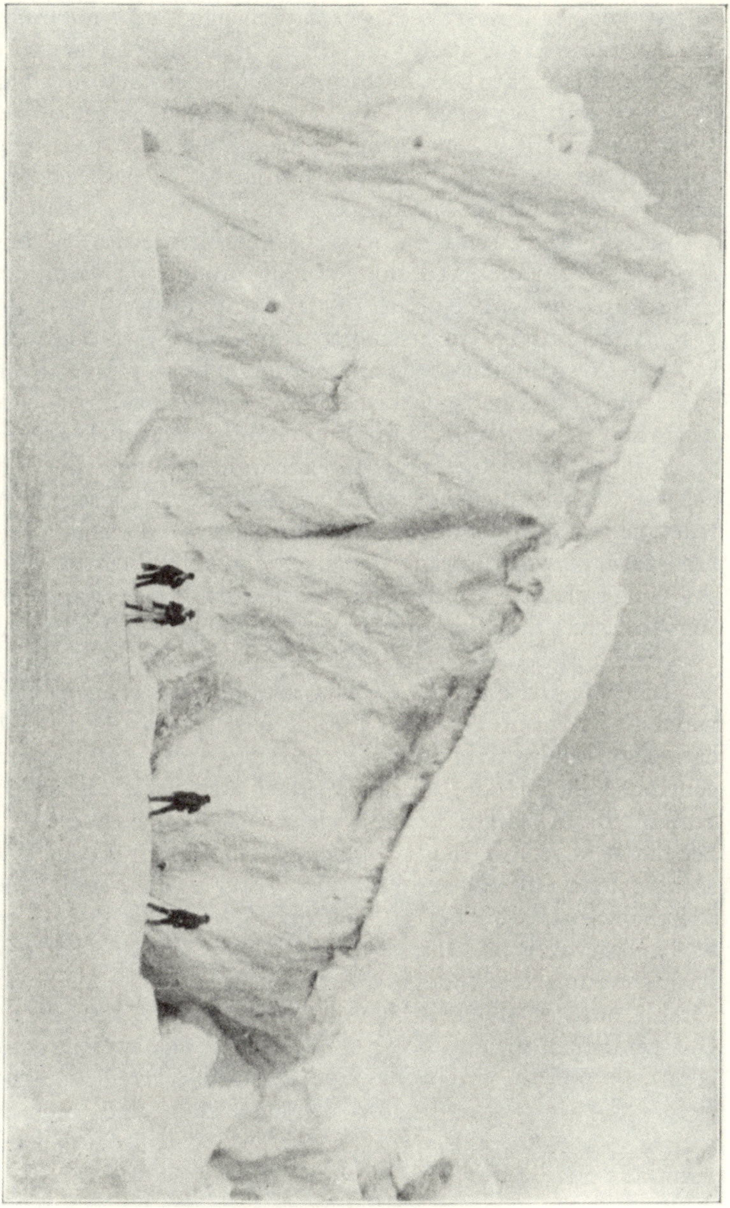

GLACIER ON MOUNT ANANEA, CORDILLERA OF ARICOMA, PERU. ALTITUDE, 17,000 FEET. [*From a Photograph.*]

of physiological research, this variation suggested some probable difference in the quality of cocaine used, which it was presumed was brought about in the process of manufacture. This varying result has since been shown to have been occasioned by a mixture, in various proportions, of the Coca bases contained in the earlier specimens of cocaine, before they had been appreciated as distinct products.

Schroff was one of the first to experiment with the new alkaloid. He observed that cocaine produces a slight anæsthesia of the tongue, and gives an agreeable sense of lightness of the mind with a condition of cheerfulness and well being, followed by lassitude and an inclination to sleep. From augmented doses he remarked giddiness, buzzing in the ears, dilatation of the pupils, impaired accommodation, headache, restlessness, and a feeling as though walking upon air. The heart was first quickened and then retarded. There was no reaction from the motor nerves, and the respiration was lowered from smaller doses.[7] Demarle, who experimented about the same time with Coca, remarked the anæsthesia from chewing the leaves and the dilatation of the pupils noticed in his own person.[8]

In 1865, Dr. Fauvel, of Paris, used a preparation of Coca which had been prepared for him by Mariani as a local application, to relieve pain in the larynx, and this treatment was continued in England by Dr. Morrell Mackenzie and in the United States by Dr. Louis Elsberg, who had remarked the beneficial effects of this application in Fauvel's clinic. It seems remarkable that no general use was made of this anæsthetic property for nearly a quarter of a century after these early observations until cocaine was adapted by Dr. Carl Koller to the surgery of the eye. A great many erroneous accounts of this adaptation have been published, but I am assured this gentleman never wrote nor authorized any writing upon cocaine except the preliminary paper and his principal paper before the *Gesellschaft der Arzte* at Vienna, and later his article in the *Reference Handbook*,[9] but in none of these is given the details which led to the surgical uses of cocaine.

[7] Schroff; 1862. [8] Demarle; 1862.
[9] *Reference Handbook of Medical Sciences*, Vol. IX, p. 175; New York, 1894.

At the period of his experiments Dr. Koller was *Sekundärarzt,* or house surgeon, on the staff of the *k. k. Allgemeinen Krankenhauses,* the largest hospital of Vienna, which serves also as a clinic for the medical faculty of the University. Through his connection with Professor Stricker he had been interested in experimental physiology and pathology and had made considerable research in the action of poisons upon the circulation. His investigations upon cocaine were therefore in a similar nature to those with which he was familiar. In August, 1884, Dr. Sigmund Freud and Dr. Joseph Breuer, of the University of Vienna, treated a prominent physiologist for morphinism by the use of cocaine, which had about then been prominently advocated in American literature. Several of the hospital staff were induced to try the effects of the alkaloid upon themselves. Among these was Dr. Koller, who, from a dose of the salt taken internally, remarked the benumbing action upon the tongue which had already been recorded by other observers. He had before been looking for a local anæsthetic, and with this in view had experimented with morphine, chloral, the bromides, and a number of other substances, so when he experienced the numbness from cocaine he realized he had found the sought-for anæsthetic, and experimented to determine its utility in ophthalmology.

It has been asserted that this discovery was made accidentally, and the story is related that a student had in mistake applied a solution of cocaine to the eye of a friend, when instead of the irritation feared from this carelessness, the property of dilatation and anæsthesia was found. Dilatation of the pupil had previously been noted from cocaine, but anæsthesia could hardly be observed accidentally, and, indeed, was determined not by local but by physiological experimentation. It had been known that the action of Coca through the circulation contracts the peripheral arteries, also that it dilates the pupil. Tschudi wrote: "After mastication of a great quantity of the Coca the eye seems unable to bear light and there is marked distention of the pupil."[10] An effect which had also been noted by many other observers.[11]

[10] Tschudi; 1840. [11] Schroff; 1862. Ott; 1876. Anrep; 1880.

Koller's experiments were carried out in the laboratory of Professor Stricker upon guinea pigs. It was found that a minute quantity of a solution of hydrochlorate of cocaine dropped in the conjunctival sac, produced such complete local anæsthesia that the cornea could be irritated with needles and electric currents and cauterized with nitrate of silver until it became opalescent. This experiment suggested that anæsthesia was not merely upon the surface but involved the entire thickness of the cornea. After experimenting upon animals the investigator applied cocaine to his own eye and examined the efficiency of the anæsthetic in diseased eyes. A preliminary paper upon the result of this discovery was sent to the annual meeting of the *Deutsche Ophthalmologiche Gesellschaft*, held at Heidelberg Sept. 15-16, 1884, which was read by Dr. Brettauer of Trieste. With this paper was a vial containing a few grammes of cocaine, which was all of the alkaloid that Merck could furnish at that time.[12] Meantime Koller continued his experiments and asked specialists in other departments to employ the alkaloid in their practice, for though satisfied that he had found a local anæsthetic adapted to the surgery of the eye, he believed that it was also suited to other special uses, a fact soon confirmed by several observers who based their researches upon this original investigation. This, briefly, is the story of the adaptation of this alkaloid of Coca to minor surgery, which is modestly all the merit of "discovery" that is claimed by the one through whom cocaine has been made a boon to suffering humanity, fully as important, and in many cases superior to the great anæsthetics, chloroform and ether.

When a two per cent. solution of cocaine is applied to the eye there is at first a slight irritation, followed by a drying of the secretions. The pupil is dilated and the eye has a staring look, occasioned from a wider opening of the lids. Anæsthesia continues for about ten minutes, followed by a stage of reduced sensibility, slowly passing into the normal condition. Dilatation reaches the highest stage within the first hour, decreases considerably in the second hour, and then soon dis-

[12] Koller; *person. com.*; Aug. 25; 1899.

appears entirely. The pupil is never at a maximum dilatation; that is, it may always be further dilated with atropine, and still responds to light and convergence. The dilating power of cocaine combined with atropine is invaluable when used in cases of iritis, the combination counteracting both the muscular spasm and the local congestion. In this condition Koller uses equal parts of a five per cent. solution of hydrochlorate of cocaine, with a one per cent. solution of sulphate of atropine. After the dilatation following a few applications the solution is used three times a day.

At first it was supposed that local anæsthesia from cocaine was due to anæmia of the minute vessels, but it was found that though anæmia followed an application of the alkaloid the anæsthesia preceded this influence.[13] That the benumbing action was not only local but might be general through the circulation was subsequently shown by the subcutaneous injection of a solution of the salt. Half a grain of hydrochlorate of cocaine so used occasioned a slight general anæsthesia,[14] while repeated injections of small doses caused a general reduction of tactile sensibility, with the sensation as though standing on cushions.[15] This was similar to the floating in the air experience of Mantegazza from large doses of Coca, and is in accord with the observation of Schroff with cocaine. The symptom is due to a lessened power of conduction in the cord.

From an injection of 0.001 gramme of hydrochlorate of cocaine under the skin of the abdomen of a monkey, not only local but general anæsthesia was produced which lasted for eighteen minutes without loss of consciousness.[16] It has been suggested that absence of tactile sensibility may give rise to the impression in the observer that consciousness in the subject is lost. From the fact that a subcutaneous injection of cocaine at any point eases pain, it has been presumed that the action must be central as well as local.[17] But general anæsthesia has been shown to follow only from very large doses.[18] While diminished sensibility may presumably be induced from a central cause,[19] the fact has been pointed out that lessened conduction in the cord is a more potent factor in

[13] Alms; 1886. [14] Da Costa; 1884. [15] Hepburn; 1884. [16] Grasset; 1884. [17] Livierato; 1885. [18] Laffont; 1887. [19] Laborde; 1885.

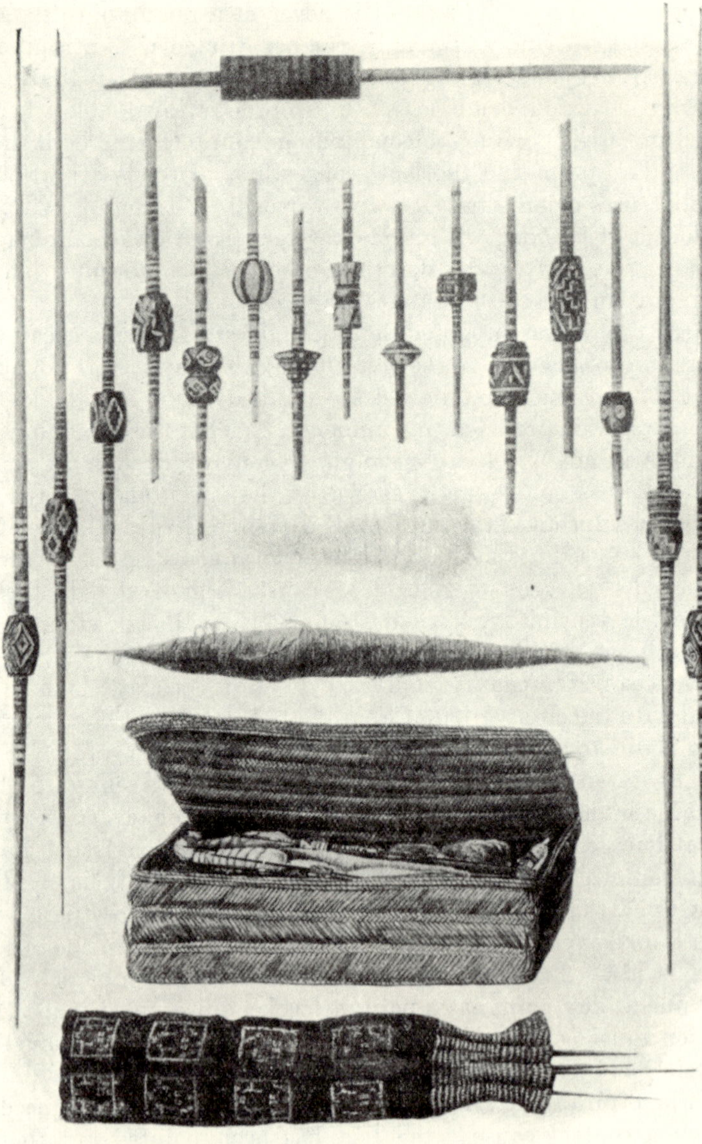

INCAN SPINNING SPINDLES AND WORK BASKET. [*Reiss and Stübel.*]

diminishing the general sensibility than any narcotic action upon the brain.[20]

Cocaine has not only the property of exciting the brain, but the special senses may be inhibited by a dose sufficient to paralyze their terminal nerve endings. Thus powdered hydrochlorate of cocaine blown into the nostrils first occasions increase and then total abolition of the sense of smell.[21] Koller observed that an injection of cocaine solution in the orbit occasioned loss of light in an eye he was about to remove.

It has been remarked by physiologists in experimenting with alkaloids that there is a relation between the constitution of the chemical molecule and the physiological action. The introduction of methyl into the molecule of strychnine, brucine and thebaine changes the convulsive action of these substances on the spinal cord to a paralyzing one exerted on the ends of the motor nerves.[22] Probably any of the organic alkaloids in which methyl and ethyl enter would paralyze both muscle and nerve, the latter before the former, the symptoms varying in accordance with the order in which different parts of the nervous system may be affected. The activity depends also upon the affinity which the substance may have for certain tissues which through alteration of function may affect the organism, and this accounts for the difference manifest between a large and a small dose. This is illustrated by atropine and by curare, either of which paralyze motor nerves, but while a very large dose of curare is necessary to paralyze the cardiac and vascular nerves a small dose paralyzes the nerves going to the muscles. On the other hand, an enormous dose of atropine is required to paralyze the motor nerves, but a very small dose is sufficient to affect the nerves of the heart and other involuntary muscles, and thus we get rapid circulation, dilated pupil and restless delirium.[23] The influence of these radicals in the Coca bases has already been referred to.*

The researches of several investigators indicate that cocaine is a protoplasmic poison, first stimulating, then paralyzing the vital functions, but it is possible to regulate this action

[20] Stockman; 1889. [21] Zwaardemaker; 1889. [22] Brunton; p. 50; 1885.
[23] *Idem;* p. 48. * See also Ehrlich; 1890; and Poulsson; 1892.

so that the functions may be either increased or held in check even in minute organisms. The motion of amœbæ in normal salt solution was stopped by a two per cent. solution of cocaine and the movement of spermatozoids and of ciliated cells was checked by stronger solutions.[24] Claude Bernard long since explained that cell metabolism in the lower organisms—in which the contractile protoplasm fulfills both the function of nerve and of muscle—may be suppressed by chloroform narcosis, the phenomenon being identical with that observed in anæsthesia of animals. In such anæsthesia there is inhibition of cell activity and not necessarily death of cell substance. He has shown by experiment upon plants that while growth and cell division ceases when under the influence of the anæsthetic, vitality is resumed when the plant is again under normal healthful conditions.[25] This influence follows upon the use of cocaine. The cell life is first stimulated and if the dose is increased there is inhibition, but activity is resumed upon the withdrawal of the drug. Similar results were obtained in my research made in the laboratory of the botanical department of Columbia University. It was found that both Coca and cocaine have a marked stimulating influence upon the lower organisms.[26]

My experiments were made with *infusoria*, yeast, *penicillium* and the aquatic plant *Elodea*, which latter forms a common substance for illustrating in the laboratory the effect of metabolism as represented by the bubbles of oxygen given off under the action of various stimuli. Portions of this plant exposed in test tubes to similar conditions of water, temperature and sunlight exhibited under the influence of Coca a stimulated metabolism as shown by the relative increase of bubbles, from twenty in twenty-eight seconds in the standard, to twenty in seven seconds in the tubes to which small portions of Coca Thé or solution of cocaine had been added. A similar result was obtained from the increased growth of the yeast plant in a solution of sugar, as indicated by the decomposition of the carbohydrate.

[24] Albertoni; 1890. [25] Bernard; 1879.

[26] In these experiments I used Coca Thé and Wine of Coca of Mariani, hydrochlorate of cocaine of Boehringer and Soehne, and cocaine of Merck.

In each of four graduated test tubes there was placed fifteen cubic centimetres of a solution of sugar and yeast. One of these was left normal. To the others there was added respectively one, two and three cubic centimetres of a one per cent. solution of cocaine. The relative activity of metabolism was increased above the standard, twenty-five per cent., fifty per cent., and twenty-five per cent., the latter indicating the excitation limit for these particular organisms had been passed.

In studying the growth of *penicillium,* upon which Dr. Curtis was then engaged in making an exhaustive series of experiments upon turgor, I had the privilege of examining specimens prepared by this skilled microscopist of drop cultures growing in a nutrient solution. There was a very marked influence to be seen in the rapidity of growth, which was readily measured under the microscope and compared with similar specimens to which no Coca had been added.

The influence of cocaine upon sensory nerves may be effected not only by local application but by a direct application to the nerve trunks, and even by an application to the nerve centres in the cortex.[27] In 1885 Dr. Corning experimented with anæsthetization of the spinal cord, and injected thirty minims of a three per cent. solution of hydrochlorate of cocaine between the spinous processes of the lower dorsal vertebræ in a subject suffering from spinal weakness. Sensibility was impaired in the lower limbs and the patellar reflexes were abolished. There was but slight dilatation of the pupils and no inco-ordination or motor impairment discernible, but the patient experienced dizziness while standing and was mentally exhilarated.[28] Dr. Bier of Kiel has recently suggested a general anæsthesia from cocaine by injecting by means of a Pravaz syringe from three to five cubic centimetres of a one per cent. solution of hydrochlorate of cocaine directly into the vertebral canal. Following the injection complete anæsthesia of the lower limbs took place within eight minutes, gradually mounting as high as the nipple; complete insensibility to pain lasted about forty-five minutes. The serious nature of this

[27] Tumass; 1887. [28] Corning; p. 91; 1885.

procedure is sufficient to condemn the process for general use, in view of less dangerous methods.

It has been suggested that as the local influence of cocaine in moderate doses is chiefly exerted upon sensory nerves, large doses occasion a sensory paralysis which may even extend to the motor branches.[29] It has been shown, however, that the motor terminals are only indirectly paralyzed either through an anæsthetic action upon the skin or from an action upon the muscle through which the nerve passes, and in this way the motor nerves may be affected.[30] A number of observers have found, from experiments upon lower animals, the motor nerves depressed,[31] or a diminution of muscle irritability[32] from cocaine only after very large doses, while others have observed muscular paralysis without previous stimulation.[33] But as alteration of sensibility always precedes the symptom of motor paralysis, the apparent lack of motion may be attributed to the former cause. Thus, Mosso describes having pressed his whole weight on the foot of a dog under the influence of a large dose of cocaine, without causing movement. Other observers have failed to note any direct effect upon muscle from cocaine.[34] The action of cocaine seems more pronouncedly upon the central nervous system, while the properties of Coca appear to be controlled by its associate alkaloids to affect muscle as well as nerve. The influence of Coca to excite muscle to energy is probably due to a direct chemical action toward the construction of proteid, as well as through the excitation of the hypothetical ferment of the contractile element, as has already been explained in the chapter upon muscle. The pronounced bearing which the associate alkaloids of Coca may exert, to maintain the balance of energy in favor of the leaf above one of its alkaloids, may be appreciated from a consideration of the distinctive physiological action of several of the more important active principles of Coca.

A physiological study of all the Coca products has not been

[29] Anrep; 1880. [30] Alms; 1886.
[31] Moréno y Maïz; 1868. Buchheim and Eisenmenger; 1870. Anrep; 1880. Mosso; 1887, *et al.*
[32] Biggs; 1885. Alms; 1886. Tumass; 1887. Stockmann; 1889, *et al.*
[33] Danini; 1873. Berthold; 1885. Sighicilli; 1885.
[34] Anrep; 1880. Kobert; 1882. Stockmann; 1889.

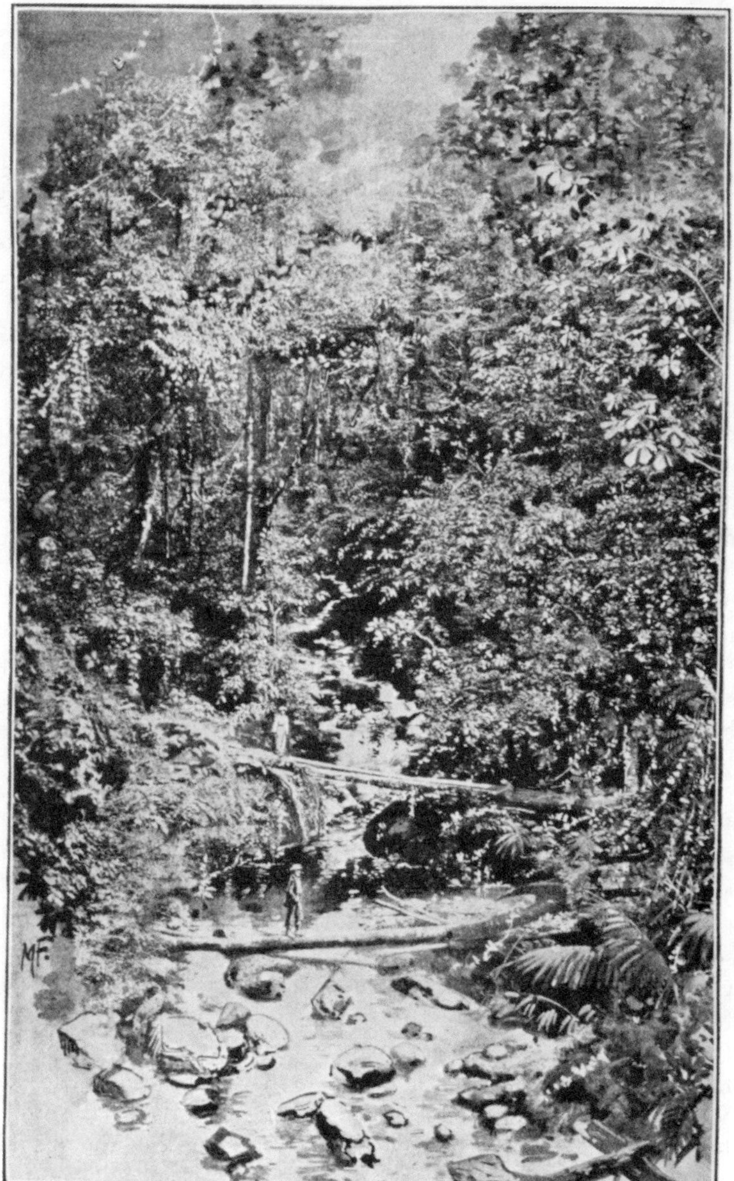

In the Heart of the Eastern Montaña. [*From a Photograph.*]

made, but Professor Ralph Stockmann* instituted an important research in this direction at the University of Edinburgh. From these experiments, it has been shown that the action of certain of the Coca alkaloids is directly upon muscular tissue; notably among these may be mentioned *ecognine, benzoyl-ecognine, cocamine* and *hygrine.* The influence of *ecgonine* upon the central nervous system is so mild that only large doses occasion slight depression, followed by increase of reflex irritability of the spinal cord which may last for several days. The substance has no anæsthetic properties, and the motor nerves are not specially influenced. There is, however, a lessening of the irritability of muscles, those having the largest blood supply being most deeply affected. When the drug was pushed to poisonous doses death followed from extension of the rigor mortis to a large number of muscles. The effect of *benzoyl-ecgonine* is directly upon muscle in a manner somewhat similar to caffeine, inasmuch as it provokes a muscular stiffness; this was followed, as late as the third or fourth day, by a slight increase in reflex excitability which upon increase of the drug tended to tetanus. This late manifestation of spinal symptoms is due to the fact that benzoyl-ecgonine has so great an affinity for muscle, that it is imbibed by adjacent muscles so thoroughly that the more distant structures receive at first very little of the drug. Non-striped muscle is not so much affected, and the heart is less involved. In cats one gramme (15.43 grains), occasioned dilatation of the pupils, great increase of the reflexes, and diarrhœa. From a poisonous dose death followed when a large number of muscles were affected, or after the spinal symptoms had been severe and long continued. The post mortem appearance revealed the remarkable influence of this alkaloid upon muscle by pronounced contractions of the intestines and bladder. *Cocamine,* which is a local anæsthetic, bears a nearer resemblance to cocaine in its action than do the other Coca alkaloids. While it exhibits the effect of a general stimulant its action is so specifically upon muscle that its influence on the spinal cord is masked. Administered to a frog the animal became

* See also Poulsson; 1892.

alert, excited, restless, and leaped in excess of its usual performance. There was an increase of the reflexes, and the signs of nervous and muscular symptoms continued for several days. The pupils, at first dilated, under an excessive dose became extremely small. The condition of the motor nerves and spinal cord was practically the same as in cocaine poisoning, though the motor nerves were more profoundly influenced. The nervous system was only affected after the alkaloid had left the muscle and entered the circulation. Cocamine, which is more lethal than is cocaine, when given in a small dose to a cat, occasioned excitement, dilatation of the pupils, twitching of the tail, ears, etc., while an increased dose caused muscular and nervous depression, vomiting, diarrhœa and weakness of gait, all of muscular origin. Death followed many hours after administration of a poisonous dose, and resulted either from rigor mortis of the respiratory muscles, or when more rapid from paralysis of the respiratory center. Post mortem there was constriction of the stomach, intestines and bladder so strongly marked as to cause hour-glass contraction. *Hygrine,* injected under the skin of a frog, occasioned depression, weakness in gait and dullness for a day or two, with tendency to starting and tremors. Its probable effect upon muscle was shown after death by hyperæmic spots, scattered throughout the muscular structure and serous membranes, where it had been carried by the circulation. Locally, to the experimenter's tongue, hygrine caused burning and tingling, the former soon passing off, but the latter lasting for an hour.

Stockmann, in experiments upon the frog, using Merck's *hydrochlorate of cocaine,* verified, or rather harmonized the accounts of numerous earlier investigators. He found that cocaine in a moderate dose created a slight torpor with depression of both brain and spinal cord, the symptoms being of sensory rather than of motor depression. The pupils were dilated. There was no stage of excitement. Under an increased dose these conditions were all exaggerated, particularly the reflex to sensory impressions, which now resembled those present in a late stage of strychnine poisoning. With excessive doses there was sensory and motor paralysis, and the pupils were contracted to mere slits. The spinal cord seemed to be given an increased excitability, its discharges being rapid, while it appeared less sensitive to stimuli from the skin and was readily exhausted. In rabbits, it was found that the convulsions occurring in cocaine poisoning could be prevented by artificial respiration.

In considering the action of any of the Coca alkaloids on man, it may be well to suggest that possibly one cause of conflicting testimony may have resulted from reporting the influence of the alkaloid upon animals, the effects of which are not always uniform with their action on man. In experiments upon animals those symptoms which follow doses full enough to create some outward sign are alone seen, while the agreeable exaltation such as would be experienced in man from a relatively much smaller dose can not be appreciated. A dose of cocaine which in one of the lower animals would cause depression, would under the controlling influence of a greater cerebral development in man occasion exhilaration, an effect probably resulting from inhibition of certain of the brain cells, thus inducing slight loss of co-ordination similar to that following a small dose of opium or alcohol. Both alcohol and opium seriously disturb the normal relations of one part of the brain with another, the nerve centers being paralyzed in the inverse order of their development. The primary exhilaration being succeeded by a narcotic action when the inhibitory paralysis permits the emotions full sway. Coca, however, appears to stimulate the brain by an harmonious influence on all the brain cells so the relation of its functions is not deranged.

The action of cocaine has been placed midway between morphine and caffeine. In man the initial effect of Coca is sedative, followed by a rapidly succeeding and long continued stimulation. This may be attributed to the conjoined influence of the associate alkaloids upon the spinal cord and brain, whereby the conducting powers of the spinal cord are more depressed than are the brain centers. In view of these physiological facts it is unscientific to regard strychnine as an equivalent stimulant to Coca or a remedy which may fulfill the same indications, as erroneously suggested by several correspondents. For immediate stimulation Coca is best administered as a wine, the mild exhilaration of the spirit giving place to the sustaining action of Coca without depression.

The action of Coca and cocaine, while similar, is different. Each gives a peculiar sense of well being, but cocaine affects the central nervous system more pronouncedly than does Coca, not—as commonly presumed—because it is Coca in a more concentrated form, but because the associate sub-

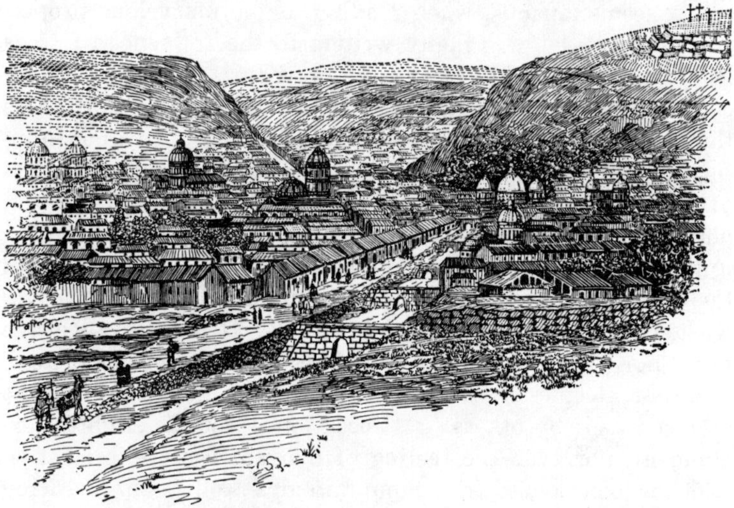

THE MODERN CITY OF CUZCO. [See page 145.]

stances present in Coca, which are important in modifying its action, are not present in cocaine. The sustaining influence of Coca has been asserted to be due to its anæsthetic action on the stomach,[35] and to its stimulating effect on brain and nervous system. But the strength-giving properties of Coca, aside from mild stimulation to the central nervous system, are embodied in its associate alkaloids, which directly bear upon the muscular system, as well as the depurative influence which Coca has upon the blood, freeing it from the products of tissue waste. The quality of Coca we have seen is governed by the variety of the leaf, and its action is in-

[35] Gazeau; 1870.

fluenced by the relative proportion of associate alkaloids present. If these be chiefly cocaine or its homologues the influence is central, while if the predominant alkaloids are cocamine or benzoyl ecgonine, there will be more pronounced influence on muscle. When the associate bodies are present in such proportion as to maintain a balance between the action upon the nervous system and the conjoined action upon the muscular system, the effect of Coca is one of general invigoration.

It seems curious, when reading of the marvelous properties attributed by so many writers to the influence of Coca leaves, that one familiar with the procedure of the physiological laboratory should have arrived at any such conclusion as that of Dowdeswell, who experimented with Coca upon himself. After a preliminary observation to determine the effect of food and exercise he used Coca "in all forms, solid, liquid, hot and cold, at all hours, from seven o'clock in the morning until one or two o'clock at night, fasting and after eating, in the course of a month probably consuming a pound of leaves without producing any decided effect." It did not affect his pupil nor the state of his skin. It occasioned neither drowsiness nor sleeplessness, and none of those subjective effects ascribed to it by others. "It occasioned not the slightest excitement, nor even the feeling of buoyancy and exhilaration which is experienced from mountain air or a draught of spring water." His conclusion from this was that Coca was without therapeutic or popular value, and presumed: "The subjective effects asserted may be curious nervous idiosyncrasies."[36] This paper, coming so soon after the publication of a previous series of erroneous conclusions made by Alexander Bennett,[37] created a certain prejudice against Coca. Theine, caffeine and theobromine having been proved to be allied substances, this experimenter proceeded to show that cocaine belonged to the same group. As a result of his research he determined that "the action of cocaine upon the eye was to *contract* the pupil similar to caffeine," while the latter alkaloid he asserted was a *local* anæsthetic; observations which have never been con-

[36] Dowdeswell; 1876. [37] Bennett; 1873.

firmed by other observers. In view of our present knowledge of the Coca alkaloids, it seems possible that these experiments may have been made with an impure product in which benzoyl-ecgonine was the more prominent base. However, the absolute error of Bennett's conclusions has been handed down as though fact, and his findings have been unfortunately quoted by many writers, and even crept into the authoritative books. Thus Ziemssen's *Cyclopædia of the Practice of Medicine*, which is looked upon as a standard by thousands of American physicians, quotes Bennett in saying: "Guaranine and cocaine are nearly, if not quite, identical in their action with theine, caffeine and theobromine."[38] The *National Dispensatory* refers to the use of Coca in Peru as being similar to the use of Chinese tea elsewhere—as a mild stimulant and diaphoretic and an aid to digestion—which are mainly the properties of coffee, chocolate and guarana, and Bennett is quoted to prove that the active constituents of all these products: "Although unlike one another and procured from totally different sources possess in common prominent principles, and are not only almost identical in chemical composition, but also appear similar in physiological action."[39] These statements, which are diametrically opposed to the present accepted facts concerning Coca, are not merely a variance of opinion among different observers, but are the careless continuance of early errors, and suggest the long dormant stage in which Coca has remained, and has consequently been falsely represented and taught through sources presumably authentic.

As may be inferred from its physiological action, Coca as a remedial agent is adapted to a wide sphere of usefulness, and if we accept the hypothesis that the influence of Coca is to free the blood from waste and to repair tissue, we have a ready explanation of its action.[40] Bartholow says:[41] "It is probable that some of the constituents of Coca are utilized in the economy as food, and that the retardation of tissue-waste is not the sole reason why work may be done by its use which can not be done by the same person without it." Stockmann considers that the source of endurance from Coca can hardly

[38] Vol. XVIII; p. 181. [39] *National Dispensatory;* 5 ed.; 1896.
[40] See page 371. [41] Bartholow, p. 467; 1885.

depend solely upon the stimulation of the nervous system, but that there must at the same time be an economizing in the bodily exchange. An idea which is further confirmed by the total absence of emaciation or other injurious consequences in the Indians who constantly use Coca. He suggests that Coca may possibly diminish the consumption of carbohydrates by the muscles during exertion. If this is so, then less oxygen would be required, and there is an explanation of the influence of Coca in relieving breathlessness in ascending mountains.

Prominent in the application of Coca is its antagonism to the alcohol and opium habit. Freud, of Vienna, considers that Coca not only allays the craving for morphine, but that relapses do not occur. Coca certainly will check the muscle racking pains incidental to abandonment of opium by an habitué, and its use is well indicated in the condition following the abuse of alcohol when the stomach can not digest food. It not only allays the necessity for food, but removes the distressing nervous phenomena. Dr. Bauduy, of St. Louis, early called the attention of the American Neurological Association to the efficiency of Coca in the treatment of melancholia, and the benefit of Coca in a long list of nervous or nerveless conditions has been extolled by a host of physicians.[42] Shoemaker, of Philadelphia, has advocated the external use of Coca in eczema, dermatitis, herpes, rosacea, urticaria and allied conditions where an application of the Fluid Extract of Coca one part to four of water lends a sedative action to the skin. The influence of Coca on the pulse and temperature has suggested its employment in collapse and weak heart as recommended by Da Costa,[43] and it has been favorably employed to relieve dropsy depending on debility of the heart, and for uræmia and scanty secretion of urine. In seasickness Coca acts as a prophylactic as well as a remedy. Vomiting of pregnancy may be arrested by cocaine administered either by the mouth or rectum. In the debility of fevers Coca has been found especially serviceable, and in this connection Dr. A. R. Booth, of the Marine Hospital Service,

[42] See Sajous' *Annual*, Vol. V, A36; 1891. [43] *Medical News*, Dec. 13, 1884.

at Shreveport, Louisiana, has written me that he considers cocaine one of the most valuable aids in the treatment of yellow fever.[44] [1] By controlling nausea and vomiting, [2] as a cardiac stimulant, [3] as a hæmostatic when indicated, [4] to hold in abeyance hunger, which at times would be intolerable but for the effect of cocaine. One who has seen a yellow fever stomach, especially from a subject who has died from "black vomit," must have been impressed with the absolute impossibility of such an organ performing its physiological functions. Dr. Booth makes it an inflexible rule, never to allow a yellow fever patient food by the mouth until convalescence is well established. In cases of fine physique he has kept the patient without food for ten or twelve days, and in two cases fourteen and fifteen days respectively, solely by the judicious administration of cocaine in tablets by the mouth. Of two hundred and six cases of yellow fever treated in this manner there was not one relapse. A similar use is made of cocaine to abate the canine hunger of certain cases of epilepsy and insanity, as well as to appease thirst in diabetes.

The Peruvian Indians employ Coca to stimulate uterine contractions and regard it as a powerful aphrodisiac. Leopold Casper, of Berlin, considers Coca one of the best of genital tonics,[45] and many modern observers concur in this opinion.[46] Vecki[47] says that cocaine internally to a man aged fifty-six invariably occasioned sexual excitement and cheerfulness. The Homœopaths who have long regarded Coca as a valuable remedy, employ Coca in sexual excesses, especially when dependent on onanism. Allen has given a "proving" of Coca that covers twelve pages, and Hering's Materia Medica gives provings by twenty-four persons, and recommends Coca in troubles coming with a low state of the barometer. Hempel says: "I have found a remarkable aversion to exertion of any kind in consequence of nervous exhaustion frequently relieved with great promptness by Coca." But it is not my intention to here enumerate the various symptoms for which Coca is regarded as a specific. I have only space to briefly suggest its

[44] Booth, *person. com.;* Jan. 15, 1898. [45] *L'Union Médicale* du Canada, p. 443; 1890.
[46] See also Hamilton, *Virginia Med. Monthly;* Oct. 1891. [47] Vecki; 1899.

possible application as a remedy. A résumé of the various conditions in which Coca has commonly been found serviceable, and its relative employment as classified from the experience of several hundred physicians, correspondents in this research, will be found tabulated in the appendix. Coca may be given in doses equivalent to one or two drachms of the

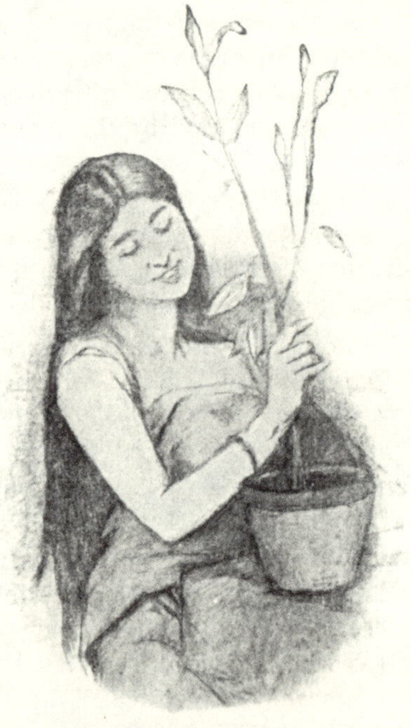

COCA MAIDEN. [*From a Drawing by Constant Mayer.*]

leaves three or four times a day, either as an infusion or as a fluid extract or wine; the latter especially being serviceable for support in acute disease as well as an adjunct indicated in those conditions where its use may tend to maintain the balance of health.

It is a noteworthy fact already referred to, that there has been no recorded case of poisoning from Coca, nor cases of Coca addiction commonly regarded as "habit." The cases of cocaine poisoning and addiction often sensationally reported are even open to grave doubt. The condition termed "cocaine habit" is not generally accepted by physicians, as shown in the specific report in the appendix. Certainly the very general use of cocaine as an anæsthetic has not resulted relatively in anything like the number of rare accidents from the use of chloroform and ether, and this fact must appear the more remarkable when it is appreciated that chloroform and ether are administered under skilled observation, while cocaine is commonly employed by hundreds of thousands—even millions—of laymen, many of whom are absolutely ignorant of its properties.

The use of any alkaloid should be with the appreciation that the factor of personal idiosyncrasy may exert an influence to occasion irregular action. A case of fatal poisoning has been recorded against cocaine from as small a dose as two-thirds of a grain of the hydrochlorate given hypodermically, and from twenty minims of a four per cent. solution (four-fifths of a grain) of the same salt injected into the urethra, and smaller doses it is asserted have produced alarming symptoms. On the other hand, numerous cases are recorded where excessive doses of the alkaloid have been continued for long periods without giving rise to serious trouble. A recovery is recorded after forty-six grains of cocaine had been taken into the stomach, and in one case twenty-three grains of cocaine was used hypodermically daily.[48]

Dr. William A. Hammond experimented upon himself by injecting cocaine subcutaneously. Commencing with one grain the dose was gradually increased until eighteen grains were taken in four portions within five minutes of each other. His pulse increased to one hundred and forty and became irregular. Five minutes after the last injection he felt elated and utterly regardless of surroundings, consciousness being lost within half an hour. The next morning on going to his study where the experiment had been performed he found the floor strewn with books of reference and the chairs overturned, indicating there had been an active mental and

[48] Mann; 1898.

physical excitement. He had turned off the gas, gone upstairs to bed, lighted the gas in his sleeping apartment and retired quite as had been his custom. At nine o'clock the following morning he woke with a splitting headache, and experienced considerable cardiac and respiratory disturbance, and for several days after felt the effects of his indiscretion by languor and indisposition to mental or physical exertion and difficulty in concentration of attention. He considered that eighteen grains of cocaine was nearly a fatal dose for him, and if he had taken it in one dose instead of within twenty minutes it might have been disastrous. This experimenter did not observe any influence upon the ganglia at the base of the brain. There was no disturbance of sensibility, no anæsthesia nor hyperæsthesia, nor interference with motility except some muscles of the face, which were subject to slight twitching. There were no hallucinations. Dr. Hammond asserted that there is no such thing as a "cocaine habit." He had given cocaine to many patients, both male and female, and never had a single objection to the alkaloid being discontinued, not as much trouble in ceasing its use, in fact, as there would have been to give up tea or coffee, and nothing like so much as to have abandoned alcohol or tobacco. He personally used for a nasal affection, during four months, from sixteen to twenty grains a day, averaging about six hundred grains of cocaine a month, applied in solution to the mucous membrane of the nose. During this period he experienced slight mental exhilaration and some indisposition to sleep. Subsequently he used nearly eight hundred grains within thirty-five days. In each instance the drug was discontinued without the slightest difficulty.[49]

Dr. Caudwell, of London, experimented upon himself with both Coca and cocaine. He took increasing doses of fluid extract of Coca until two ounces were taken at a dose. From this he experienced giddiness with unsteadiness of gait, followed by sensations of mental and physical activity when it seemed any exertion could have been undertaken without difficulty. Under cocaine, in doses of one grain he ex-

[49] Hammond; 1887-88.

perienced drowsiness, followed by sleep, and then persistent insomnia. Two and a half grains produced frontal headache, mental excitement and marked insomnia. Three grains after abstinence from food for twenty-four hours produced drowsiness, slight vertigo and wakefulness with a sense of well being. On the following morning five grains produced giddiness with a supra-orbital headache and a sense of weight at the pit of the stomach, while the pupils were widely dilated, and there was inability for exertion. All unpleasant sensations following this experiment had passed in two hours, though dilatation of the pupils lasted for six hours.[50] Professor Bignon, of Lima, considers that the Peruvian Indians consume daily an amount of Coca which represents from thirty to forty centigrammes—[4.5 to 6. grains] of cocaine. He regards ten centigrammes of that alkaloid per day [1.5 grains] a good average dose for those unaccustomed to its use. The average initial dose of cocaine hypodermically should not exceed a quarter of a grain. Under a moderate dose of cocaine, the central nervous system is stimulated through a direct action on the nerve cells. There is psychic exaltation, with increased capacity for mental work, which passes off in a few hours and is followed by complete restoration to the normal condition without after depression. Indeed, whatever depression there may be precedes the exaltation. From larger doses, the medulla and the sensory columns of the spinal cord may be directly affected, but only after very large doses is there weakness and lassitude, and general anæsthesia can only follow from an excessive dose.

Under a poisonous dose of cocaine there is an initial increase of respiration and of the heart beat, both of which soon slow under the influence of paralysis of the vaso motor center, this effect of cocaine upon respiration and the circulation being similar to that from atropine. The pupils are widely dilated and do not respond to light. Involuntary movement of the muscles of mastication, as in chewing, and rotation of the head or body has been noted in animals. There may be epileptiform attacks, clonic convulsions or tetanus. The most

[50] Caudwell; 1885.

common symptoms of cocaine poisoning are those of profound prostration, with dyspnœa, pallor, cyanosis and sweat. When the drug has been taken by the stomach that organ should be evacuated and washed out, while in any case stimulants may be indicated, such as nitrite of amyl, ammonia, ether hypodermically, chloroform to check spasm of the respiratory muscles and even artificial respiration may be indicated. After the severe symptoms have passed chloral may be administered. Both chloral and morphine are regarded as antagonistic to cocaine. Recovery may take place even after a long period of unconsciousness. I was called in one case to a dentist's office to resuscitate a patient after his careless injection of an unknown quantity of cocaine, and we labored over the subject eight hours before consciousness was restored.

Mosso puts the lethal dose of cocaine at 0.03 per kilogramme, in animals, and in man it is probably less. Mannheim,[51] from a collection of about a hundred cases of cocaine poisoning—of which nine were fatal—has determined that one gramme [15.43 grains], of the alkaloid may be considered a fatal dose in man. A "cocaine habit," as already referred to, is not generally accepted. Yet symptoms presumably due to the excessive use of large doses of cocaine are described. These embrace frequency of pulse, relaxation of the arterial system, profuse perspiration, rapid fall of flesh and hallucinations of sight or feeling.[52] A peculiar symptom of chronic cocaine poisoning is that known as Magnan's symptom, after the name of the describer. It is an hallucination of sensation in which the patient complains of feeling a foreign body under the skin. While other hallucinations are common from poisons this is said to be distinctive of cocaine.

There is but one further feature in the physiological study of Coca that we have to consider, and that is the manner of its elimination from the body. From experiments of Dr. Helmsing[53] it was long since determined that cocaine is very difficult of detection in animal tissues. This may be appreciated when the important rôle which it is possible that Coca plays

[51] Mannheim; 1891. [52] Obersteiner and Erlenmeyer; p. 483; 1896.
[53] *Thesis*, Dorpat; 1886.

in assimilation is considered. When taken into the stomach Coca soon disappears from the alimentary canal, being decomposed and gradually setting free the products to which its physiological action is due. As these several alkaloids are carried through the tissues, they enter into further chemical change whereby they are still further broken down, and only soon after the administration of a very large dose is it possible to recover the bases from the alkaline urine with benzoyl. Immediately after a poisonous dose of cocaine given to a cat there was found a distinctive reaction in the urine and blood, but a diminished dose gave after a longer interval only faint tracings, which gradually disappeared.[54] Because of this difficulty of detection the decomposition products of Coca, chiefly as ecgonine, are determined post-mortem by a process of assay. The comminuted tissue is mixed with two parts of acidulated alcohol and digested at 60° in a reflux condenser, the process being repeated with fresh alcohol and the filtrates evaporated to almost dryness. The residue is taken up with water, and the solution shaken out with ether, the residual concentrated liquid being precipitated with baryta and extracted repeatedly with ether. The ethereal solution is then evaporated in a vacuum and the residue tested for the alkaloid.[55]

The fact that the Coca products are so thoroughly consumed in the body indicates the important influence these substances exercise in nutrition, the philosophy of which has been more fully detailed in other chapters.

[54] *Journn. Chem. Soc.;* 1891. [55] Mussi; 1889.

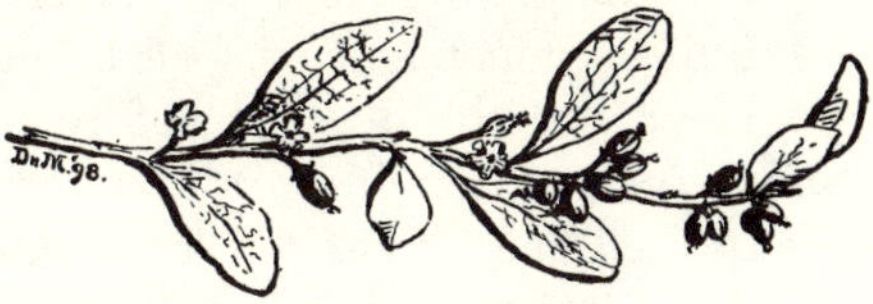

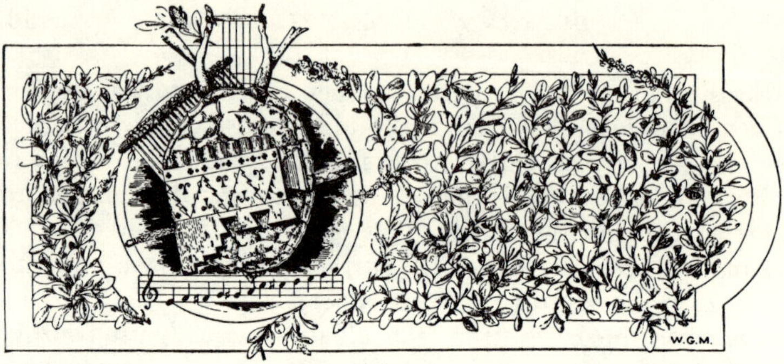

CHAPTER XV.

ADAPTATION OF COCA TO VOICE PRODUCTION.

"Music, the greatest good that mortals know,
And all of Heaven we have below."
—Addison, *Song for St. Cecilia's Day;*
(about 1700.)

SO much has been written in regard to the action of Coca in voice production, that it may be said its praise and its effects have literally been sung. Its use has been so pronouncedly successful in the treatment of laryngeal troubles generally that it seems appropriate to say something as to the organs which govern voice and of the application of Coca to their benefit.

Darwin supposed the progenitors of the human race employed musical sounds before articulate language, for musical feeling is quite independent of speech, and so children are often able to sing before they can talk. The fact of this manifestation in childhood or among those not especially educated has suggested that musical expression may be a separate sense which in some cases is phenomenally developed, while in others it remains dormant. Musical perception is found throughout the animal world, and Professor Owen describes among the apes of the family of gibbons, the rendition of a series of musical sounds, which in their shrill pitch of *oa-oa* ranges through one octave, the scale both upward and downward being sung in the same tones.

The untutored aboriginal peoples had a music of their own, which though differing in method belonged to the great family of sentiment. Whether of poet or peasant, music is the one universal language which appeals to the soul of all without the necessity for translation. We may trace its harmonies through the religion of the Hindus, the Chinese, the Japanese and the Incas during thousands of years. Subsequently it was developed by the Greeks, among whom it was used in the declamation of their epic poems, as was also the custom among the early Peruvians. Since these days the traditions of every nation have furnished examples of folk songs through their past antiquity. The Celts made great progress in these and were noted for their musical culture. The French have their *chansons*, the Italians their *canzonetti,* and the Germans have their *volkslieder*. The early Hebrews adapted their music from the Egyptians, though sacred history tells us that Jubal was the father of all such as handle the harp and organ.[1]

There are many references throughout the Scriptures to the association of music with worship and also with ceremonial entertainment, and its influence on the emotions was recognized as soothing or inspiring in accordance with its application. Thus when Saul was troubled with an evil spirit, his servant sought out a cunning player on the harp who might cure him, and we learn with what success David played for his refreshment.[2] Singers are frequently spoken of in the Old Testament and all sorts of musical instruments are enumerated, such as the cornet, cymbals, dulcimer, harp, organ, pipe, psaltery, sackbut, tabret, timbrel, trumpet and viol, so that we should have to look further back to find the first traces of musical conception.

Of the more crude instruments, the trumpet is frequently

[1] *Genesis;* IV., 21. [2] *First Samuel;* XVI., 14-23.

mentioned in the sacred writings. Commonly this was employed for signalling, and it was used among the Romans to proclaim the watches of the day and night. In the *Metamorphoses* Ovid describes Jupiter—when the world was overflowed by the deluge—as commanding Triton to blow his trumpet as a signal for the mighty waters to recede, and tradition has ever pictured the vast and weird harmony of the sea as controlled by a god blowing through a shell, just as it has associated the proclamation of eternity with the trumpeting of the Angel Gabriel. Misenus, who was a trumpeter in the

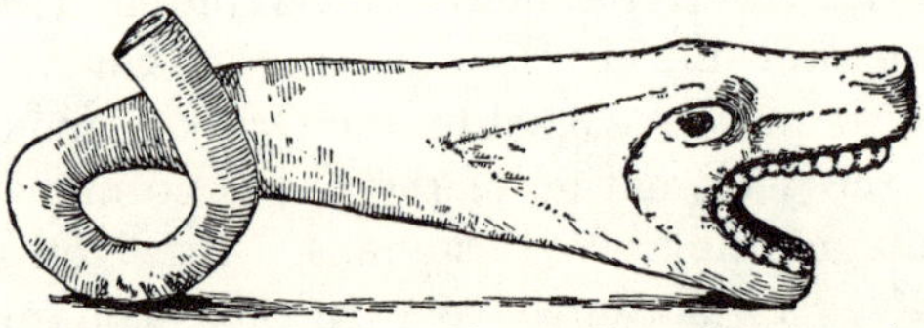

PERUVIAN CLAY TRUMPET. [*Metropolitan Museum of Art.*]

Trojan war, was so proud of his skill as to challenge the god of the waters to a contention for which his bravado was immortalized by Virgil:

"But while the daring mortal o'er the flood
Rais'd his high notes and challenged every god,
With envy Triton heard the noble strain
And whelmed the bold musician in the main."
—*Æneid* VI, 163.

The shell trumpet has long been in use among the Peruvian Indians; the Spanish named it *bosina,* from the sound produced by blowing into it having a suggestive resemblance to the roar of a bull. The Indians use it for signalling and it is employed in their celebration of the festival of the Coca harvest, when its braying reaches far over the hills.

From the use of music upon occasions of religious ceremonial it was but natural to associate it with all emotional functions, whether in times of reverential awe or during a period of danger as a means to divert fear. Thus battles were fought to the sound of the lute, or even the viol or harp, and we know with what utter abandon Nero fiddled away Rome, for music has ever been a natural accompaniment to passionate appeal or to the melancholy of despair.

Professor W. Max Mueller has recently completed a collection of the ancient love songs of Egypt of forty centuries or more ago, in which though the poetry may seem strange, the feeling expressed is that of to-day, just as we find modern sentiment among the early Peruvian songs. The melodies of the Incas were composed in measured thirds and for the most part are written to celebrate amorous passions, expressive of joy, of sorrow, of kindness or the cruelty of some fair one to whom the enamored strains were poured forth. Some of these ancient airs are still sung among the Indians. One from Rivero's collection will serve to illustrate their melody which, though rambling and formless as compared to our musical ideas, is full of feeling. Of course it has been transcribed phonetically to the modern musical notation.

Professor Louis Mounier, of Vineland, New Jersey, to whom I submitted this example, believes that its arrangement has been made by some musician acquainted with the classic style of the period in which Haydn, Mozart and the few French followers of the German school flourished. He says: "I should be very much surprised to find the rigid forms, from which Beethoven, Schumann and Wagner tried to escape, adhered to by people with an oriental turn of mind, or at least of a totally different civilization." Mr. Samuel Sosnowski, a finished pianist conversant with classic interpretation, regards this particular piece as suggesting the early Italian school, such as that of Scarlatti. In any case it exhibits a weird example of Peruvian melody considered to be aboriginal. (*See page* 440.)

The Incas had regularly appointed musicians to the court who accompanied the *haravis,* or love songs, on the native Pandean pipes such as are still in use throughout the Sierra. "The players were Indians, instructed for the amusement of the King and for the lords his vassals, and although their music was so simple it was not generally practiced, but was learned and done by study."[3] These pipes were made of

[3] Garcilasso; 1609.

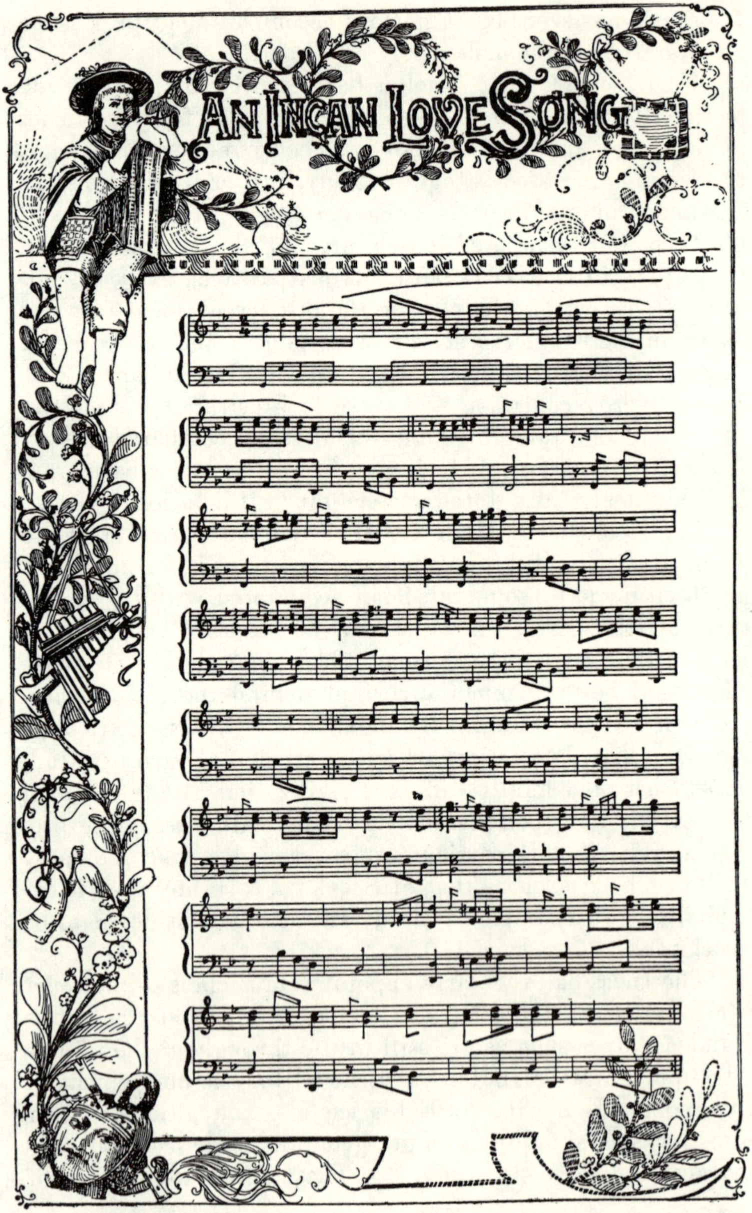

ANCIENT INCAN HARAVI. [*Rivero and Tschudi.*]

joints of bamboo or from reeds of different lengths arranged in a row or in parallel pairs, forming a set with a scale of ten notes. Sometimes they were made of stone, and in the museum at Berlin there is a cast of such an instrument, the original having been made of a species of talc of greenish color. This example is five and three-eighth inches high and six and one-quarter inches wide, containing eight short pipes. Four of the pipes are stopped by small lateral finger holes opening on the second, third, fifth and seventh. When these holes are open the tones are raised half a tone, while the closed tubes have unalterable tones.*

The Peruvians appear to have used different orders of intervals for different kinds of melodies, in a way similar to that in vogue among certain Asiatic nations. "Each poem, or song, had its appropriate tune, and they could not put two different songs to one tune; and this was why the enamoured gallant, making music at night on his flute, with the tune which belonged to it, told the lady and all the world the joy or sorrow of his soul, the favour or ill-will which he possessed; so that it might be said that he spoke by the flute."[4] In a similar manner the Hindus have certain tunes for certain seasons and fixed occasions, and likewise a number of different modes, or scales, used for particular kinds of songs.[5]

Some of the Peruvian reed pipes are fastened together in sets of four, each reed being of different length, one set adapted for high notes, another for different notes of the scale, so that the four natural voices—soprano, tenor, contralto and bass—might be represented by four sets of reeds. When an Indian played on one of these instruments he was answered by some other Indian at a distance playing a fifth above, and these by another, who might rise to higher notes or descend the scale, but always in tune. In the musical collection of the New York Metropolitan Museum of Art there is shown a variety of Peruvian instruments, among which are a number of specimens of these pipes, some made with but a few reeds, others with twenty or more bound together. Some of these are in a double row arranged side by side, while others are in

* See headpiece, p. 436. [4] Garcilasso; p. 193; 1609. [5] Carl Engel; 1874.

a single row of varying length, the pipes being either open or closed at the lower end.

Besides the Pandean pipes the Incans had horns on which four or five notes might be made, as the flageolet, *huayllaca,* and the *ccuyvi,* while others only made one note, as the *pincullu.* Both of these instruments are still used among the Andean Indians. In addition to these the early Peruvians also had instruments known as the *chhilchiles,* and castanets —*chanares,* timbrels, bells, *huancar*—a drum, *tinya*—a guitar of five or six chords, and the *queppa*—a sort of oboe—trumpet, which Rivero describes as emitting lugubrious sounds which fill the heart with an indescribable sadness capable of bringing involuntary tears into the eyes. This is probably the *jaina,* which is still used by some Indian tribes in Peru, and which was termed by the early Mexicans *chayna.* While these ancient instruments make seemingly crude music to refined ears they were probably effective in rendering the sort of melody the people desired, and their employment presumably dates from a very early period.

Castlenau discovered in an ancient Peruvian tomb a flute made of a human bone. It has four finger holes at its upper end and appears to have been blown into at one end like a horn. Two similar examples, each about six inches long, are in the British Museum. Each is provided with five finger holes; one which is ornamented with some simple designs in black, has all the holes at its upper side and one of the holes is considerably smaller than the rest. This same construction, still followed in the bone flutes of Guiana, was common, for Alonso de Ovalle, writing of the Indians in Chili, says: "Their flutes which they play upon in their dances are made of the bones of the Spaniards and other enemies whom they have overcome in war. This they do by way of triumph and glory for their victory. They make them likewise of bones of animals, but the warriors dance only to the flutes made of their enemies." This, however, was not an Incan custom, but may have been practiced among some savage Peruvian tribes. Garcilasso, writing some years after leaving Peru, said that in 1560 but five Indians in Cuzco played the flute well from any music book for the organ that might be placed before them. At present throughout the Sierra every *arriero* and herdsman plays upon the pipe, and that instrument is as much a portion of the every-day paraphernalia of the Indian in his lonely tramps over the mountains as is his pouch of Coca.

Looking back for the inception of our modern music, it appears to have developed with the Church. In early days, before there was a method for recording melodies, they were preserved by oral tradition through ages just as were the Homeric poems and the Vedas. The first attempt at musical notation—long before the staff was employed—consisted of the letters of the Greek alphabet, to which signs were added to indicate the inflection of the voice. Subsequently Roman letters and syllables were used, written in an undulating way, to show a rise and fall, without indicating fixed notes. In early manuscripts syllables are employed to represent the first six notes of our present scale. These were adapted from the lines of an ancient hymn to Saint John the Baptist, their first use being attributed to the Benedictine monk, Guido of Arezzo, in the eleventh century:

> *Ut* queant laxis *Re*sonare fibris
> *Mi*ra gestorum *Fa*muli tuorum,
> *Sol*ve polluti *La*bii reatum.
> —*Sancte Johannes.*

Afterwards these syllables were altered by the Italian school to the present notation. These names do not indicate any certain pitch, but merely the fixed ratios; once the first note—or tonic—is determined the others ascend in regular order.

Franco, of Cologne, in the twelfth century is said to have been the first writer to systematize "measured music," designating the length of notes, but division into bars and accent was not adapted until several centuries later. Before this, written music was described as of "perfect" or "imperfect time," and such ancient manuscripts are consequently found exceedingly difficult of transcription.

The progress of music was earlier and greater in England

than elsewhere, until its rise in Flanders in the fifteenth century, when the Flemish established schools and gave impetus to the art in Germany and in Italy. But the greatest factor in the development of music was the Church, and as Rome was the ecclesiastical centre, musicians of all lands flocked there for study, where every effort was made at perfection in religious uses, authority and sanctification even being granted for the perpetuation by surgical means of the treble voice of youth throughout manhood. With the increase of learning music became an essential part of education, and among the knights in the age of chivalry skill in verse and a melody to "my ladye faire" was regarded as a fitting accompaniment to heroic exploits at arms. Such a race of knightly musicians were the *minnesingers* of Germany, who set so great value on the invention of new metre that he who produced one with a melody to suit it was called a *meister*—master, while he who cast his verse in a previously accepted metre, or adapted them to a known melody, was styled *tondieb*—a tone thief.[6]

At the commencement of the sixteenth century the Madrigal form of composition was introduced, constructed on the form of the *canon* and abounding in imitations of one part of the melody by another; this chiefly flourished in England, and later gave rise to the part-songs of Germany. At this period the oratorio originated from a simple arrangement of short hymns to the gradual development of a sort of religious drama, and the opera now sprang into life after its long dormant period since the early Greek tragedies. So great became the impetus to musical composition that musical instruments began to assume a new importance and were perfected in accordance with requirements of the composer or the skill of the performer, in which harmony began to be regarded as a greater factor than loudness.

Luther has been credited with adapting metrical verse on sacred subjects to the language of the people. Sometimes these were set to ancient church melodies, or again to tunes of secular songs, the object being to put the choral singing of the Church within the lips of the masses. Yet the psalmody of

[6] Macfarren; 1885.

the ancient Hebrews had been of a similar nature centuries before, when the doings of the people were recounted in song with the greatest poetic beauty, and a similar custom was practiced among the Incans. Indeed, it is remarkable how close some of the songs of the Incas are by comparison to the psalms of the Old Testament, not only in their metrical arrangement, but in form of expression, as for example with the Song of Solomon, that "Song of Songs."

The great advance of orchestration during the seventeenth and eighteenth centuries, the development of the symphony and opera elaborated through a host of phenomenal composers —several of whom are accredited with having written every possible combination of notes—has enabled a modern civilization to enjoy the refinement of the highest type of musical culture, beyond which further progress seems almost incredible. But that which concerns us chiefly in musical production is the formation of voice.

Marin Mersenne explained in his universal harmony, in 1636, that the string of a musical instrument when struck yields other tones than that to which its entire length is tuned. Before then musical sound had been only a phenomenon of observation rather than of precise knowledge, but from this the science of harmonics and the laws of melody were evolved.

If an open vibrating string be stopped at any part of its length its vibrations will be broken into quickened waves of a length equal to that of the first division. Thus, if a string be stopped at one-half its length there will be two equal waves, each vibrating twice as rapidly as the open string, or if stopped at one-third its length there will be three shorter waves, each vibrating three times as rapidly as did the unstopped string, the vibrations increasing and giving forth a higher tone in proportion to the shortness of the waves. This same law is true of the sound produced from a column of air passing through a tube, and the influence of stopping the tube on the formation of notes is similar. The point of stoppage between the waves is termed a node and the swell of vibrating string between the nodes is termed a loop. The open string vibrating through its whole length gives a sound which is termed fundamental, while the sound produced from each of the nodal divisions—originally known as a harmonic—is termed a partial tone, or over-tone. This observation was almost immediately recorded by Dr. Cowley, who will be recalled as having written so charmingly of Coca:

> "Thus, when two brethren strings are set alike,
> To move them both, but one of them we strike."
> —*The Troubles of David.*

When the string of a musical instrument is sounded the overtones are united in a complex wave with the fundamental tone. Just as periodicity in vibration distinguishes a musical sound from a mere noise, so this harmonic blending of tones—the *klang* of the Germans—distinguishes a note from a simple sound, and gives rise to the varied quality or timbre —the *klangfarbe*—of notes of the same pitch in different instruments.

Harmony has been compared with color, through the analogy between the blending of the seven primary colors in their production of light and similar vibrations of the seven notes of the gamut in the production of tones; but Helmholtz has shown that if the lavender rays beyond the violet in the spectrum be included, light has an octave and a quarter instead of one octave. From this similarity of vibration it was long since suggested, as referred to by Dr. Haweis,[7] that a symphony might be reproduced in color. This experiment was done, I believe, by a priest in France some years since.

Music is to be regarded then as due to rhythmical vibration, whether this be produced through the chirp of insects or the roar of cataracts in the wide area of nature, or by a mere attempt to interpret through artifice those harmonies constantly displayed about us, for as was taught by Pythagoras two centuries and a half ago:

> "From heavenly harmony
> This universal frame began."
> —Dryden, *An Ode for St. Cecilia's Day;* (1687.)

[7] Haweis; 1873.

The organ of voice—one of the greatest gifts to man—is a natural instrument to which cleverness and skill may only hope to harmonize other musical instruments. And just as we have seen, there has been a gradual growth of musical expression as the development of musical taste and knowledge was improved, so the singing voice has been slowly evolved with the scientific unfolding of the principles of tone formation which has been marked by the elaboration of fixed means of musical expression.

In a similar manner to that in which a vibrating string gives forth a note, the human voice produces tones by the vibration of two membranous folds—really the ligamentous edges of two muscles. These are attached at their outer borders, while their free margins—pearly white in color—are movable, and may be approximated or opened more widely, leaving a narrowed slit between, termed the *rima glottidis,* or "vocal chink." In the adult man these folds—or vocal cords, are about three-quarters of an inch in length, and in women they are some quarter shorter, while situated on a higher plane. To this variation in size and position, as well as to a slight difference in the shape of the vocal box, is due the range and quality between the male and the female voice. The female voice has three registers, while the male voice has but two, though having the greater number of over-tones.

The delicate cords which give rise to voice are within the larynx, a triangular cartilaginous box constituting the protuberance in the neck known as "Adam's apple." This vocal box is between the pharynx above and the trachea below, surrounded by muscles and lined with mucous membrane which is closely adherent to the vocal cords, and is continuous with that lining the entire respiratory tract. Because of this continuity when any part of this membrane is diseased other parts of the respiratory tract may suffer. This indicates why applications to the cavity of the nose may improve voice, or why sipping Coca wine, as commonly advocated among vocal instructors, will give tone to the vocal cords although not actually coming in contact with them.

The walls of the larynx are not rigid, and the two little

elbow-like cartilages to which the cords are attached are so placed that they seemingly are pivoted at the angle upon which they swing and so may bring the cords parallel or extend them wider apart. In quiet breathing the space between the cords is elliptical, or shaped like a narrow V, with the point of the V in front, the space opening a little at each inspiration, while in a forced effort the V is bowed and widely dilated. At the moment of the emission of sound the "vocal chink" becomes narrowed by the pivoting of the cartilages, to which are attached the posterior ends of the cords, and by thus swinging about the edges of the vocal bands are approximated and made parallel. The result of this movement occasions a fixation and increased tension and the note rendered is of higher pitch, just as it would be from the string of any musical instrument similarly made tense.

Voice has *pitch*—produced by the rapidity of vibration of the vocal bands, *intensity* of tone—governed by the force of the expiratory blast of air, and *timbre*—wholly an individual peculiarity dependent upon the number of over-tones accompanying the fundamental, which is governed by the anatomical construction and integrity of the parts involved in tone formation. The particular kind of voice being due neither to highness, lowness, nor loudness, but upon the length of the vocal cords and the distances of these from the upper resonant chambers—the pharynx, mouth and nose—each of which serves as a factor of individual quality. Vocal gymnastics is not music. Patti is recalled by her clear tones in the middle register, a quality more greatly admired by musical critics than would be the endurance displayed by the Salvation Army adjutant who is recorded as singing fifty-nine hymns in fifty-eight minutes.

The normal compass of the voice is some two octaves, the principal difference between registers being one of pitch, occasioned by the anatomical peculiarities of the individual larynx. The lowest note of the average female voice is about an octave higher than the lowest of the male voice, while the highest note of the female is an octave above the top note of the male. The average bass voice ranges from *f* (176) to *d*

(594), though some famous basses even take the low *c* of the cello, and Bastardella is said to have sung notes vibrating from forty-four to one thousand seven hundred and eighty.[8] Composers have often written for certain phenomenal singers, thus Meyerbeer in "Robert le Diable" (1831), in "Les Huguenots" (1833) and "Le Prophète" (1849) wrote *b* flat for the bass voice. A good soprano ranges from *b* (495) to *g* (1584), and Nilsson used to take *f* (2816) in "The Magic Flute." Mozart is said to have heard at Parma, in 1770, an Italian songstress whose voice had the extraordinary range from *g* (396) to *c* (4224), three and a half octaves.[9] But these are the exception and not the rule. A phenomenally high range among voices of the present day is

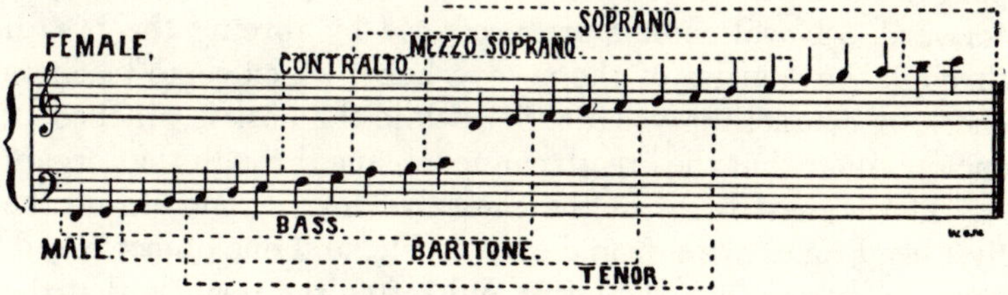

RANGE OF HUMAN VOICE.

that of Miss Yaw, which reaches the second *d* above the staff, a compass due to an unusual arrangement of the vocal cords.

There are sounds too grave and too acute for perception by the human ear. Helmholtz's investigations show that from thirty to forty vibrations per second are the lowest ordinarily audible and thirty-eight thousand are the highest. Other experimenters have varied a little to either extent of these limits. The generality of vibrations which are musical range from forty to four thousand, while an average of human voices would indicate a range from fifty to one thousand eight hundred. Among all voices the classic sopranos seem to have an advantage in number: Albani, Calvé, Eames, Gadsky, Juch, Melba, Nordica and Sembrich—whom I have purposely enumerated alphabetically, reserving for my readers a classification in accordance with individual ideas of great-

[8] Browne and Behnke; 1886. [9] Martin; p. 603; 1881.

ness—are not paired by modern tenors of equal prominence. Among some of the great tenors of the past are Rubini, Mario, Duprez, Wachtel, Campanini, Ravelli, Gayarre, and Massini. Tamberlik was regarded as the most famous tenor, basing that indication upon the reach of voice in pure chest tones of the upper register.

Chest tones are produced by sending forth the breath in such manner that in its passage it sets up a vibration of the entire length of the vocal cords while not striking against any part of the vocal tract which would alter the resultant tone. Head sounds are made by directing the breath towards the frontal sinus, and throat sounds—always faulty, are occasioned by pressing the tongue backwards or against the lower part of the mouth instead of keeping it suspended and a little forward. Nasal sounds are produced by forcing the breath through the cavities of the nose, a habit which some teachers check by compelling vocalization while the nose is pinched in such manner that the breath cannot escape through that organ.

The highest tones of the chest are very strong, while the first head tones are soft and even feeble, and one object in culture is to strengthen the latter and soften the former, that the sounds of one register may glide imperceptibly into those of the other, though the chest notes of bass voices are too strong to smoothly blend with those of the head. To form the voice it is desirable to sing on the vowel *a*—vocalizing as it is termed, which exposes errors which might be masked if an attempt were made to utter words. In singing not only musical tones are to be produced, but these must be accompanied by words, the articulation of which occasions such a series of movements in the muscles of the tongue, soft palate and lips as to considerably influence the character of the tube through which voice is sent forth. Because of these technical difficulties there is a need for proper instruction and training, for while science has done much to point out the basis of voice production the rational cultivation of the singing voice is an art which cannot be elaborated through any fixed rules.

Though voice is the essential element in the art of singing, yet it does not always reach that quality naturally in all who wish to sing; indeed, there are many *virtuosi* in whom it would have been impossible to have foretold any vocal achievements, either from an examination of their vocal cords or from a conclusion based upon their earlier opportunities. Wachtel, of high *c* fame, was originally a cab driver; Sellier, of the Paris Opera, was a sailor, and, without knowledge of music, was compelled to learn his pieces by ear, and Campanini was a blacksmith before his qualities were developed. Rossini used to say it takes three things to make a singer: "*voce, voce, voce*"—voice, voice, voice, but Francesco Lamperti, the famous *maestro,* said it required—"*voce, talento e criterio*"—voice, talent and judgment. The great Garcia told Jenny Lind that of one hundred qualities which constitute a great singer, one who has a good voice has ninety-nine. The foundation of voice, however, must be a proper physical development.

It seems surprising that any one with a sufficient knowledge to understandingly follow musical instruction should be mistaken as to their vocal register. The voice of each person is dependent upon the anatomical—one might almost say mechanical, construction of their larynx and vocal cords. It would be just as sensible for one to ordinarily attempt to give a violin solo on a double bass viol as for one with a bass voice to attempt to sing tenor. But as "there is no new thing under the sun," this has been attempted. Bottesini, a celebrated Italian player, used to charm his auditors by the exquisitely soft tones of his bass viol in imitation of the violin. Yet this is not an example within the rule. But I would impress that register is not a matter of individual choice nor cleverness in technique. A soprano is such because her vocal apparatus has been made for a soprano voice and it would be wholly impossible to make her a contralto through any natural means. Mistakes of a misplaced voice are, however, of frequent occurrence, not only among those who are uneducated in music but among those who are artists. The principles of the voice are so mysterious, says Stephen de la Madelaine,[10] that it is easy to mistake not only the nature of the

[10] Reclus; 1895.

voice but the voice itself. Specialism has so divided all teaching that there are now masters who devote themselves exclusively to voice placing, which is recognized as a pre-requisite to any attempts at vocal culture. Tamberlik was at first a *tenor serio,* but after a stay in Portugal his voice changed and became much higher, when he was classed as *tenor sfogato.* It is said that Jean de Reszké, the famous tenor, was at one time almost equally famous as a baritone until the error of register was shown, when his voice was cultivated as a tenor. There are some artists who have so phenomenal a range that their voice overlaps both above and below into other registers. Madame Scalchi is the possessor of such an organ, and while nominally a contralto, her voice seems to command the entire scale from a deep bass to high soprano, which she pours forth in a peculiar richness.

Knowledge, exercise, and cultivation will bring out the most favorable qualities of the voice, and will improve those factors which may have remained dormant through improper use, just as any musical instrument may be more artistically manipulated by a skilled performer. But just as it would be impossible to add additional notes to an instrument of fixed tones, so it is even more impossible to add one note either to the high or low register of the voice. I once listened to a young man attempting to sing a tenor solo which he struggled with in a very strained and unnatural way, who when asked, did not know the range of his voice, which a trial proved to be bass of little power. Upon surprise being expressed that he should attempt to sing tenor songs with a bass voice, he said: "My brother sings bass; I want to sing tenor." Register is dependent upon the range of pitch of the chest tones and mistakes of register are dependent upon a false rendition, so that strained and throaty tones are produced, or even those which are falsetto, occasioned by some mal-position of the cords, or by a vibration of merely their anterior ends instead of their entire length.[11]

The direct influence of Coca upon the mucous membrane of the larnyx long since gave it importance as a tensor of the

[11] Vacher; 1877.

vocal cords,[12] and in throat troubles generally it has received a wide application among professional singers and speakers. It is used as a tonic to the mucous membrane[13] and to render tone more clear,[14] giving an improved quality to the upper voice,[15] as well as to sustain tone.[16] Several correspondents report the beneficial action of Coca in aphonia,[17] a result that has been attributed to general improvement of health following its use.[18]

One of the most pronounced influences of Coca is its power upon respiration. In considering this action, it may be well to briefly review the anatomical and physiological factors engaged in this function.

The air in its entrance to the lungs passes the larynx and through the trachea—or windpipe. The latter, after its entrance into the chest divides into the right and left bronchial tube, and each of these divides again into two, and still again and again until the smallest terminations are reached, which end in minute sacculated dilatations known as air cells. These delicate little pouches—which might represent a cluster of bubbles blown at the end of a minute tube—are so extremely small that one hundred and twenty-five of them would go within the space of an inch, and upon the thin epithelial wall composing these the finest capillaries are distributed as a network of blood vessels.

The function of respiration is purification of the blood by an interchange of gases; in the lungs this occurs directly through the walls of the air cells, oxygen being introduced at each inspiration and carbonic acid being carried off as a product of combustion at each expiration. The oxygen of the air is taken up by a crystallizable element of the blood known as *hæmoglobin*, which is carried by the red corpuscles, and thus the circulation is enabled to convey this purifying gas to the various tissues of the body, where in the thin-walled capillaries another interchange of gases takes place.

In the lungs oxygen is added to the blood stream and carbonic acid is given off. In the other organs of the body car-

[12] Fauvel; also *Collective Investigation;* 511. See Appendix.
[13] *Idem;* 143, 289, 366, 563, 593, 658, 1131. [14] *Idem;* 311. [15] *Idem;* 148, 537.
[16] *Idem;* 274, 1074. [17] *Idem;* 339, 365, 982. [18] *Idem;* 629.

bonic acid is added to the blood and the oxygen is given off to the tissues, while the venous blood charged with waste matter is sent to the lungs for purification through healthful respiration. This illustrates why as more waste material is thrown out from the tissues during exertion the necessity for respiration increases, because of an increased call upon the blood for a purifying influence. It also emphasizes the necessity for a constant supply of pure air to replace that which has been breathed, and as combustion of any sort—whether by fire or respiration—consumes oxygen, this should be regarded when considering appropriate ventilation. The drowsiness and feeling of fatigue experienced when on a shopping tour in stores which are crowded, and similar feelings of lethargy and tire suffered in assemblies, are but illustrations of the necessity for a purer air. The condition is allied to that of bodily fatigue occasioned when the blood is loaded with waste material. It is not that expired carbonic acid gas is alone poisonous, but when in addition the air is filled with organic substances resulting from the excretion of countless tissues or the volatile exhalations from decomposing particles of food, there should be no surprise at headache or sore throat.

The mechanical act of respiration is eminently a muscular one, of considerable effort—though nominally performed unconsciously. The cycle being put in action involuntarily by a double nerve centre supposedly situated in the medulla; normally automatic in its action, though, it is capable of being influenced through the will and of being excited reflexly. This centre is stimulated by a venous condition of the blood, under which it may become so active as to excite the extraordinary muscles of respiration. Such labored breathing—due to deficient aeration of the blood—is called *dyspnœa;* while, if the blood be too highly charged with oxygen, as may occur in artificial respiration, the centre is not stimulated, and breathing ceases under the condition termed *apnœa.* The cycle, or rhythm of respiration, consists of inspiration, expiration and pause.

The number of respirations in one resting quietly varies greatly and it is difficult to fix a fair average, the frequency

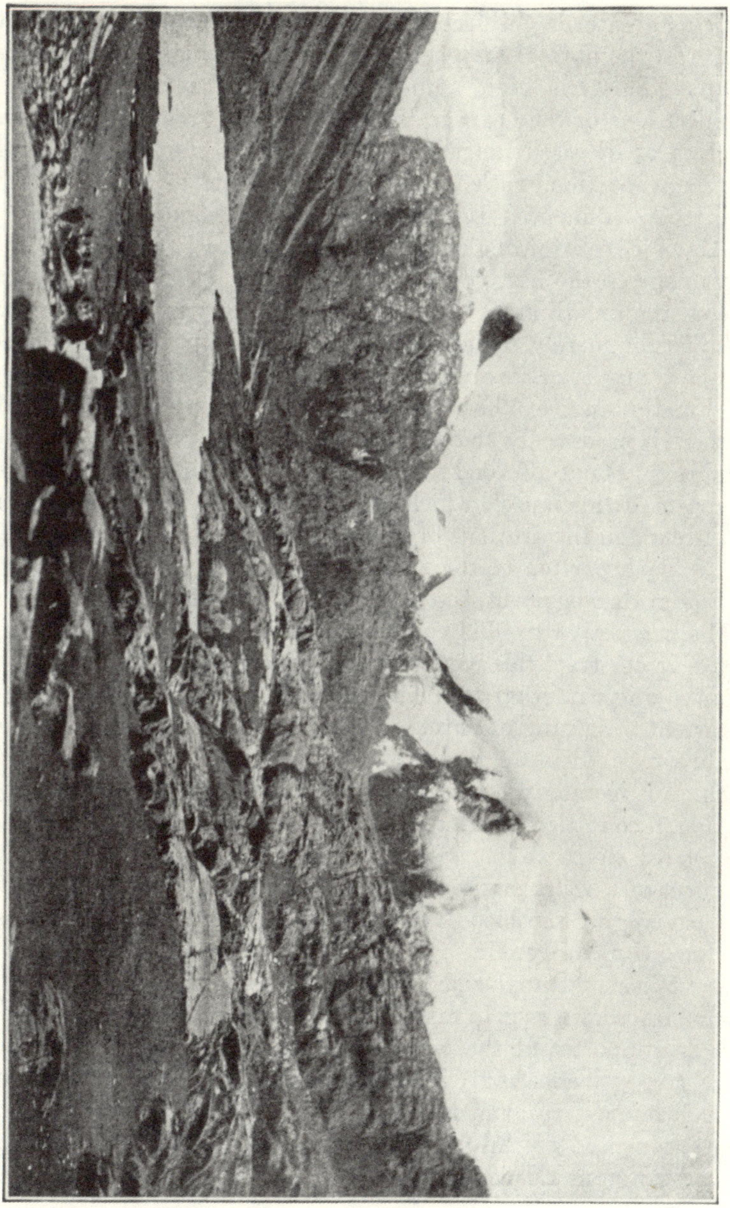

LAKE ARICOMA, ALTITUDE 14,800 FEET, ABOVE TITICACA, PERU. See page 141. [*From a Photograph.*]

being greater in children than in adults. For a healthy adult at rest the normal may be from fourteen to eighteen per minute. This has been found to correspond relatively to the pulsations of the heart in the ratio of about one to four. In cases of diseased lungs the respiratory act increases beyond this proportion, while in affections in which the heart is more directly influenced the pulse relation becomes more rapid. An exact control of the respiratory muscles is of decided advantage to the best vocal effort, though it should be recalled that the breath must be delivered to the larynx in a quantity sufficient merely to set the vocal cords in appropriate vibrations, any excessive effort occasioning the fault known as "breathiness." When the abdominal organs are distended there is necessarily an oppression in the chest, because the diaphragm is not afforded a free opportunity for descent. It is spasm of this muscle which constitutes the annoying factor in the sudden inspirations of hiccough, sobbing and laughing.

Each portion of the respiratory tract is liable to its particular derangement, the most common of which results from the congestive trouble commonly termed catching cold. In the upper tract this condition is frequently manifest through annoying catarrhal troubles, probably resulting from a persistent relighting of chronic local derangement in the nose or throat, or from an acute congestion. As a consequence the mucous membrane is swollen and gives out an increased secretion, a condition which may even be conveyed through continuity of tissue to the larynx or bronchial tubes. Here the effect of Coca is marked in lessening the profuse secretion by constringing the blood vessels, while the muscular system is toned to favor repair.

When the malarial-bone-racking accompaniment of influenza known as grip raged, Coca was found the most serviceable supporter of the organism during an attack. The use of a grog made from "Vin Mariani" and hot water taken at bed time was recommended abroad by Dr. H. Libermann, surgeon-in-chief of the French army, and in the United States by Dr. Cyrus Edson.[19] Personally, I advocate in this affection

[19] Edson; p. 39, 1891.

quinine combined with phenacetine—three grains of each, repeated at intervals of two or three hours, with at the same time a tablespoonful to a wineglassful of the wine already mentioned. Quinine has a very depressing influence upon many patients and is apt to check the flow of bile as well. Coca, on the other hand, is mildly laxative, and while furthering the action of the antifebrile remedies, it antagonizes the disease, buoys the patient and serves as a nutrient when food and even a milk dietary is distasteful. When the acute condition has passed the Coca wine used less frequently may wholly replace other medication, checking the fearful incidental despondency and toning up the patient to recovery.

Asthma is an exceedingly unfortunate affliction which may exhibit no local signs between the attacks. It is occasioned by a spasm of the minute tubes set up reflexly either by trouble in the upper air passages, or wholly from a nervous influence, and an attack is often precipitated by worry or some unusual nervous strain. The source of trouble is well prevented by the judicious use of Coca, not only acting beneficially upon the mucous membrane, but through a sedative influence upon nervous tissue and as a tonic support to the muscular system generally.

A cough may have its seat in the trachea, the explosive manifestation being an effort to clear the tract of some foreign body, which may be either simply the swollen mucous membrane or the excessive secretion from its congestion. The deeper such a trouble is carried along the respiratory tract the more serious it is, whether a bronchitis—affecting only the larger tubes, or a more profound catarrh of the smaller ones intimately associated with the air cells—capillary bronchitis —or a congestion of the air vesicles themselves, when their capacity is encroached upon by the products thrown out by inflammation, as in pneumonia. In phthisis so destructive is the prolonged consuming congestion that several of these air cells may be broken together and coalesce as one cavity.

An appropriate method of breathing, while absolutely necessary to the professional singer or speaker, is desirable to improve the organism generally. Commonly we are apt to breathe too shallow, and in such cases a sort of respiratory gymnastics is desirable. Such an exercise may best be taken standing, with the clothing loosed. The breath should now be drawn in slowly and the chest gradually expanded to its full capacity, the shoulders being raised to admit of every available space in the lungs being filled with air. After a short retention the breath may be permitted to escape slowly. Then, after a few ordinary respiratory movements, another enforced respiration should be taken, and so on during a period of ten minutes, the exercise being repeated two or three times each day. By such a method lungs of moderate capacity may be cultivated to breathe more deeply, and enabled to maintain a tone from twenty to thirty seconds. All sorts of devices have been designed to entertain the patient while bringing about this result, one of which is a little tube which is blown into. In doing this the lungs are emptied by an enforced expiration, which necessitates an increased inspiration.

This breathing exercise may well be done while counting mentally and uniformly so many seconds for an inspiration, so many while the breath is held, and so many counts during the period of expiration. While at commencement the respiratory cycle may not be prolonged to exceed ten or twelve seconds, after a short practice the time may be doubled. The rationale of all exercise is to make breathing deeper and so to purify the blood and tissues. It is, therefore, desirable that all exercise shall be taken where the air is comparatively pure. I commonly instruct my patients to accustom themselves to deep breathing during their out-of-door walks, selecting a given point up to which the inspiration is taken and an equally distant point up to which the breath is slowly let out. With such a guide there is often an incentive to perform the exercise properly. Professional singers well understand the importance of this quality of deep breathing and of the control of a supply of wind in the bellows—as in this instance we may term the accessory apparatus of the lungs—which may gradually be let out to excite the vocal bands to vibration, and some phenomenal renditions have been related of great capacity. The tenor Gunz is said to have been able to take sufficient air at one inspiration to sing all of Schumann's "The Rose, the Lily," and an Italian songstress is mentioned who could trill up and down the chromatic scale through two octaves with one breath.

Artists who appreciate the importance of a sound body in order to render desirable tones take especial care to carry out a line of general exercise which, while improving the physique, may be recreative. Following the idea that work, not idleness, is the more restful, a change of occupation is sought, and the same impulse which led Gladstone to tree chopping for his rest has prompted several prominent singers to stock farming. Professional singing is not the dreamy, idle life which the poetry of music suggests, but calls forth all the powers of a sound organism. Indeed, the exertion, and consequent exhaustion of both nerve and muscle, is greater than commonly supposed in all prolonged use of the voice, either in singing or speaking. Meyerbeer was termed a voice breaker as far back as 1837, since his day the task of such artists as sing the Wagnerian music is really phenomenal, and they deserve credit as noble examples of endurance quite as much as for their cultivated rendering of harmony. It is not unusual for singers to break down physically, so the professional singer's care is constantly excited to the preservation of health. A story is related of a lady who went to Bayreuth to rehearse under Wagner the part of one of the flower girls in "Parsifal." The great composer told her to sing the high note loud and take the next deep note, which immediately followed, from the chest. She replied: "Why, *Meister,* if I do, I will have no voice left in two years," to which it is said Wagner replied: "Well, do you expect to sing any longer than that?"

From the particular strain put upon the vocal organs through prolonged periods there is a constant liability among those who use their voice in such a way, to "relaxed throat" and hoarseness, and this, with tonsillitis and sore throat, which may be prompted by either a climatic change or any personal indiscretion, is the *bête noire* of the professional singer and speaker. Perhaps greater prominence has been given Coca preparations for the treatment of such functional derangements of the throat and voice than its application to any other use. Years before cocaine came into general utility Dr. Charles Fauvel, of Paris, directed attention to the importance of Coca for laryngeal troubles, while its use was speedily advanced in England by Dr. Morell Mackenzie and in the United States by Dr. Louis Elsberg, the father of American laryngology. Both of these gentlemen were in the clinic of Fauvel, and their methods were soon adopted by a host of skillful workers. Among those quoted as having used Coca successfully in laryngeal troubles are Lennox Browne, Beverley Robinson, Jarvis, H. H. Curtis, E. Fletcher Ingals, Solis Cohen, Sajous, Bosworth, Rice, and a host of other prominent laryngologists.[20] As has been shown, however, the effect of Coca is not in any sense merely a local one, but systemic, and its benefit is wholly dissimilar to that resulting from the topical application of cocaine, for Coca not only acts as a purifier of the blood, but through this influence as a nerve and muscle tonic.[21] This is exhibited through the empirical use of Coca long resorted to in mountain climbing.

The condition termed mountain sickness, experienced by travelers in high altitudes, is commonly supposed due to defective oxygenation of the blood. M. Jourdanet some years since explained that as there is less weight of oxygen in each inspiration the blood suffers from impoverishment exactly the same as though its percentage of red corpuscles had been reduced. Added to this difficulty is the intense cold and the bodily heat is used up more rapidly than the organism can supply it. M. Paul Bert more recently is of the opinion that man ordinarily inhales more oxygen than he actually requires, and just as one may accustom himself to a diet below that ordinarily consumed, so at the expense of some temporary suffering he could exist without the amount of oxygen normally taken. He has proposed an acclimating period, united with cultivating the number of red corpuscles, whereby

[20] Sajous' *Annual*, Vol. V, A35; 1891.
[21] Santa; 1891. See also *Collective Investigation*, in Appendix.

their capacity for absorbing a larger relative amount of oxygen is increased.[22] In this he has been supported by some experiments of Mosso, who has explained that the condition is due to a chemical influence upon the nerve centres, and suggests that cocaine in small doses increases the chemical processes of the body and augments respiration.[23] This is in full accord with our knowledge of the practical uses of Coca among the Andeans, united with facts of modern physiology.

The severity of mountain sickness is well illustrated through a recent attempt of Mr. Edward A. Fitz Gerald to reach the highest point of the Andes, at Aconcagua, twenty-three thousand and eighty feet above the sea, in the Argentine Republic; though an experienced Alpine traveller, he was obliged to abandon this feat himself and to be content with such laurels as he might reap through sending his Swiss guide, Zurbriggen, over the peak. Fitz Gerald was completely overcome when a few hundred yards from the top, beyond which it was impossible for him to proceed, through the severity of symptoms occasioned in the rarefied atmosphere. He says: "I tried more than once to go on, but was only able to advance two or three steps at a time and then had to stop, panting for breath, my struggles alternating with violent fits of nausea. At times I would fall down, and each time had greater difficulty in rising; black specks swam across my sight; I was like one walking in a dream, so dizzy and sick that the whole mountain seemed whirling round with me."[24]

The symptoms of mountain sickness often present themselves suddenly and without premonition. The guides commonly advise those unaccustomed to high altitudes not to go to sleep at night, for often the most oppressing symptoms occur, when the organism is lowered during sleep, and one will awaken as from a horrible nightmare, gasping for breath in terrible apprehension. The Indians prepare a Coca tea, which they administer for this condition. It affords relief that is so instantaneous as to appear magical, and accepting the inference of Mosso that the cause of mountain sickness is of a chemico-nervous origin, there is a further suggestion that

[22] Whymper; 1892. [23] Mosso; 1890. [24] Fitz Gerald; 1899.

whether the condition combated be muscular tire, nerve exhaustion from worry, or a physical incapacity due to chemical changes in the blood, the action of Coca is depurative.

It is a modern scientific theory that most functional derangements are due to a loading up of impurities from the blood or stored in the tissues, which have originated from a long-continued impropriety in living, and are made manifest through some aggravating indiscretion. If the hypothesis be true that Coca frees the blood of products of waste, this affords ample explanation of properties attributed to Coca which have hitherto appeared phenomenal, and its widespread usefulness and seemingly contradictory action over a host of apparently dissimilar conditions may be well understood. Whether the relief sought be for a simple vocal strain, for rheumatism, or for mountain sickness, nervous irritability or muscular fatigue, the conditions are of common origin. Coca simply makes better blood and a healthy blood makes healthy tissue.

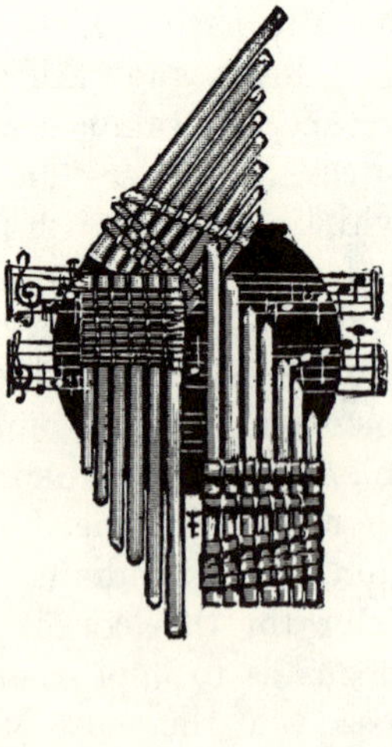

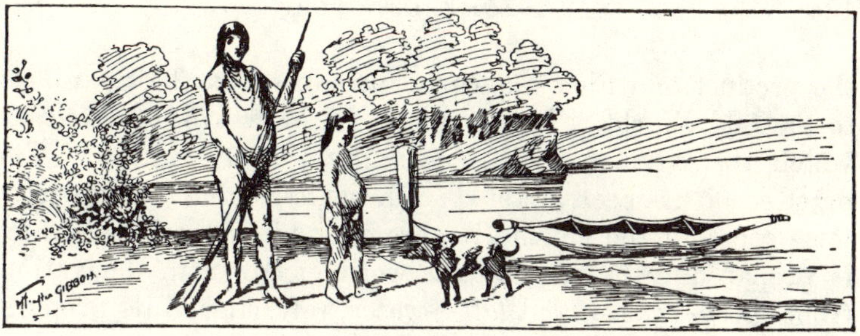

CHAPTER XVI.

THE DIETETIC INFLUENCE OF COCA.

"Each Leaf is Fruit, and such substantial Fare,
No Fruit beside to rival it will dare."

—Cowley.

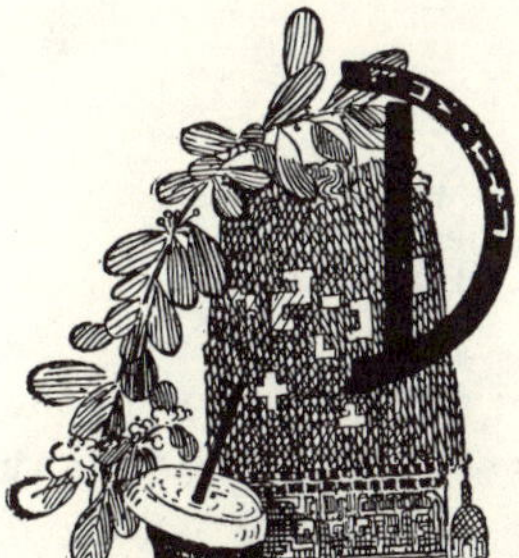

DURING the ages that Coca has been employed, its use as a source of energy and endurance without other means of subsistence, long since gave rise to the problem whether Coca can rightly be considered a food. Associated with this thought, there has apparently been suggested to the minds of some a name of similar sound of more common usage. The mention of Coca in a food connection has at once recalled to them cocoa and chocolate, which, though often components of an excellent dietary, are in no manner whatever related to Coca even by the most distant ties of kinship. This similarity of names has occasioned amusing errors, some of which are related—without reflection on their authors---to impress the distinction.

Cocoa is prepared from the roasted seeds of the palm *Theobroma Cacao,* Linn., an ancient tree of tropical America, the product of which was early introduced by the Spaniards to the Old World. It belongs to the order *Sterculiaceæ*, of which the African kola—(*Sterculia*), is a relative. The name cocoa has been adapted from the less euphonious specific term cacao of the genus *Theobroma*, while chocolate—which is prepared from cacao—is a word of Mexican derivation, from *choco*—cacao, and *latl*—water, referring to its preparation as a beverage. From cocoa there is obtained an active principle present in the proportion of about two per cent. This, first described by Woskresensky in 1845, was named theobromine, and though not identical, has been found closely allied to caffeine. From phonetic semblance Coca has been erroneously associated with cocoa or with the coconut, just as these latter two have been misquoted by the unthinking. Thus Dr. Johnson in his *Dictionary* published in 1755, confounded them, as emphasized in the following quotation which he has given under *cocoa:*

> "Amid those orchards of the Sun,
> Give me to drain the *cocoa's* milky bowl,
> And from the palm to draw its freshening wine!"
> —Thomson, *Seasons*, (Summer); line 677.

Those who have followed the history of Coca, and the story of the gradual unfolding of its leaves to usefulness, may express a cunning surprise that so careless a confusion of terms is possible. Some may consider that such knowledge is purely technical and hardly to be expected of the laity, yet very many of the medical profession are apparently among those who are uninformed. To an exceedingly large class Coca means simply chocolate, while the coconut is erroneously regarded as belonging to the same botanical group. Certain knowing ones there are who appreciate that cocoa seeds yield chocolate; yet among these some few are content in a belief that the leaf of the cocoa plant is the Coca chewed by the Andean Indians. It is hardly to be expected that physicians, who are commonly regarded as well informed, would continue an ignorance on this subject, in view of the very wide interest awakened by the application of cocaine.

In spite of the antiquity of centuries, the fact remains that Coca is not well known. This has been emphasized in the present inquiry. That this is not a mere apparent error, through hasty or illegible orthography, may be assured from the fullness of certain replies. Some of these, after describing the physiological action and therapeutic uses of Coca, have displayed a confusional state of knowledge by saying they have used some preparation of breakfast cocoa in place of tea or coffee at meals, or in greater detail have said: "I never use the liquid preparations—I prefer chocolate." One enthusiast, from a personal examination of cocoa with a microscope, pronounced "it free from adulteration," and another busy practitioner who uses "the ordinary cocoa of commerce for drinking at the table," and to whom some vague recollections of former readings has entwined the change of Coca by age with an awe inspiring potency of its active principle, says: "It should be seen to that it is fresh; age causes it to deteriorate," and concludes: "It is a dangerous remedy, which should be used with caution." One has answered my physiological question: "From memory, of the personal effects from the use of sweet chocolate." Another really kindly disposed gentleman regrets: "The great diversity of opinion regarding the effects in the application of the medicine," and as an explanation of his own neglect cites as illustration: "I am very unpleasantly affected by coffee or tea, presumably by caffeine. It depresses my heart's action and delays digestion. Ordinarily breakfast coffee for two mornings makes my pulse intermit; strong tea the same. Cocoa or chocolate is something worse. It does not digest, causing unpleasant eructations and a heavy, sour feeling in my stomach. Most people like cocoa, or especially chocolate, and prefer it when ill to coffee. From personal dislike I never recommend it and have never investigated the good qualities ascribed to it."

Amidst such a jumble resulting from an investigation among those especially educated to be observers it seems easier to believe with what seriousness the article was written some few years ago on *Cocoa and Cocaine,* a title which might be overlooked as a typographical error were it not for the statement that "cocoa contains two alkaloids, theobromine and cocaine,"[1] while a further muddle is possible through the recent introduction of a cocoa preparation by an English firm called "Cocoaine." There is always confusion unavoidable in the gradual evolvement of any remedy to usefulness; in the present instance this has not been confined to any one department, but has extended through each branch of research from the doings of the early Spanish historians to the botanists, the chemists, physiologists and physicians.

All the accounts of the early writers of Andean travel indicate that Coca has a phenomenal effect upon endurance, so great, indeed, that many of these accounts have been regarded as simply fabulous; but as we have considered the possibilities of Coca through the potential energy hidden in its leaf, it is very easy to trace the foundation of truth from these stories. The Indians were described as relying upon Coca for food and drink, with no other resource. "If you ask them why they thus continually keep Coca in the mouth and venerate it, they will answer you that its use prevents the feeling of hunger, thirst, and loss of strength, as well as preserves them in health."[2] Cieza refers to Coca as a most marvellous panacea "against hunger, or any need of food or drink."[3]

There was early desire on the part of the Church to discountenance the use of Coca, whether it contained food properties or not, because of its superstitious associations. Its use must be prohibited because it was a substance "which is connected with the work of idolatry and sorcery, strengthening the wicked in their delusions, and asserted by every competent judge to possess no true virtues; but on the contrary, to cause the deaths of innumerable Indians, while it ruins the health of the few who survive."[4] So that in order to restore the usefulness of Coca to the Indian, to whom it was found a necessity by his Spanish masters, this law was repealed after it had been demonstrated for politic reasons that Coca could not be a food. Some of the earlier writers presumed that any sustaining action must be due to some starchy or mucilaginous properties in the leaf, and to maintain this hypothesis it was

[1] Foy; 1886. [2] Monardes; 1580. [3] Cieza (Hakluyt); 1864. [4] *Ordinance;* 1567.

asserted that every ounce of leaves yielded a half ounce of gum. Poeppig, who has written many hasty conclusions of Coca, denied this, because from repeated analysis he found such a small portion of mucilage in the leaf that its food properties must be slight. He said: "The saliva of the Coca chewer is thin and watery, like that which flows from the chewing of tobacco, and it betrays not the least trace of sugar to the palate."[5]

Through all obstacles of prejudice or doubt the facts of the sustaining influence of Coca are so apparent as to be undeniable, and skepticism must be carried very far to now doubt the effect of Coca on nutrition. As Dr. Weddell has said: "One of two things is certain. Either the Coca contains some nutritive principle which directly sustains the strength or it does not contain it, and therefore simply deceives hunger while acting on the system." He was of the opinion that the nutritive principle of Coca might be due to the presence of a notable quantity of nitrogen, together with assimilable carbonized products.

This same hesitancy between acknowledging effects which are apparent to all observers, united with a preformed prejudice without the weight of scientific evidence, is still intermixed in the confusion of our own time. An indication of the readiness with which opinion is swayed may be inferred from some of the letters received in my investigation. One physician writes: "I quit the use of Coca after some publications in the journals. I was scared off too soon, probably." This conservatism, born of timidity, is shown through many replies similar to the following: "I scarcely ever prescribe a medicine unless it has been done by others more venturesome than myself; I think the hesitancy in prescribing Coca was owing to the numerous reports of the cocaine habit contracted by patients which have been published from time to time;" yet such so-called "habit," as elsewhere shown, is not proven.

We have seen under what difficulty the Andeans were permitted to continue the use of Coca as a means of sustenance, and from that early superstition to the subsequent prejudice

[5] Poeppig; 1835.

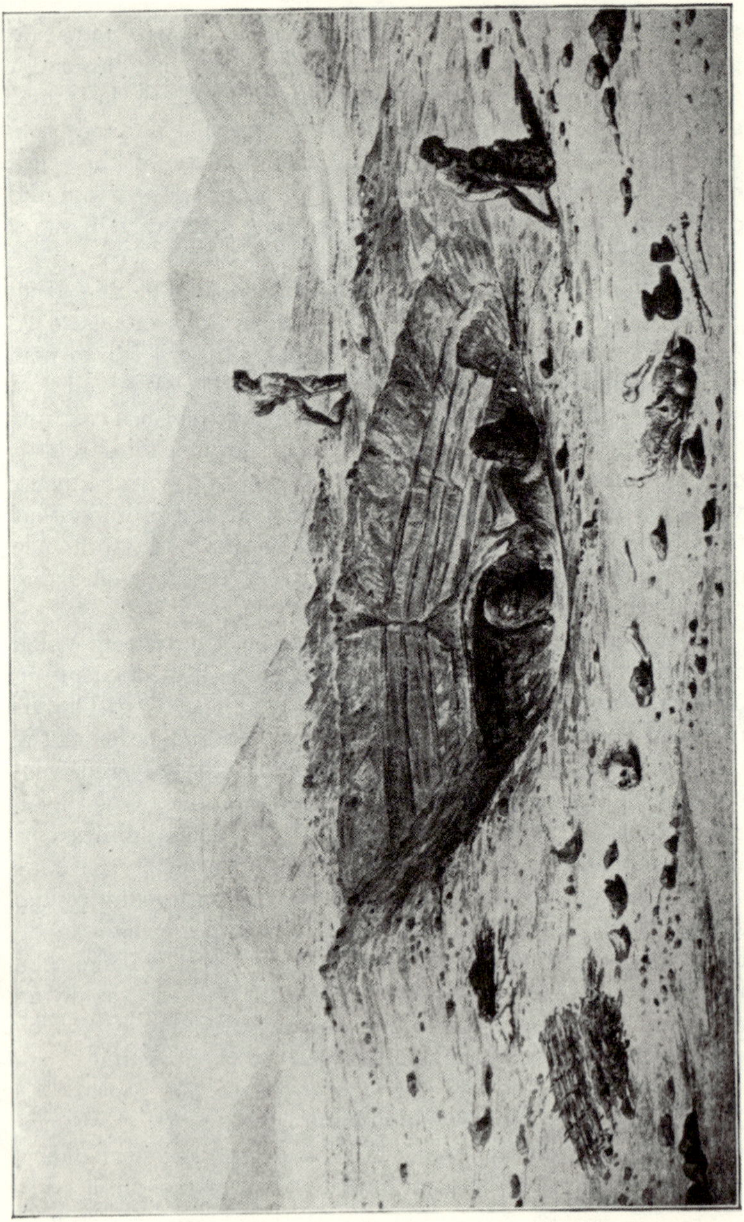

Opening Incan Graves. Coast of Ancon, Peru. [*Reiss and Stübel.*]

and confusion, which has continued even to our own time, it is not at all surprising that Coca has been little understood, wrongly applied, or has occasioned little thought toward its application as a food.

The popular idea of the term food may possibly be embodied in the one word—repletion—without regard to whether the substance consumed is capable in itself to sustain the bodily functions. It is such a thought perhaps which prompted the reply to my inquiry as to the dietetic uses of Coca: "This is all a terrible mistake—cocoa is used as food, but Coca, never!" The misconception of the term food, as well as the mistaken application arising from this, has laid the foundation for many a disease. Scientists well know that there is no one article of food that will supply all the requirements of the organism. Nature demands a certain quantity of chemical elements, properly apportioned and combined, which shall go to repair the tissues. It is by this repeated aid that the complex process of living in the struggle for the maintenance of supremacy or of even mere existence, is continued.

The whole matter of dietetics is little understood—not among those whose duty it is to explain such matters, but among the people who eat indiscriminately of whatever may be offered so long as it shall be of tempting form and palatable, and to whom the ponderable is commonly the more potent. This is often the occasion for much resultant misery, poor health, and consequent unhappiness, generated through an improper use of those blessings which are given to enjoy. It is use without abuse that should be impressed—not abstinence, and yet not unbridled indulgence. Some who look at this narrowly are apt to moralize, as did the little chap when deprived of his sweets and forced to castor oil: "All the good things *is* bad, and all the bad things *is* good." The fact is we become so familiarized with ordinary functions that their performance is often lightly dismissed as instinctive—something which every one should know for himself. As a result few care to read physiology while well, and when they are ill it is too late.

In a modern civilization desire is apt to seek indulgence in proportion to opportunity. There is a privilege in wealth, increase of which usually suggests freer methods, and greater comforts, which often point toward sensual indulgence rather than to any philosophy of living. Then follows not only luxuriance, but an extravagance and ultimate *dis*-ease, a veritable want of ease and comfort. This has ever been the cycle since the world began, and it rolls on so easily and quickly that before excesses are even dreamed of much constitutional harm is done. But: "the doctors are here to attend to such little matters; let them do the worrying, we will continue our enjoyment."

The history of all aboriginal peoples indicates a simple dietary of natural products, a thought from which our vegetarian friends doubtless find much prestige:—

> "The field as yet untilled, their feasts afford
> And fill a sumptuous and unenvied board."

sang Hesiod. We have seen how the Incans lived largely upon maize or the starchy food of various tubers; yet while the common herd must find content in these, the nobility enriched their feasts with game and the various productions from the hot valleys and stimulated their desires or allayed the effects of over indulgence by Coca. Even fresh fish was served at the royal tables, brought by rapid runners, who by a special grant of a few handfuls of Coca were enabled to make a trip of several hundred miles from the sea to the imperial city of Cuzco in a single day.[6]

It is curious to consider how the first blind selections of foodstuffs may have been made in the early days when there were no botanists, chemists nor cooks. Many must have chosen wrongly and suffered for their boldness, for we know that similar errors are occurring about us everywhere and with equally unfortunate results. These early errors gave rise to the necessity for a more careful choice—for an elective knowledge, and we who followed long ages after, while continuing to profit by the methods of these early specialists benefit through their method of natural selection. We owe gratitude for a multitude of important and what are now consid-

[6] Prescott; I; p. 70; 1848.

ered absolutely necessary foodstuffs which have been preserved and improved for us through a refinement of cultivation and are now universally used. Among these we have examples in those Peruvian products, Coca, maize and the potato, which have been so long cultivated that the most profound research has not been enabled to determine their original home in the wild state.

We have seen why it is probable that aboriginal peoples were vegetarians, and we know through the ancient historians that the use of meat was often considered unlawful or unholy. Possibly the use of meat may be associated with the stimulus demanded in the incessant struggle for supremacy in the larger cities where statistics show its greater consumption than among agricultural people. Homer alludes to the moderate use of meat among his heroes, a chine of beef roasted being a favorite dish not often indulged in. Boiled meats and broths seem to have been among the earlier means of using flesh, but as tastes change, so these early simple methods soon gave place to greater variety. Then—as the senses have ever led the judgment—we read of wealthy gourmands who vied with each other in serving absurd and often disgusting dishes as epicurean delights. Apicius—who wished for the neck of a stork that he might longer enjoy the delights of deglutition—dissolved pearls and offered them in wine to his guests, and after squandering a fortune in dining killed himself because he had but a paltry eighty thousand pounds left.

Among some of the dainty relishes served during the early Grecian period was the dormouse, the hedgehog and puppies, while the flesh of the young ass was considered a delicacy. Peacocks were regarded as essential to every well ordered banquet, and Aufidius Lures is said to have derived an income of many thousands of dollars from the sale of these at a price of seven to eleven dollars apiece. Such fabulous sums were spent for single entertainments that Seneca, who was himself enormously wealthy, refers to the profusion of dishes and extravagance of the times when he alludes to:

> "Vitellius' table which did hold
> As many creatures as the ark of old."

The Middle Ages were scarcely better in habits of indulgence; swans, peacocks and the wild boar continued among the delicacies of the table until long after the reign of Edward the Fourth, while Charles the Fifth of Germany was a royal gourmand who delighted in dishes quite as extravagant as any of those that graced the tables of the Greeks or Romans, some of his viands being lizard soup, roast horse and cats in jelly, which were washed down with deep draughts of Rhine wine.

We have seen that among the Incas hospitality was considered so essential as to demand a law necessitating and governing its practice. On all state occasions the monarch feasted the nobles at a banquet, where important consumma-

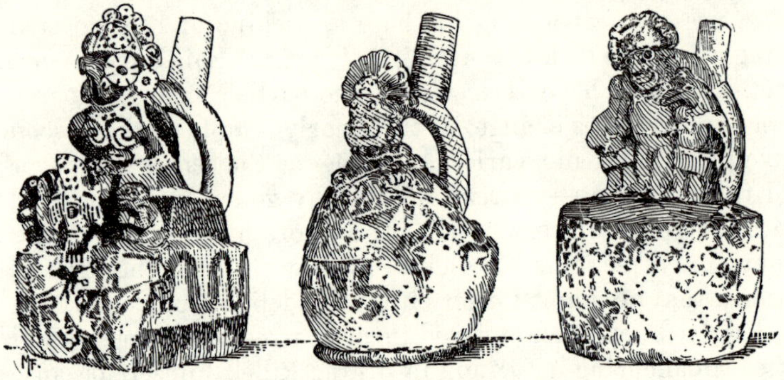

PERUVIAN VASES. [*Tweddle Collection.*]

tions were solemnized by royal bumpers of the native *chicha* quaffed from golden goblets. Among the masses the usual hours for eating were eight or nine in the morning and at sunset; these latter periods Garcilasso says were sometimes turned into a veritable revelry extending far into the night, a custom which has not been wholly neglected among the modern Andeans, who were quick to adopt the *fiesta* which is prompted on slight impulse in all Spanish countries.

If we review the history of dietetics we shall find it fluctuating between indulgence and satiety, with an occasional interim of enforced fasting through necessity. During the last century many were actually starved through the return wave of abstemiousness, because of the scientific efforts of their medical advisers, many of whom—like Dr. Sangrado,[7] urged copious draughts of hot water with liberal blood letting, or insisted on some rigid dietary for all, unmindful of the fact that what might be advisable for a sick man may not prove desirable to one in health. Thus matters dietetical have largely balanced themselves through appetite and opportunity, while physicians have too commonly followed the methods of the masses and suffered or benefited in accordance with the resources of their environment.

With such changes between excess and abstemiousness—of too much or too little advice—popular views have naturally been unsettled or indifferent on the diet question. It is unanimous upon one point, however, and as Sancho Panza,[8] after he became Governor of the Island of Barataria—"Having appetite, must eat something." It is to teach what this something may be which proves the great stumbling block. It can only be broadly done in any book, the individual necessities must be the subject of personal attention.

One value of knowledge is to recognize error; it is negative as well as affirmative. In matters dietetic there should be sufficient preliminary education to understand more closely not only what to eat with advantage but what to avoid in order to make better citizens. We are at present in an age of preventive methods of many things, and it would seem that the modern physician—he who aims more especially to guide his patients so as to keep them from becoming ill, rather than he who confines his problems to curing them when prostrate—may find the greatest and most profitable solution in the maintenance of health through an appropriate and well directed dietary. Without necessarily following we can adapt the means of others which seem desirable to our own necessities. If in this adaption prejudice be set aside and the possibilities of Coca shall be considered, there will occur opportunities which must ultimately result in a more pronounced benefit to overworked and overtired humanity.

[7] Le Sage; *Gil Blas.* [8] Cervantes; *Don Quixote.*

It is only within the last fifty years that our chemico-physiologic knowledge in dietetics has developed from the foundation laid by Liebig, the work since his time tending chiefly to clearing up errors or explaining his theories, which are not yet fully accepted. From a review of the opinion of many physiologists it is difficult to give a concise definition of a food. In accordance with the theory here advocated I will thus define it: *Food is any substance taken into the body which maintains integrity of the tissues and creates the energy we term life.* With such a definition in view, it may the more readily be appreciated that it is not necessarily what is eaten but what is assimilated that is beneficial. It is somewhat as Froude has said of knowledge: "The knowledge which a man can use is the only real knowledge." So the food which the body utilizes is the only real food. This of necessity must vary with conditions and environment, and as civilization tends to shape all things to her own demands, it is the object of dietetics to adapt the varying possibilities to man's requirements.

It is a common assertion advanced in all seriousness that one partakes of the nature of the food eaten. The vegetarian claims to see in the meat eater the ferocity of the carnivorous animal. The pugnacious beef-eating Briton and the seemingly docile Chinese rice-eater are sometimes cited as examples. Aside from the effect on the emotions as a result of companionship there can be no weight to the homely saying: "He who drinks beer thinks beer." Again, the idea that: "Every part strengthens a part" is another common error, for physiologically we know that bone does not make bone nor does fat make fat. There are many who presume that vegetables are the only appropriate food for man. Plutarch tells us that Grillus—who, according to the doctrine of transmigration, had at one time been a beast—describes how much better he fed and lived when an animal than when he was turned again to man. It is not necessary to accept this literally, but it suggests the fact that all flesh is grass and emphasizes the indestructibility of matter. But man need not eat grass as did Nebuchadnezzar, for when he eats animal flesh he virtually eats the very elements which are comprised in the vegetable kingdom and which have been appropriately elaborated.

Our tissues are a combination of chemical elements, chief among which are carbon, hydrogen, oxygen and nitrogen, with some minor ones present as salts in small proportions. These elements compose all animal cells, just as we have seen their presence is essential in vegetable structures. In order that the integrity of the tissues shall be maintained these principles must be introduced into the organism. It has been estimated that the average daily loss of these consists of carbon, 281.2 grammes; hydrogen, 6.3 grammes; oxygen, 681.41 grammes; nitrogen, 18.8 grammes,[9] so that the selection of any dietary should be made to approximate this proportionate loss in order to balance waste. These elements are not of themselves food, nor can they synthetically be built into a food in the laboratory.

Chemistry teaches us that energy is liberated by every chemical union, and so it is the conversion of the food materials taken and containing these chemical elements which liberates the energy essential to continue the cell growth which constitutes existence. The body is but a colony of cells through which the several elements pass after an elaboration from inorganic compounds through vegetable and animal tissue. After their property is exerted to the maintenance of a higher organization they are cast aside, only to again pass through the cycle of elaboration and to be again consumed and so on for innumerable times without ultimate loss, but in each interchange yielding the energy we term life.

Food substances according to variation of primal elements are embraced in two groups: The nitrogenous—of which albumen is the type—containing carbon, hydrogen, oxygen and nitrogen, comprises the proteids of which muscle and the structure of the body generally is formed, which among foods is represented by the lean of meat, fish and poultry, casein of milk and cheese, albumen of eggs, gelatin, gluten of cereals and the albuminous substance contained in such vegetables as peas, beans and lentils. The second class, the non-nitrogenous

[9] Kirkes'; p. 212; 1884.

—technically known as the carbohydrates—contains carbon, hydrogen and oxygen and embraces the sugars and starches, however derived, and the oils and fats whether of cream, flesh, fish or fowl.

The nitrogenous group constitutes the incombustible framework of the body, in which, according to Liebig, the second class—the combustible non-nitrogenous—fuel foods are consumed. It seems strange to speak of combustion, which is suggestive of fire, as going on within the body, but the process of chemical conversion within is akin to that of combustion without, and before food can reach its ultimate end in the repair of tissue, internal oxidation is essential to create heat, which is an index of the available force for work. The deprivation of food is chiefly made manifest through heat loss, and starvation has been paralleled to death by cold, while in restoration from prolonged lack of food the application of warmth is at first really more essential than is food.

From various physiological experiments it has been shown that animals fed exclusively on a non-nitrogenous diet speedily emaciate and die, as though from starvation, and experimentally life is more prolonged in those fed with nitrogenous than in those fed upon non-nitrogenous food, while animal heat is maintained fully as well by the former as by the latter.[10] Most of the evils of mankind are due to mal-nutrition, whereby the body undergoes changes which are comparable to those resulting either from starvation or from overproduction. Changes which are really induced not necessarily by taking too much or too little food, but from taking improper proportions of the two broad classes, or due to a lack of stimulus to a proper conversion. At times the excess will pass through the alimentary canal unchanged or remain in the intestine unabsorbed, undergoing a slow decomposition setting free gases and inducing various digestive disturbances.

The carbohydrates are readily converted into storage food, which, under certain conditions, may be transformed into fat, and this may so clog the working of the organs as to prove a

[10] Kirkes'; p. 221; 1884.

decided detriment to the body rather than a source of strength. It is commonly considered, however, that an excess of nitrogenous food is the chief source of trouble in overfeeding, and possibly, because of concentration, this class of food may the more readily be eaten in excess unthinkingly.

There is a vast physiological importance to the alimentary canal, for through it is introduced all the material which goes to build up the organism, including every chemical element of the body except oxygen. Hippocrates considered that the stomach bears the same relation to animals as soil does to plants, a parallel which leads a modern writer[11] to say: "A man whose digestion is defective is comparable to a tree which planted in sterile soil finishes by withering and perishing." The alimentary canal, however, does not end at the stomach, an organ which is really a mere expanded reservoir for the digestive tract. The fact that conversion and absorption takes place through almost the entire extent of this canal is not commonly considered. There seems to prevail a popular idea that it is the stomach only which is responsible in preparing food for assimilation. This opinion was so prevalent in the time of Dr. William Hunter that he remarked the error by saying to his class: "Gentlemen, physiologists will have it that the stomach is a mill; others that it is a fermenting vat; others again that it is a stew-pan; but in my view of the matter it is neither a mill, a fermenting vat nor a stewpan, but a stomach, gentleman, a stomach."

To effect the proper conversion of food its minute division is essential in order that the several digestive substances with which the bolus comes in contact in its passage through the alimentary canal may act upon the different parts for which they have an elective affinity. By the action of these enzymes, or ferments as they are termed, the food is rendered soluble, and so made capable of absorption. A substance taken as food which remains insoluble is virtually out of the body so far as nutrition is concerned and is really only an irritant. The whole process of digestion is one of solution so that the food may pass through the tissues into the blood. Ab-

[11] Beau; *Traité de la Dyspepsie.*

sorption takes place in every part of the digestive tract and as the unabsorbed mass is passed onward different ferments act upon different portions of the bolus to prepare it for solution. The process of mastication when properly performed not only breaks up the food and softens the mass with saliva ready for its transit, but sets free a ferment which changes the insoluble starchy particles into a soluble sugar. The flow of saliva is increased by the act of chewing, or may even be effected reflexly by the emotions through the sympathetic nerve, either of which causes increases the blood supply to the secreting gland.

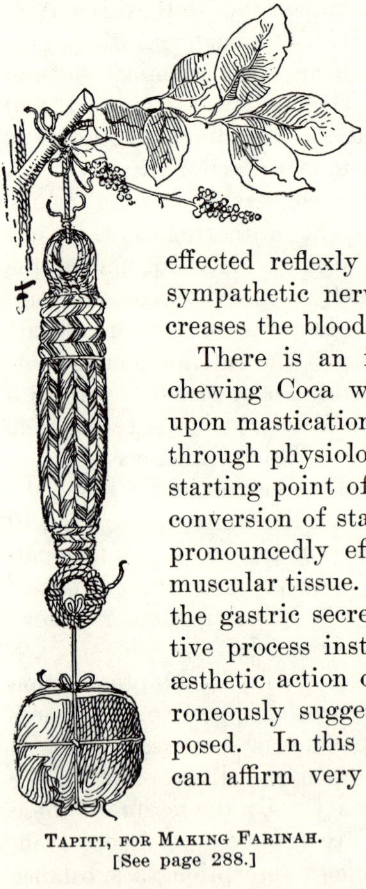

TAPITI, FOR MAKING FARINAH.
[See page 288.]

There is an increased flow of saliva from chewing Coca which is not wholly dependent upon mastication, but the function is increased through physiological action. This may be the starting point of its beneficial influence in the conversion of starchy foods which is ultimately pronouncedly effective in the building up of muscular tissue. Then through its action upon the gastric secretions Coca furthers the digestive process instead of checking it by any anæsthetic action on the stomach, as has been erroneously suggested and as is commonly supposed. In this relation Dr. Weddle says: "I can affirm very positively that Coca, as it is taken habitually, does not satiate hunger. This is a fact of which I have convinced myself by daily experience. The Indians who accompanied me on my journey chewed Coca during the whole day, but at evening they filled their stomachs like fasting men, and I am certain I have seen one devour as much food at a single meal as I should have consumed during two days."

A host of modern observers have recognized the true food value of Coca in nutrition, particularly serviceable in the emergency of protracted fevers or in debility until other food may take its place, and life has been prolonged for long periods under the exclusive use of Coca during the enforced abstinence from other food.* Rusby found that Coca allays the hunger sense, but does not suspend ability, being really a tonic to digestion, while Reichert, from laboratory experiments, concluded that Coca might not only replace food, but "in cases of restricted diet, or even in the entire absence of food, will enable the individual to perform as much or even more work than under ordinary circumstances."[12]

There has been an attempt to explain this influence of Coca upon the sense of hunger through an anæsthetic action on the mucous membrane of the stomach, which seems parallel to the idea that tobacco abolishes the sense of hunger through disgust by prostrating nervous action. But as Anstie says: "It is wholly improbable that agents having a depressing influence on the nervous system, such as antimony and ipecac, would relieve the feeling of weakness occasioned through hunger and fatigue."[13] It should be recalled that the sense of hunger is not local, but general. It is the demand of the system for nourishment, a call for fuel in order to supply energy. The sensation is experienced by the stomach reflexly, but the demand may be fulfilled by the introduction of food into the organism through any channel. Thus the sensation of thirst which is commonly referred to a dryness in the throat may be relieved by the addition of fluid to the blood by any method. The probability is that Coca through its nitrogenous influence so affects metabolism as to enable the organism to utilize substances which might otherwise pass off as waste. Just as we have seen in plant structures a similar influence under well-apportioned nitrogenous substances.

The local effect on the stomach by the introduction of food is to cause the mucous membrane to become reddened through an increased blood supply. This stimulates the gastric secretion of watery fluid, salts, pepsin and the acids which

* See Food Uses, *Collective Investigation* in Appendix.
[12] Reichert; October, 1890. [13] Anstie; 1864.

render that ferment active. The action on starch which commenced in the mouth is now checked and the solution of saline particles of the food is continued, while the insoluble nitrogenous bodies are converted into soluble peptones. The gastric juice also acts by retarding decomposition in bodies which are prone to this change in the presence of warmth and moisture.

From the stomach the food mass passes to the small intestine, where the influence of the gastric fluid ceases and a new process is commenced by the bile, intestinal juice, and the secretions of the pancreas, acting in an alkaline fluid. Here the albuminous materials which have escaped the former processes are converted into soluble peptones, while any starchy matters which have not been converted by the ptyaline of the saliva are also acted upon and changed into glucose. The pancreatic juice also emulsifies the oils and fats, splitting them up into their fatty acids and glycerine to enable their more ready absorption by the lacteals of the intestine and by the blood vessels.

Food does not pass through the digestive tract just as a weight might be dropped through a tube, but having once entered the œsophagus it is propelled by a peculiar undulating movement termed peristalsis—a motion similar to the method by which an angle worm creeps along. The muscular fibres contract and draw a portion of the tube over the mass to be propelled, elongation then takes place and a succession of such waves rather draws the substance down than presses it on, while at the same time it is checked from too rapid passage, so that digestion may proceed. As the mass reaches the large intestine there is probably no digestive process continued, though assimilation may take place through the absorption of some portion of the fluids which have been carried there. This peristaltic motion throughout the digestive tract is governed by certain muscular fibres, physiologically influenced by the action of Coca, which accounts for its beneficial effect in overcoming constipation.

The average time of the passage of food along the alimentary canal is about twenty-four hours, during which transit it is augmented by several gallons of fluids or juices which are concerned in the process of digestion. There is a constant interchange of these juices from the tissues of the digestive tract and the blood vessels which supply them, absorption taking place wherever there are blood vessels with their accompanying lymphatics, and the tissues of the body are bathed in a sort of lymph at all times even outside of the vessels. Such fluid as may not be directly absorbed into the blood is carried towards the heart and soon becomes part of the circulation, while the refuse is passed off as excreta.

To the liver, which is the largest glandular organ of the body, is attributed a marked influence upon the emotions, an effect really dependent on the fact whether the excreta of the blood are properly converted and eliminated or not. As Henry Ward Beecher said: "When a man's liver is out of order the kingdom of heaven is out of joint," and I presume he knew. Certain it is that there has always been associated with the imperfect action of this organ the idea of despair, which the Greeks presumed due to "black bile" and hence named melancholia *μελας*—black, *χολη*—bile. The liver forms an important function in nutrition not only in the elaboration and purification of the blood, but also in a peculiar property of forming glucose—or a substance akin to sugar or to the starch of plants—which is stored up in the liver cells[14] to be doled out as occasion may demand for the purpose of combustion or the formation of fat.[15] So active is this function that the liver even continues after death to make glycogen, as is termed this first product in its sugar formation.

This animal starch is elaborated chiefly from saccharine or starchy foods, though it is also made from proteids, which are split up into glycogen and urea—a striking example of direct conversion within the body from nitrogenous into a non-nitrogenous substance. The readiness with which the liver forms sugar indicates the possibility of its over production, which is indeed what takes place in glycosuria when the increase of the small amount of sugar which may normally be found in the blood is probably augmented through some nervous impulse and excreted by the kidneys.

[14] Bernard; 1877. [15] *Idem;* 1853.

The influence of Coca upon nutrition is markedly evidenced by its physiological action, and specifically by the effect of cocaine on glycogen conversion, as demonstrated by the experiments of Ehrlich[16] on the cells of the liver of mice, which under cocaine resembled stuffed goose livers. It should be recalled that the food must be rendered soluble before it can enter the circulation, and once in the blood, if the soluble products of starch—grape sugar, and the soluble peptones from proteids can not be converted into insoluble products they will be swept out of the body through the kidneys. This is precisely what occurs in certain forms of albuminuria and glycosuria. The conversion of similar substances in plant structures under the influence of nitrogenous compounds strongly suggests the utility of the nitrogenous Coca in the conversion of these soluble products into less soluble glycogen and proteids, and indicates a possible application of Coca to the relief of diabetes and albuminuria, disorders in which it has already been employed empirically with advantage.

Man's chief desire is to acquire strength and energy for the furtherance of his ambition, be that of a physical or mental nature. The intelligent being should base his sustenance upon this hopeful instinct. One engaged in active work in the open air usually finds appetite for the food presented without being over fastidious. Throughout the greater part of British India and China the majority of the people live largely upon rice stimulated in its conversion to muscle energy through the nitrogenous influence of a liberal tea drinking. Diametrically opposite on the globe, amidst the cold and rigors of the higher altitude of the Andes the Indian finds his powers effectively sustained by a diet of maize and nitrogenous Coca leaves. Science has verified this crude empirical experience by proving that carbohydrates contribute force when properly converted and that Coca not only creates mental energy, but muscular power through an actual change within the tissue cells. These are facts which it is well to remember.

Every one realizes that active muscular work provokes

[16] Ehrlich; p. 717; 1890.

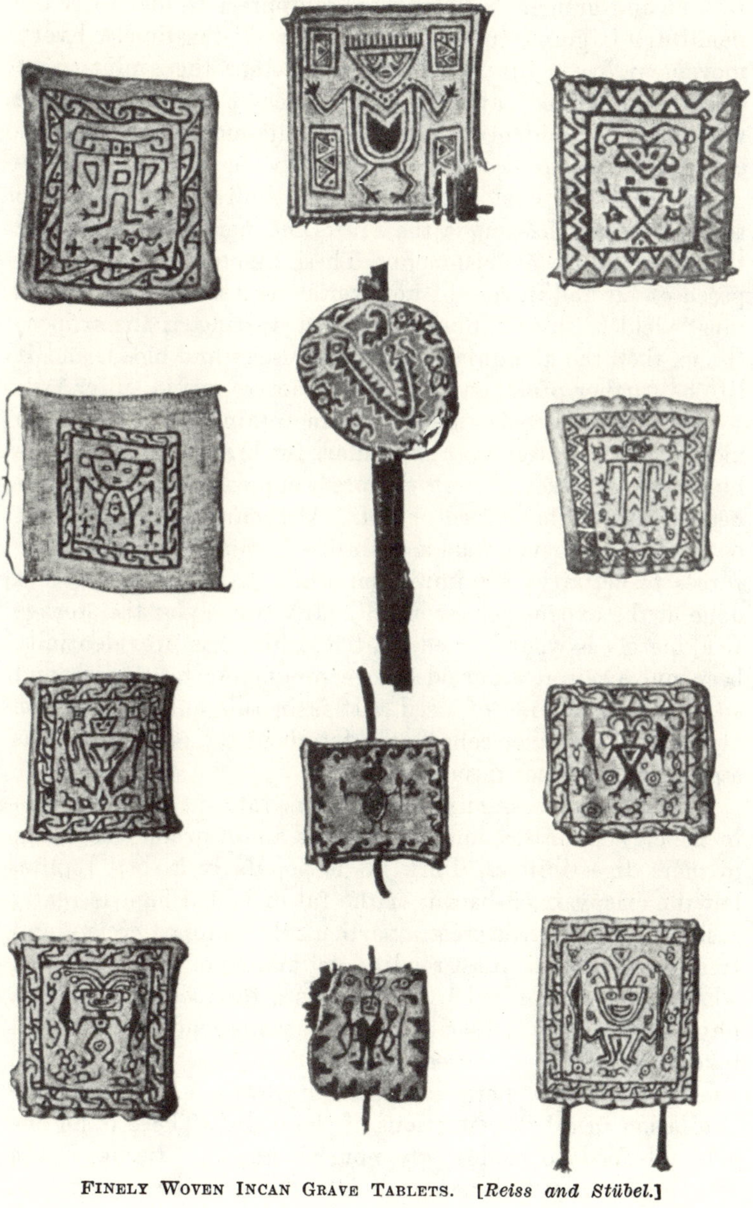

Finely Woven Incan Grave Tablets. [*Reiss and Stübel.*]

fatigue and hunger, but few seem to appreciate that force expenditure is going on within the body all the time. Every movement, be it the most simple, whether the evolution of gentle thought in prayer, the turbulence of passion, even the vital changes incidental to existence, although performed unconsciously, each occasions a conversion of tissue which demands repair. That these functions shall be performed to the end nature has made the brain and nerves imperious in their demand for nourishment. These tissues are chiefly composed of fat and in case of impoverishment every other tissue must yield to their support. First a wasting of the adipose tissue, then the glandular, then the muscles and blood, and if life be further prolonged, brain and nerves would suffer last.

Food therefore is essential to maintain bodily repair in mental work as well as in muscular, for brain work indeed is hungry work, even though the pre-occupied worker may forget whether he has dined or not. At such times what might be termed emergency food is desirable to stimulate the flagging forces to activity; a stimulation which we have seen is not done at the expense of essential bodily tissue, for the storage food merely is what is used up, that which has providentially been put away at a period of overproduction to nourish and support in the time of need. It is in this quality that the glycogen in the liver cells or the fat about the muscles acts as a preserver of other tissue.

Fat is not necessarily created from fat, but has its origin in the carbohydrates, and certain fats are desirable according to their digestibility. Pork fat is popularly in bad repute, but the crispy fried bacon, or the fat of boiled ham is really easily digested, while cream, particularly whipped cream, and fresh butter are the most readily assimilated of all edible fats. The chief value of cod liver oil is as a fat food and modern physicians do not prescribe it for patients who can and will take other and more agreeable fats.

Strength and energy are the outgrowths of a proper assimilation in all the functions of the body. There is no one class of food to exclusively nourish any one tissue, but a complex dietary embracing a wide variety is demanded, and is as absolutely necessary for the development of muscle, or brain, or nerve as it is for mere existence itself, for life implies unanimity between all the cells which form the colony of the organism. It is in this sense that Coca is to be regarded as having an important bearing upon nutrition and hence worthy to be ranked among the highest type of stimulants. It is a stimulant to energy, though it does not supply in itself the whole force any more than any other one food can do. In this sense, to borrow an apt simile suggested by Gubler, Coca may be compared to the fulminate of a cartridge, which, though not in itself the force, yet it excites the energy which propels the bullet.[17] As a nitrogenous fulminate is essential to cause the powder to act, so, too, nitrogenous substances are necessary in all metabolism, whether of plant or animal life to provoke nourishment, to stimulate repair and to convert the stored-up substances to activity and usefulness.

There is a foundation of truth when in training a meat diet is adopted—not to make muscle because the meat itself is muscle, but to excite the conversion of stored-up tissue into energy. For this reason during such a diet flesh is often lost through the using up of stored supplies—but not necessarily of frame work tissue, for the muscles become firmer as the fat is taken from them. It is true that an injudicious dietary may so completely use up this stored tissue that instead of strength there is a lack of power and endurance. This is one example of how mischief may be done by limiting food supplies to one class, which is always an unwise course to follow as a matter of choice for any length of time.

It would seem that the whole idea of "wear and tear" has been popularly misconstrued, and through this misunderstanding there has resulted much mischief. "The body does not waste because it works, but works because it wastes."[18] There is certainly a constant decomposition—a wear and tear—going on in every cell of the tissues, and the more actively these are exercised—within physiological limits—the more rapidly they are renewed. This renewal through activity means life and is absolutely essential to existence.

[17] Gubler; 1881. [18] Martin; p. 290; 1881.

Food may be stored up, but without its proper conversion there can be no energy and our cells would be simply storehouses of supplies hoarded in a miserly way to no purpose, while death would certainly follow from the encumbrance of surfeit and consequent inertia.

Unfortunately the body supplies have often been compared to the money saved in a bank, and the excitation to energy through stimulus has been allied to the withdrawal of a certain amount of capital, which, if not immediately returned, must result in impoverishment. This is only theoretical, for if it were literally true the more work the human machine performed the sooner it would be used up, while all know that work—activity—is essential to life and well being, even to rejuvenation and happiness.

If the bodily energies must be compared to a saved-up fund it should be recalled that a bank carries on its affairs by the stimulus of the moneys which pass through it. It does all its work, gives forth an energy of interest, yet holds the capital unimpaired. So the tissues of the human organism are maintained by the stimulus of food, from which there is given forth an interest in energy, while the capital is not necessarily consumed. The mistake, it seems, has arisen from the supposition often advanced that each being is born with a certain life force, just as a steam engine is created capable of a certain amount of work, which may be all consumed in a day or gradually used through a period of years. The modern physiology of cell life emphatically contradicts such a supposition.

The question of the daily amount of food necessarily is a relative one, to be determined by physical development, and the work to be performed. The average amount has been calculated from the daily loss of elements and the proportion of these in the various foodstuffs, a balance being maintained in the relation of the nitrogenous to non-nitrogenous substances, as one to four. It has been estimated that a man weighing one hundred and fifty pounds and in moderate activity will lose somewhere about three hundred grammes of carbon and twenty grammes of nitrogen a day. Constructing a theoretical diet on this basis the amount of food is selected to approximate this loss. The common error arises in an excess of one or the other of these substances, rather than in too much food, and as satiety gives a sense of satisfaction, the mischief is apt to be overlooked. Every kind of food is capable of maintaining the body for a time and man's high organization admits of ready adaptability, but the necessity for a mixed dietary is founded upon scientific fact. With this thought in view more good may be done by the shaping of an appropriate diet in health than may be accomplished by the most clever wielding of potent remedies in disease.

There is one other factor allied to this matter of dietetics quite as important in regulating assimilation as is the proportion of elements or of comparative digestibility. As all processes and actions are governed by brain power, controlled through nerve conduction, it is essential that the several organs shall not only be fitted, but unimpeded for their functions. In large cities the feverish struggle of daily life more closely concerns money-getting than any elective dietary. This constant nervous tension is a primal cause of digestive disturbance and the long train of evils which follow. Business men as a rule do not take sufficient time to eat, as may be seen in any one of the great restaurants in this city, where the entire feeding of coming and going thousands is sustained in a period almost too brief to admit of enjoying an appropriate meal. The excitement, the hurry and bustle is contagious and the nervous strain reflected is too great to permit of proper digestion. The food is hurried to the stomach improperly prepared, where it must remain as an irritant both to that organ and the nervous system.

A brain engaged in deep thought cannot properly attend to the digestion of a hearty meal, nor encompassing a hearty meal will the digestive tract permit a brain to give forth its clearest work, both processes must be imperfectly performed when attempted together. The best after dinner speakers commonly only make a pretense of dining when they anticipate that their oratorical efforts are to be called for, while those who, like the Romans, have "dined to the full," fall into that unargumentative ecstatic condition which dominates a good listener.

Let it be remembered that as the nervous system is first to suffer from a faulty dietary, so, too, a disordered nervous organization is prone to derange the digestive functions. Modern usage has happily appointed the principal meal after the care and worry of the day is over. Pleasant surroundings at meals stimulates appetite and conversation facilitates digestion, because, aside from the emotional influence, the time is prolonged and eating is done more deliberately.

Perhaps better judgment does not commonly go far astray in these matters, still a reiteration of truths is desirable to impress the greatest good, and if anything is evolved from this chapter in dietetics it should be the fact that food is better than medicine, and that Coca is not only theoretically but practically a food. Coca, indeed, is a food not only serviceable in emergency, but a desirable adjunct to the accustomed dietary, in order to provoke an effective conversion of other food supplies into vigor and happiness.

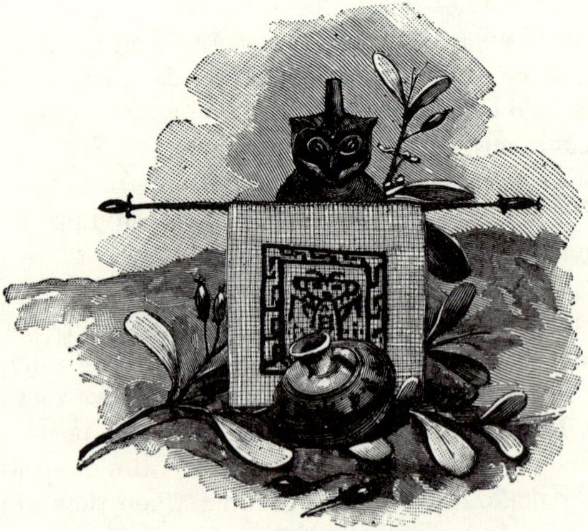

APPENDIX

A COLLECTIVE INVESTIGATION AMONG SEVERAL HUNDRED PHYSICIANS ON THE PHYSIOLOGICAL ACTION AND THE THERAPEUTIC APPLICATION OF COCA

APPENDIX

A COLLECTIVE INVESTIGATION UPON THE PHYSIOLOGICAL ACTION AND THERAPEUTIC APPLICATION OF COCA, AMONG SEVERAL HUNDRED PHYSICIANS.

The method of this investigation was to address an autograph letter to a selected set of physicians, principally teachers in the different medical colleges, who, being informed of the nature of the inquiry, were asked to give the result of their personal observations upon the uses of Coca. With this letter was enclosed a blank of questions for convenience of recording information and a stamped envelope for reply. Five thousand such letters were sent out during the year 1897.

As a great majority of those addressed made no response at all, an additional communication was sent, the entire inquiry and correspondence numbering upward of ten thousand letters. The total of replies received from all sources was twelve hundred and six. Of this number forty-four had failed to obtain results from the preparations of Coca hitherto used by them, while many had never employed it in their practice, either because they were not familiar with it or from some vague fear or prejudice, the nature of which they could not explain. In the compilation of this report all observations, whether in favor of or opposed to Coca, are given equal prominence, for in such an investigation the negative side is quite as valuable as is the affirmative testimony. The principal objections against the use of Coca which have been advanced, are a supposed inertness of Coca through confounding it with cocoa and chocolate, or to the other extreme attributing its potency to cocaine, which was to be regarded as a subtle poison, the continuance of even the most attenuated doses of which must result in a demoralizing habit beggaring description.

The reason for this confusion has already been shown. There has been a want of direct knowledge upon Coca, for as ancient as is its use in history its scientific employment is comparatively recent, having been admitted to the United States Pharmacopœia in 1882, and to the British Pharmacopœia in 1885. The text books are filled with inaccuracies concerning Coca, and in many instances reflect the old superstitions and prejudices of some of the early chroniclers. It is not then suprising that we find in the writings of some clever authors allusions to Coca as though not only similar to, but identical with, certain narcotic drugs. Thus Kipling, who is said to carefully study the subjects on which he writes—when describing preparation of opium in an Indian factory—says the opium is assayed for "morphine and cocaine, etc."* Such errors appearing in lay writings are

* *City of the Dreadful Night.*

usually passed unchallenged, yet they engender a false impression, while those errors of Poeppig, who attributed a perniciousness to the use of Coca comparable to opium, and of Dowdeswell, who declared it inert and without the exhilaration of a breath of mountain air or a draught of spring water, and the physiological conclusions of Bennett, who identified the action of Coca with caffeine, are for some unknown reason repeated as authoritative in spite of their falsity as against the testimony of many more careful observers. This misinformation must necessarily require a considerable period of time to correct. It is hoped that the earnestness and broad thoroughness of the present investigation, will establish an ample foundation of scientific fact which shall tend to place Coca in general usage.

Physiologically, Coca has been shown to be as mild as tea and coffee, while without the disadvantage of those substances, which load the blood with uric acid derivatives. Coca frees the blood of impurities and chemically exerts an influence in the formation of energy. While sufficiently mild to be popularly employed, its well directed medicinal use must prove a boon to the weak and depressed, as divine as its substance was held among the Incas.

The twelve hundred and six letters returned in answer to this inquiry were numbered consecutively as received. Of the entire list of correspondents, three hundred and sixty-nine gave some record of their observations on the physiological action and therapeutic application of Coca from experiences in their practice. In the following compilation these reports are referred to by numbers to avoid repetition of names. A comparison of any number with the corresponding number in the subjoined list of correspondents, will give the name of the author of the report.

PHYSIOLOGICAL ACTION OF COCA.

REPORT FROM 369 CORRESPONDENTS.

[The numbers refer to letters of correspondents whose names may be found in the appended list.]

Appetite Diminished.

141	153	195	199	204	229	280	298
318	422	429	438	452	481	490	507
537	631	752	758	763	825	839	889
896	921	1065					**27**

Appetite Increased.

16	34	38	41	54	82	92	107
108	112	130	138	143	150	163	175
182	188	194	198	215	225	234	245
248	265	267	270	274	281	286	289
293	297	304	312	319	333	358	359
365	377	384	387	390	392	393	400

401	402	405	421	422	423	426	439
450	454	456	457	469	479	483	492
520	553	554	564	629	636	641	642
662	665	683	686	691	692	694	695
716	718	725	732	769	802	806	814
815	829	842	855	864	865	867	894
901	913	920	987	1001	1004	1042	1058
1072	1074	1084	1101	1135	1144	1159	1166
1171							**113**

Blood Pressure Raised.

46	54	108	112	138	174	175	194
215	234	248	265	267	270	280	286
293	298	312	319	327	335	356	358
359	363	384	387	390	392	393	400
402	405	421	423	426	438	439	450
452	456	469	479	481	492	507	532
536	538	564	582	631	636	641	642
665	691	692	694	695	708	725	732
752	758	806	814	825	826	829	830
839	870	889	911	950	952	1001	1004
1065	1072	1074	1085	1135	1147	1166	1171
							88

Blood Pressure Lowered.

537	894						**2**

Circulation Stimulated.

16	46	92	107	108	112	130	138
146	174	175	204	215	225	229	234
238	248	258	267	274	280	286	293
298	299	312	333	335	356	359	363
364	384	387	388	390	393	400	401
402	421	422	439	450	456	469	479
481	483	488	492	507	532	536	537
538	564	582	636	641	642	646	653
662	665	683	691	692	694	695	708
718	725	752	758	769	802	806	814
815	825	826	830	839	842	864	865
870	889	913	950	952	987	1001	1004
1042	1065	1072	1074	1084	1085	1135	1144
1147	1166	1171					**107**

Digestive Functions Improved.

38	54	92	108	130	138	146	150
163	175	188	194	215	225	229	234
245	248	265	267	274	280	281	286
293	297	312	319	333	339	357	358
359	375	377	390	393	401	402	405
421	423	426	439	446	450	452	454
456	457	469	483	490	492	507	520

554	564	582	631	636	641	642	653
662	665	683	686	691	692	694	695
708	716	718	732	752	769	802	806
814	815	842	855	863	864	865	894
901	913	987	1001	1004	1042	1053	1072
1084	1101	1135	1144	1147	1159	1166	1183
							104

Digestive Functions Impaired.

153	204	438	537	758	763	896	921
							8

Heart Strengthened.

34	35	38	46	92	108	112	138
174	175	194	195	198	199	215	229
232	234	238	248	258	265	267	270
274	280	286	289	296	298	304	312
318	335	339	356	358	359	363	364
375	377	384	387	390	392	393	400
401	402	421	422	423	426	438	439
446	450	452	456	457	469	479	483
488	490	507	514	532	536	537	553
564	582	631	642	646	653	662	665
686	692	694	695	708	718	725	752
758	769	802	814	839	842	855	863
864	865	870	879	894	901	911	920
952	1001	1004	1065	1074	1084	1085	1135
1147	1159	1166	1171	1183			**117**

Heart Made Irregular.

645	763	827					**3**

Heat of Skin Raised.

92	130	174	188	234	248	265	267
280	286	298	335	359	364	387	423
438	479	492	507	641	646	691	694
708	725	732	752	758	889	1001	1042
1065	1074	1085	1135				**36**

Heat of Skin Lowered.

896							**1**

Mind Stimulated.

38	46	68	82	92	138	143	146
174	175	180	185	194	195	199	204
215	229	232	234	238	248	258	265
267	280	286	289	296	297	298	312
327	329	335	356	357	359	365	366
377	384	390	392	400	405	421	426
429	438	439	450	452	456	457	479

481	483	492	520	532	537	582	631
636	641	642	646	653	662	665	683
686	691	694	695	708	725	732	735
752	758	769	806	842	864	865	867
870	889	894	911	950	952	985	987
1001	1004	1027	1065	1072	1084	1085	1101
1147	1159	1166	1171	1183			**109**

Mind Depressed.

488	564	641					**3**

Muscles Stimulated.

46	82	92	102	108	153	174	175
194	204	229	232	234	248	265	267
280	286	295	296	298	312	318	335
356	357	358	366	375	377	384	387
390	405	421	422	429	439	446	450
456	479	481	492	507	534	564	636
641	642	653	662	665	686	692	695
718	725	732	752	758	771	802	815
825	842	863	867	879	894	911	950
952	1004	1027	1072	1085	1101	1135	1147
1166	1171						
							82

Muscles Depressed.

532							**1**

Nerves, Sedative to.

34	130	232	258	327	356	377	401
423	439	564	641	642	686	718	814
825	826	911	950	1042			**21**

Nerves Stimulated.

46	102	175	188	194	204	229	234
248	280	289	296	298	304	312	319
375	378	384	387	388	393	439	446
450	452	456	479	481	492	507	514
532	536	538	631	642	691	692	725
732	758	771	839	864	867	870	879
894	913	921	1004	1074	1085	1135	1147
1166	1171						
							58

Nutrition Improved.

34	82	107	108	130	138	150	153
163	174	175	185	198	229	234	265
267	274	280	286	289	329	333	335
339	359	363	371	377	378	384	388
390	392	393	401	405	421	429	439
450	456	457	492	520	538	554	582
636	641	642	646	662	665	686	691

692	694	695	708	718	725	732	752
769	802	814	825	842	855	863	865
867	901	913	950	952	1004	1042	1072
1074	1084	1144	1147	1175			**85**

Nutrition Impaired.

536	758	763	896				**4**

Peripheral Sensations Diminished.

304	536	642	725	735	752		**6**

Peripheral Sensations Increased.

188	234	488	691	692	758	802	1147
							8

Pupils and Vision Enlarged.

174	194	234	267	270	421	537	631
642	691	708	752	826	870	896	911
950	1074	1085	1135	1171			**21**

Pupils Contracted.

318	377	532	636	1004			**5**

Secretions Increased.

146	450						**2**

Bowels Constipated.

304	305	438	439	708	1147		**6**

Bowels Relaxed.

108	146	174	194	234	280	631	665
732	863	865	894	896	950	1004	1072
1135							**17**

Mucous Surfaces, Secretion Increased.

234	274	280	304	421	422	686	732
894	1004	1072	1135				**12**

Mucous Surfaces Constringed.

827	911						**2**

Skin Activity Increased.

68	146	194	280	335	708	732	752
870	894	1072	1135	1171			**13**

Skin Activity Lessened.

127							**1**

Urine Increased.

46	107	174	175	194	215	238	248
270	274	286	298	335	357	390	392
421	426	438	439	452	456	479	483
492	537	631	683	695	725	732	752
771	802	814	826	864	865	870	889
894	952	1004	1072	1135			**45**

Urine Lessened.

153	267	318	636	708			**5**

Respiration Deeper.

68	229	234	258	274	339	377	641
642	842	863	1072	1074	1147		**14**

Respiration Increased.

46	108	174	194	248	265	267	274
280	286	312	318	375	405	421	422
438	452	479	481	507	631	665	694
695	708	725	752	825	855	870	901
911	913	952	1004	1084	1085	1171	1183
							40

Respiration Lowered.

304	335	384					**3**

Sexual Functions Stimulated.

34	46	108	130	141	174	175	229
234	245	248	267	280	286	289	295
304	312	339	359	365	377	378	390
392	400	405	421	439	454	481	490
492	520	532	537	564	582	631	636
683	686	692	708	725	735	802	839
865	894	901	913	1004	1072	1084	1085
1135	1147	1166	1183				**60**

Sexual Functions Depressed.

501	752	870	896				**4**

Sleep Improved.

16	34	38	92	102	107	108	130
138	141	175	188	198	225	245	258
289	293	297	305	329	333	364	377
390	392	401	402	405	421	423	439
450	483	536	537	538	564	582	636
662	665	686	692	695	752	802	806
815	826	839	864	867	894	901	913
1065	1074						**58**

Sleep Prevented.

68	194	199	204	229	234	248	267
280	295	298	312	318	365	481	488
694	708	725	735	758	826	870	896
911	952	1004	1147	1166	1183		**30**

Temperature Increased.

248	267	280	421	507	537	631	665
708	725	735	752	913	1085		**14**

Temperature Lowered.

384	763	896					**3**

Temperature Negative.

483	802	901					**3**

Saliva Secretion Diminished.

393	631	826					**3**

THERAPEUTIC APPLICATION OF COCA.

REPORT FROM 369 CORRESPONDENTS.

Fail to Get Results.

14	39	74	78	173	178	206	235
264	267	300	338	351	367	380	406
410	453	466	495	591	666	685	727
760	793	811	821	873	879	882	891
921	934	956	982	1019	1073	1098	1102
1120	1129	1137	1200				**44**

Considered as a Stimulant.

111	176	187	202	231	242	253	261
315	332	382	412	476	556	563	671
706	709	731	889	960	1025	1041	1102
1112	1153	1162					**27**

Considered as a Tonic.

15	26	202	272	332	535	543	544
554	562	564	589	696	706	889	936
1080	1102	1115	1139	1150	1153		**22**

TENDENCY TO A "COCA HABIT"?

No.

3	16	26	35	38	46	54	82
83	107	108	112	130	138	141	150
153	174	175	179	182	183	185	188
190	195	198	201	204	213	229	238
248	254	258	261	265	270	274	275
283	285	286	293	297	300	304	305
311	312	318	319	325	327	329	333
335	356	357	358	359	361	364	365
371	373	374	378	384	387	388	390
392	393	401	405	409	414	422	423
426	434	438	439	446	450	452	469
479	483	492	495	496	502	507	511
514	520	537	538	552	554	562	564
572	582	607	629	636	642	646	653
658	662	665	683	686	692	694	695
708	716	718	732	735	763	765	769
771	776	802	806	815	825	826	829
830	842	855	863	864	865	867	868
870	887	889	894	901	911	920	921
933	935	952	985	987	1001	1004	1027
1042	1078	1084	1116	1144	1159	1171	**167**

Yes.

92	199	251	267	289	296	350	400
454	490	559	604	631	725	752	758
798	814	896	1065	1072			**21**

IF SO, IN NEUROTIC SUBJECTS?

Yes.

92	199	267	400	490	559	604	631
725	752	814	896	1065	1072		**14**

Antagonistic to Other Drugs, as Alcohol and Opium.

68	108	118	174	175	350	352	388
469	492	515	537	631	692	695	708
725	735	826	836	1171			**21**

Assists Action of Other Drugs.

450							**1**

Against Alcoholism.

7	46	108	130	138	141	174	175
188	190	204	248	265	267	285	286
296	327	357	365	371	373	375	377
384	390	392	400	405	407	409	414

426	450	469	475	481	490	492	511
514	515	536	537	554	564	604	631
638	642	658	662	683	686	695	708
725	732	735	752	758	764	794	806
814	825	826	855	865	867	870	889
894	901	911	913	952	1017	1072	1074
1144	1147	1171	1183	1206			**85**

Anœmia.

7	16	34	92	153	174	201	248
265	267	274	275	285	286	312	358
359	384	393	400	402	407	421	457
483	490	510	537	554	564	582	604
631	642	662	665	683	686	694	695
725	732	758	802	814	825	855	863
865	867	987	1001	1004	1074	1085	1135
1143	1144	1147					**59**

Angina Pectoris.

92	188	274	450	483	504	537	564
695	1072	1074	1135				**12**

Asthma.

46	68	92	107	108	130	190	195
312	358	361	377	390	400	407	421
492	504	507	536	537	564	642	662
692	695	758	763	1166	1171		**30**

Brain Troubles.

7	38	108	174	188	194	198	215
227	245	254	267	275	358	364	375
377	400	405	407	423	439	450	479
490	492	504	536	537	631	642	683
695	725	814	825	865	867	868	870
887	901	911	913	1004	1027	1147	1166
1171							**49**

Bronchitis.

68	92	215	257	280	358	374	405
407	520	537	554	604	631	642	662
695	725	752	825	911	1072	1135	**23**

Debility.

1	3	7	26	34	46	49	68
82	92	102	107	108	112	130	138
150	153	163	174	185	194	195	204
205	215	229	248	257	258	265	267

270	272	274	275	281	285	286	293
312	319	325	327	333	339	352	357
358	361	364	365	375	377	384	390
393	400	401	402	407	409	414	421
422	429	446	450	452	454	456	481
483	490	511	520	536	537	552	553
559	563	564	572	582	593	604	629
631	641	642	646	662	665	686	692
694	695	702	708	716	718	725	732
758	802	806	814	815	819	825	826
829	842	855	863	864	867	868	870
901	913	987	1001	1004	1025	1074	1078
1079	1085	1101	1126	1135	1143	1144	1147
1159	1166	1170	1171	1183			**141**

Exhaustion.

3	7	16	26	34	46	54	68
82	92	102	107	108	112	130	138
150	153	174	175	185	188	194	195
202	204	215	225	229	238	248	257
258	265	267	274	275	281	285	286
293	296	304	312	318	319	327	333
339	352	356	357	358	361	364	365
371	373	377	387	390	393	400	401
402	407	409	414	423	426	439	446
450	452	454	456	483	492	514	520
521	536	537	538	553	564	582	593
604	631	642	662	665	686	692	694
695	708	716	718	725	735	758	778
806	814	825	826	829	830	855	864
867	868	901	911	913	1001	1004	1065
1072	1074	1085	1101	1116	1126	1135	1143
1144	1147	1166	1170	1183			**133**

Fever.

7	174	183	215	245	248	267	274
319	335	358	363	375	387	388	407
426	450	496	507	514	551	559	631
641	642	694	695	708	716	758	802
814	893	958	1065	1070	1074	1078	1079
1126	1147						**42**

As a Heart Tonic.

7	92	108	190	204	215	265	267
275	283	335	356	364	377	387	405
407	421	450	535	537	564	582	604
631	642	662	695	718	758	787	814
825	865	920	1001	1028	1074	1116	1135
1144	1147						**42**

Kidneys.

35	204	286	421	492	537	604	695
758	814	887	1135	1147			**13**

La Grippe.

26	35	38	87	92	138	174	183
188	194	202	204	215	248	257	265
275	293	305	318	327	339	352	358
361	364	375	387	393	405	407	414
450	481	483	490	504	536	538	554
564	582	629	631	642	646	662	686
695	716	718	725	752	758	765	802
814	815	825	826	829	870	879	901
911	936	952	987	1004	1012	1042	1053
1072	1074	1135	1147	1170			**77**

Lungs.

68	202	248	254	267	274	286	358
387	390	393	407	423	454	520	536
537	554	564	604	642	695	708	725
758	802	825	936	1001	1065	1072	1147
							32

Melancholia.

3	26	38	46	92	107	108	138
175	185	194	198	248	275	304	352
364	373	377	400	402	405	407	409
414	429	450	456	483	490	496	504
515	520	536	537	552	564	582	604
631	642	662	686	694	695	725	732
735	752	758	806	855	865	867	870
896	911	913	1004	1074	1116	1147	1166
							64

Muscle.

4	108	130	153	174	175	187	191
195	213	225	234	245	275	285	296
304	366	387	407	421	422	502	535
536	537	538	564	586	604	631	642
665	667	686	695	716	718	735	758
777	812	825	863	867	899	901	924
1004	1027	1072	1085	1101	1135	1147	**55**

Nerve.

108	130	141	146	153	175	187	188
191	215	245	254	258	275	285	301
304	318	353	358	373	387	392	407
422	440	450	483	492	520	536	537

538	564	604	631	642	671	683	686
695	732	758	794	825	863	867	870
901	913	924	1004	1025	1042	1053	1065
1078	1085	1089	1101	1135	1144	1147	1149
1162							**65**

Neurasthenia.

7	16	26	34	46	54	68	82
92	102	108	112	118	150	185	188
194	195	198	201	205	234	240	245
248	258	265	267	270	272	281	285
286	289	297	312	319	327	339	350
358	359	361	364	365	390	393	400
401	402	405	409	414	422	426	454
456	479	481	483	490	501	504	511
520	535	536	537	538	554	564	582
604	631	646	653	662	665	686	692
694	695	708	716	718	725	732	752
758	787	801	802	806	814	825	826
829	830	836	867	870	889	896	901
911	913	920	942	952	987	1001	1004
1012	1017	1065	1070	1074	1101	1116	1135
1144	1147	1166	1183				**124**

Nutrition.

34	54	107	108	118	130	174	175
201	242	275	285	286	312	319	327
335	358	364	371	387	388	392	393
407	421	450	456	496	511	537	554
564	593	604	631	642	646	662	686
695	716	718	725	732	740	758	802
814	855	865	867	901	913	924	1001
1004	1028	1056	1072	1074	1079	1101	1115
1147	1149						**66**

Overwork.

3	26	34	46	82	102	107	108
112	118	130	138	141	150	153	175
185	215	234	238	245	248	258	274
281	285	286	296	298	312	318	319
329	339	357	358	359	361	364	371
374	375	387	390	400	409	421	423
426	429	450	479	481	490	492	511
520	535	536	537	538	552	554	564
582	629	631	642	653	662	665	692
694	695	716	718	725	732	752	758
778	814	826	867	868	870	879	885
901	911	913	987	1001	1004	1065	1070
1074	1085	1101	1135	1143	1144	1147	1166
1170	1183						**106**

Sexual Exhaustion.

7	108	118	130	141	174	175	188
194	195	201	215	229	234	245	248
254	272	285	286	289	312	327	339
352	357	359	364	365	377	378	390
400	407	438	439	450	454	481	490
496	504	515	520	537	564	604	631
653	662	665	692	695	708	725	732
758	764	802	865	867	879	901	911
913	935	963	1001	1004	1065	1072	1084
1101	1135	1147	1166	1183			**77**

Shock.

108	141	377	402	537	564	593	642
694	695	716	758	814	855	865	952
1004	1072	1074	1147				**20**

Stomach.

141	174	179	182	185	190	248	265
283	358	361	364	370	375	388	393
409	421	426	439	446	450	457	507
537	564	631	662	683	686	695	716
758	764	802	825	865	901	963	1025
1053	1079	1147					**43**

Throat.

185	215	274	285	293	305	339	352
364	374	390	393	400	407	481	536
537	552	593	631	642	686	695	814
819	911	952	1147	1183			**29**

Voice.

83	102	108	143	148	180	204	234
245	265	267	274	285	289	293	327
339	352	359	364	365	366	374	390
400	407	421	423	464	481	483	504
511	536	537	552	562	593	629	642
686	692	694	695	735	758	778	819
870	911	920	952	1074	1085	1147	1166
1171	1183						**58**

Convalescence.

7	183	202	204	270	327	390	421
484	537	554	559	631	752	801	825
							16

RÉSUMÉ OF THE ACTION AND USES OF COCA.

Each observer did not note every physiological action nor specify the method of using Coca medicinally, but from the reports of the three hundred and sixty-nine correspondents who gave any detailed information the following classification is made:

Physiological Action.

Appetite—	
diminished	27
increased	113
Blood pressure—	
raised	88
lowered	2
Circulation—	
stimulated	107
depressed	0
Digestive functions—	
improved	104
impaired	8
Heart—	
strengthened	117
irregular	3
Heat of skin—	
raised	36
lowered	1
Mind—	
stimulated	109
depressed	3
Muscles—	
strengthened	82
weakened	1
Nerves—	
stimulated	58
sedative	21
Nutrition—	
improved	85
impaired	4
Peripheral sensations—	
diminished	6
increased	8
Pupils and vision—	
enlarged	21
contracted	5
Secretions—	
increased	2
Bowels—	
constipated	6
relaxed	17
Mucous surfaces, secretion—	
increased	12
constringed	2
Skin activity—	
increased	13
lessened	1
Urine—	
increased	45
lessened	5
Respiration—	
deeper	14
increased	40
lowered	3
Sexual functions—	
stimulated	60
lowered	4
Sleep—	
improved	58
prevented	30
Temperature—	
increased	14
lowered	3
not influenced	3
Saliva—	
diminished	3

Therapeutic Application.

Fail to get results with Coca	44
As a stimulant only	27
As a tonic	22
Have you noticed a tendency to formation of "habit" from the use of Coca?	
No	167
Yes	21
If so, was the patient subject to the formation of habit or neurotic?	
Yes	14

Antagonistic to other drugs (opium or alcohol)	21
Assists action of other drugs	1
Alcoholism	85
Anæmia	59
Angina pectoris	12
Asthma	30
Brain	49
Bronchitis	23
Convalescence	16
Debility	141
Exhaustion	133
Fever	42
Heart	42
Kidneys	13
La Grippe	77
Lungs	32
Melancholia	64
Muscle	55
Nerve	65
Neurasthenia	124
Nutrition	66
Overwork	106
Sexual exhaustion	77
Shock	20
Stomach	43
Throat	29
Voice	58

FOOD VALUE OF COCA.

Among the reports of these three hundred and sixty-nine investigators seventy-seven (20.86 per cent. of the observers) recognize the food value of Coca and have employed it as a nutrient, chiefly serviceable in wasting diseases, in the typhoid condition and in convalescence, as shown by the following answers:

Have You Employed Coca as Food?

[The smaller numbers refer to the period of observation; ^{5} five years or less; ^{10} five to ten years; ^{15} ten to thirty years.]

YES.

16^{10}	92^{10}	174	175^{15}	179^{5}	198^{15}	202	205
213	215^{15}	242	245^{5}	248^{10}	258^{5}	261^{10}	264^{5}
265	267^{15}	275^{10}	280	285^{15}	286^{5}	289^{10}	304^{5}
319^{15}	335^{10}	356^{10}	358^{15}	371^{10}	374^{10}	384^{10}	400
407^{15}	421^{5}	422^{10}	475	483^{5}	492^{15}	496^{5}	504^{10}
507^{10}	511^{15}	532^{5}	536^{10}	537	553^{15}	572^{15}	593^{15}
642^{10}	667	683	695^{15}	702	708^{15}	709	716^{15}
732^{15}	752^{15}	802^{5}	814^{10}	825^{5}	839^{15}	855^{5}	889^{15}
894	896^{15}	901^{15}	911^{10}	1001	1065	1072^{15}	1074^{10}
1078^{15}	1085^{15}	1101^{10}	1116^{15}	1175^{5}			**77**

Of this number seven have used Coca exclusive of all other food during emergency, varying in time from three to twenty-one days, as indicated by the replies:

How Long Supported on Coca Exclusively?

3 days; 407^{15}; (F. W.)
7 days; phthisis; 593^{15}; (W.)
8 days; pneumonia and typhoid; 1072^{15}; (F.)
9 days; gastric carcinoma; 507^{10}; (F. W.)
10 days; gastric carcinoma; 179^{5}; (F.)
10 days; intestinal constriction; 1004^{15}; (W.)

21 days; gastric carcinoma; 179[5]; (F.)
Several months; cancer of pharynx, etc.; 537 (F. W.)

(F.) Fluid Extract; (W.) Wine.

In the case of intestinal constriction reported with recovery: "No food, either solid or liquid, was given during a period of ten days, excepting small and repeated doses of Wine of Coca."

One hundred and thirteen have found Coca to increase appetite, and one hundred and four that it improves digestion, while eighty-five find it has a direct influence on nutrition. This is largely confirmed through its physiological action on the blood vessels and heart. One hundred and seven recognize that Coca stimulates the circulation, eighty-eight find it raises the blood pressure, and one hundred and seventeen that it strengthens the heart.

A direct influence of Coca on the brain and nervous system is recorded in one hundred and nine observations upon its action on the mind, forty-nine on functional brain troubles, seventy-nine on its application to the nervous system, one hundred and twenty-four in neurasthenia, while sixty find Coca a stimulant to the sexual system and seventy-seven have employed it more or less successfully in the treatment of sexual exhaustion.

A very suggestive fact, in view of the prejudice often asserted from irresponsible sources against Coca, is the positive statement of one hundred and sixty-seven observers, who state they have never seen any tendency to habit formation from its use. Of twenty-one who believe they have seen such a tendency, fourteen of the cases were subjects prone to habit formation. One hundred and six have especially emphasized the utility of Coca in the treatment of habitués of alcohol and opium.

Other uses of Coca not tabulated which have been advocated are following surgical operation (543, 593, 856), in seasickness (537), at the climacteric (195, 1079), and in uterine inertia (496), in each of which the physician may recognize the ready adaptability of Coca from its physiological action.

An important matter to the statistician which must add much weight to this report is the period of observation during which these cases were noted and the preparation of Coca employed. Regard should be had, too, for the manner in which the testimony is given. In no case is it the result of any special experimentation wherein certain theories may have influenced the observation, nor has there been any effort to draw any biased testimony; but in each instance the account is taken from the case book of a physician in active practice. Eighty-one have made observations during five years or less, fifty-four during a period from five to ten years, and seventy-one from ten to thirty years, not always continuously but at intervals during the time mentioned.

Two hundred and seventy-six observers have specified in detail the form of Coca used, not in all cases confining themselves exclusively to any one preparation, though in a majority of instances the wine prepared by Mariani has been particularly referred to as embodying the true qualities of Coca.

PREPARATION OF COCA USED.

[AS REPORTED BY 276 PHYSICIANS.]

[The smaller figures refer to the period of observation; ^{5} five years or less; ^{10} five to ten years; ^{15} ten to thirty years.]

Tincture.

14	180^{5}	446^{5}	495^{10}				**4**

Infusion.

7^{15}	108^{10}	225^{15}	490^{15}	732	1074^{10}	1102^{15}	**7**

Solid Extract.

175	194	201	213	280	450	511^{15}	593
641	683	725	732^{15}	894	896^{15}	2867^{10}	**15**

Leaves.

7^{15}	130^{10}	174	198^{15}	205	423	450^{10}	466
502	563^{15}	586	593	653^{15}	667	735^{15}	758^{15}
794	924	1143	1171^{15}				**20**

Fluid Extract.

4	46^{5}	68	87^{5}	102^{15}	108^{10}	141	174
175^{15}	179^{5}	182^{5}	185	187	188^{5}	195^{5}	229^{10}
248^{10}	254^{15}	257	258^{5}	270^{5}	272^{15}	274^{10}	293^{10}
296^{15}	311	318^{5}	329^{5}	335^{10}	352	357^{15}	365^{15}
377^{5}	378^{10}	380^{5}	382^{5}	384^{10}	390^{10}	405^{5}	407^{15}
409	414^{15}	421^{5}	429^{15}	450^{10}	469^{5}	479^{10}	485
496^{5}	507^{10}	511^{15}	515	520^{10}	536^{10}	537	552
556	563^{15}	564^{5}	604^{15}	607	631	653^{15}	665^{10}
691^{15}	692^{5}	695^{15}	702	708^{15}	725^{5}	732^{15}	735^{15}
752^{15}	758^{15}	763^{10}	821	826^{15}	863^{5}	865^{5}	867
889^{15}	894	896^{15}	901^{15}	911^{10}	933	935	952^{15}
1001	1042^{5}	1072^{15}	1074^{10}	1078^{15}	1101^{10}	1102^{15}	1135^{15}
1147^{10}	1149	1159^{5}	1166^{10}	1171^{15}	1175^{5}	1183^{10}	1200
							104

Wine.

1	7^{15}	14	16^{10}	26	34	35^{10}	46
54^{15}	68	82^{5}	83^{15}	92^{10}	101	107^{10}	111
112	118	130^{10}	141	143^{5}	148^{10}	150^{10}	153^{5}
163^{5}	173^{5}	174	175^{15}	176	183^{5}	185^{10}	188^{5}
190	194^{5}	195^{5}	199^{5}	201	202	204^{10}	205
213	215^{15}	225^{15}	229^{10}	234^{5}	240	245^{5}	248^{10}
257^{10}	258^{5}	261^{10}	264^{5}	265	267^{15}	270^{5}	274^{10}
280	281^{5}	283	285^{15}	286^{5}	289^{10}	293^{10}	296^{15}
297	300^{5}	304^{5}	305^{5}	312^{15}	319^{15}	325^{10}	327^{10}
335^{10}	352	353	356^{10}	357^{15}	358^{15}	359	361
363^{5}	364^{15}	366	370^{5}	371^{10}	374^{10}	375^{5}	378^{10}
384^{10}	388^{5}	390^{10}	393	400	401^{10}	402^{5}	405^{5}
407^{15}	409	414^{15}	421^{5}	422^{10}	423^{10}	426^{5}	429^{15}

438^{15}	440	450^{10}	452	454^{5}	456^{5}	464	469^{5}
475	481^{15}	483^{5}	484	488^{5}	492^{15}	496^{5}	502
504^{10}	507^{10}	532^{5}	536^{10}	537	538^{15}	543	551
552	554^{10}	559	562	564^{5}	572^{15}	582^{15}	589
593^{15}	604^{15}	609	629^{5}	636^{15}	641	642^{10}	646^{5}
653^{15}	662^{15}	665^{10}	667	683	685	686	694^{15}
696	706	708^{15}	716^{15}	718	725^{5}	732^{15}	735^{15}
758^{15}	763	769	771	787	794	802^{5}	811^{5}
814^{10}	815	819	821	825	826^{15}	829^{10}	836^{5}
839^{15}	842^{10}	855^{5}	864	868^{15}	870	879^{15}	893
894	896^{15}	901^{15}	911^{10}	913	920^{5}	921^{5}	935
936	942	950	952^{15}	985	987^{15}	1001	1004^{15}
1025	1027^{10}	1028	1042^{5}	1053^{15}	1065	1070	1074^{10}
1078^{15}	1079	1084^{10}	1085^{15}	1102^{15}	1115	1116^{15}	1135^{15}
1143	1144^{5}	1147^{10}	1149	1150	1159^{5}	1162	1166^{10}
1170^{15}	1171^{15}	1175^{5}	1183^{10}	1206			**229**

Preparations mentioned as employed by 276 physicians:

Tincture, used by 4 (1.44 per cent.). Infusion, used by 7 (2.53 per cent.). Solid Extract, used by 15 (5.43 per cent.). Leaves, used by 20 (7.24 per cent.). Fluid Extract, used by 104 (37.67 per cent.). Wine, used by 229 (82.97 per cent.).

CORRESPONDENTS.

THE COLLECTIVE INVESTIGATION EMBRACES REPORTS FROM THE FOLLOWING PHYSICIANS, RECEIVED DURING THE YEARS 1897, 1898 AND 1899.

[The attached numbers are used to avoid repetition of names.]

1. Coffin, John L., Boston, Mass.
3. Jackson, J. Henry, Barre, Vt.
4. Colby, Edward P., Boston, Mass.
7. Cobb, C. H., Boston, Mass.
14. Tyson, James, Philadelphia, Pa.
15. Vischer, Carl V., Philadelphia, Pa.
16. Reeves, J. M., Philadelphia, Pa.
26. Butler, W. K., Washington, D. C.
34. Guest, James W., Louisville, Ky.
35. Crutchfield, Eugene Lee, Baltimore, Md.
38. Bushnell, Chas. H., Chicago, Ill.
39. Morgan, W. B., St. Louis, Mo.
41. Allen, H. C., Chicago, Ill.
46. Robinson, Paul S., New Haven, Conn.
54. Boldt, H. J., New York, N. Y.
68. Prentiss, D. Webster, Washington, D. C.
74. Douglas, O. B., New York, N. Y.
78. Curtis, F. C., Albany, N. Y.
82. Dowling, J. W., New York, N. Y.
83. Harrison, Wallace K., Chicago, Ill.

87. Taylor, Wm. H., Cincinnati, O.
92. Hopkins, H. R., Buffalo, N. Y.
102. Hayward, J. W., Boston, Mass.
107. Hooper, E. D., Boston, Mass.
108. Thurston, J. M., Richmond, Ind.
111. Dunlevy, Rita, New York, N. Y.
112. Osborne, O. T., New Haven, Conn.
118. Steele, D. A. K., Chicago, Ill.
130. Perry, Joseph R., Indianapolis, Ind.
138. Yarrow, Harry Crécy, Washington, D. C.
141. Smith, Nelson G., Columbus, Ind.
143. Parker, Edward F., Charleston, S. C.
146. Wirt, Wm. E., Cleveland, O.
148. Rice, George B., Boston, Mass.
150. Wood, Alfred C., Philadelphia, Pa.
153. Meyer, Max, New York, N. Y.
163. Lytle, Albert T., Buffalo, N. Y.
173. Smith, Joseph T., Baltimore, Md.
174. Clarke, Augustus P., Cambridge, Mass.
175. Glenn, W. Frank, Nashville, Tenn.
176. Phillips, Lincoln, Hartwell, O.
178. Steele, N. C., Chattanooga, Tenn.
179. Goldman, Gustav, Baltimore, Md.
180. Harris, Raymond J., Philadelphia, Pa.
182. Ussery, W. C., St. Louis, Mo.
183. Waters, George M., Columbus, O.
185. Foote, Charles J., New Haven, Conn.
187. Mulhall, J. C., St. Louis, Mo.
188. Jerowitz, H. D., Kansas City, Mo.
190. Caillé, A., New York, N. Y.
191. Davis, N. S., Chicago, Ill.
194. Gayle, Virginius W., Kansas City, Mo.
195. Schultz, H. H., Seward, Neb.
198. Williamson, A. P., Minneapolis, Minn.
199. Goldsmith, A. E., Home City, O.
201. Coutter, F. E., Omaha, Neb.
202. Linthicum, G. Milton, Baltimore, Md.
204. Laidlaw, Geo. Fred., New York, N. Y.
205. Larrabee, Jno. A., Louisville, Ky.
206. Inglis, David, Detroit, Mich.
213. Kuh, Sydney, Chicago, Ill.
215. Nelson, H. Payton, Chicago, Ill.
225. Talbot, I. T., Boston, Mass.
227. Williams, Robert F., Richmond, Va.
229. Powell, C. H., St. Louis, Mo.
231. Smith, Andrew H., New York, N. Y.
232. Foster, Jno. M., Denver, Col.
234. Seebass, Alfred, Denver, Col.
235. Lockwood, George Roe, New York, N. Y.
238. Hall, J. N., Denver, Col.

240. Whitney, H. B.,
Denver, Col.
242. Ohmann-Dumesnil, A. H.,
St. Louis, Mo.
245. Wiggers, H. H.,
Cincinnati, O.
248. Lillie, C. W.,
Staunton, Ill.
251. Bauduy, J. K.,
St. Louis, Mo.
253. Van Sweringen, B.,
Ft. Wayne, Ind.
254. Johnson, J. H. S.,
Chicago, Ill.
257. Lynds, J. G.,
Ann Arbor, Mich.
258. Bernard, Chas. C.,
Chicago, Ill.
261. Booth, David S.,
St. Louis, Mo.
264. Spalding, S. K.,
Omaha, Neb.
265. Upshur, J. M.,
Richmond, Va.
267. Stephens, Ernest L.,
Ft. Worth, Tex.
270. Potts, Chas. S.,
Philadelphia, Pa.
272. Taylor, R. W.,
New York, N. Y.
274. Kuyk, D. A.,
Richmond, Va.
275. Reading, Arthur H.,
Chicago, Ill.
280. Saunders, C. B.,
Chicago, Ill.
281. Fort, Sam'l J.,
Ellicott City, Ind.
283. Grundmann, F. W.,
St. Louis, Mo.
285. Neumeister, Anton E.,
Kansas City, Mo.
286. Duffield, Geo.,
Detroit, Mich.
289. Southwick, George R.,
Boston, Mass.
293. McNaught, F. H.,
Denver, Col.
295. Burt, F. L.,
Boston, Mass.
296. Baumgarten, G.,
St. Louis, Mo.
297. Ravogli, A.,
Cincinnati, O.
298. Capps, E. D.,
Ft. Worth, Tex.
300. Fleischner, H.,
New Haven, Conn.
301. Stemen, George C.,
Ft. Wayne, Ind.
304. Whitford, H. E.,
Chicago, Ill.
305. Twitchell, Herbert F.,
Portland, Me.
311. Gleason, E. B.,
Philadelphia, Pa.
312. Harris, W. John,
St. Louis, Mo.
315. Mosher, Eliza M.,
Ann Arbor, Mich.
318. Hazzard, T. L.,
Allegheny, Pa.
319. Irving, P. A.,
Richmond, Va.
325. Lewis, W. Milton,
Baltimore, Md.
327. Moody, H. A.,
Mobile, Ala.
329. Pollock, Robert,
Cleveland, O.
332. Ross, Geo.,
Richmond, Va.
333. Blake, Jno. D.,
Baltimore, Md.
335. Smith, Andrew J.,
Metamora, Ind.
338. Holman, S. A.,
Pittsburgh, Pa.
339. Young, James K.,
Philadelphia, Pa.
350. Adolphus, Joseph,
Atlanta, Ga.
351. Handerson, H. E.,
Cleveland, O.
352. Moore, W. Oliver,
New York, N. Y.
353. Foster, Charles Wm.,
Woodfords, Me.
356. Griffin, J. M.,
Detroit, Mich.

357. Salomon, Lucien F., New Orleans, La.
358. Parra, H. A., New Orleans, La.
359. Bozon, Henry, New Orleans, La.
361. Caron, George G., Detroit, Mich.
363. Perrier, J., Cleveland, O.
364. Dreifus, E., New Orleans, La.
365. Billé, Waldemar, New Orleans, La.
366. Fitch, J. E., New Orleans, La.
367. Dana, Charles L., New York, N. Y.
370. Patterson, C. E., Grand Rapids, Mich.
371. Dees, C. J., Detroit, Mich.
373. Scroggy, G. H., Garland, Tex.
374. Welsh, Dennett, Grand Rapids, Mich.
375. Macduirnied, G. A., New Orleans, La.
377. Innis, J. H., Grand Rapids, Mich.
378. Cox, W. G., Detroit, Mich.
380. Hubbard, C. W., Detroit, Mich.
382. Egan, W. L., Detroit, Tex.
384. Slaight, John L., Hot Springs, Ark.
387. Bruce, W. J. E., Little Rock, Ark.
388. Phenix, N. J., Alvin, Tex.
390. Kingsley, B. F., San Antonio, Tex.
392. Porter, Phil, Detroit, Mich.
393. Burg, S., San Antonio, Tex.
400. Roman, Chas. V., Dallas, Tex.
401. Corcoran, John P., Detroit, Mich.
402. Florence, J. H., Dallas, Tex.
405. Dunaway, W. C., Little Rock, Ark.
406. Wallace, H. C., Hot Springs, Ark.
407. Goddard, Andrew, Waco, Tex.
409. Chase, E. D., Galveston, Tex.
410. Nonette, Geo. N., New Orleans, La.
412. Stell, Geo. S., Paris, Tex.
414. Wallace, D. R., Waco, Tex.
421. Porter, Edwards H., Detroit, Mich.
422. Brown, Owen C., Detroit, Mich.
423. Ross, W. H., Grand Rapids, Mich.
426. Peyser, Mark W., Richmond, Va.
429. Mitchell, J. H., Dallas, Tex.
434. Birdsong, M. J., Greenville, Tex.
438. Griswold, Wm. Henry, San Francisco, Cal.
439. Anthony, J. C., San Francisco, Cal.
440. Webster, L. R., Oakland, Cal.
446. Bradley, E. W., Oakland, Cal.
450. Day, B. W., Los Angeles, Cal.
452. Phipps, Gordon, Corsicana, Tex.
453. Millard, F. R., San Diego, Cal.
454. Lewis, W. M., Los Angeles, Cal.
456. Hill, H. B., Austin, Tex.
457. McTaggart, J. E., Syracuse, N. Y.

464. Joachim, O., New Orleans, La.
466. Davidson, A., Los Angeles, Cal.
469. Borders, J. M., Ft. Worth, Tex.
475. Weathers, L. V., Davenport, Tex.
476. Hazlewood, Arthur, Grand Rapids, Mich.
479. Sexton, L., New Orleans, La.
481. Mayer, C. R., New Orleans, La.
483. Spencer, Ralph H., Grand Rapids, Mich.
484. Boice, Jno., Denver, Col.
488. Hitchcock, Chas. W., Detroit, Mich.
490. Gereaux, F., New Orleans, La.
492. Sears, J. H., Waco, Tex.
495. Strader, H. W., Sacramento, Cal.
496. Harcourt, L. A., Sacramento, Cal.
501. Webster, Alfred M., Grand Rapids, Mich.
502. Leach, Reginald Barkley, Minneapolis, Minn.
504. Taylor, Harry, Honey Grove, Tex.
507. Ahlborn, Augustus, Detroit, Mich.
510. Cornell, G. L., Detroit, Mich.
511. Shoemaker, John V., Philadelphia, Pa.
514. Andrews, M. H., Detroit, Mich.
515. Moffat, Walter, Grand Rapids, Mich.
520. Neagle, J. H., Sacramento, Cal.
521. Southworth, M. A., San Jose, Cal.
532. McElure, L. C., St. Louis, Mo.
535. French, Hayes C., San Francisco, Cal.
536. MacKinnon, G. W., Oxford, Mich.
537. Docking, T., San Diego, Cal.
538. Pierce, R. E., San Jose, Cal.
543. Mayer, Oscar J., San Francisco, Cal.
544. Bucknall, Geo. J., San Francisco, Cal.
551. Taylor, Richard H., Hot Springs, Ark.
552. Chaney, Willard, Detroit, Mich.
553. Cruthers, T. D., Hartford, Conn.
554. Johnston, J. N., San Jose, Cal.
556. Harkness, Geo. S., Stockton, Cal.
559. Paterson, E. M., Oakland, Cal.
562. Gordon, W. A., San Jose, Cal.
563. Simpson, William, San Jose, Cal.
564. Long, S. F., San Francisco, Cal.
572. Bellows, H. P., Boston, Mass.
582. Bryce, C. A., Richmond, Va.
586. Stevens, Rollin H., Detroit, Mich.
589. Mason, A. L., Boston, Mass.
591. Schwatka, J. B., Baltimore, Md.
593. Cohn, J. E., Berkeley, Cal.
604. Dabney, T. S., New Orleans, La.
607. Buckland, Owen, San Francisco, Cal.
629. Wheeler, John Brooks, Burlington, Vt.
631. de Corval, E. Lorentz, San Francisco, Cal.

636. McGork, Thos.,
Galveston, Tex.
638. Collings, S. P.,
Hot Springs, Ark.
641. Anderson, Charles,
Santa Barbara, Cal.
642. Hamilton, H. J.,
Laredo, Tex.
646. Wright, H. J. B.,
San Jose, Cal.
653. Price, Eldridge C.,
Baltimore, Md.
658. Wheeler, Frank H.,
New Haven, Conn.
662. Rutherford, Frances A.,
Grand Rapids, Mich.
665. Miller, C. S.,
Toledo, O.
666. Watson, Arthur W.,
Philadelphia, Pa.
667. Nichols, Charles L.,
Worcester, Mass.
671. Hearn, N. Joseph,
Philadelphia, Pa.
683. Dunham, John M.,
Columbus, O.
685. Atkinson, R. C.,
St. Louis, Mo.
686. Tagert, Adelbert H.,
Chicago, Ill.
691. Rice, John P.,
San Antonio, Tex.
692. Osborne, W. C.,
Viesca, Tex.
694. Dannaker, C. A.,
Kansas City, Mo.
695. Eaton, O. P.,
Detroit, Mich.
696. Hall, P. Sharples,
Philadelphia, Pa.
702. Davison, W. M. W.,
Chicago, Ill.
706. Stelwagon, Henry W.,
Philadelphia, Pa.
708. McNary, W. T.,
San Jose, Cal.
709. Roy, G. G.,
Atlanta, Ga.
716. Casseday, Frank F.,
Minneapolis, Minn.
718. Gaston, J. McFadden,
Atlanta, Ga.
725. Horwitz, D.,
Philadelphia, Pa.
727. Benedict, A. L.,
Buffalo, N. Y.
732. Boteler, Wm. C.,
Washington, D. C.
735. Waugh, Wm. F.,
Chicago, Ill.
740. Stark, S.,
Cincinnati, O.
752. Brower, Daniel R.,
Chicago, Ill.
758. Logan, M. H.,
San Francisco, Cal.
760. Stites, Ida M.,
Stockton, Cal.
763. Kelly, L. E.,
Oakland, Cal.
764. Mackay, J. H.,
Norfolk, Neb.
765. Bishop, A. B.,
Los Gatos, Cal.
769. McPheeters, W. M.,
St. Louis, Mo.
771. Benson, O. D.,
Des Moines, Ia.
776. Anderson, C. L.,
Santa Cruz, Cal.
777. Putter, W. H.,
Pasadena, Cal.
778. Ellis, H. Bert,
Los Angeles, Cal.
787. Truitt, Wm. John,
Naperville, Ill.
793. Johnston, William W.,
Washington, D. C.
794. De Saussure, P. Gourdin,
Charleston, S. C.
796. Leavitt, H. H.,
Minneapolis, Minn.
801. Sloan, R. T.,
Kansas City, Mo.
802. Staples, Loren H.,
Buffalo, N. Y.
806. Stoner, C. E.,
Des Moines, Ia.
811. Schooler, Lewis,
Des Moines, Ia.

812. Rogers, Edmund J. A.,
Denver, Col.
814. Reynolds, Otero C.,
Lincoln, Neb.
815. Scarborough, J. G.,
Little Rock, Ark.
819. Merrick, S. K.,
Baltimore, Md.
821. Winterberg,
San Francisco, Cal.
825. Jones, I. J.,
Austin, Tex.
826. Brown, Henry M.,
Cincinnati, O.
829. Eichberg, Joseph,
Cincinnati, O.
830. Taylor, T. E.,
Denver, Col.
836. Shotwell, C. H.,
Gainesville, Tex.
839. Lennox, L. J.,
Detroit, Mich.
842. Wilson, Frank C.,
Louisville, Ky.
855. Axtell, E. R.,
Denver, Col.
856. Bernays, Augustus C.,
St. Louis, Mo.
863. Weir, F. A.,
Pasadena, Cal.
864. Shurly, E. L.,
Detroit, Mich.
865. Locher, Henry E.,
Grand Rapids, Mich.
867. Delamater, N. B.,
Chicago, Ill.
868. Herrick, S. S.,
San Francisco, Cal.
870. Hubbard, T. V.,
Atlanta, Ga.
873. Williams, J. O.,
Houston, Tex.
879. Goldmann, Edw.,
Wrights P. O., Cal.
882. Aikin, J. M.,
Omaha, Neb.
887. Stockton, Chas. G.,
Buffalo, N. Y.
889. Parsons, G. L.,
Boston, Mass.
891. Keith, W. E.,
San Jose, Cal.
893. Lusson, P. M.,
San Jose, Cal.
894. Williams, M. Hilton,
Los Angeles, Cal.
896. Chittick, W. R.,
Detroit, Mich.
899. Peabody, James H.,
Omaha, Neb.
901. Burton, H. G.,
Los Angeles, Cal.
911. Wilson, J. T.,
Sherman, Tex.
913. Hale, Morris,
Hot Springs, Ark.
920. Cutter, Ephraim,
New York, N. Y.
921. Clark, E. Willard,
Los Angeles, Cal.
924. James, Frank L.,
St. Louis, Mo.
933. Taylor, John J.,
New Orleans, La.
934. Keiller, William,
Galveston, Tex.
935. French, F. L.,
Little Rock, Ark.
936. Red, S. C.,
Houston, Tex.
942. Manton, W. P.,
Detroit, Mich.
950. Poole, W. H.,
Detroit, Mich.
952. Hasencamp, O.,
Toledo, O.
956. Canfield, William B.,
Baltimore, Md.
958. Alderman, H. L.,
Detroit, Mich.
960. Weidenthal, N.,
Cleveland, O.
963. Burton, S.,
Waco, Tex.
982. Bigg, Arthur H.,
Detroit, Mich.
985. Cree, Walter J.,
Detroit, Mich.
987. Smith, Julia Holmes,
Chicago, Ill.

1001. Neumann, M.,
San Francisco, Cal.
1004. Pasco, M. H.,
Grand Rapids, Mich.
1017. Avery, Alida C.,
San Jose, Cal.
1019. Cook, F. C.,
San Francisco, Cal.
1025. Hughes, Chas. H.,
St. Louis, Mo.
1027. Smith, Asbury G.,
Los Angeles, Cal.
1028. Deacon, Geo.,
Pasadena, Cal.
1041. Michael, W. L.,
Sherman, Tex.
1042. Bailey, Sara Brown,
San Jose, Cal.
1053. Mauzy, W. P.,
Oakland, Cal.
1056. Strong, C. G.,
San Francisco, Cal.
1065. West & Davis,
Dallas, Tex.
1070. Snead, A. H.,
Waco, Tex.
1072. Clark, H. H.,
Santa Cruz, Cal.
1073. Bleecker, J. J.,
Pasadena, Cal.
1074. Thompson, Wesley,
San Bernardino, Cal.
1078. Sanders, A. F.,
Hot Springs, Ark.
1079. Aronson, E.,
Dallas, Tex.
1080. Muffe, Frederick P.,
San Francisco, Cal.
1084. American, S.,
San Francisco, Cal.
1085. FitzGerald, O. D.,
Los Angeles, Cal.
1089. Beach, Eliza J.,
Pasadena, Cal.
1098. Cole, Geo. L.,
Los Angeles, Cal.
1101. Gaff, John V.,
Tucson, Ariz.
1102. Turner, Wm. D.,
Pasadena, Cal.
1112. Knox, S. B. P.,
Santa Barbara, Cal.
1115. Summers, Thomas O.,
St. Louis, Mo.
1116. Overend, Edmund J.,
San Francisco, Cal.
1120. Newkirk, A. B.,
Los Angeles, Cal.
1126. Wheeler, A. E.,
Los Angeles, Cal.
1129. Gibbons, Henry, Jr.,
San Francisco, Cal.
1135. Ellis, L. E.,
Detroit, Mich.
1137. Watts, Pliny R.,
Sacramento, Cal.
1139. Bunch, W. J.,
Hot Springs, Ark.
1143. Hinds, Harriet C.,
East Orange, N. J.
1144. Ross, Thos.,
Sacramento, Cal.
1147. Simot, J. Moore,
New Orleans, La.
1149. Johns, P. W.,
Hot Springs, Ark.
1150. Campbell, Mary Page,
San Francisco, Cal.
1153. Bishop, Seth Scott,
Chicago, Ill.
1159. Foster, N. K.,
Oakland, Cal.
1162. Reynolds, Dudley S.,
Louisville, Ky.
1166. Jones, Allen A.,
Buffalo, N. Y.
1170. Gilbert, John,
Fall River, Mass.
1171. King, Frank B.,
Houston, Tex.
1175. Arndt, Leroy M.,
Detroit, Mich.
1183. Fouchy, A. D.,
Alameda, Cal.
1200. Bressler, Frank C.,
Baltimore, Md.
1206. Hay, E. C.,
Hot Springs, Ark.

Total, 369.

BIBLIOGRAPHY

OF TITLES CONSULTED OR REFERRED TO

AND AN

INDEX AND GLOSSARY

TO THE VOLUME

BIBLIOGRAPHY

[No effort has been made to include here all the titles upon Coca or upon the Incas, but the writings quoted have been referred to in the preparation of the present volume.]

ACOSTA, JOSÉ DE: *Historia natural y moral de las Indias;* Sevilla, 1588. Translated into French by Robert Regnault, Paris, 1616. Translated into English by Clements R. Markham, C.B., F.R.S. (Hakluyt Society), London.

ALBERTONI, PIETRO: *Azione della cocaina sulla contractilita del Protoplasma; Annales de Chimie;* p. 305; Paris, 1890.

ALCEDO, ANTONIO DE: *Diccionario geografico historico de las Indias occidentales ó America;* fol. 93. Appendice au t. V, *Vocabulario de las voces provinciales de la America;* (Art. *Hayo*), 5 vols., 8vo.; Madrid, 1788.

ALLEN, ALFRED H.: *Commercial Organic Analysis;* III, Part II, (*Vegetable Alkaloids*). 2 ed., 8vo.; Philadelphia, 1892.

ALLEN, TIMOTHY F., A. M., M.D.: *Encyclopedia of Pure Materia Medica;* III, pp. 369-381; 8vo.

ALMS, H.: *Die Wirkung des Cocaïns auf die peripherischen Nerven; Archiv für Physiologie,* [Suppl-band.] p. 293; Leipzig, 1886.

ANGRAND, LÉONCE: *Note sur la Coca in Pérou avant la conqûete espagnole;* Ernest Desjardins; 8vo.; p. 60; Paris, 1858.

ANREP, B. VON: *Ueber die physiologische Wirkung des Cocaïn; Archiv für die gesammte Physiologie,* XXI; Bonn, 1880. Also *Journal Medecine de Chirurgie, et de Pharmacologie,* IXX; Bruxelles, 1880.

ANSTIE, FRANCIS E.: *Stimulants and Narcotics; Their Mutual Relations, with special researches on the Action of Alcohol, Ether and Chloroform on the Vital Organism;* 8vo.; Philadelphia, 1865.

ANTRIK, OTTO: *Das optische Verhalten des Cocaïns und eine Methode zur Prüfung seines salzsauren Salzes auf Reinheit; Berichte der chemischen Gesellschaft, Jahrg.* XX; 1; p. 310, Feb. 14; Berlin, 1887.

ARANGO, A. P.: *Note sur la Coca; Bulletin général de therapeutique,* IXXX; Paris, 1871.

ARRIGA, JOSÉ DE: *Estirpacion de la Idolatria del Peru;* Lima, 1621.

AUBREY, GEORGES: *Contribution à l'étude de la Coca du Pérou, et de la cocaïne.* 2 pl., 4to.; Nancy, 1885.

AVILA, DR. FRANCISCO DE: *A Narrative of the Errors, False Gods, and Other Superstitious and Diabolical Rites in Which the Indians of the Provinces of Huarochiri, Mama, and Chaclla Lived in Ancient Times;* MSS., 1608. Translated and edited by Clements R. Markham, C.B., F.R.S. (Hakluyt Society); London, 1873.

BAILLON, M. H.: *Dictionnaire de Botanique;* 4to.; Paris, 1886.

BAKER, A. R.: *The Coca Leaf and Its Alkaloid; Cincinnati Lancet-Clinic* (n. s.), XIII; Cincinnati, 1884.

BAKER, SIR G.: *Medical Tracts;* London, 1818.

BALBOA, MIGUEL CAVELLO: *Miscellanea Austral;* Quito, (about) 1580. Translated by Ternaux Compans; Paris, 1840.

(Part Third treats of Peru.)

BALFOUR, JOHN HUTTON, M.D.: *A Manual of Botany;* London, 1849.

BALFOUR, EDWARD: *Cyclopedia of India and Eastern and Southern Asia;* 3 vols., 3 ed.; London, 1885.

BARHAM, DR. HENRY: *Hortus Americanus;* Kingston, Jamaica, (about) 1795.

(Containing an account of the trees, shrubs and other vegetable products of South America, etc.)

BARTHOLOW, ROBERTS, M.A., M.D., LL.D.: *A Practical Treatise on Materia Medica and Therapeutics;* 5 ed.; New York, 1885.

BAUHINUS, GASPARDUS: *Pinax theatri botanici;* 4to.; Basileæ Helvetorum, 1623.

BEARD, GEORGE M., M.D.: *Neurasthenia; Boston Medical and Surgical Journal*, April, 1869.

Same: *Treatise on Nervous Exhaustion;* New York, 1880.

Same: *Sexual Neurasthenia;* Edited by A. D. Rockwell, A.M., M.D., 2 ed.; New York, 1886.

BEAU, J. H. S.: *Traité de la Dyspepsie;* 8vo.; Paris, 1866.

BELL, JOHN: *Regimen and Longevity;* Philadelphia, 1842.

BELL, J. A.: *Use of Coca; British Medical Journal*, London, 1874.

BENDER: *Year Book of Pharmacy;* London, 1886.

BENNETT, A.: *An experimental inquiry into the physiological action of theine, guaranine, cocaine, and theobromine; Edinburgh Medical Journal*, XIX; Edinburgh, 1873.

Same: *The physiological action of Coca; British Medical Journal*, I; London, 1874.

BENTHAM, G., and HOOKER, J. D.: *Genera Plantarum ad exemplaria imprimis in herbariis Kewensibus servata de linita*, 8vo.; Londini, 1862-67.

BENTLEY, W. H.: *Erythroxylon Coca; Therapeutic Gazette;* (n. s.), I; Detroit, 1880.

Same: *Erythroxylon Coca in the opium and alcohol habits; Therapeutic Gazette*, 253; Detroit, 1880.

BENTLEY and TRIMEN: *Medicinal Plants;* 4 vols., 8vo.; London, 1880.

BENZONI, HIERONYMUS: *De Peruanis, l'Historia del Mundo nuovo;* III; Venezia, 1565. Translated into French by Urbain Chauveton, 8vo.; Avignon, 1579.

BERNARD, CLAUDE: *Nouvelle Fonction du Foie;* Paris, 1853.

Same: *Leçons sur le Diabète;* Paris, 1877.

Same: *Leçons sur les phenomènes de la vie communs aux animaux et aux végétaux;* Paris, 1878-79.

BERNARD, W.: *Observations on the effects of Cuca leaves; British Medical Journal*, I; London, 1876.

BERNEAUD, THIEBAUT DE: (About) 1830. (Art. *Coca*), in Larousse, *Dictionnaire Universel*, IV; p. 498, Paris, 1869.

BERTHOLD, E.: *Zur physiologischen Wirkung des Cocaïns; Centralblatt für die medicinischen Wissenschaften;* Berlin, 1885.

BEUGNIER-CORBEAU: *Recherches historiques, expérimentales et thérapeutiques sur la Coca et son alcaloïde; Bulletin général de thérapeutique*, CVII; Paris, 1884.

BIANCHI, A.: *La Coca e la cocaina, loro azione fisiologica e terapeutica; Sperimentale*, LVIII; Firenze, 1886.

BIBRA, DR. ERNST FREYHERR VON: *Die Narkotischen Genussmittel und der Mensch.* (Art. *Coca*), pp. 151-174; Nürnberg, 1855.

BICHAT, M. F. X.: *Physiological Researches on Life and Death.* Translated by F. Gold, London, 1799.

BIGGS, H. M.: *The Physiological Action of Cocaine on the Common Frog, with Special Reference to its Action on Organs and Tissues; Journal American Medical Association;* Chicago, 1885.

BIGNON, A.: *A New Method of Preparing Cocaine. L'Union Pharmac.*, XXVI; p. 456. *American Journal of Pharmacy;* p. 607, Dec.; Philadelphia, 1885.

Same: *Note on the Properties of Coca and Cocaine;* [Nouveaux Remèdes]; *Pharmaceutical Journal and Transactions;* Sept. 26, London, 1885.

Same: *Acción fisiológica de la cocaina; Bol. Acad. de Med.*, de Lima, I; 319-339, 1885-86.

Same: *Des Propiétes toxiques de la Cocaine; Bulletin Génerale de Thérapeutique*, II; Paris, 1886.

Same: *Sobre el valor comparativo de las cocainas; Bol. Acad. de Med.*, de Lima, II; 37-39, 1886-7.

BINZ C.: *Ueber die Einwirkung des Chinin auf die Protoplasma Bewegungen; Archiv für mikroskopische Anatomie*, III; Bonn, 1867.

BLAKE, JOHN: *Reports of the Peabody Museum of American Archæology and Ethnology;* II, 1876-79; Cambridge, 1880.

BOCQUILLON, H.: *Manuel d'Histoire Naturelle Médicale;* 12mo.; Paris, 1871.

BOERHAAVE, HERMANN: *Institutiones Medicæ;* Leyden, 1708.

BOLLAËRT, WILLIAM: *Antiquarian, ethnological and other researches in New Grenada, Ecuador, Peru and Chile;* pp. 163-168, 8vo.; London, 1860.

BONNYCASTLE, R. H.: *Spanish America; History of Peru;* 2 vols.; London, 1818.

BORDIER, A.: *Dictionnaire, Encyclopêdique des sciences médicales*, XVIII; (Art. *Coca*), 161-170, Paris, 1875.

BRAID, JAMES: *Neurypnology, or the Rationale of Nervous Sleep considered in Relation with Animal Magnetism*; London, 1843.

BRETTES, COMTE JOSEPH DE: *Six Ans d'Explorations chez les Indiens du Nord de la Colombie;* (Voyage executé en, 1890-1896), *Le Tour du Monde*, 38; Paris, 1898.

BREWSTER, DAVID: *Edinburgh Encyclopedia*, IV; (Art. *Botany*), part

III, *classification.* (Art. *Erythroxylon Coca*), 18 vols., 4to.; Edinburgh, 1830.

BRINTON, DANIEL G., M.D., LL.D.: *Myths of the New World;* 12mo.; Philadelphia, 1868.

BROADBENT, SIR W. H., M.D., F.R.C.P.: *The Pulse;* London.

BROCA: *Les Ossements des Eyxiès;* Paris, 1868.

BROWNE, LENNOX, and EMIL BEHNKE: *Voice, Song and Speech,* 2 ed.; 1886.

BROWNE, PATRICK, M.D.: *The Civil and Natural History of Jamaica;* folio, p. 278; London, 1756.

BRUCE, J. MITCHELL, M.D.: *Materia Medica,* 12mo.; Philadelphia, 1884.

BRUNTON, T. LAUDER, M.D., F.R.S., etc.: *Pharmacology, Therapeutics and Materia Medica; Adapted to the U. S. Pharmacopœia* by Francis H. Williams, M.D., 8vo.; Philadelphia, 1885.

BUCHHEIM UND EISENMENGER: *Beiträge zur Anatomie und Physiologie,* V; 1870.

BURCK, DR.: (Buitenzorg, Java), *Coca Plants in Cultivation; Pharmaceutical Journal and Transactions* (3 s.), XXII; pp. 817-848; London, 1892.

CALANCHA, DE LA FR. AUGUSTIN: *Coronica moralizada de la Orden de San Augustin en el Peru;* Barcelona, 1639.

CALDERON ET ROBLES: *Traité sur les plantes du Pérou;* Paris, 1790.

CALMELS, G., and GOSSIN, E.: *Comptes rendus de l'Académie des Sciences;* 100; Paris, 1885.

CANSTATT, G.: *Jahres Bericht über die Fortschritte der gesammten Medicin in allen Ländern;* IV; p. 560; Erlangen, 1843.

CARTER, W.: *The use of Coca; British Medical Journal,* I; London, 1874.

CAUDWELL, EBER, M.D.: *The physiological action of Cuca and cucaine; British Medical Journal,* Jan. 3, London, 1885.

CAVANILLES, ANTOINE JOSÉ: *Monadelphiae classis; Dissert.,* VIII; p. 399, 4to.; Parisiis, 1789.

CELEDON, RAFAEL: *Gramática de la lengua Goajira;* Paris, 1878.

Same: *Gramática de la lengua Köggaba;* Paris, 1886.

CHAIX, PAUL: *Histoire de l'Amérique méridionale au seizième siècle;* Premiere Partie, *Pérou,* 2 vols., 8vo.; Genève, 1853.

CHAPPELL: *The History of Music;* 4 vols.; London, 1874.

CHISHOLM: *Hand Book of Commercial Geography.*

CHRISTISON, SIR ROBERT, M.D.: *The effects of Cuca or Coca: The leaves of Erythroxylon Coca; Address before the Royal Botanical Society of Edinburgh,* April 13, 1876, *on the restoration and preservative virtues of the Coca leaf against bodily fatigue; Pharmaceutical Journal and Transactions,* (3 s.), VI; also *British Medical Journal,* I; London, 1876.

CIEZA DE LEON, PEDRO: *The Second Part of the Chronicles of Peru;* Translated and Edited with Notes and an Introduction by Clements R. Markham, C.B., F.R.S. (Hakluyt Society); London, 1883.

CISNEROS, CARLOS B.; y GARCIA, ROMULO, E.: *Geografia Comercial de la América del Sur;* Lima, 1897.

CLEMENS, T.: *Erfahrungen über die therapeutische Verwendung der Cocablatter; Deutsche Klinik,* XIX; Berlin, 1867.

CLEMENT, FELIX: (Art. *Music*) in Larousse, *Dictionnaire Universel;* Paris, 1869.

CLUSIUS, CAROLUS: (Atrebatis): *Exoticorum,* libri decem. I, pp. 177-540, folio; Antverpiae, 1601-1605. Translated into French by Anthoine Colin; Lyons, 1602.

(See Monardes.)

Cocoa: All About It, by "Historicus," 12 mo., III.; London, 1896.

Coca du Pérou: Bulletin général de thérapeutique, 458-460; Paris, 1867.

COCHET, ALEXANDRE: *Note sur la culture et les usages de la Coca; Journal de chimie médicale, de pharmacie, de toxicologie,* VIII; p. 475; Paris, 1832.

COLE, R. FITZ-ROY: *The Peruvians at Home;* 12mo.; London, 1884.

COLLIN, R.: *De la Coca et ses véritables propriétés thérapeutiques; L'Union médicale* (3 s.), XXIV; Paris, 1877.

COLMAN: *Myths of the Hindus.*

COLOMBE, GABRIEL: *Etude sur la Coca et les sels de cocaïne;* 4to.; Paris, 1885.

CORNING, J. LEONARD, M.D.: *Brain Exhaustion;* 8vo.; New York, 1884.

Same: *Brain-Rest: A disquisition on the curative properties of prolonged sleep;* 2 ed., 12mo.; New York, 1885.

Same: *Local Anæsthesia in General Medicine and Surgery;* 8vo.; New York, 1886.

COWLEY, ABRAHAM, M.D.: *Poems; Four Books of Plants;* London, 1721.

("Botany in the mind of Cowley turned into poetry," said Dr. Johnson.)

CRESPO, PEDRO NOLESCO: *Memoria sobre la Coca;* 8vo.; Lima, 1793.

CRUM-BROWN, and FRASER: *Transactions Royal Society of Edinburgh;* XXV.

CURTIS, CARLTON C., A.M., Ph.D.: *A Text-Book of General Botany;* 8vo.; London, 1897.

CUTTER, EPHRAIM, M.D.: *Erythroxylin Coca as a Heart Tonic; Journal American Medical Association;* p. 1277; Chicago, 1898.

DA COSTA, J. M., M.D., LL.D.: *Some observations on the use of the Hydrochlorate of Cocaine: especially its hypodermic use; Medical News,* XIV; Philadelphia, 1884.

DALECHAMP, JACQUES: *Histoire générale des plantes; tom.* 11, CXXXV, p. 745, 2 vols., folio; Lyons, 1663.

DANA, CHARLES L., M.D.: *Urinology of Neurasthenia; Post Graduate,* IV; New York, 1888-89.

DARWIN, CHARLES: *Narrative of the Surveying voyages of His Majesty's ships Adventure and Beagle between the years 1826-1836;* 3 vols., 8vo.; London, 1839.

Same: *On the Origin of Species by means of Natural Selection;* 6 ed., 8vo.; London, 1872.

Same: *The Expression of the Emotions in Man and Animals;* 8vo.; London, 1872.

Same: *Insectivorous Plants;* 8vo.; London, 1875.

Same: *The Movements and Habits of Climbing Plants;* 2 ed.; London, 1875.

Same: *The different forms of flowers on plants of the same Species;* 8vo.; London, 1877.

Same: *A Biographical Sketch of an Infant; Mind,* II; 1877. Also *Revue Scientifique,* XIII; 1877.

Same: *The Descent of Man;* 2 vols., 2 ed., 8vo.; London, 1883.

Same: *The Variation of Animals and Plants under domestication;* 2 vols., 2 ed., 8vo.; London, 1885.

DA SILVA, FERREIRA: *Sur une reaction caracteristique de la cocaine; Comptes rendus de l'Académie des Sciences,* CXI; p. 348; Paris, 1890. Also, *Med. Contemp.;* Lisbon. Also, *Chicago Medical Times,* XXVII; 365-367; Chicago, 1895.

DAVENPORT, C. B., and NEAL, H. V.: *Studies in Morphogenesis, V. on the acclimatization of organisms to poisonous chemical substances; Archiv für Entwickelungswech,* II; 1896.

DAY, ALFRED: *Treatise on Harmony;* 1845.

DEANE: *Serpent Worship.*

DE BRY, THEODORIUS: *American Voyages,* 3 vols., folio; Frankfort, 1600.

(Full of Quaint Illustrations.)

DE CANDOLLE, ALPHONSE: *Origin of Cultivated Plants;* 12mo.; New York, 1886.

DE CANDOLLE, PYRAMUS: *Prodromus systematis naturalis, regni vegetabilis;* I, pp. 574-575, 8vo.; Paris, 1824.

DE CASTELNAU, FRANCIS: *Expédition dans les parties centrales de l'Amérique du Sud: Histoire du voyage;* III; p. 348, IV; pp. 282-285; 6 vols., 8vo., Paris, 1850-51.

(The last volume written by his assistant, Dr. H. A. Weddell.)

DE LA CONDAMINE, M.: *Journal d'un Voyage fait par ordre du roi;* Paris, 1751.

(A Voyage to measure an arc of the meridian on the plain of Quito, S. A. The expedition occupied nine years.)

DELANO, AMASA: *Narrative of Voyages and Travels in the Northern and Southern Hemispheres: Comprising Three Voyages around the World;* 8vo.; Boston, 1817.

DE LOS RIOS, J. A.: *Sobre la Coca de Peru;* 4to.; Lima, 1868. Also in *Gaceta médica de Lima,* XII; Lima, 1867-68.

DEMARLE, L. G.: *Sur la Coca;* 4to; Paris, 1862.

DESJARDINS, E.: *Le Pérou avant la Conquête Espagnole;* Paris, 1858.

DEVILLE, CH. STE. CLAIRE: *Voyage dans l'Amérique méridionale; le Magasin pittoresque,* M. Charton; 4to.; Paris, 1851.

D'ISRAELI, ISAAC: *Curiosities of Literature;* (Art. *Tea, Coffee and Chocolate*), London, 1823.

D'ORBIGNY, ALCIDE DESSALINES: *L'Homme Américain,* 2 vols.
Same: *Voyage dans l'Amérique méridionale; Relation historique,* II; 9 vols., 4to.; Paris, 1839-45.
DORVAULT: *L'officine ou Répertoire général de pharmacie pratique;* 5me edit., 8vo.; Paris, 1858.
DOWDESWELL, G. F.: *Observations on the properties and action of the leaf of the Coca plant, Erythroxylon Coca, made in the physiological laboratory of University College; Lancet,* I; London, 1876.
DROUIN DE BERCY: *L'Europe et l'Amérique comparées;* Paris, 1818.
Dublin Medical Press: On the Coca leaves, a new stimulant; Aug. 28, Dublin, 1861.
DUJARDIN-BEAUMETZ: *Diseases of the Stomach and Intestines;* Translated by E. P. Hurd, M.D.; 8vo.; New York, 1886.
Same: *New Medications;* (Art. *Coca*), Translated by E. P. Hurd, M.D.; Detroit, 1886.
DULAURE: *Phallic Worship.*
DURET, CLAUDE: *Histoire admirable des plantes et herbes esmerveillables et miraculeuses en nature;* Paris, 1605.
(Extracts from the works of Benzoni, Monardes, Oviedo, Acosta, Cieza and Fuchs.)
DYER: *The Folk-Lore of Plants.*
EDSON, CYRUS, M.D.: *La Grippe and its Treatment;* 12mo.; New York, 1891.
EHRLICH: *Studien in der Cocainreihe; Deutsche medicinische Wochenschrift,* 32; Berlin, 1890.
EINHORN, ALFRED: *Ueber Ecgonin; Berichte der chemischen Gesellschaft,* XX; 1, p. 1221; Berlin, 1887.
Same: *Beitrage zur Kenntniss des Cocaïns; idem;* XXI; 1, p. 47, see also, 3335, 1888.
Same, und ALBERT MARQUARDT: *Zur Kenntniss des Rechtscocaïns und der homologen Alkaloide; idem;* XXIII; 1, p. 979; 1890.
EMMET, THOMAS ADDIS, M.D.: *The Principles and Practice of Gynæcology;* (Art. *Principles of General Treatment*), Philadelphia, 1879.
EMMERLING: *Landwistschaft Versuchsstationen,* 34, 109; 1887.
ENGEL, CARL: *A Descriptive Catalogue of Musical Instruments in the South Kensington Museum;* London, 1874.
ENGLEMANN, TH. W.: *Ueber die Flimmerbewegung; Jenaische Zeitschift für Naturwissenschaft,* IV; Leipzig, 1868.
ENGLER, A., und PRANTL, K.: *Die Natürlicher Pflanzenfamilien;* (in several volumes in course of publication.) K. Reiche, (Art. *Erythroxylaceæ*), 8vo.; Leipzig, 1897.
ERB, WILHELM HEINRICH: *Neurasthenia Spinalis; Ziemsen's Cyclopædia,* XIII; p. 369; New York, 1878.
ERNST, M.: *De L'emploi de la Coca dans les Pays Septentrionaux de l'Amérique du Sud; Comptes rendus, Congrès International des Américanistes;* Berlin, 1890.
ESPINOSA: *Edinburgh Medical Journal,* XXI; II, 1151; 1876.

EUSEBIUS NIEREMBERGIUS, JOHANNES: *Historia naturæ, maximæ peregrina*, IV; XXV, fol. 304-305; Antverpiae, 1635.

FAVRE-CLAVAIROZ, LÉON: *La Bolivie, son présent, son passé et son avenir.* Dans les livraisons 118, 119 et 120 de la *Revue contemporaine;* Paris, 1857.

FEIGNEAUX, A.: *L'Érythroxylum Coca; la coca et la cocaine, Historique, physiologie, thérapeutique;* Ixelles, 1885.

FERGUSON, JAMES: *Rude Stone Monuments.*

Same: *Tree and Serpent Worship, or Illustrations of Mythology and Art in India;* large 8vo.; London, 1868.

FICK and WISLICENUS: *On the Origin of Muscular Power; Philosophical Magazine*, XXXI; London, 1866.

FIGUEROA, DIEGO DAVALOS Y: *Miscellanea Austral;* Lima, 1602.

FITZ GERALD, EDWARD A.: *The Highest Andes;* 8vo.; New York, 1899.

FLEISCHER, R.: *Ueber die Einwirkung des Cocainum muriaticum auf das Nervensystem und den thierischen Stoffwechsel; Deutsches Archiv für klinische Medicin*, XLII; pp. 82-90; Leipzig, 1887-1888.

FLETCHER, DR. ROBERT: *Prehistoric Trephining and Cranial Amulets;* V; *Smithsonian Report;* Washington, 1882.

FLINT, AUSTIN, JR., M.D.: *On the Physiological Effect of Severe and Protracted Muscular Exercise*, etc.; 8vo.; New York, 1871.

FLÜCKIGER, F. A.: *Note on Cocaine and Atropine; Pharmaceutical Journal and Transactions*, XVI; March 20, London, 1886.

FOSTER, FRANK P., M.D.: *An Illustrated Encyclopædic Medical Dictionary;* (Art. *Coca*), II; p. 1066; 4 vols.; New York, 1890.

FOSTER, MICHAEL, M.A., M.D., F.R.C.S.: *Text Book of Physiology*, 4 ed.; London, 1880.

Same: *Lancet*, I; London, 1893.

FOY, G.: *Cocoa and cocaine; Medical Press and Circular* (n. s.), XLI; London, 1886.

FRAGOSO, JOHAN: *Catalogus simplicium medicamentorum;* 8vo.; Compluti, 1566.

Same: *Discursos de las cosas aromaticas que se traen de la India oriental;* 8vo.; Madrid, 1592.

(Also in Latin; Argentinæ, 1601.)

FRAMPTON, JOHN: *Joyful Newes out of the Newe Founde Worlde, wherin is declared the Virtues of Hearbes, Treez, Oyales, Plantes and Stones;* London, 1596.

FRANCK ET BRASSAUD: *Marey's Travaux;* III; Paris, 1877.

FRANKL, J.: *Mittheilung über Coca; Ztschrift d. k. k. Gesellschaft d. Aerzte zu Wien*, XVI; Vienna, 1860.

FRANKLAUSER, W.: *Coca as a stimulant; American Medical and Surgical Bulletin*, VII; New York, 1894.

FREUD, S.: *Coca; Centralblatt für die gesammte Therapie;* Wien, Translated by S. Pollak, *St. Louis Medical and Surgical Journal*, XLVII; St. Louis, 1884.

Same: *Beiträge zur Kenntniss der Cocawirkung; Wiener medizinische Wochenschrift*, XXXV; Vienna, 1885.

Same: *Ueber Coca; Neu durchgeseh. u. verm. Sep.-Abdr. aus dem Centralblatt für die gesammte Therapie;* Vienna, 1885.

Same: *Bemerkungen über Cocaïnsucht und Cocaïnfurcht; Wiener Medizinische Wochenschrift,* XXXVII; 929-932; Vienna, 1887.

Frézier, A. F.: *Relation du voyage de la Mer du sud aux côtes du Chili et du Pérou, fait en 1712, 1713 et 1714;* 4to; Paris, 1732-41.

Fristedt, R. F.: *Om Cocabladen såsom njutnings. och läkemedel. Upsala Läkaref.* III; 1867-68.

Fronmuller sen: *Coca und Cat; pharmakologische Studien Vrtljschr. f. d. prakt. Heilk.,* LXXIX; Prag., 1863.

Fuchs, Leonhard: *De historia stirpium,* XVIII; Basileæ, 1542.

Fuentes, Manuel A.: *Guia historico—descriptiva, administrativa, judicial y de domicilio de Lima;* Lima, 1860.

Same: *Mémoire sur le Coca du Pérou;* Paris, 1866.

Gaedcke, F.: *Archives de Pharmacie,* LXXXII; Paris, 1855.

Gage, Simon H.: *Reference Hand Book of the Medical Sciences,* V; p. 72; New York, 1887.

Galt, F. L., M.D. (Lynchburg, Va.): *The Indians of Peru; Smithsonian Report;* pp. 308-315; Washington, 1877.

Garcia, E.: *Erythroxylon Coca, ó Coca del Perú; Gaceta del hospital,* I; 108, 128, 180, 200; Valencia, 1882.

Garcia, Gregorio: *Orígen de los Indios del Nuevo Mundo é Indias occidentales;* p. 92, 4to.; Madrid, 1729.

Garcilasso de la Vega: *Commentarios Reales,* primera y secunda parte, 2 vols., small folio; Lisboa y Cordova, 1609-17. Translated into French by Baudoin, 2 vols., 4to.; Amsterdam, 1737.

Same: *The First Part of the Royal Commentaries of the Yncas;* 1609. Translated and edited with notes and Introduction by Clements R. Markham, C.B., F.R.S. (Hakluyt Society); 8vo.; London, 1871.

Gattel, Dr. Felix: *Ueber die sexuellen Ursachen der Neurasthenic und Angstneurose;* Berlin, 1898.

Gazeau, C.: *Nouvelles recherches expérimentales sur la pharmacologie, la physiologie et la thérapeutique du Coca;* 4to.; Paris, 1870. (Also in *Courrier Médical;* Paris, 1871.)

Gélineau, E.: *Des peurs maladies ou phobies;* Paris, 1894.

Gentleman's Magazine and Historical Chronicle: London, 1751, 1795, 1814. *The Incas of Peru;* 1751. *Coca,* 1795-1814.

Gibbs, Benjamin F., M.D. (Surgeon U. S. N.): *Report on Coca; Sanitary and Medical Report, U. S. Navy,* p. 675, 1873-74; Washington, 1875.

Gibbs: *The Coca plant; Leonard's Illustrated Medical Journal,* VII, 24; Detroit, 1886.

Giesel, F.: *New Test for Cocaine; American Journal of Pharmacy;* (From *Pharmaceutische Zeitung;* Feb. 27, p. 132; Berlin, 1886); LVIII; p. 247; May, Philadelphia, 1886.

Same: *Chemisches Centralblatt,* II; Berlin, 1889.

Same: *Berichte der chemischen gesellschaft;* XXIV; p. 2336; Berlin, 1891.

Same: (See Liebermann.)

GILLESPIE, A. LOCKHART: *The Natural History of Digestion;* 12mo.; London, 1898.

GINTLER, J.: *Ueber Coca, Extractum der Coca und Cocain; Wiener medizinische Wochenschrift,* XII; Vienna, 1862.

GOMARA, FRANCISCO LOPEZ DE: *Historia de las Indias; in Historiadores primitivos de las Indias occidentales;* II; pp. 178-179; Madrid, 1749.

GOODALE, GEORGE LINCOLN: *Address before American Association for Advancement of Science;* Washington, 1891.

GOSSE, L. A. (Genève): *Monographie de L'Erythroxylon Coca; Présentée à l'Académie royale de Belgique,* le 3 mai, 1861; 8vo., 2 pl.; Bruxelles, 1861.

(Extrait du tome XII des mémoires de l'Académie royale de Belgique.)

GRANDIDIER, ERNEST: *Voyage dans l'Amérique du Sud, Pérou et Bolivie,* pp. 70, 109-116, 8vo.; Paris, 1861.

GRASSET, J.: *Sur l'action anesthésique cutanée du chlorhydrate de cocaïne; Comptes rendus de l'Académie des Sciences;* XCIX; p. 1122; Paris, 1884.

GRAY, J. L.: *Erythroxylon Coca; Journal American Medical Association,* IV; 455-458; Chicago, 1885.

GRIFFITHS, A. B., Ph.D., F.R.C.S., etc.: *Researches on Micro-Organisms;* 12mo.; London, 1891.

GRIFFITHS, R. EGLESFELD, M.D.: *Medical Botany;* 8vo.; Philadelphia, 1847.

GUBLER, ADOLPHE, M.D.: *Principles and Methods of Therapeutics.* English translation; Philadelphia, 1881.

GUENTHER, F.: *Berichte Deutsche Pharm. Gesellschaft,* IX; p. 38, Feb. 2, 1899.

GUIBOURT: *Histoire naturelle des drogues simples,* III, p. 545, 4me édit., 8vo.; Paris, 1850.

GUNN, ALEXANDER, F. C. S.: *The Determination of Total Alkaloids in Coca Leaves; Pharmaceutical Journal and Transactions;* (4), III; Sept. 19; p. 249; London, 1896.

HAIG, ALEXANDER, M.A., M.D., etc.: *Uric Acid as a Factor in the Causation of Disease;* 4 ed., 8vo.; London, 1897.

HALL, CAPTAIN BASIL (Royal Navy): *Extracts from a Journal written on the coasts of Chili, Peru and Mexico in the years 1820-21-22;* 2 vols.; London, 1825.

HALLER, C.: *Notizen über die Coca; Ztschrift d. k. k. Gesellschaft der Aerzte zu Wien,* XVI; Vienna, 1860.

HAMMOND, WILLIAM A., M.D.: *Sleep and its Derangements;* Philadelphia, 1869.

Same: *Diseases of the Nervous System;* 8vo.; New York, 1886.

Same: *Coca; its preparations and their therapeutic qualities, with some remarks on the so-called cocaine habit; Virginia Medical Monthly,* XIV, 598-612; Richmond, 1887-88.

HANANSECK, DR. T. E.: *Pharm. Rundschau,* April, 1885.

HAWEIS, REV. HUGH R.: *Music and Morals;* 12mo.; London, 1873.

HEBBING, H., F.C.S.: *Materia Medica;* 3 ed., 12mo.; London, 1892.

HEDBOM, K.: *Om kokabladen och kokaïnet; Lakäreförenings förhändlingar;* XX; Upsala, 1884-85.

HEINIGKE, DR. CARL: *Pathogenetic Outlines of Homœopathic Drugs;* New York, 1880.

HELMHOLTZ, HERMANN, L.F.: *On the sensations of tone as a physiological basis of the theory of music.* Translated by Alexander J. Ellis; 3 ed.; London, 1895.

HELMSING, DR.: *Thesis;* Dorpat, 1886.

HELPS, ARTHUR: *The Spanish Conquest in America and Its Relations to the History of Slavery and to the Government of Colonies;* 4 vols.; London, 1855.

HEMPEL, CHARLES J., M.D.: *Materia Medica and Therapeutics;* 8vo.; Chicago, 1880.

HEPBURN: *New York Medical Record;* II; New York, 1884.

Herbarium, Columbia University: *Plantæ Bolivianæ; Erythroxylaceæ;* collected by Miguel Bang, Yungas, Bolivia, 1890. (Distributed by Drs. Britton and Rusby.)

HERMANN: *Die Ergebnisse Neurer Unters aus dem Gebiet der thierisch. Electricität;* 1878. See also *Journal Physiology*, I; London, 1878.

HERNANDEZ, FRANCISCO: *Rerum medicarum Novae Hispaniae thesaurus;* 4to.; Romae, (about) 1551.

HERNDON, WILLIAM LEWIS, and LARDNER GIBBON, Lieutenants, U.S.N.: *Exploration of the Valley of the Amazon; made under Direction of the Navy Department;* 2 vols., 8vo.; Washington, 1853-54.

HERRERA, ANTONIO DE: *Historia general de los hechos de los Castellanos en las Islas y tierra firme del Mar Oceano;* V, VI, VII, VIII; 4 vols., folio; Madrid, 1730.

HERTWIG, O. and R.: *Ueber den Befruchtungs und Theilungsvorgang des thierischen Eies unter dem Einfluss aüsserer Agentien; Jenaische Zeitzchift für Naturwissenschaft;* XIII; 1887.

HESSE, O.: *The Alkaloids of Coca Leaves; Pharmaceutische Zeitung;* July 16, Berlin, 1887. *American Journal of Pharmacy;* Philadelphia, 1887. *Pharmaceutical Journal and Transactions;* (3 s.), Nov., 1887; *ibid*, Aug. 8, London, 1891.

HIGGINS: *Celtic Druids.*

HOLMES, E. W.: *Erythroxylon Coca and its alkaloid cocaine; Therapeutic Gazette* (3 s.), II; Detroit, 1886.

HOOKER, SIR JOSEPH DALTEN, M.D.: *Erythroxylon Coca; Curtis's Botanical Magazine*, comprising Plants of the Royal Gardens of Kew; L; (3 s.), 8vo.; London, 1894.

HOOKER, W. J., LL.D., etc.: *Companion to the Botanical Magazine;* I, p. 161; II, p. 25, with plates; London, 1835-36.

HOWARD, WILLIAM C., Ph.D.: *Separation of Hygrine from Cocaine; Pharmaceutical Journal and Transactions;* (3 s.), p. 71 July 23, London, 1887.

HUMBOLDT, ALEXANDRE DE, et AIMÉ BONPLAND: *Voyage aux regions équinoxiales du nouveau continent;* 15 vols.; Paris, 1817-31.

Same: *Personal Narrative of Travels to the Equinoctial Regions of the New Continent, etc., during the Years 1799-1804;* 8 vols.; London, 1849.

Same: Bonpland et Kunth: (See Kunth.)

HUNTER, JOHN: *Works edited by Palmer;* 4 vols.; London, 1839.

HUSE, E. C.: *Coca-Erythroxylon; A new cure for the opium habit; Therapeutic Gazette* (n. s.), I; Detroit, 1880.

INWARDS, RICHARD: *The Temple of the Andes;* London, 1884.

ISAACS, JORGE: *Estudios sobre las tribus indigenas del Estado Magdalena, antes Provincia de Santamarta;* (*anales de la Instruccion publica en los Estados Nuidos de Colombia*, VIII); 1884-87.

JABLONOWSKI, W.: *Liscie zwane "Coca" i spór o pierwszeństwo otrzymania "Kokainy."*

(The leaf called coca, and the contest of priority of the discovery of cocaine.) *Czasopismo*, XIV; 98, 117, 132; Lwow, 1885.

JACKSON, JOHN R., A.L.S.: *Commercial Botany of the Nineteenth Century;* 12mo.; London, 1890.

JANEWAY, E. G., M.D.: *Some Reflections upon Therapeutics, Transactions, New York Academy of Medicine*, XII; p. 79; New York, 1897.

JAUCOURT, LE CHEVALIER DE: (Art. *Coca*), dans *l'Encyclopédic francaise ou dictionnaire raisonné des sciences, des arts et des métiers*, III, p. 557, folio; Paris, 1753.

JOHNSTON, J. F. W.: *Report British Association Advancement of Science;* London, 1853.

JOHNSTON, JOHANN: *Historia naturalis de arboribus et plantis*, V, p. 33, 2 vols., 4to.; Heilbronn, 1768.

JOLYET: *Recherches sur l'action physiologique de la cocaïne; Comptes rendus Société de biologie;* Paris, 1867-69.

JULIAN, PADRE ANTONIO: *Disertacion sobre Hayo o Coca dans la Perla de la America;* Lima, 1787

JURIST, DR. LOUIS: *On the substitution of the preparations of Coca for cocaine; College and Clinical Record*, VI; 8vo.; Philadelphia, 1885.

JUSSIEU, ADRIEN DE: (Art. *Coca et Érythroxylées*)*;* dans le *Dictionnaire universel d'histoire naturelle;* D'Orbigny, Charles; IV: p. 41; V; p. 425; 13 vols., 8vo.; Paris, 1848-49.

JUSSIEU, ANTOINE LAURENT DE: (Art. *Coca*)*;* dans le *Dictionnaire des sciences naturelles*, IX, p. 487; 8vo.; Paris, 1817.

JUSSIEU, JOSEPH DE: *Réflexions sur deux espèces de quinquina; Histoire de la Société de médecine de Paris*, pp. 252-263; Paris, 1779.

KATSIN, M. B.: *Coca and its preparations; Vestnik. obsh. hig., sudeb. i prakt. med.*, XXVII; 193-232; St. Petersburgh, 1895.

KAVANAGH: *Origin of Language and Myths.*

KELLER, FRANZ: *The Amazon and Madeira Rivers;* 4to.; New York, 1874.

KING, C. W.: *The Gnostics and their Remains, Ancient and Mediæval;* London, 1864.

KIRKES': *Handbook of Physiology;* by W. Morrant Baker, F.R.C.S., and Vincent Dormer Harris, M.D.; 11 ed.; London, 1884.

KNIGHT, RICHARD PAYNE: *An Inquiry Into the Symbolic Language of Ancient Art and Mythology; Being Vol. II of Specimens of Ancient Sculpture;* large folio, III; London, 1835.

Same: *Discourse on the Worship of Priapus, and its connection with the Mystic Theology of the Ancients;* London, 1865.

KOBERT, E. R.: *Ueber den Einfluss verschiedener pharmakologischer Agentien auf die Muskelsubstanz; Archiv für experimentelle Pathologie und Pharmakologie;* XV; p. 22; Leipzig, 1882.

KOLLER, CARL, M.D.: *Ueber die Verwendung des Cocaïn zur Anästhesirung am Auge; Wiener Medizinische Wochenschrift;* p. 1307; Vienna, 1884.

KOSMOS: *Die Coca und ihr Einfluss; Zeitschrift für angewandte Naturwissenschaft;* 4me année, No. 11, p. 185; Leipzig, 1860.

KOZLOWSKI, W. M.: *The Primary Synthesis of Proteids in plants; Bulletin,* Torrey Botanical Club, XXVI; New York, 1899.

KRAFT-EBING, R. VON: *Psychopathia Sexualis;* Translated by Charles Gilbert Chaddock, M.D.; 8vo.; Philadelphia, 1892.

KUNTH, CAROL SIGISM: *Nova genera et species plantarum, quas in peregrinationibus orbis novi colligerunt descripserunt partim adumbraverunt Amat.* Bonpland et Alex. de Humboldt; Paris, 1825.

LABORDE, J. V.: *Note préliminaire sur l'action physiologique de la cocaïne et ses sels; Tribune médicale* XVI; Paris, 1884.

Same: *De l'action physiologique de la cocaïne amorphe et de la cocaïne liquide (de Duquesnal) comparée à l'action de la cocaïne cristallisée; Comptes rendus Société de Biologie* (8), II; 241; Paris, 1884.

Same: *Étude expérimentale de l'action physiologique de la cocaïne et de ses sels; Deuxième note, ibid,* XVII, 3-8; Paris, 1885.

LADENBURG and BUCHKA: *Cocaine Relationship to Atropine; Pharmaceutical Journal and Transactions;* (3 s.), June 28, London, 1890.

LAET, JOHANNES DE: *Novus Orbis, seu descriptiones Indiae occidentalis;* XII, folio, Lugd.; Batavorum, 1633.
(Extracts from works of Monardes, Acosta and Garcilasso.)

LAFFONT, M: *The action of cocaine on the Sympathetic Nervous System; Comptes rendus Société de Biologie,* Dec. 3, 1887.

Same: *The analgesic action of cocaine; ibid,* Dec. 17, 1887.

Same: *Étude physiologique sur la Coca et sels de Coca; Comptes rendus Société de Biologie, Académie de Médecine,* Jan. 4, Paris, 1888.

Same: *Erythroxylon Coca; its value as a medicament; New York Medical Journal,* I; 623; New York, 1889. *Maryland Medical Journal,* XXII; 272-274; Baltimore, 1889-90. See also Sajous' *Annual,* V; A34; 1891.

LA HARPE, J. F.: *Abrégé de L'Histoire Générale des Voyages,* XIII, XV; Paris, 1814.

LAMARCK, J. B. P. A.: (Art. *Coca*); dans *l'Encyclopédie méthodique, Dictionnaire de Botanique,* II, p. 393, 4to.; Paris, 1786.

LAROUSSE, P.: (Art. *Coca*), *Dictionnaire Universel du XIX Siècle;* IV, 498; Paris, 1869.

LEARED, A.: *The use of Coca; British Medical Journal,* I; 272; London, 1874.

LEEBODY, J. R.: *The action of Cuca; British Medical Journal,* I; 750, London, 1876.

LE MAOUT and DECAISNE: *Traité Générale de Botanique;* Paris, 1876. Also translated by Hooker; 8vo.; London.

LEON, PEDRO CIEZA DE: (See Cieza.)

LE PÉROU: *Société Franco-Peruvienne des mines d'or de la province de Carabaya;* Paris, 1853.

LE PLONGEON, AUGUSTUS: *Sacred Mysteries among the Mayas and Quiches, 11,500 years ago;* 8vo.; New York, 1886.

LESZYNSKY, WILLIAM M., M.D.: *Coffee as a beverage, and its frequent deleterious effects upon the nervous system; Medical Record;* January 12, New York, 1901.

LEVILLAIN, D. FERNAND: *La Neurasthénie;* Paris, 1891.

LEVINUS-APOLLONIUS: *De Peruviae regionis, inter Novi-orbis provincias celeberrimæ, inventione et rebus gestis,* I, 8vo.; Antverpiae, 1557.

LIEBERMANN, C.: *Nebenalkaloïd des Cocaïns, das Isatrophylcocaïn; Berichte der chemischen Gesellschaft;* XXI; 2, p. 2342; Berlin, 1888.

Same: *Ueber Cinnamylcocaïn; idem,* XXI; 2, p. 3372; Berlin, 1888.

Same, und F. GIESEL: *Ueber eine neue technische Darstellungsart und theilweise Synthese des Cocaïns; idem,* XXI; 2, p. 3196, also, XXII; 3, p. 522; see also, XXII; 1, pp. 130, 672, 675; 2, pp. 2240, 2261; Berlin, 1889.

Same: *On the History of Coca bases; Pharmaceutical Journal and Transactions;* (3 s.), XXII; pp. 61-101; London.

LIEBIG: *Animal Chemistry or Chemistry in its Application to Physiology and Pathology;* London, 1843.

Same: *The Source of Muscular Power; Pharmaceutical Journal and Transactions;* (3 s.), London, 1870.

LINDLEY, JOHN, Ph.D.: *The Vegetable Kingdom;* 8vo.; London, 1853.

LINNÆUS, CAROLUS: *Systema Naturae;* London, 1768.

LIPPMANN, E.: *Étude sur la Coca du Pérou;* These de Strasbourg; 1868.

LIVIERATO, P.: *Contribuzione allo studio dell' azione biologica e terapeutica della cocaina; Salute Italia Med.,* XIX; p. 209-217; Genova, 1885.

LOSSEN, W.: *On Cocaine, the active Principle of Coca; Inaugural Dissertation,* Gottingen, 1862; *Journal de Pharmacie;* Juin, Paris, 1862. Also *American Journal of Pharmacy;* Philadelphia, 1862. *Annalen der Chemie und Pharmacie,* CXXI; Leipzig; *ibid,* CXXXII; p. 351; Leipzig, 1865.

LUDEWIG: *Literature of American Aboriginal Languages.*

LYONS, A. B., M.D.: *Notes on the Alkaloids of Coca Leaves; American Journal of Pharmacy;* LVII; p. 466, Oct., also p. 596, Dec.; Philadelphia, 1885.

Same: *A Study of the Use of Mayer's Reagent in the Estimation of Alkaloids.* [Read before the Michigan State Pharmaceutical Association, Oct., 1886.]

Same: *Manual of Practical Pharmaceutical Assaying,* 12mo.; Detroit, 1886.

Same: *Note on Estimation of Cocaine by Mayer's Reagent; American Journal of Pharmacy;* Philadelphia, 1886.

Macedo, Dr.: *Comparison of Incan and Aztec Civilization; Proceedings of Numismatic and Antiquarian Society;* Philadelphia, 1883.

McBean, S.: *Erythroxylon Cuca in the treatment of typhus and typhoid fevers, and also of other febrile diseases; British Medical Journal,* I; 291; London, 1877.

Macfarren, G. A.: *Musical History,* 12mo.; New York, 1885.

Maclagan: *Journal de Chimie et de Pharmacie,* XXXIX; Paris, 1857.

McLaumaille: *Paris to Vienna by Bicycle;* London, 1875.

Magnan et Saury: *Trois cas de cocainisme chronique; Comptes rendùs Société de Biologie;* p. 60; Paris, 1889.

Mahomed, F. A., M.D.: *The effect of Prolonged Muscular Exertion on the Circulatory System; British Medical Journal;* March 18, London, 1876.

Maimonides: *De Idolatria.*

Maisch, John M., Ph.M., Ph.D.: *Translation of Niemann's original dissertation,* from *Wittstein's V. Schrift.;* IX; pp. 489-524. *American Journal of Pharmacy;* IX; p. 496; Philadelphia, 1861.

Same: *On Coca leaves; Medical and Surgical Reporter* (n. s.), VI, 399; Philadelphia, 1861.

Same: *A Manual of Organic Materia Medica,* 5 ed., 12mo.; Philadelphia, 1892.

Mann, J. Dixon, M.D.: *Forensic Medicine,* 2 ed., 8vo.; London, 1898.

Mannheim, Paul: *Ueber das Cocaïn und seine Gefahren in physiologischer, toxicologischer und therapeutischer Beziehung; Zeitschrift für klinische Medicin;* XVIII; 3, 4, p. 380; Berlin, 1891.

Mantegazza, Dr. Paola: *Ymportancia dietetica y medicinal de la Coca; El commercio Journal;* Jan. 14, Salta, 1857.

Same: *Sulle virtio igieniche e medicinale della Coca, a sugli alimenti nervosi in generale;* (Prize Essay), Milan, 1859.

Marcoy, Paul: *Scènes et paysages dans les Andes,* I, pp. 66-289; II, pp. 81, 91, 210; 2 vols., 8vo.; Paris, 1861.

Same: *Voyage à travers L'Amérique du Sud. De L'Océan Pacifique à L'Océan Atlantique,* Illustré de 626 vues, Types et Paysages par E. Riou, et accompagné de 20 cartes gravées sur les dessins de l'Auteur, 2 vols., 4to.; Paris, 1869.

(Paul Marcoy was the *nom de plume* of the Frenchman, Lorenzo St. Criq.)

Mariani, Angelo: *La Coca du Pérou; Revue de thérapeutique médi-*

co-chirurgicales, 148-152; Paris, 1872. *Monde pharm.*, IV; 25; Paris, 1875.

Same: *La Coca du Pérou; botanique, historique, thérapeutique;* Paris, 1878.

Same: *La Coca et la cocaine;* Paris, 1885.

Same: *La Coca et ses applications thérapeutiques*, 8vo.; Paris, 1888.

Same: *Coca and its Therapeutic Application*, 3 ed., 8vo., III; Paris, 1896. Translated by J. N. Jaros; New York, 1896.

MARKHAM, CLEMENTS, C. B., F. R. S.: *Cuzco; a Journey to the Ancient Capital of Peru; With an Account of the History, Language, Literature and Antiquities of the Incas, with Illustrations and Map*, 8vo.; London, 1856.

(Mr. Markham translated and edited most of the works of the earlier Peruvian historians which are published by the Hakluyt Society, London.)

Same: *Travels in Peru and India*, with Maps and Illustrations, 8vo.; London, 1862.

Same: *Ollantay, an Ancient Ynca Drama.* Translated from the Original Quichua, 12mo.; London, 1871.

Same: *Narrative of Rites and Laws of the Yncas.* (Hakluyt Society); London, 1873. (Embracing the Manuscript Translations of Santa Cruz, Molina, Avila and Ondegardo.)

Same: *A Memoir of the Lady Ana de Osorio, Countess of Chinchon and Vice-Queen of Peru, with a plea for the correct spelling of the Chinchona genus;* Map and Illustrations, 4to.; London, 1874.

Same: *Peruvian Bark; A popular account of the introduction of cinchona cultivation into British India;* 12mo., XV; pp. 145-153; *Coca cultivation;* London, 1880.

Same: *A History of Peru;* Chicago, 1892.

MARTIN DE BORDEAUX: *Notice sur la Coca du Pérou*, dans les *Actes de l'Académie des sciences et arts de Bordeaux*, pp. 185-207; Bordeaux, 1841.

MARTIN DE MOUSSY: *Description géographique et statisque de la confédération Argentine;* I, p. 194, 3 vols., 8vo.; Paris, 1860.

MARTIN, H. NEWELL, M.D., etc.: *The Human Body*, 12mo; New York, 1881.

MARTIN, STANISLAS: *Journal de Pharmacie;* Paris, 1859.

MARTINDALE, W.: *Coca, cocaine and its salts; their history, medical and economic uses, and medicinal preparations*, 12mo.; London, 1886.

MARTINS: *Annales de Science Natural* (3 s.), V; Paris, 1846.

MARTIUS, C. F. P. DE: *Beiträge zur kenntniss der gattung Erythroxylon;* in *Abhandl. d. Math.-phys. Kl. d. Acad. d. Wiss.;* München, 1840.

Same: *Systema Materia Medica Braziliensis*, 8vo.; Leipzig, 1843.

Same: *Flora Braziliensis*, XII; Part I; p. 130, *et seq.*, *Erythroxylaceæ.* (In many vols.) Large folio; 1878. (See Peyritsch.)

MASON, A. P.: *Erythroxylon Coca: its physiological effects, and especially its effects on the excretion of urea by the kidneys;*

(*Graduation thesis*), *Boston Medical and Surgical Journal*, CVII; 221-223; Boston, 1882.

MAYO: *Mythology of Pagan World.*

MAYS: *Therapeutic Gazette;* June, Detroit, 1885.

MERAT ET DE LENS: *Dictionnaire universel de matière médicale et de thérapeutique générale.* (Art. *Erythroxylon.*) III, p. 148, 7 vols., 8vo.; Paris, 1831.

MERCK, C. E.: *Zur Kenntniss des Ecgonins; Berichte der chemischen Gesellschaft*, 19; 2; p. 3002; Berlin, 1886.

MERCK, E.: *Cocaine and Its Salts; Pharmaceutical Journal and Transactions;* (3 s.), Nov. 29, London, 1884.

MERCK, W.: *Ueber Benzoyl Ecgonin; Berichte der chemischen Gesellschaft;* XVIII; 1, p. 1594; *Künstliches Cocaïn; idem;* 2, p. 2264. *Ueber die künstliche Darstellung von cocaïn und seinen Homologen; idem;* 2, p. 2952; Berlin, 1885.

Mercurio Peruano: Contains many important Contributions on the History, Botany, Topography, etc., of Peru. Lima.
(Dr. Unanue contributed to its columns during 1791-1794.

MILLER, JOHN: *Memoires of General Miller in the service of the Republic of Peru;* 2 vols., 8vo.; London, 1828.

MITCHELL, S. WEIR, M.D.: *Fat and Blood*, 4 ed., 12mo.; Philadelphia, 1884.

MOLINA, CHRISTOVAL DE: *The Fables and Rites of the Yncas* (MSS. 1570-1584). Translated and edited by Clements R. Markham, C.B., F.R.S. (Hakluyt Society); London, 1873.
(The original Peruvian manuscript was translated and published in French by Ternaux Compans in 1840.)

MONARDES, NICOLAUS: *Historia medicinal de las cosas que se traen de las Indias occidentales que sirven al uso de Medicina*, 4to.; Seville, 1580. (Translated into Latin by Clusius under the title *Simplicium medicamentorum ex novo orbe delatorum historia*, 4to.; Antverpiae, 1582.)

MONEY, ANGEL: *Physiology of Infancy; Keating's Encyclopedia of Diseases of Children*, 4 vols.; Philadelphia, 1889.

MONTENEGRO, ALONZO DE LA PEÑA: *Itinerario para Parochos de Indios;* IV, t. V, sec. VII, p. 570, 4to.; Amberes, 1754.

MONTESINOS, FERNANDO: *Memoires Historiques sur l'ancien Pérou*, Ternaux Compans; Paris, 1840.
(Montesinos gives a long list of Peruvian sovereigns prior to the accepted Incan period.)

MOORE, W. O., M.D.: *The physiological and therapeutical effects of the Coca leaf and its alkaloids; New York Medical Journal*, XLI, 19-22; New York, 1885.

MORÉNO Y MAÏZ, T.: *Recherches chimiques et physiologiques sur l'Erythroxylon Coca du Pérou, et la cocaine*, 4to.; Paris, 1868. Also translated *Gaceta médica de Lima*, II; 58, 70, 78, 88, 95, 101, 109, 117, 124, 134, 141; Lima, 1876.

MORRIS, D.: *Proceedings Linnæan Society*, XXV; pp. 381-384, December, 1888.

MORTON, W. J., M.D.: *Tea Drinkers' Disorder, or Toxic Effects of*

Tea; Journal of Nervous and Mental Diseases; Oct., New York, 1879.

Mosso, Ugolino: *Archiv für experimentelle Pathologie;* XXIII; Leipzig, 1887.

Same: [*Physiological research on Cocaine.*] *Giornale della reale Accademia di Medicina;* XXXVIII; pp. 65, 297, 444; Torino, 1890. [An extract of this article appears in Sajous' *Annual;* V; B23; Philadelphia, 1891.]

Same: *La Fatica;* Milano, 1891.

Motta, E.: *Do Erythroxylon Coca; Journal de Sociedade das sciencies medicas de Lisbon* (2 s.), XXVI; 257, 307, 325; Lisbon, 1862.

Moxon, Walter, M.D.: *Influence of the Circulation upon the Nervous System; British Medical Journal,* I; London, 1881.

Müeller, Baron Ferd.: *Select Extra Tropical Plants readily eligible for Industrial Culture or Naturalization;* 7 ed., 8vo.; Melbourne, 1888.

Muñiz, Manuel Antonio; and W. J. McGee: *Primitive Trephining in Peru; Sixteenth Annual Report of the Bureau of American Ethnology,* 1894-95, 8vo.; Washington, 1897.

Murchison: *Clinical lectures on Diseases of the Liver,* 3 ed.; New York, 1885.

Muscle, Influence of Exercise on the Metabolism of; J. C. Dunlop, M.D., F.R.C.P.; Nöel Paton, M.D., F.R.C.P.; R. Stockman, M.D., F.R.C.P., and Ivison Maccadam, F.R.S., Experimental research of British Medical Association; *Journal of Physiology,* XXII, p. 68; London, 1897-98.

Mussi, W.: *Ricerche chimico-legali sull' avvelenamento acuto per cocaina;* 8vo.; Firenze, 1888.

Same: *Zur Abscheidung des cocaïns aus Leichentheilen; Zeitschrift für Analytische Chemie;* Wiesbaden, 1889. *Separation of Cocaine from Animal remains; Chemical News;* London, 1890.

Nadaillac, Marquis de: *Prehistoric America.* Translated by N. D'Anvers, edited by W. H. Doll, 8vo.; London, 1885.

Same: *Manners and Monuments of Prehistoric Peoples.* Translated by N. D'Anvers, 8vo.; New York, 1892.

Neudorfer J.: *Die Coca; Allgemeiner Mil-ärztl Zeitung;* 377-380; Vienna, 1870.

Nevinny, Dr. Jos.: *Das Cocablatt eine Pharmakognostiche Abhandlung;* Wien, 1885.

Niemann, A.: *Ueber eine neue organische Base in den Cocablättern,* Inaugural dissertation, *Viertel Jahreschrit für practische Pharmacie;* Gottingen, 1860.

Nikolski, M.: *Materialî dlya rïesheniya Voprosa o vliyanii kokaïna na zhivotnîy organizm;* 8vo.; St. Petersburg, 1872. [The influence of cocaine on animal organisms.]

Norris, William F., A.M., M.D.; and Charles A. Oliver, A.M., M.D.: *Text Book of Ophthalmology,* 8vo.; Philadelphia, 1893.

Novy, Frederick G., M.S.: *Cocaine and Its Derivatives;* 12 mo.; Detroit, 1887.

NUÑEZ DEL PRADO, E.: *Estudio sobre la Coca; Gaceta médica de Lima*, I; 238, 246, 254, 262, 271, 279; Lima, 1875.

NYSTEN: *Dictionnaire de médecine, de chirurgie et de pharmacie*, par Littré et Robin, I, 2 vols., 4to.; Paris, 1858.

OBERSTEINER und ERLENMEYER: *Deutsche medizinal Zeitung;* Berlin, 1896.

ODIN, M.: *Des propriétés toniques et stimulantes de la Coca; France Med.*, II; 1738, Paris, 1884.

OESTERLEN, FR.: *Handbuch der Heilmittellehre*, 6 ed., 8vo.; Tübingen, 1856.

OLIVEIRA, HENRIQUE VELLOSO DE: (Art. *Coca*), *Systema de materia medica vegetal brasileira;* Rio de Janeiro, 1854.

OLIVER, REV. GEORGE, D.D.: *The History of Initiation*, 8vo.; New York, 1888.

ONDEGARDO, POLO DE: *Report of the Lineage of the Yncas and How They extended their Conquests* (MSS., about 1560). Translated and edited by Clements R. Markham, C.B., F.R.S. (Hakluyt Society); London, 1873.

ORTEGA, CASIMIRO: *Resumen historico del primar viaje hecho al rededor del mundo por Hernando de Magellanes;* 8vo.; Madrid, 1769.

OSMA, DON PEDRO DE: *Histoire naturelle du Pérou;* Lima, 1638.

OTT, ISAAC: *Physiological action of the leaves of the Erythroxylon Coca on the excretion of urine; Medical Times*, I; Philadelphia, 1870-71.

Same: *Cocain, veratria and Gelsemium; Toxicological studies*, 12mo.; Philadelphia, 1874.

Same: *Coca and its alkaloid, cocaine; Medical Record*, II, 586; New York, 1876.

OVIEDO, GONZALO-FERNANDEZ DE OVIEDO Y VALDEZ: *Historia general y natural de las Indias, islas y tierra ferme del Mar Oceano*, II, V, folio; Salamanca, 1547.

(Translated into French by Jean Poleur; Paris, 1556.)

PALMER, E. R.: *Coca in fatigue; American Practitioner*, XXXI; 69-74, Louisville, 1885.

PARIS, J. A., M.D., F.R.S.: *Pharmacologia;* 9 ed., Charles A. Lee, M.D., 8vo.; New York, 1846.

PARKES: *Proceedings of Royal Society*, Nos. 89-94, XV, XVI; London, 1867, also 1871.

PAUL, B. H.: *Cocaine Benzoate; Pharmaceutical Journal and Transactions*, Oct. 17, 1885, March 27, London, 1886.

Same, and A. J. COWNLEY: *Cinnamylcocaine in Coca Leaves. Pharmaceutical Journal and Transactions;* [3] XX; p. 166; 1889, *idem;* [4] p. 587; London, 1898.

PAVY, F. W., M.D., F.R.S.: *A Treatise on Food and Dietetics*, 2 ed., 8vo.; London, 1875.

PAZ-SOLDAN, D. D. MATEO: *Geografia del Peru, obra postuma; Corregida y aumentada por su hermano Mariano Felipe Paz Soldan;* Publicada á expensas del gobierno Peruano; Paris, 1862.

PERCY, S. R., M.D.: *Transactions New York Academy Medicine;* November, New York, 1857.

PEYRITSCH, J.: *Erythroxylaceæ;* in Martius, *Flora Braziliensis,* XII, Part I; 1878.

PFEIFFER, H. T.: *Chemiker-Zeitung,* XI; 783, 818; Cöthen.

PFLÜGER: *Die Quelle der Muskelkraft; Archiv für der gesammte Physiologie,* L; p. 98; Bonn, 1891.

Same: *Ueber Fleisch. und Fettmastung,* LII, pl., *ibid;* 1892.

Pharmacopœia of the U. S. of America; 7th decennial revision, 1891; Philadelphia, 1893.

PIEDRAHITA, LUCAS FERNANDEZ: *Historia de las Conquistas del Nuevo Reyno de Grenada;* Antwerp, 1688.

PIÉTRA-SANTA, P. DE: *Erythroxylon Coca; therapeutic, hygienic; New York Medical Journal,* LIII, 748, 1891.

PINELO, ANTONIO DE LEON: *Question sobre el chocolate; L'Epitome de la biblioteca oriental y occidental, nautica y geografica,* secunde parte, 2 vols., folio; Madrid, 1737.

PINKERTON: *General Collection of Voyages and Travels;* London, 1813.

PLOSS, H.: *Vergiftungsversuch durch Cocain; Zeitschrift für Medicin Chirurgie u. Geburtsh.,* n. f., II; 222, 227; Leipzig, 1863.

PLUKENETII, LEONARDI: *Phytographia;* Mantissa 25 (Art. *Coca*); London, 1692.

POEPPIG, EDUARD VON: *Reise in Chile, Peru und auf dem Amazonen Strohme wahrend der Jahre 1827-32;* Leipzig, 1836.
(An extract is contained in the *Companion to the Botanical Magazine of Hooker;* I; p. 161; London, 1835; also *Foreign Quarterly Review,* 33.

POIZAT, C. H.: *The Erythroxylon Coca; Medical and Surgical Reporter,* XLV; 418; Philadelphia, 1881.

POMET, PIERRE: *Histoire générale des drogues;* p. 160; Paris, 1694.

PORRES, MATHIAS DE: *Fruits et plantes du Pérou;* Lima, 1621.

POULSSON, E.: *Beiträge zur Kenntniss der pharmakologischen Gruppe des Cocain; Archiv für experimentelle Pathologie und Pharmakologie,* XXVII; p. 301; Leipzig, 1892.

PRADIER: *Extrait d'un voyage dans les mers du Sud en 1831, 1832, et 1833; Bulletin de la société des sciences, arts et belles-lettres,* I; p. 548; Toulon, 1833.

PRESCOTT, WILLIAM H.: *History of the Conquest of Peru, with a Preliminary View of the Civilization of the Incas;* Edited with notes by John Foster Kirk, 2 vols.; Philadelphia, 1848.

PURCHAS, SAMUEL: *Pilgrimes; containing a History of the World in Sea voyages and Lande travels;* 5 books, large folio; London, 1625-26.

RAIMONDI, DON ANTONIO: *El Perú;* 8vo., 3 vols.; Lima, 1874.
(An elaborate work of Peruvian history and customs. Since the death of the author the Geographical Society has undertaken its completion.)

RANKE: *Tetanus eine Physiologische Studie;* Leipzig, 1865.

RAU: *The Stock in Trade of an Aboriginal Lapidary; Smithsonian Report;* Washington, 1877.

RAYNAL, GUILLAUME THOMAS: *Histoire philosophique et politique des établissements et du commerce européen dans les deux Indes;* II; 4 vols., 4to.; Genève, 1780.

RECLUS, ELISÈE: *Nouvelle Géographie Universelle;* XVIII; p. 489, *et sec.;* Paris, 1895.

REICHE, K.: *Erythroxylaceæ,* Contrib. June, 1890, in Engler und Prantl, *Die Natürlicher Pflanzenfamilien;* Leipzig, 1897.

REICHERT, EDWARD T.: *Action of cocaine on animal heat; University Medical Magazine,* May, Philadelphia, 1889.

Same: *The Action of Drugs which are believed to conserve the Tissues: Alcohol, Tea, Coffee, Coca, Maté, Kola, Guarana, Hemp, Tobacco, Opium,* etc.; *University Medical Magazine,* October, Philadelphia, 1890.

Same: *Influence of caffeine upon animal heat; New York Medical Journal,* April 26, New York, 1890.

Same: *Action of Alcohol on animal heat; Therapeutic Gazette,* Feb. 15, Detroit, 1890.

REINKE: *Studien über das Protoplasma;* Berlin, 1881.

REISS and STÜBEL: *The Necropolis of Ancon in Peru, a Contribution to our Knowledge of the Culture and Industries of the Incas.* Translated by Professor A. H. Keane, B.A., F.R.G.S., 3 vols., large folio; Berlin, 1880-87.

(A magnificent work of beautifully lithographed plates in color illustrating objects found in Incan tombs at Ancon.)

RITTER: *History of Music in the Form of Lectures,* 2 vols.; 1871-74.

RIVERO, MARIANO EDWARD; and TSCHUDI, JOHANN JACOB VON: *Antigüedades Peruanas;* large folio, Ill.

Same: *Peruvian Antiquities.* Translated by Francis L. Hawks, D.D., LL.D.; New York, 1854.

ROBERTSON: *History of America.*

ROBINSON, BEVERLEY, M.D.: *Heart Strain and Weak Heart; Medical Record,* Feb. 26, New York, 1887.

ROSSIER, DR. H. (DE VEVEY EN SUISSE): *Sur l'action physiologique des fuilles de Coca; l'Echo medical,* No. 8, pp. 193-198; Avril, Neuchatel, 1861.

RUIZ, DON HIPOLITO: *Quinologia, ó tratado del árbol de la Quina o Cascarilla;* Madrid, 1792.

RUSBY, HENRY H., M.D.: *The Cultivation of Coca; Therapeutic Gazette;* January, p. 14, Detroit, 1886.

Same: *Coca at home and abroad; Therapeutic Gazette;* (3 s.), IV; pp. 158-165; also 303-307; Detroit, 1888.

RUSSELL, J. RUTHERFORD, M.D.: *The History and Heroes of the Art of Medicine,* 8vo.; London, 1861.

SACHS: *Botanische Zeitung;* 1862.

SAJOUS, CHARLES E., M.D.: *Annual of the Universal Medical Sciences; A Yearly Report of the Progress of the General Sanitary Sciences throughout the World;* 8vo.; Philadelphia.

SANTA CRUZ, DON JUAN DE: *An Account of the Antiquities of Peru;*

Six Spanish Chapters from MSS. about 1620. Translated and edited by Clements R. Markham, C.B., F.R.S. (Hakluyt Society); London, 1873.

SANTILLAN, FERNANDO DE: *Relacion*, 1570, edited by Don Marcos Jimeñes de la Espada, 1879. (Referring to Incan Government.)

SCAGLIA: *Le Coca et ses applications thérapeutiques; Gazette des hôpitaux*, I; 427; Paris, 1877.

SCHERZER, DR. KARL: *Reise von Valparaiso nach Lima und über den Isthmus con Panama nach Europa; Ausland*, No. 7; p. 151; Stuttgart, Augsberg, 1860. (Report to the Imperial Academy of Sciences of Vienna.)

Same: *Uber die Peruanische Coca; Ausland*, No. 50, p. 1199; December; Stuttgart, Augsberg, 1860.

Same: *The Voyage of the Novara;* London, 1863.

SCHIEFFERDECKER: *Uber die Coca Pflanze. Schriften der Königlichen physikalisch aeconomischen Gesellschaft zu Königsberg, Berichte;* p. 22; Konigsberg, 1860-61.

SCHIMPER: *Botanische Zeitung;* 1888.

SCHLÖSING und MÜNTZ: *Comptes rendus de l'académie des sciences*, LXXXIX; Paris, 1879.

SCHMIDT: *Jahrbücher der in und ausländischen gesammten Medicin*, 7me vol., p. 44, 8vo.; Leipzig, 1851.

SCHNEIDER, ALBERT, M.D., Ph.D.: *Coca Leaves; The Western Druggist*, December, Chicago, 1898.

SCHOOLCRAFT, HENRY R., LL.D.: *History, Condition and Prospects of the Indian Tribes of the United States*, 5 vols., 8vo.; Philadelphia, 1853.

SCHRENK, DR. JOSEPH: *American Druggist;* 1887.

SCHROFF, C.: *Vorläufige Mittheilungen über Cocaïn, Wchnbl. d. k. k. Gesellsch. d. Aerzte in Wien*, XVIII; 233, 241, 249, 268; Vienna, 1862.

SCHULTZE and UHRICH: *Landwirtschaftliche Versuchsstationen*, 18, 20; 1875, 1877.

SCOTT, SAMUEL MATHEWSON: *La Goya;* (A Short Tale illustrative of Peruvian Life); London.

SCRIVENER, J. H.: *On the Coca leaf, and its uses in diet and medicine; Medical Times and Gazette*, II; London, 1871.

SEARLE, W. S., A.M., M.D.: *A new form of nervous disease; together with an essay on Erythroxylon Coca*, 12mo.; New York, 1881.

SELER, DR.: *Peruanische Alterthümer; Königliche Museen zu Berlin;* folio; Berlin, n. d.

(64 plates, 47 of which relate to Peru, comprising specimens of the collection of *Centeno, Macedo, Ruiz and others.*)

SHELLY, C. E.: *Note on the astringent action of Coca and of castor oil; Practitioner*, XXXV; 401-406; London, 1885.

SHOEMAKER, JOHN V., A.M., M.D.: *A Practical Treatise on Materia Medica and Therapeutics;* Philadelphia, 1893.

SHUTTLEWORTH, E. B.: *On Some Preparations of Erythroxylon*

Coca; Canadian Pharmaceutical Journal; November, 1874, *ibid*, August, 1877.

SIEVEKING, E. H.: *Coca; its therapeutic use; British Medical Journal*, I; 234; London, 1874.

SIEVERS, W.: *Reisen in der Sierra Nevada de Santa Marta;* Leipzig, 1887.

Same: *Die Sierra Nevada de Santa Marta die Sierra Peiyá; Zeitschrift der Gesellsch. für Erdkunde zu Berlin*, XXIII; pp. 1-158; Berlin, 1887.

SIGHICELLI, C.: *Contributo allo studio dell' azione fisiologica della cocaina; Annali di chimica medico-farmaceutica e di farmacologia;* Milano, 1885.

SIMMONDS, P. L.: *The Commercial Products of The Vegetable Kingdom;* London, 1854.

SIMONS, F. A. A.: *On the Sierra Nevada of Santa Marta and its watershed; Proceedings of the Royal Geographical Society and Monthly Rec. of Geograph.;* December; London, 1881.

Same: *An explanation of the Goajira Peninsula, ibid;* December; London, 1885.

SKINNER, JOSEPH: *The Present State of Peru*, 8vo.; London, 1805. (See Sobreviela.)

SKRAUP, ZD. H.: *Ueber Benzoylecgonin und dessen Ueberführung in Cocaïn; Berichte der chemischen Gesellschaft;* XVIII; 3, p. 635; Berlin, 1885.

SMITH, ARCHIBALD, M.D.: *Peru as it is;* London, 1839.

SMITH, JOHN, A.L.S.: *Dictionary of Economic Plants*, 8vo.; London, 1882.

SOBREVIELA, MANUEL P. P.; y BARCELO, NARCISO: *Mercurio Peruano.* (Translated into English under the title of *The Present State of Peru*, by John Skinner. Translated into French, with notes by P. F. Hardy, under the title of *Voyages au Perou faits en 1791 et 1794*, I; 2 vols., 8vo.; Paris, 1809.)

SOLORZANO, JUAN DE: *Politica Indiana*, I, 2 vols., 4to.; Madrid, 1756.

SOUDÉE, L.: *Étude synthétique sur le Coca*, 4to.; Paris, 1874.

SPIX und MARTIUS: *Reise in Brasilien*, I, p. 548; III, pp. 1180-1196, with plates and atlas, 3 vols., 4to.; München, 1831.

SQUIBB, E. R., M.D.: *Coca at Source of Supply; Ephemeris*, May, 1880; *ibid*, 1884, 1885, 1887, 1888; Brooklyn, N. Y.

Same: *Cocaine Assay; Proceedings American Pharmaceutical Association*, XXXVIII, p. 678.

SQUIRE, E. GEORGE, M.A., F.S.A.: *Antiquities of Nicaragua; Smithsonian Report;* Washington, 1850.

Same: *The Serpent Symbol and the Worship of the Reciprocal Principles of Nature in America*, Ill., *American Archæological Researches*, No. 1, 8vo.; New York, 1852.

Same: *Ancient Peru, Its People and Monuments, Harper's Magazine*, VII; 1853.

Same: *The Primeval Monuments of Peru Compared with those in other parts of the world; American Naturalist;* 1870.

Same: *Peru, Incidents of Travel and Exploration in the Land of the Incas*, Ill., 8vo.; New York, 1877.

Same: *Among the Andes of Peru and Bolivia; Harper's Magazine*, XXXVI, XXXVII.

STEVENSON, W. B.: *Historical and Descriptive Narrative of Twenty Years' Residence in South America*, 3 vols., 8vo.; London, 1825.

STEWART, F. E.: *Coca leaf cigars and cigarettes; Philadelphia Medical Times*, XV; 933-935; Philadelphia, 1884-85.

STIMMEL, A. F.: *Coca in the opium and alcohol habits; Therapeutic Gazette;* (n. s.), II; Detroit, 1881.

STOCKMAN, RALPH, M.D., F.R.C.P.: *The Action of Benzoyl-ecgonine; Journal of Anatomy and Physiology;* XXI; 46; London, 1886.

Same: *Amorphous Cocaine; Pharmaceutical Journal and Transactions;* (3 s.), XVII; 861; London, 1887.

Same: *Note on Hygrine; Pharmaceutical Journal and Transactions;* (3 s.), XVIII; London, 1888.

Same: *Report on the Coca alkaloids; British Medical Journal*, I; pp. 1043, 1108, 1158; London, 1889.

STOCKWELL, G. A.: *Erythroxylon Coca; Boston Medical and Surgical Journal*, XCVI; 399-405; Boston, 1877.

STÜBEL und UHLE: *Die Ruinenstaette von Tiahuanaco im hochlande des Alten Peru;* large folio; Breslau, 1892.

STÜBEL, REISS und KOPPEL: *Kultur und Industrie südamerikanischer völker nach den im Besitze des Museums für völkerkunde zu Leipzig;* Text und Beschreibung der Tafeln von Max Uhle, 2 vols., large folio; Berlin, 1890.

SUTCLIFFE, THOMAS: *Sixteen Years in Chile and Peru;* London, 1841.

TANNER, W.: *Erythroxylon Coca; Medical and Surgical Reporter*, XXXVI; 327; Philadelphia, 1877.

TEMPLE, EDMUND: *Travels in Various Parts of Peru*, 2 vols.; London, 1830.

THORPE: *A Dictionary of Applied Chemistry*, III, 3 vols. (Art. *Cocaine*), p. 914; London, 1893.

THUDICHUM, J. L. W.: *On the Coca of Peru and its immediate principles; their strengthening and healing powers;* London, 1885.

TORQUEMADA, JUAN DE: *Monarquia Indiana*, 3 vols., folio; Madrid, 1723.

TRIANA, et PLANCHON: *Prodromus Floræ Novo Granatensis;* Paris, 1862.

Same: *American Sciences Nat.*, XVIII; 338.

TSCHUDI, JOHANN JACOB VON: *Die Kechua Sprache*, 3 pts. in 2 vols., 8vo.; Vienna, 1853.

Same: *Reise in Brasilien, u. s. w., aus den Jahren 1839-42;* St. Gallen, 1840.

(A translation of this work has been made by Thomasino Rosa, published in 8 vols., Ill.; London, 1847.)

Same: *Ueber die Urbewohner von Peru;* Müller's *Archiv für Physiologie*, pp. 98-109.

Ttahuantin-Suyu, or the Empire of the Yncas in its Four Great Divisions; with Map (Hakluyt Society), London.

TUKE, D. HACK, M.D., F.R.C.P., LL.D.: *The Influence of the Mind upon the Body in Health and Disease*, 2 ed., 8vo.; Philadelphia, 1884.

Same: *A Dictionary of Psychological Medicine*, 2 vols., 8vo.; London, 1892.

TUMAS: *Ueber die Wirkung des salzsauern cocaïns auf die Psychomotorischen Centren; Archiv für experimentelle Pathologie und Pharmakologie;* XXII; Leipzig, 1887.

TURNBULL, L.: *Coca and cocaine; Therapeutic Gazette;* (3 s.), I; 226-228; Detroit, 1885.

ULLOA, JUAN JORGE, y ANTONIO DE: *Relacion historica del viage a la America meridional;* 5 vols., 4to.; Madrid, 1798.

Same: *Nouveau dictionnaire d'historie naturelle* (Art. *Coca, et Erythroxylon Coca*), V, pp. 90 et 556, 8vo.; Paris, 1803.

Same: *Noticias Secretas de América;* folio; Londres, 1826.

Same: *Secret Expedition to Peru undertaken in 1735;* translated in 1851. (See Pinkerton's Voyages.)

UNANUE, HIPOLITO: *Disertacion sobre el aspecto, cultivo, commercio y virtudes de la famosa planta del Peru nombrada Coca; Mercurio Peruano;* XI, pp. 205-250; Lima, 1794.

Same: *Communication to Mr. Mitchil*, February, 1821; *American Journal Sciences and Arts*, III; p. 397; New Haven, 1821.

(Dr. Unanue was born at Arica, Peru, in 1755.)

URICOECHEA: *Gramatica Vocabulaire*, etc., *de la Lengua Chibcha;* Paris, 1871.

URSEL, COMTE D': *Sud Amérique;* Paris, 1879.

VACHER: *De la Voix;* Paris, 1877.

VALDEZ Y PALACIOS, JOSÉ MANOEL: *Viajem da cidade do Cuzco a de Belem da grao Para, pe los rios Vilcamayu, Ucayale e Amazonas;* p. 79, 8vo.; Rio Janeiro, 1844-46.

VALERA, BLAS: *Laws, Vegetable Products and Medicinal Plants of Peru;* Edited by Garcilasso de la Vega, and Contained in his "*Commentarios Reales*." 1609.

VECKI, VICTOR G., M.D.: *The Pathology and Treatment of Sexual Impotence*, 12mo.; Philadelphia, 1899.

VEGA, GARCILASSO INCA DE LA: (See Garcilasso.)

VELASCO, JUAN DE: *Historia del Reino de Quito; Ternaux Compans;* Paris, 1840.

VERWORN, MAX, M.D., Ph.D.: *General Physiology.* Translated by F. S. Lee, Ph.D.; 8vo.; London, 1899.

VILLAFANE: *Oran y Bolivia a la margen del Bermejo;* Salta, 1857.

VINES, SYDNEY HOWARD, F.R.S.: *Lectures on the Physiology of Plants*, 8vo.; London, 1886.

Vishnu Purana. (For Comparison of Eastern Religions.)

VOIT: *Ueber den Einfluss des Kochsalzes des caffee's;* etc.; München, 1860.

WACKENRODER, H.: *Archiven de Pharmacie;* July; Paris, 1853.

WAITZ, T.: *Anthropologie der Naturvölker,* III; 6 vols.; Leipzig.

WARD, G. A.: *The uses of Coca in South America; Medical Record,* XVII; 497; New York, 1880.

WARDEN, C. J. H.: *Note on Erythroxylon Coca grown in India; Journal Agricultural and Horticultural Society of India,* VIII; Part II.

WATTS: *Dictionary of Chemistry* (Art. *Cocaine*), II; p. 230, 4 vols.; London, 1889.

WEDDELL, H. A.: *Notice sur la Coca sa culture, sa préparation, son emploi et ses propriétés* dans les *Mémories de la Société impériale et centrale d'agriculture;* 1re partie; p. 141, Paris, 1853.

Same: *Voyage dans le nord de la Bolivié,* etc.; Paris, 1853.

WESTMARK, EDWARD: *The History of Human Marriage;* 8vo.; London, 1894.

WHYMPER: *Travels in the Great Andes of the Equator;* New York, 1892.

WIENER, CHARLES: *Essai sur les Institutions Politiques, Religieuses Économiques, et Sociales de L'Empire des Incas;* 4to.; Paris, 1874.

Same: *Pérou et Bolivié; récit de voyage suivi d'études archéologiques et éthnographiques et des notes sur l'écriture et les langues des populations Indiennes,* 8vo.; Paris, 1880.

WILDE, W. R.: *Catalogue of the Museum of the Royal Irish Academy;* Dublin, 1857.

WILSON, ALBERT, M.D.: *The Brain Machine,* 8vo.; London, 1899.

WILSON, DANIEL, LL.D., F.R.S.E.: *Prehistoric Man. Researches into the Origin of Civilization in the Old and the New World;* 2 vols., 3 ed.; London, 1876.

WOEHLER, F., und W. HEIDINGER: *Ueber das Cocaïn, eine organische Base in der Coca,* 8vo.; Wien, 1860. Also *American Journal of Pharmacy,* under title of *A New Alkaloid in Coca,* XXXII; Philadelphia, 1860.

Same; und LOSSEN, W.: *Annalen der Chemie und Pharmacie,* CXXI; 372; Leipzig, 1860; *ibid,* 1862.

WRIGHT, G. FREDERICK: *Man and the Glacial Period;* New York, 1892.

XERES, FRANCISCO DE: Seville, 1535. *Narrative on the Discovery of Peru;* (Hakluyt Society); London, 1872.

(Xeres was the Secretary of Pizarro and wrote on the spot at the time of the Conquest.)

ZARATE, AUGUSTIN DE: *Historia del descubrimiento y de la conquista del Peru,* 8vo.; Amberes, 1555.

(Zarate was accountant to the first Viceroy to Peru, Blasco Nuñez Vela.)

ZWAARDEMAKER, H.: *Cocain-anosmie; Fortschritte der Medic*[illegible] July 1, Berlin, 1889.

INDEX AND GLOSSARY

A

B

C

D

H

I

J

K

N

O

Q

R

S

T

U